HEIRS OF HIPPOCRATES

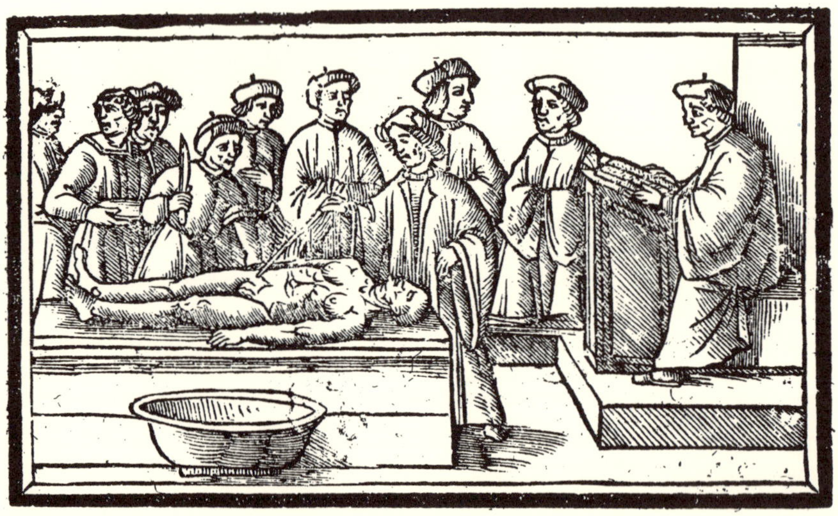

ʽΟ βίος βραχύς, ἡ δὲ τέχνη μακρή, ὁ δὲ καιρὸς ὀξύς, ἡ δὲ πειρα σφαλερή, ἡ δὲ κρίσις χαλεπή. δεϊ δὲ οὐ μονον ἑωυτὸν παρέχειν τὰ δέοντα ποιέοντα, ἀλλὰ καὶ τὸν νοσέοντα καὶ τοὺς παρεόντας καὶ τὰ ἔξωθεν.

HEIRS OF HIPPOCRATES

THE DEVELOPMENT OF MEDICINE IN A CATALOGUE OF HISTORIC BOOKS IN THE HEALTH SCIENCES LIBRARY, THE UNIVERSITY OF IOWA

FRIENDS OF THE UNIVERSITY OF IOWA LIBRARIES IOWA CITY
1980

Greek quotation on title page:

No. 2. Hippocrates. *Aphorismi Hippocratis Graecè & Latinè una cum Galeni commentariis.*

Hippocrates' first aphorism from the recto of the first leaf. Francis Adams's translation from No. 7, p. 697: "Life is short, and the Art long; the occasion fleeting; experience fallacious, and judgment difficult. The physician must not only be prepared to do what is right himself, but also to make the patient, the attendants, and the externals cooperate."

Illustration on title page:

No. 92. Berengario. *Anatomia.*

A typical anatomical lesson of the Middle Ages. From his elevated podium, the teacher reads from a text, most likely Galen, while assistants dissect the cadaver.

Library of Congress Cataloging in Publication Data

Iowa. University. Health Sciences Library.
Heirs of Hippocrates.

Includes index.
1. Medicine—Bibliography—Catalogs. 2. Medicine—History—Sources—Bibliography—Catalogs. 3. Iowa. University. Health Sciences Library—Catalogs. I. Title. [DNLM: 1. Bibliography of medicine—Catalogs. 2. Libraries, Medical—Iowa—Catalogs. 3. Rare books—Catalogs. Z 675.M4 U645h]
Z6676.I68 1980 [R129] 016.61 80-26503
ISBN 0-87414-016-1

HEIRS OF HIPPOCRATES

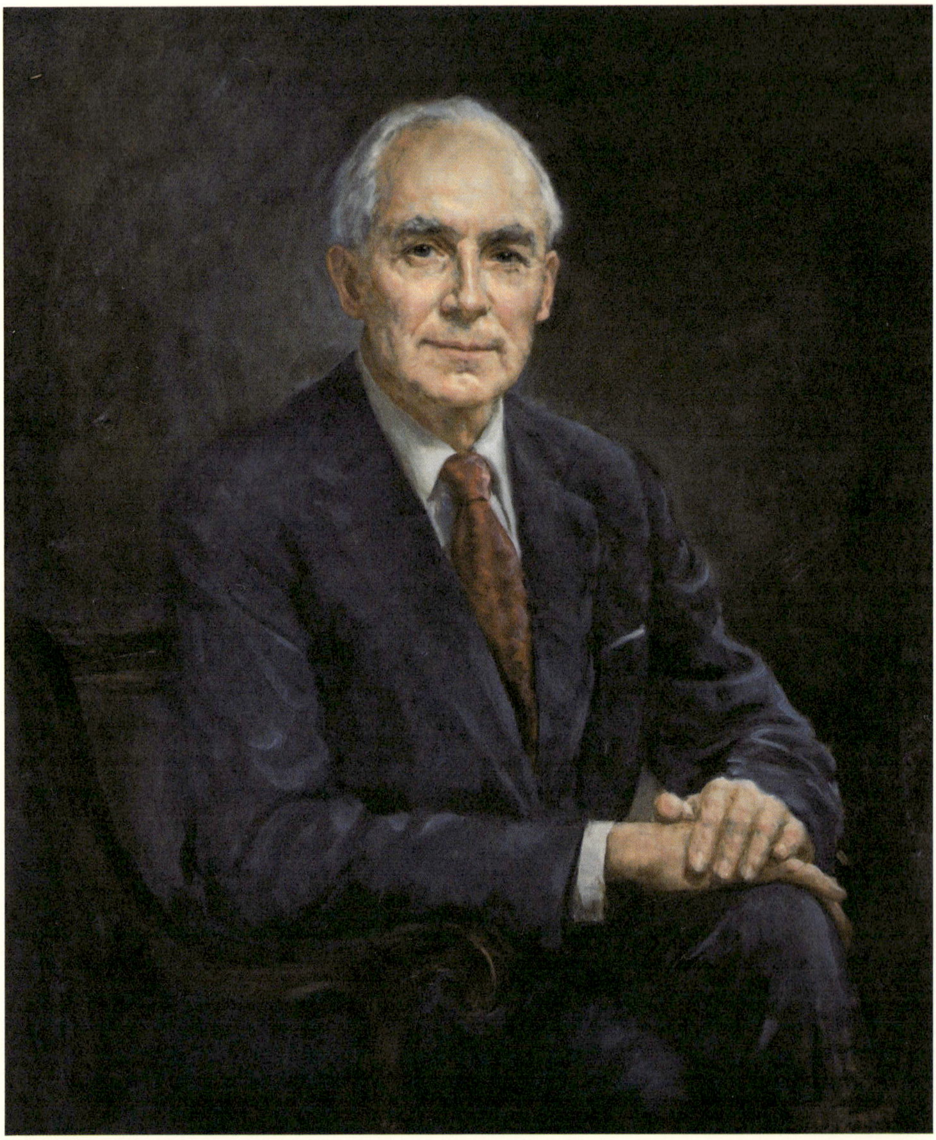

John Martin, M.D.

For Paul and Elynor Carney, with grateful thanks for their friendship.
John Martin
23 April '81

11 Sept. 1993

Dear Elynor,

Your sad letter which came yesterday was shocking, but not altogether surprising to me. I knew Paul was not well, for he had told me some of his problems, bbt he never did indicate that he had a lung malignancy. Well, that was to be his destiny, I guess, and I am only grateful, with you, that he did not have to suffer a long, lingering, and paknful illlness, nor lie a vegetable for months. He is released, at peace. This I truly believe.

I have known Paul since 1930. We were medical school classmates, fraternity brothers, and friends from "day one". I always enjoyed his bright Irish spirit and his comments on the world and the people around him. I will miss his letters. I had not heard from him for some time and about two weeks ago it occured to me that he might be seriously ill. I wanted to write, but thought it might not be wise to do so if he really were seriously ill, or pre-terminal. I definitely had a hunch that something serious was wrong. No, I'm not superstitious, but it does seem that sometimes these premonitions come true.

I know you will have a difficult period of adjustment, but how fortunate you are to have children, grandchildren and good friends. I know you can meet these difficult time head on!

With my love and sympathy,

John

FOREWORD

LIBRARIANS ARE prone to characterize catalogues which cover a field comprehensively as "monumental," and this one deserves that characterization as the word is commonly used and in the restricted sense of a work undertaken to memorialize the labors and benefactions of a collector and donor, in this case Dr. John Martin, neurosurgeon of Clarinda, Iowa. As a medical student, John Martin frequented bookshops in Chicago and became aware that he suffered from the incurable disease known as "bibliomania." After a time the disease "was complicated by collective fever, a happy combination." "Happy," indeed, for the institution which receives as a gift the books acquired during most of a lifetime spent in healing the sick and in learning about the development of his profession.

Dr. Martin, whose portrait in the John Martin Rare Book Room in the Health Sciences Library is reproduced as a frontispiece in this volume, concluded about ten years ago that his books, not limited to the field of medicine, belonged in the library of a teaching institution, and visits to Clarinda by faculty members of the College of Medicine, Dr. William Bean and Dr. Robert Hardin, and by librarians on our staff induced him to bestow his favors on The University of Iowa. This he has done with princely largesse. A catalogue of 394 books in the John Martin Rare Book Room, most of which came from Dr. Martin, was published in 1974 to mark the opening of a new Health Sciences Library building. In the years since, Dr. Martin has sought out, acquired, and presented to The University of Iowa hundreds of books important in the history of medicine, and he established in 1979 an endowment which ensures that his admirable work will be continued. Dr. Martin was recognized most appropriately in 1976 as a recipient of an award made to a "Distinguished Friend of The University of Iowa," and the publication of this "monumental catalogue" presents a detailed picture of Dr. Martin's learning and scholarship.

Each book presented to the University by Dr. John Martin is indicated by an asterisk before an entry, and the other donors of works described herein are named at the end of entries. The work of compilation was done largely by members of the staff of the Health Sciences Library, in particular by Richard Eimas and Edwin Holtum, and the Health Sciences Librarian, David Curry, chaired the committee which carried the project to completion. Other members of this *ad hoc* publication committee were Frank Hanlin and John Martin, compilers of the edition of *Heirs of Hippocrates* published in 1974, Norman Sage, who helped immensely in shaping this book, Wayne Rawley, and the undersigned. Dr. Martin's role in the preparation of this catalogue was singular in that he was the only member of the publishing committee competent to determine the contribution of a particular book to the development of medicine and the other health sciences, including dentistry, nursing, and pharmacy, so it fell to him to delineate these particulars in the notes. Dr. Martin performed this essential scholarly work as a regular member of the team and never requested special consideration. To be sure, his admiration for the "monumental" anatomical atlases which were published in the late sixteenth and early seventeenth centuries in Padua by Vesalius and his followers understandably led Dr. Martin to want to include in this catalogue more reproductions of notable illustrations than some of us believed we could afford, yet in such discussions Dr. Martin graciously deferred to his lay collaborators.

Dr. Martin has been an active member of the Friends of the University of Iowa Libraries, and other members of the organization who have become acquainted with him at meetings know and appreciate how much he has enriched the collections of the University of Iowa Libraries. Single-handedly he raised our modest holdings in the history of medicine to the prominent position which will be achieved by the publication of this catalogue. In the midst of his labors in our behalf, Dr. Martin has become a valued friend to many faculty members and librarians at The University of Iowa (especially to the writer), and our many associations with him during the last decade have permitted us to enjoy his thoughtful courtesies and his profound knowledge of the development of the history of medicine.

It would be easy to say too many nice things about Dr. John Martin; it is better now to direct your attention to his living monument which is defined for the present in the pages which follow.

Leslie W. Dunlap
Dean of Library Administration

June 19, 1980

PREFACE

THIS CATALOGUE contains descriptions of 1,196 of the 1,600 books in the John Martin Rare Book Room in the Health Sciences Library. Works were chosen for the catalogue which seemed to illustrate best the history of medicine, are most representative of a particular author, or presented a particular topic not otherwise treated even though the work is not of great importance. Because scientific periodicals became the primary medium for publishing original research in the late nineteenth century, it was necessary to limit selections from this voluminous literature. However, seventeen journal articles, reprints, or offprints were chosen for the catalogue because they are key contributions to the developing story of medicine in the late nineteenth and early twentieth centuries.

The arrangement of this catalogue is chronological by year of birth of the authors whose works are included. An exception is made for books with no attributable author which are entered under the date of their first publication. Another exception is made for serial titles which are entered under their first year of publication. Multiple works by an individual author are arranged under his name by date of publication. In the case of joint authors, entry is by year of birth of the first author with a cross reference from the other author or authors. In instances where an author's year of birth or death is not known, a "flourished" date was established based on the publication date of an author's work.

Each entry follows the following format: item number; author with year of birth and death; title; edition statement (infrequent); number of volumes if more than one; place of publication (standardized to modern usage); publisher; year of publication; pagination; presence of plates, illustrations, figures, maps, etc. as appropriate; height of title page in centimeters; and sometimes notes on binding, condition, paper, inscriptions, etc. An annotation follows, usually consisting of a brief note about the author and about the work itself. If more than one work of an author is entered, biographical notes ordinarily are given in the first entry. Birth and death dates usually are given for individuals the first time they are mentioned in an annotation. Birth and death dates are not given in an annotation for authors whose works appear elsewhere in the catalogue, or for royalty, other figures of state, and other well-known individuals. After the annotation, references are usually made to one or more bibliographies, catalogues of other collections, or other published works which refer to the annotated work. A bibliography of works cited follows this preface.

Facsimiles are not included in the catalogue unless they reproduce manuscripts or are facsimiles of books of which very few copies are extant. Bibliographies, histories, biographies, ephemera, and items of state or local interest are not included.

An asterisk (*) preceding the item number indicates that the book is a gift from Dr. John Martin. Sources of other gifts are noted at the ends of entries.

ABBREVIATIONS AND SYMBOLS

b.	born
ca.	circa
cm.	centimeter
col.	colored
d.	died
diagr., diagrs.	diagram, diagrams
ed.	edition
facsim., facsims.	facsimile, facsimiles
fig., figs.	figure, figures
fl.	flourished
fold.	folding
front.	frontispiece
illus.	illustrations
incl.	includes
l., ll.	leaf, leaves
n.d.	no date
n.p.	no place
n. publ.	no publisher
p., pp.	page, pages
port., ports.	portrait, portraits
pt., pts.	part, parts
vol., vols.	volume, volumes

[ ] Square brackets enclosing numbers of pages or leaves indicate that the pages or leaves are not numbered but are determined by count. Brackets enclosing an author's name indicate that the work was published anonymously or pseudonymously. Brackets enclosing a date, place of publication, or publisher indicate that this information was obtained from a source other than the title page.

* An asterisk preceding an item number indicates a gift of Dr. John Martin.

LIST OF REFERENCES CITED

Austin	U.S. National Library of Medicine. *Early American Medical Imprints; Guide to Works Printed in the United States, 1668–1820,* by Robert Austin. Washington, D.C.: U.S. Dept. of Health, Education, and Welfare, Public Health Service, 1961.
Choulant-Frank	Choulant, Johann Ludwig. *History and Bibliography of Anatomic Illustration. Translated and edited . . . by Mortimer Frank.* Chicago: University of Chicago Press, 1920.
Cushing	Yale University. School of Medicine. Library. *The Harvey Cushing Collection of Books and Manuscripts.* New York: Schuman's, 1943.
Cushing Vesalius	Cushing, Harvey. *A Bio-bibliography of Andreas Vesalius.* New York: Schuman's, 1943.
Durling	U.S. National Library of Medicine. *A Catalogue of Sixteenth Century Printed Books in the National Library of Medicine.* Compiled by Richard J. Durling. Bethesda, Maryland: National Library of Medicine, 1967.
Garrison-Morton	Garrison, Fielding H., and Lester T. Morton. *A Medical Bibliography: an Annotated Check-list of Texts Illustrating the History of Medicine.* 3rd ed. Philadelphia: Lippincott, 1970.
GKW	*Gesamtkatalog der Wiegendrucke.* Vols. 1–7 (A-Eig). Leipzig: Hiersemann, 1925–
Goff	Goff, Frederick R., ed. *Incunabula in American Libraries; a Third Census of Fifteenth-century Books.* New York: Bibliographical Society of America, 1964.
Hain-Copinger	Copinger, Walter A. *Supplement to Hains' Repertorium bibliographicum.* 2 vols. in 3. London: Sotheran, 1895–1902.

Keynes	Keynes, Sir Geoffrey. *A Bibliography of the Writings of Dr. William Harvey, 1578–1657.* 2nd ed. Cambridge: University Press, 1953.
Klebs	Klebs, Arnold C. *Incunabula scientifica et medica.* In *Osiris,* Vol. 4 (1938), pp. 1–359.
Lindeboom	Lindeboom, Gerrit A., *Bibliographia Boerhaaviana.* Leyden: E. J. Brill, 1959.
Osler	Osler, Sir William. *Bibliotheca Osleriana: a Catalogue of Books Illustrating the History of Medicine and Science, Collected, Arranged and Annotated by Sir William Osler, bt., and Bequeathed to McGill University.* Oxford: at the Clarendon Press, 1929.
Russell	Russell, Kenneth F. *British Anatomy, 1525–1800, a Bibliography.* Parkville: Melbourne University Press, 1963.
Sudhoff	Sudhoff, Karl. *Bibliographia Paracelsica.* [Reprint of Berlin, 1894 ed.] Graz: Akademische Druck- u. Verlagsanstalt, 1958.
Waller	Uppsala. Universitet. Bibliotek. *Bibliotheca Walleriana; the Books Illustrating the History of Medicine and Science Collected by Dr. Erik Waller and Bequeathed to the Library of the Royal University of Uppsala.* 2 vols. Stockholm: Almqvist, 1955.
Wellcome	Wellcome Historical Medical Library, London. *A Catalogue of Printed Books.* 3 vols. (A–L). London: Wellcome Historical Medical Library, 1962–

THE CATALOGUE

*1. HIPPOCRATES (ca. 460 B.C.–ca. 368 B.C.). *Aphorismi, cum Galeni commentariis, Nicolao Leoniceno interprete. Praedictiones, cum Galeni commentariis, Laurentio Laurentiano interprete.* [n.p., n. publ.] 1527. [19] 283 *ll.* 14.6 cm. Newly rebound in green morocco.

Very little is known about Hippocrates, the man; he was born in Greece and died there at a very old age; he traveled widely in the eastern Mediterranean; he was a physician who practiced and taught medicine. A highly respected teacher, his influence was immediate and long-lasting. Much, probably most, of what has been ascribed to Hippocrates in what is called the Hippocratic Collection of writings is by other members of his school or by later writers. But none of the writings is inconsistent with his empirical method or with his high ethical standards. The most celebrated physician of his time and, indeed, of all time, he is appropriately called "the father of medicine." The Hippocratic Oath has been taken in spirit if not in precise form by medical students for more than two thousand years.

The *Aphorisms*, the best known work of the Hippocratic Collection, are probably genuinely Hippocratic, at least in part. They are here presented with the commentaries of Galen, both of which are in Latin translation. The well-known aphorism "Vita brevis, ars vero longa" (Life is short, but art is long) opens the book.

The second work which, too, is probably a genuinely Hippocratic work, *Praedictiones* (or, in Greek, *Prognostika*), with Galen's commentaries, is also present here in Latin translation.

This edition, one of dozens appearing during the early years of printing, seems to be little known. It was probably printed in Paris by the editor, Simon Sylvius, though neither the place nor the publisher is indicated.

Durling 2382; Wellcome 3191.

2. ———. *Aphorismi Hippocratis Graecè & Latinè una cum Galeni commentariis: interprete Nicolao Leoniceno Vincentino.* Paris: Ex officina Carolae Guillardae, 1542. [viii] 186 [2] *ll.* 16.2 cm.

Another of the great number of editions of the *Aphorisms.*

Durling 2358; Wellcome 3211.

———. *In septem Aphorismorum Hippocratis particulas commentaria.*

See No. 147.

3. ———. *Les sept livres d'aphorismes . . . en latin et en françois . . . Par Me Michel le Long.* Paris: Chez Nicolas & Jean de la Coste, 1645. [8] 954 [37] pp. 22.8 cm. Old vellum.

In this edition of Hippocrates' well-known work, each aphorism is given first in Latin and then in French. The editor and translator, Michel le Long (fl. 1633–1643), has also included a lengthy commentary and discussion with each aphorism.

Wellcome III, p. 273.

*4. ———. Επιδημιῶν τὸ πρῶτον, καὶ τὸ τρίτον. *De morbis popularibus liber primus, & tertius. His accomodavit novem de febribus commentarios Johannes Freind.* London: Impensis Gul. Innys, 1717. xxix [3] 119 [3] 174 pp. 21.9 cm. Vellum.

These two books, of the total of seven on epidemics, were probably from Hippocrates or from his pupils. They are here in the Greek text with Latin translations accompanied by a commentary by John Freind (see No. 490).

Osler 179; Wellcome III, p. 271.

———. *De natura pueri.*

See No. 84.

*5. ———. *Octaginta volumina, quibus maxima ex parte, annorum circiter duo millia Latina caruit lingua, Graeci vero, Arabes, & prisci nostri medici, plurimis tamen utilibus praetermissis scripta sua illustrarunt, nunc tandem per M. Fabium Caluum . . . Latinitate donata . . . ac nuncprimum in lucem aedita. . . .* [Rome: Ex aedibus Francisci Minitii Calvi, 1525]. [lxxxiii] dccxxxiii [ii] pp. 28.1 cm.

Although various fragments of Hippocrates' works had been published earlier in Greek and Arabic versions, these eighty works, translated for the first time from the Greek texts into Latin by Marco Fabio Calvo (d. 1527), form the first so-called "complete" Hippocrates. The *editio princeps* of the Greek texts was published in 1526. These eighty texts, the most familiar of which is the *Aphorisms*, were probably written by a number of authors, but all are in the Hippocratic tradition. This historically important book, along with the massive French translation of Littré (see No. 6) in the nineteenth century, must be regarded as the definitive Hippocrates.

Durling 2320; Osler 149; Waller 4495; Wellcome 3177.

———. *De victus ratione in morbis acutis librum.*

See No. 138.

*6. ———. *Oeuvres complètes. Traduction nouvelle avec le texte grec.* Par É. Littré. 10 vols. Paris: J. B. Baillière, 1839–1861. 21 cm.

The large body of medical writings attributed to Hippocrates and his school were first definitively edited in the third century B.C. for the library of Alexandria. Some manuscript fragments of works dating from the tenth, eleventh, and twelfth centuries still exist but the first printed Latin edition did not appear until 1525 (see No. 5). Various selections from the body of these works have been printed many times since then. Émile Littré's (1801–1881) monumental work, said to have occupied him for twenty-two years, is the modern source for the entire Hippocratic Collection. His objective was to make the Hippocratic works as easily readable and understandable as a contemporary book and his French translation confirms that hope. The vast size of the work and the extensive notes and references make this a monument to his industry and scholarship.

Garrison-Morton 13; Osler 147; Waller 4494; Wellcome III, p. 269.

7. ———. *The genuine works of Hippocrates.* 2 vols. London: Printed for the Sydenham Society, 1849. Vol. I: x, 466 [2] pp., 2 plates; Vol. II: vi [467]–872 [2] pp., 6 plates. 20.8 cm.

This important and valuable translation by Francis Adams (1796–1861) includes only those works that can definitely be attributed to Hippocrates. A competent and skilled translator, Adams also translated works by Aretaeus and Paulus Aegineta (see No. 32).

Cushing H344; Garrison-Morton 14; Osler 151; Waller 4501; Wellcome III, p. 270.

*8. ARISTOTELES (384 B.C.–322 B.C.). *De natura animalium. De partibus animalium. De generatione animalium.* Venice: Bartholomaeus de Zanis, for Octavianus Scotus, 1498. [6] 89 *ll.*, woodcuts: initials, publisher's device. 31.7 cm. Contemporary uncovered wooden boards with blind-stamped polished calf spine and remnants of four clasps.

So great was the influence of Aristotle that his teachings and thought were accepted and enlarged upon for nearly two millenia. He was acquainted with more than five hundred species of animals and had dissected and investigated in detail at least fifty kinds, ranging over the entire animal kingdom. Despite the fact that many of his conclusions now appear fanciful and primitive, others have stood the test of time. Among them may be mentioned his descriptions of the mechanisms of locomotion, of the process of digestion in ruminants, of the habits of bees, of the mechanism of animal reproduction; his exposition of analogous structures in living bodies; and his methods of biological classification.

The works included in this volume constitute three of Aristotle's five principal works on biology. They are here presented in the Latin translation of Theodorus Gaza (1398–1478).

The first page of this incunable is decorated with a handsome illuminated border and capital initial, the colors remarkably preserved.

GKW 2353; Goff A 976; Hain-Copinger 1703; Klebs 85.4; Wellcome 427.

POLYBUS (fl. 380 B.C.). *De salubri victus ratione privatorum.*

See No. 14.

C. PLINIUS SECUNDUS (23–79). *De re medica.*

See No. 112.

*9. AULUS CORNELIUS CELSUS (25 B.C.–50 A.D.). *De medicina.* Venice: Philippus Pincius, for Benedictus Fontana, 1497. xci [3] *ll.*, woodcut: publisher's device. 30.1 cm. Eighteenth century half calf and floral boards.

"The *De medicina* is the oldest medical document after the Hippocratic writings. It was written about 30 A.D. After the invention of printing it was still considered important, being one of the first medical books to be set up in type. Celsus has left the best account of Roman medicine; he was the first important medical historian. The manuscript of the *De medicina* was lost during the Middle Ages and rediscovered in Milan in 1443" (Garrison-Morton 20).

Celsus was probably not a professional physician, and his work seems to be a compilation of the work of others, echoing the Greeks and especially Hippocrates. Nevertheless, it is an extremely able and interesting history of medicine and surgery, including descriptions of symptoms and treatment of disease as well as descriptions of plastic surgery, goiter operations, tonsillectomies, treatment of fractures, and dental procedures.

Cushing 33; GKW 6459; Goff C 367; Hain-Copinger 4838; Klebs 260.4; Osler 290; Waller 47; Wellcome 1394.

*10. ———. *Medicinae libri. VIII.* [Venice: In aedibus Aldi, et Andreae Asulani soceri, 1528). [8] 164 *ll.* 20.7 cm. Blind-stamped calf, rebacked.

Celsus' work has gone through many editions, translations, expansions, and adaptations since its first appearance in print in Florence in 1478. This is the first Aldine edition published by the well-known Manuzio family of printers who issued many works of the classical Greek and Roman authors and were responsible for introducing small pocket editions which became known as "Aldines."

Quintus Serenus Sammonicus' *Liber de medicina et ipsa castigatiss* (see No. 23) is also included in this edition.

Cushing C147; Durling 908; Osler 291; Wellcome 1397.

11. ———. *De re medica libri octo. Accessere in primum eiusdem, Hieremiae Thriveri Brachelii commentarii doctissimi: in reliquos verò septem, Balduini Ronssei Gandensis, enarrationes.* Leiden: Ex officina Plantiniana, apud Franciscum Raphelengium, 1592. [24] 752 [15] pp. 21.6 cm. Vellum, rebacked.

This edition contains commentaries of Jérémie de Dryvère (1504–1554) and Boudewijn Ronsse (1525–1597), two Dutch physicians.

Durling 921; Waller 1851; Wellcome 1405.

*12. ———. *De medicina libri octo, brevioribus Rob. Constantini, Is. Casauboni aliorumque scholiis. . . . Cura & studio Th. J. ab Almeloveen.* Amsterdam: Apud Joannem Wolters, 1687. [48] 574 [25] pp., illus., port. 13.9 cm. Vellum.

This revision and expansion by Theodoor Jansson van Almeloveen (1657–1712) of an edition of 1657 contains a biography of Celsus as well as a three-page bibliography of the editions of Celsus to 1687.

Osler 295; Wellcome II, p. 318.

13. ———. *De medicina libri octo.* Jena: Apud Joannem Felicem Bielckium, 1713. [24] 590 [72] pp., front. (port.). 16.7 cm.

This edition of Celsus' *De medicina* was prepared by the noted Swiss physician, Georg Wolffgang Wedel (1645–1721). Wedel was a well-known clinician and chemist whose many publications and interests also included medical history.

*14. SCRIBONIUS LARGUS (fl. ca. 40 A.D.). *De compositione medicamentorum liber, iampridem Jo. Ruellii opera è tenebris erutus, & à situ vindicatus.*

ANTONIO BENIVIENI (1443–1502). *De abditis nonnullis ac mirandis morborum & sanationum causis.*

POLYBUS (fl. 380 B.C.). *De salubri victus ratione privatorum, Guinterio Joanni Andernaco interprete.* [Basel]: Apud Andream Cratandrum, 1529. [16] 318 [2] pp. 15.2 cm. Half calf.

This small book contains works by Scribonius Largus, Antonio Benivieni, and Polybus.

Scribonius Largus was one of the more important physicians of the early Roman Empire and was the first medical author of note after Celsus. In all probability he was a freedman, perhaps a Greek, who took the name of his patron. He was physician to the Empress Messalina and is known to have accompanied the Emperor Claudius on his expedition to Britain in 43 A.D. This collection of 271 remedies, nostrums, and recipes is here edited by the French physician, Jean Ruel (1479–1537), who made the first Latin translation of Dioscorides. The work is arranged from "head to foot," an arrangement that was especially favored during the late Middle Ages. Scribonius traveled widely and used his journeys to extend his pharmaceutical knowledge and add to his personal pharmacopoeia. He described a primitive type of electrotherapy for headaches and similar nervous afflictions which employed a living black torpedo (ray fish). Scribonius was also the first to mention opium as an extract and is the earliest known writer to mention the Hippocratic oath. An advocate of polypharmacy, many of his remedies are fantastic and of a magical nature. Nevertheless, his work was basically a sound and valuable collection of recipes and remained popular and authoritative for hundreds of years.

Antonio Benivieni (see No. 79) achieved lasting fame from his *De abditis nonnullis ac mirandis morborum et sanationum causis*, the first work on pathological anatomy.

Osler observed that "The special interest of the work is that here, for the first time in modern literature, we have reports of post-mortem examinations made specifically with a view to finding out the exact cause of death" (Osler 3951).

Polybus (fl. 380 B.C.), Hippocrates' son-in-law, and Hippocrates' sons, Thessalus and Draco, founded the School of Dogmatism, a medical sect which based its teachings on Hippocrates' aphorisms. They emphasized the importance of investigating not only the obvious, but also the underlying and hidden causes of disease, which eventually led to meaningless philosophical speculation. Polybus is reputed to have been a quiet and studious individual who devoted himself to the study of anatomy and physiology. Aristotle attributes at least two works dealing chiefly with physiology to him. In the present work, edited by Joannes Guinterius (see No. 154), Polybus expounds on his regimen for attaining good health.

Durling 4168; Garrison-Morton 1785 (1528 ed.); Osler 3951; Waller 8785; Wellcome 5894.

———. *De compositione medicamentorum* [Selections].

See No. 73.

QUINTUS REMMIUS PALAEMON (fl. 48 A.D.). *De ponderibus et mensuris.*

See No. 23.

*15. DIOSCORIDES PEDANIUS (fl. ca. 50 A.D.) *[De materia medica] Libri octo Graece et Latine. Castigationes in eosdem libros.* Paris: Apud Petrum Haultinum, 1549. [20] 392 *ll.* 16.8 cm. Blind-stamped calf.

Dioscorides, a Greek citizen of Cilicia, accompanied the Roman armies as physician through many countries. While on his journeys he collected information on plants which he compiled into *De materia medica* which was considered authoritative on both botany and medicine for nearly sixteen hundred years. This present edition, one of many published after its first printing in 1478, is remarkably detailed and accurate and contains parallel Greek and Latin texts. The editor, Jacques Goupyl (ca. 1525–1564), is said to have produced, in this edition, the best of this work to date. The *Castigationes* which conclude the work are by Goupyl.

Durling 1135; Wellcome 1779.

16. ———. *De materia medica libri VII. Accedunt Nicandri et Eutecnii opuscula medica. Codex Constantinopolitanus saeculo X. exaratus et picturis illustratus olim Manuelis Eugenici, Caroli Rinuccini Florentini, Thomae Phillipps Angli, nunc inter thesauros Pierpont Morgan Bibliothecae asservatus.* 2 vols. in 4. Paris: n. publ., 1935. 385 *ll.* 48.3 cm. In portfolios. A facsimile.

This great work of Dioscorides had no illustrations when it was first written. Illustrations, which aided greatly in identification, were probably added in revisions made during the third or fourth century. In addition to descriptions of the medical properties of six hundred plants, the book contains some important early material on chemistry as well as descriptions of chemical compounds. In his classification, Dioscorides recognized natural families of plants long before Caspar Bauhin (see No. 246) and Carl von Linné (see No. 552). The Codex Constantinopolitanus was created in the tenth century and this facsimile is from MS. 652 in the Pierpont Morgan Library, New York. Other manuscripts of equal interest are one from the ninth century in the Bibliothèque Nationale and sixth century Vienna and Neapolitan codices in the library of St. Mark's, Venice.

*17. ARETAEUS (ca. 81–ca. 138). *Περὶ αἰτίων καὶ σημεῖων ὀξέων καὶ χρονίων καθῶν, βιβλία τέσσαρα. Περὶ θεραηεῖασ ὀξέων καὶ χρονίων καθῶν, βιβλία τέσσαρα. De causis et signis acutorum, et diuturnorum morborum libri quatuor. De curatione acutorum, et diuturnorum morborum libri quatuor.* Leiden: Apud Janssonios Vander Aa, 1735. [10] 604 pp. 40.2 cm. Contemporary vellum.

All that is known of Aretaeus with certainty is that he was a Greek physician from the Roman province of Cappadocia in Asia Minor who described diseases in excellent, stylistic Greek. He studied medicine in Alexandria and is believed to have practiced there and in Italy, perhaps at Rome. Aretaeus was a follower of the pneumatic school and left many descriptions of disease that are unsurpassed for their accuracy and elegance. The present books on acute and chronic diseases are all that remain of his works and, in them, Aretaeus discusses the causes, symptoms, and therapy for a wide variety of diseases. These works contain his fine descriptions of tetanus, epilepsy, asthma, migraine, jaundice, diarrhea, dropsy, elephantiasis, dysentery, diabetes, pneumonia, and an early account of diphtheria. The works are here edited by Hermann Boerhaave (see No. 474) and contain the Greek and Latin text in parallel columns. Boerhaave published the first edition of this work in 1731 and the present work is a reprint of that edition with an altered title page. It is an important critical edition and contains the notes and commentaries of Pierre Petit (1617–1687), John Wigan (1695–1739), and Daniel Wilhelm Triller (1695–1782), and is indexed by Michael Maittaire, a noted French classicist.

Lindeboom 557; Osler 330; Waller 461; Wellcome II, p. 54.

SORANUS, of Ephesus (ca. 98–ca. 138). *In artem medendi isagoge.*

See No. 112.

APULEIUS Madaurensis (fl. 2nd century). *De herbarum virtutibus.*

See No. 112.

*18. GALENUS (ca. 130–ca. 200). *Operum omnium sectio prima [-octava] Illustriores quàm unquam antea prodeunt in lucem omnes hi Galeni libri.* 8 vols. in 10. Venice: [Apud Joannem de Farris, et fratres de Riuoltella] 1541–1545. Illus., 56 plates. 16.4 cm. Old vellum over boards.

Next to Hippocrates, Galen was the most noted physician of antiquity. Born in Pergamon, he received his formal medical education in Smyrna, after which he

834 GAL. IN HIPP. LIB. DE FRACT.

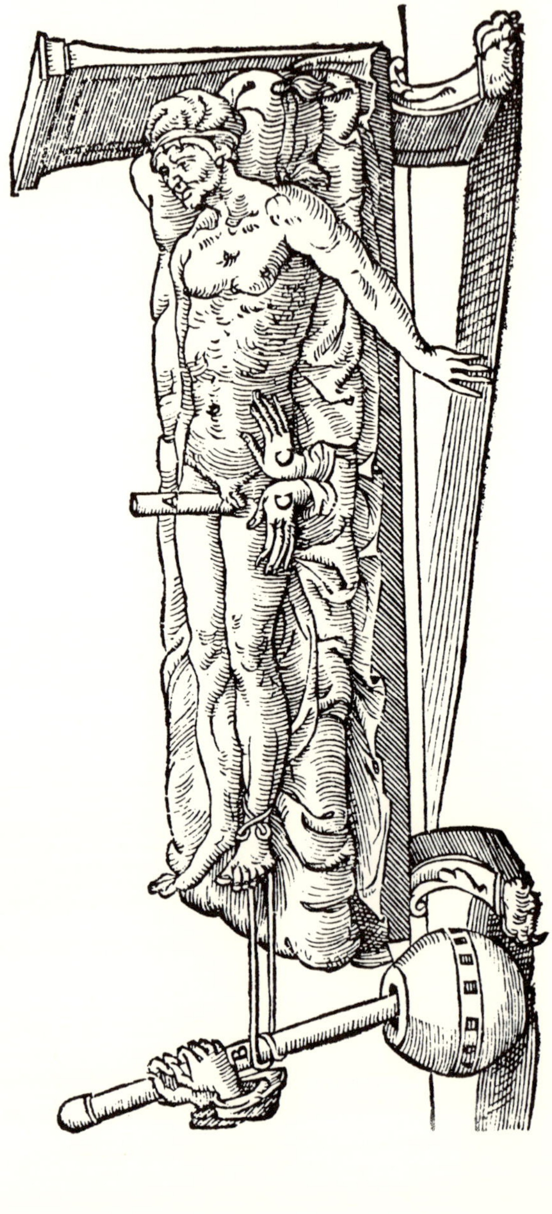

No. 18. Galen. *Operum Omnium*. Reduction of a fractured femur.

traveled widely in Asia Minor and to Alexandria to extend his medical knowledge. He settled in Rome where he carried on a large practice, attracting patients from all over the empire. His influence was enormous, and for centuries his writings were accepted as authoritative by Greek, Roman, and Arabic physicians, reaching a zenith in the Middle Ages.

The first Latin translation of Galen's works was published late in the fifteenth century. However, the Aldine text of 1525, the Basel edition of 1539 (both in Greek), and the nine editions of the Latin text published by the Giunta family between 1541 and 1625 are among the more important editions of Galen's complete works. This extremely rare complete edition was edited by Vittore Trincavelli (1496–1568) and Agostino Ricchi (1512–1564). The fifty-six plates in the set deal primarily with anatomical figures and scenes of orthopedic treatment.

Durling 1752 (incomplete); Wellcome 2513.

*19. ———. *Omnia quae extant opera in Latinum sermonem conversa.* 5th ed. 12 vols. in 4. Venice: Apud Juntas, 1576–1577. Illus. 34.3 cm.

This fifth Giunta edition, edited by Girolamo Mercuriale (see No. 223), is of special interest because it contains Andreas Vesalius' (see No. 171) 1541 translation of the nine books on anatomy, appearing here in Part IV. It also includes the exhaustive index done by Antonio Musa Brasavola (see No. 134).

Durling 1760; Osler 355; Waller 3390.

———. *De inaequali intemperie.*

See No. 108.

———. *De differentiis febrium.*

See No. 161.

———. *De humoribus.*

See No. 214.

20. ———. *Delli mezzi, che si possono tenere per conservarci la sanita. Recato in questa lingua nostra da M. Giovanni Tarcagnota.* [Venice: per Michele Tramezzino, 1549]. [8] 165 (misnumbered 157) *ll.* 15 cm. Vellum.

Galen's work on hygiene, *De sanitate tuenda*, has here been translated into Italian by Giovanni Tarcagnota (d. 1566). Galen did not write this book for the common man but addressed it to a small, cultured upper-class who had the time and means to follow his recommendations and regimen. It provides an interesting insight into how much more highly developed and sophisticated personal hygiene had become since the time of Hippocrates.

Durling 1933; Wellcome 2617.

1294 GALENI LIBER

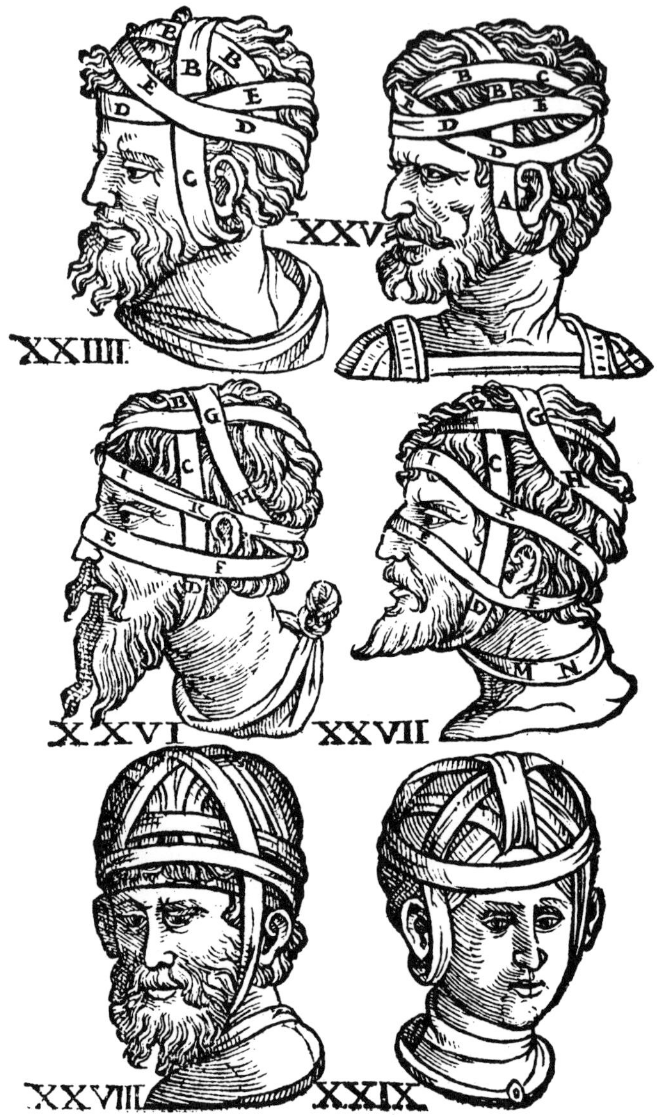

No. 18. Galen. *Operum Omnium.* A few of the many bandages for various types of head wounds.

*21. ———. *De ossibus Graecè & Latinè. Accedunt Vesalii, Sylvii, Heneri, Eustachii, ad Galeni doctrinam exercitationes. Ex bibliotheca Joannis van Horne.* Leiden: Apud Danielem vander Boxe, 1665. [12] 276 pp. 12.7 cm. Vellum. Bound with No. 336.

This work on the bones is one of Galen's more important works. Galen had done little dissection except on animals but he mentions having studied an actual human skeleton in Alexandria. To this work of Galen are added extracts from anatomical works of Vesalius, Dubois, Eustachius, and others in disputation or support of Galen, as well as excerpts from Hippocrates and Celsus. The work was edited by Joannes van Horne (see No. 342).

Cushing G48; Waller 3362; Wellcome III, p. 82.

22. ———. *Oeuvres anatomiques, physiologiques et médicales.* 2 vols. Paris: J. B. Baillière, 1854–1856. Vol. I: [4] xvi, 706 [2] pp.; Vol. II: [4] 786 [2] pp., illus. 20.9 cm.

The medical, physiological, and anatomical works of Galen are here translated into French by Charles Victor Daremberg (1817–1872). Daremberg, perhaps the most distinguished French medical historian, held the chair of medical history at Paris and was an expert on Greek and Roman medicine.

Osler 364; Waller 3389.

23. QUINTUS SERENUS SAMMONICUS (d. 211 or 212). *De medicina . . . per D. Caesarium . . . Item Q. Rhemnii Fannii Palaemonis, De ponderibus & mensuris.* Paris: Apud Simonem Colinaeum, 1533. 30 *ll.* 17.1 cm.

A father and son named Quintus Serenus Sammonicus lived during the late second and early third centuries. Few details regarding their lives are available but it is known that the father was put to death by the Emperor Caracalla purportedly for the use of magic in his medical practice. Although much research has been done, it has not been possible to ascertain which of the two actually wrote the present work.

A medical poem of 1,115 hexameters, it is primarily a compendium of remedies for the poor, many of which were taken from the writings of Pliny and Dioscorides. The first part of the poem consists of remedies for various disorders arranged *a capite ad calcem,* the popular head to foot arrangement favored during the late Middle Ages. The remainder of the poem contains recipes for such medical problems as fever, fractures, insomnia, epilepsy, jaundice, warts, as well as many others. Although many of the remedies are practical and useful, others are disgusting and border on the superstitious. A popular book, it was printed in Leipzig as late as 1786. The poem is here edited by Johannes Caesarius (1468?–1550). Caesarius, a physician and philosopher at Cologna, also edited and prepared commentaries on the works of Celsus and Pliny.

Also included with Serenus Sammonicus' poem is *De ponderibus et mensuris.* Attributed to Quintus Remmius Palaemon (fl. 48 A.D.), it is a short poem on weights and measures.

Cushing S109; Durling 4190; Wellcome 5938.

———. *Liber de medicina et ipsa castigatiss.*

See No. 10.

*24. ORIBASIUS (325–403): *Synopseos ad Eustathium filium libri novem.* Venice: [Apud Paulum Manutium, Aldi filium, 1554]. 216 *ll.* 15.8 cm. Limp vellum.

Oribasius, born in Pergamon (as was Galen) and a pupil of Zeno in the medical school of Alexandria, became physician to Emperor Julian, the nephew of Constantine. He was one of the most important medical figures of the Byzantine period and was responsible for preserving the writings of many medical authorities of antiquity in his *Synagogae medicae*. In this seventy-volume encyclopedia of medicine, of which only one-third has been preserved, he carefully translated and excerpted the works of such notable authors as Archigenes, Rufus, Aristotle, Heliodorus, Soranus, Antyllus, and Galen.

This volume, an epitome of his works written at the request of his son Eustachius, demonstrates his clear judgment in the treatment of such matters as diet in pregnancy, the choice of nurses, and diseases of children.

Cushing O43; Durling 3411; Osler 433 (Paris, 1554 ed.); Waller 7004; Wellcome 4648.

*25. ———. *Opera, quae extant omnia, tribus tomis digesta.* Vol. 1 (of 3 vols.). Basel: Apud Michaëlem Isingrinium, 1557. 336, 104 [126] pp., illus. 16.1 cm.

This volume of Oribasius' three-volume *Opera* contains his *Synopseos* (see No. 24), here translated by Giovanni Battista Rasario (1517–1578), and *De laqueis* and *De machinamentis,* two well-illustrated shorter works translated by Guido Guidi (see No. 158). Oribasius excerpted *De laqueis,* a work on knots and harnesses designed to immobilize limbs, from the writings of Heracleides of Tarentum (fl. 75 B.C.) and, from the work of Heliodorus (fl. 100 A.D.), *De machinamentis,* a tract on mechanical devices used by surgeons to set broken limbs and reduce dislocations.

Durling 3403.

———. *De victus ratione.*

See No. 112.

*26. AËTIUS OF AMIDA (502–575). *Contractae ex veteribus medicinae tetrabiblos.* Basel: [Impensis Hier. Frobenii et Nic. Episcopii] 1542. [10] 932 [30] pp. 31.9 cm. Contemporary blind-stamped calf, rebacked.

Aëtius studied in Alexandria and lived in Byzantium where he was court physician under the Emperor Justinian I. He was held in great repute by Renaissance physicians and his translator here, Janus Cornarius (1500–1558), regarded him as the greatest of the medical writers. His *Tetrabiblos* (so called because the text, as here, is divided and subdivided into four parts each) is a compilation which remains the chief source of knowledge for the works of Rufus of Ephesus and Leonides in surgery, and of Soranus and Philumenos in gynecology and obstetrics. Aëtius gives his own description of diseases of the eyes, ears, nose, throat, and teeth and includes good accounts of goiter, rabies, diphtheria, and various surgical procedures, such as tonsillectomy, urethrotomy, and the treatment of hemorrhoids.

Durling 46; Garrison-Morton 33 (1534 ed.); Waller 238; Wellcome 50.

*27. ALEXANDER Trallianus (525–605?). *Libri duodecim. Razae de pestilentia libellus. . . . Conversi, multisque in locis restituti & emendati, per Joannem Guinterium Andernacum.* Venice: Apud Hieronymum Scotum, 1555. [8] 274 [1] *ll.* 15.5 cm. Limp vellum, tape ties.

One of the leading Alexandrine physicians, Alexander of Tralles possessed a scanty knowledge of anatomy and physiology, but he was nonetheless a very keen observer of clinical conditions and his descriptions of pleurisy and other chest conditions are remarkably accurate. After Paul of Aegina and Alexander, Byzantine medicine went into decline, although their works were much used in the East and the West. This translation is by Joannes Guinterius of Andernach (see No. 154).

Rhazes' (see No. 34) treatise on smallpox and measles is of great importance in early epidemiology.

Durling 150; Osler 436 (1556 ed.); Waller 347; Wellcome 211.

*28. ———. *De lumbricis epistola.* Venice: Apud Paulum & Antonium Meietos Fratres, 1570. [10] *ll.* 19.7 cm.

This highly original work on intestinal parasites, one of the earliest on the subject, was a chapter in the author's *Practica,* first printed in Lyons in 1504. Girolamo Mercuriale (see No. 223) later included the Greek text and his own Latin translation as an addition at the end of his *Variarum lectionum libri quatuor* of 1570 and 1571. It is usually found with Mercuriale's work but occasionally, as here, it is a separate.

See Durling 3110.

*29. PAULUS AEGINETA (625?–690?). *Opus de re medica nunc primum integrum.* Cologne: Opera et impensa Joannis Soteris, 1534. [52] 507 pp. 27.9 cm. Calf, in slipcase.

Paul of Aegina was the last of the great Byzantine physicians, the last important product of the school of Alexandria, and a compiler whose works were consulted well into the Renaissance. He was a skilled surgeon and was especially eminent in obstetrics and in surgery of the genitalia. He also devoted much attention to diseases of the heart. The present book is Paul's only remaining complete work. A Latin translation had appeared in print as early as 1489 but the present translation is based on the first Greek Aldine edition of 1528. The translator and editor is Joannes Guinterius of Andernach (see No. 154), one of the best-known humanists of his day and a teacher of Vesalius at Padua. This edition was first published in

Practi. Jo. Serap.

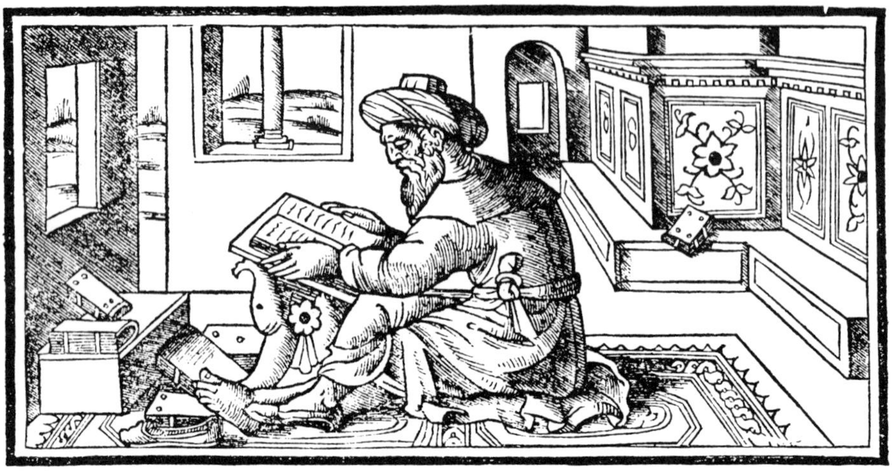

Necessarium ac perutile opus totius medicine Practice/
Profundissimi ac antiquissimi Arabis dñi Joãnis filij Serapionis/ In quo nõ
solum habetur Breuiarium totam Practicam sub breuitate continens/ Verũ/
etiam Librum copiosum de Simplici medicina/ Diligenti ac nouo examine
correctum/ Pulchrisq; ac vtilibus Annotationibus exornatum/ vna cum pluri/
mis huic spectantibus nouissime additis.
¶ Practica etiam breuis Dñi Joannis Plateari Salernitani vtilissima.

MD 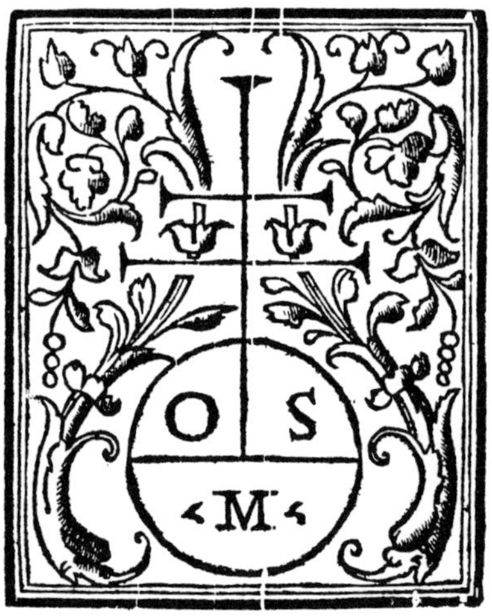 XXX

No. 33. Serapion, the Elder. *Practica*. Title page with illustration of Arabian scholar and device of the printer, Octavianus Scotus of Venice.

1532 and contains extensive commentaries by the translator. Paul's work is valuable for the light it throws on medicine and surgery of the seventh century. He covers eye surgery, trephining, military surgery, obstetrics, dentistry, and numerous other subjects.

Cushing P156; Durling 3552; Osler 438 (1528 Greek ed.); Wellcome 4866.

*30. ———. *[De re medica.] Libri septem . . . per Albanum Torinum Vitodurensem partim recogniti, partim recens Latinitate donati.* Basel: [Per Balthasarem Lasium] 1538. [44] 637 [11] pp. 20.9 cm. Blind-tooled pigskin with metal clasps and catches.

The present translation, also based on the Greek Aldine edition of 1528 is by Alban Thorer (Torinus), professor of medicine at Basel.

Durling 3553; Osler 439 (1532 ed.); Wellcome 4864.

*31. ———. *Opera, a Joanne Guinterio Andernaco . . . conversa.* Strasbourg: Per Vuendelinum Rihelium, 1542. [36] 489 [3] pp., 40 (misnumbered 39) [1] *ll.* 30.4 cm. Limp vellum.

Another Latin translation of Paul of Aegina's works, this one by Joannes Guinterius of Andernach.

Durling 3554; Osler 439 (1532 ed.); Waller 7247 (1551 ed.); Wellcome 4868.

*32. ———. *The seven books of Paulus Aegineta.* Translated from the Greek. . . . By Francis Adams. 3 vols. London: Printed for the Sydenham Society, 1844–1847. Vol. I: xxviii, 683 pp.; Vol. II: xi [1] 511 pp.; Vol. III: viii, 653 pp. 22.1 cm.

Francis Adams' commentary on *De re medica* gives a fuller account of Greek and Roman medicine than is elsewhere accessible in English or perhaps in any modern language. We are indebted to Adams, a Scottish physician and classical scholar, for his important translations and contributions in the history of Greek medicine. This is the first English translation of *De re medica* and was Adams' major work.

Cushing P158; Garrison-Morton 36; Osler 441; Wellcome II, p. 13.

*33. SERAPION the Elder (9th century). *Practi[ca].* [Venice: Impressum mandato & expensis heredum Octaviani Scoti ac sociorum, 1530]. 211 *ll.* 30.4 cm.

By the ninth century, nearly all of the important Arabian medical works were derived from Greek writers and translated into Arabic. In the Renaissance they were then translated into Latin from Arabic and erroneously taken to be Arabian works. Such is the case with Serapion the Elder, a Syriac Christian, whose principal work, called *Aphorisms,* was used for centuries in the Arabian medical schools. Originally written in Syriac, then translated into Arabic and eventually into Latin, it was first printed in 1479.

The shortened version of his work, variously called the *Practica, Breviarium, Pandectae,* or *Aggregator,* is an encyclopedic work which was a frequent source of quotation by men of science and medicine during the Renaissance. It is here accompanied by the *Practica brevis* of Joannes Platearius (fl. ca. 1100). Platearius was one of the seven chief masters of the school of Salerno and his synopsis of medical thought and practice was one of the outstanding works of the period.

Durling 4777.

*34. RHAZES [ABŪ BAKR MUHAMMAD IBN ZAKARĪYĀ, al-Rāzī] (865–925). *Opera parva.* Lyons: [Impressa per Gilbertum de Villiers, impensis Johannis de Ferrariis, alias de Jolitis, ac Vincentii de Prothonariis, 1511]. [8] cclxxxiv *ll.* 15.5 cm. Blind-stamped half vellum and wood boards.

Rhazes (commonly so called from his birthplace in Persia) was one of the great Persian physicians in this period when Arabian medicine was flourishing and when independent thought, especially as to therapeutics, was leading away from fixed dogma and Galenic rules. Rhazes had a thorough liberal education before deciding, at the age of thirty, to devote himself to medicine. He studied medicine at Baghdad, where he later gained fame as director of the hospital, teacher, and court physician. He was a pure Hippocratist, yet his inquiring mind and his writings covered the fields of medicine, philosophy, religion, mathematics, and astronomy. Of his more than two hundred writings, however, the majority have been lost. Of his medical writings, the most important are his *Kitab al-hawi,* an immense collection of excerpts and notes from classical physicians and from his own practice, which might have served as an encyclopedia of medicine had it been organized and completed; and *Almansor* (see No. 36). His most important individual work is his vivid description of smallpox, clearly distinguishing it from measles, with which it had earlier been confused.

The present work is an anthology of various of Rhazes' shorter writings on medicine and surgery and includes parts of the *Almansor* and *Aphorisms.* Although apparently complete, it lacks the final two works listed in the lengthy subtitle which serves as a table of contents.

Durling 3312; Garrison-Morton 41 (1510 ed.); Wellcome 5459.

*35. ———. *Opera exquisitiora. . . . Per Gerardum Toletanum medicum Cremonensem . . . Andream Vesalium . . . Albanum Torinum . . . latinitate donata, ac iam primum quàm castigatissimè ad vetustum codicem summo studio collata & restaurata.* Basel: In officina Henrichi Petri [1544]. [47] 590 pp. 27.4 cm.

This is the first of Rhazes' collected works to contain the ninth book of the *Almansor,* which was the source of therapeutic knowledge until long after the Renaissance. The work was edited by Alban Thorer (see No. 112) who also translated the tenth book. Andreas Vesalius (see No. 171) translated the ninth book and this was his first published work. Gerardus Cremonensis (1114–1187) made the translations of the remaining eight books of the *Almansor* and Giorgio Valla (see No. 154) translated the *Liber de pestilentia.*

Cushing R130; Durling 3313; Wellcome 5460.

*36. ———. *Almansoris liber nonus cum expositione Sillani Papiensis: & cum Receptis Petri de Tussignano supra eundum*. [Venice: Impensis heredum . . . Octaviani Scoti: ciuis Modoetiensis ac sociorum, 1517]. 90 *ll*. 28.5 cm.

The *Almansor*, so called because of its being dedicated to al-Mansur, prince of Bokhara, is an encyclopedic general review of medicine. It is divided into ten parts; the first six treat physiology and dietetics, the seventh surgery, the eighth poisons, the ninth pathology, and the tenth the doctrine of fevers. It is the ninth book which was long used in the West as the foundation of academic instruction on therapeutics and was often translated and commented upon, as in the present volume. The extensive commentary here is by Syllanus de Nigris, an early fifteenth-century Pavian physician. Added at the end of the book is a collection of "recipes" by Pietro da Tossignano (fl. 1376–1410), professor of medicine at Bologna and Padua in the latter part of the fourteenth century.

Cushing R129.

———. *De pestilentia*.

See No. 27.

*37. AHMAD IBN IBRĀHĪM (d. ca. 1009). *Études sur le traité de médicine d'Abou Djáfar Ah'mad*. Paris: Imprimerie impériale, 1853. 67 pp. 21.3 cm.

This brief treatise on the life and works of Ahmad ibn Ibrāhīm was prepared by Gustave Dugat (1824–1894), a member of the Société Asiatique. Ahmad ibn Ibrāhīm, called Ibn al-Jazzār, was a physician of North Africa to whom is ascribed the authorship of a medical compendium and a treatise on pharmacology. Dugat has here translated two chapters from the Arabic manuscript of al-Jazzār's medical compendium selecting chapters on the "disease" of love and hydrophobia. Dugat has also included a list of the complete contents of al-Jazzār's medical compendium and a list of the works cited in the compendium.

*38. ABŪ AL-QĀSIM (d. 1013?). *Liber theoricae necnon practicae Alsaharavii*. [Augsburg: Impensis Sigismundi Grimm, & Marci Vuirsung, 1519]. [6] clix [1] *ll*. 29.5 cm. Modern half vellum.

Abū al-Qāsim (or Abulcasis, or Albucasis, as he is variously known), a native of Cordova in Moorish Spain, may be classed with Avicenna in the importance of his great medical encyclopedia, *al-Tasrif*. It was published in three parts after the invention of printing: the pharmaceutical part in 1471, the surgical in 1497, and the present volume, the part on general medicine, in 1519, edited by the Augsburg physician and printer Sigismund Grimm (fl. 1519). The work was known to physicians and surgeons in the West as well as in the Moslem world.

The woodcut vignette on the title page, showing six physicians animatedly examining a large tome, is signed HB, for Hans Burgkmair (1473–1531), the famous sixteenth-century painter and printmaker of Augsburg, although it may

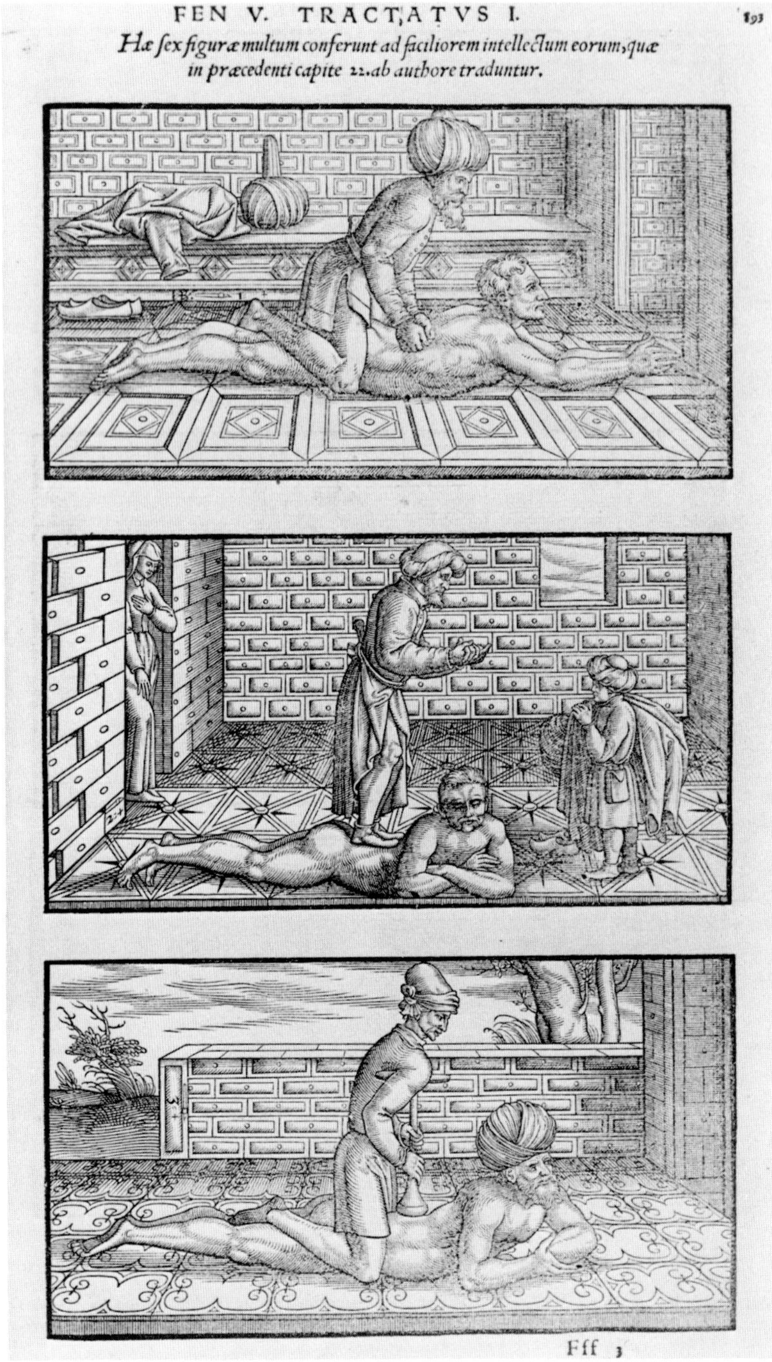

FEN V. TRACTATVS I. 193

Hæ sex figuræ multum conferunt ad faciliorem intellectum eorum, quæ in præcedenti capite 22. ab authore traduntur.

Fff 3

No. 40. Avicenna. *Liber Canonis.* Therapeutic methods for mild sprains and dislocations.

have been cut by the Petrarca Master, whose splendid woodcut printer's device appears on the last leaf.

Cushing A16; Durling 21; Garrison-Morton 3048; Waller 175; Wellcome 11.

———. *Medendi methodi libro II.*

See No. 228.

*39. AVICENNA (980–1037). *Canon medicinae.* 4 vols. in 3. Lyons: Johannes Trechsel, completed by Johannes Clein, 1498. Vol. I: [452] *ll.*; Vol. II: [380] *ll.*; Vol. III: [358] *ll.*; Vol. IV: [142] *ll.* 39.8 cm. Contemporary three-quarter blind-stamped pigskin, vellum sides painted black.

Avicenna needs little or no introduction to those familiar with the history of medicine. Known in the Persian world as the Chief or the Second Doctor (Aristotle having been the first), Avicenna was an accomplished physician as well as a noted philosopher. He wrote widely on theology, metaphysics, astronomy, philosophy, law, and medicine, and it has been estimated that he was the author of more than one hundred books. The present work was his greatest medical compilation and "stands for the epitome of all precedent development, the final codification of all Graeco-Arabic medicine" (Max Neuburger, *History of medicine*, translated by Ernest Playfair. London, 1910. Vol. I, p. 368). A large encyclopedic work on medicine, it is, for the most part, based on the writings of Hippocrates and Galen although Avicenna included many original observations and noteworthy clinical descriptions. It went through many editions and was a dominant force in medical thought, practice, and writing for more than five centuries. This massive and beautiful incunable is the first edition of Avicenna to have been printed in France and is a landmark in the history of French printing. These three large volumes, printed on heavy paper, were rubricated throughout in red and blue.

GKW 3127; Goff A 1428; Hain 2214; Klebs 131.13.

*40. ———. *Liber canonis, De medicinis cordialibus, et Cantica.* Basel: Per Joannes Heruagios, 1556. [44] 1104 (misnumbered 2004) [38] pp., illus. 37.4 cm. Nineteenth century blind-stamped calf.

This later edition of Avicenna's *Canon* was edited by Benedictus Rinius (1485–1565) and translated by Gerardus Cremonensis who is best known for his many translations of such Arabian physicians as Rhazes, Serapion the Elder, Mesuë, and Abulcasis. The version of *De viribus cordis* in this edition is by Arnaldus de Villanova (ca. 1240–1311) and that of the *Cantica* by Armengandus Blasii (fl. 1280). The biography of Avicenna was translated by Niccolò Massa (see No. 113). The six woodcuts illustrating the treatment of dislocations were drawn by the famous German artist, Hans Burgkmair.

Durling 386; Wellcome 578.

41. IBN BUTLĀN (d. ca. 1068). *Theatrum sanitatis, codice 4182 della R. Biblioteca casanatense.* Rome: La Libreria dello stato, 1940. 523 pp., 208 plates and portfolio (34 col. plates). 40.2 cm. A facsimile: No. 264 of 500 copies.

Ibn Butlān was a Christian-Arab physician of Baghdad, and this sumptuous work is an example of the service which the Arabs, at the time of their greatest cultural activity, rendered to posterity. The present work is a reproduction of the illuminated manuscript Codex 4182 in the Casanatensis Library in Rome, and it contains 208 facsimile plates in black and white with a portfolio of 34 colored facsimile plates. The scenes portrayed in the book are of everyday life, industry, navigation, vegetation, medicinal herbs, illness, wounds, and medical treatment.

*42. ———. ———. 3 vols. Parma: F. M. Ricci, 1970–1971. Vol. I: 201 pp., plates; Vol. II: 149 pp., plates; Vol. III: 160 [2] pp., plates. 35 cm. Each volume in slipcase. A facsimile.

This important work was reprinted again in the early 1970's under the editorship of Franco Mario Ricci. Here in three volumes are 412 brilliantly colored reproductions, each hand mounted, with explanatory text, of Ibn Butlān's manuscript.

TROTULA (fl. 1050). *De passionibus mulierum.*

See No. 228.

COPHO (ca. 1110). *Anatomia porci.*

See No. 139.

JOANNES PLATEARIUS (fl. ca. 1100). *Practica brevis.*

See No. 33.

*43. *Regimen sanitatis Salernitanum.* Strasbourg: Georg Husner, 1491. 80 *ll.* 20.5 cm.

Authorities disagree even as to the approximate date of the original composition of this poem, but a date near 1100 would probably not be far wide of the mark, although it seems not to have been widely known until the middle of the thirteenth century. It is believed to have emanated from the school of Salerno; at least, that school's chief claim to popular fame rests with this long didactic poem which sums up most of the practical medical literature up to its time. The work itself is actually a catch-all of advice and instruction on how to preserve health, rules of hygiene and diet, simple therapeutics, and other instruction intended more for the laity than for the medical profession. It was committed to memory by thousands of physicians and, after the invention of printing, was published in nearly three hundred editions, in Latin as well as in several vernacular languages. Numerous variations and additional verses which accrued through the years have doubtless obscured the original state of the *Regimen,* but this collective effort remains one of the most revealing medical works of the Middle Ages.

Goff R 73; Ḣain-Copinger 13758; Klebs 830.10; Wellcome 5369.

44. ———. *Conservandae sanitatis praecepta saluberrima, regi Angliae quondam à doctoribus scholae Salernitanae versibus conscripta.* Frankfurt: Apud haeredes Chr. Egen-[olphi] 1559. [12] 279 *ll.*, illus. 16.5 cm. Decorated paper wrapper.

Commentaries on the *Regimen* were common and one of the most famous of these is that of Arnaldus de Villanova, included in the present work, edited by Joannes Curio (d. 1561), a German physician. Interspersed throughout the text are rather crude but interesting small woodcuts of homely subjects: mealtime, milking cows, bathing, etc.

Durling 3812; Waller 7819; Wellcome 5376.

45. ———. *De conservanda bona valetudine, opusculum Scholae Salernitanae . . . cum Arnoldi Novicomensis . . . enarrationibus.* Venice: Apud Petrum Marinellum, 1587. [12] 271 [4] *ll.* 13.6 cm.

Another of the many editions of this medical vade mecum with the commentaries of Arnaldus de Villanova and edited by Curio.

Durling 3831.

*46. MESUË the Younger (fl. ca. 1200?). *Canones universales.* [Venice: [n. publ.] 1502]. 355 *ll.* 28.9 cm. Limp vellum.

Masawayh al-Mardini (known in the West as Mesuë the Younger) is supposed to have been a Jacobite Christian who lived in the tenth century. Since none of his writings has been found in its original language and no Arabian historian or bibliographer seems to know him, it is now believed that a Latin author (perhaps an Italian) of the early thirteenth century assumed the name of Mesuë, hoping thereby to gain ready recognition for his works under the guise of the ninth century Syrian physician who wrote in Arabic. At any rate, his writings were accepted as genuinely Arabian and held such a place of importance that they went through more than a dozen editions between their first printing in 1471 and 1500.

The work contains the whole of the Pseudo-Mesuë's writings, consisting of three works: one on laxatives; an antidotarium, or apothecary's manual, which was the most popular handbook of drugs in medieval Europe; and an incomplete manual of special therapeutics. In addition, there are commentaries of Mondino dei Luzzi (see No. 54) and additional works by Pietro d'Abano (see No. 51), Nicolaus Salernitanus (fl. 1140), and others.

Cushing M318 (1510 ed.); Durling 3121; Osler 3400 (1510 ed.); Wellcome 4276.

*47. ———. *De re medica libri tres. Jacobo Sylvio medico interprete.* Paris: [n. publ.] 1553. 248 [4] *ll.* 15.8 cm.

Another of the more than forty works attributed to Mesuë the Younger, this one deals with the principles of medicine and the use of drugs, laxatives, and antidotes. It was an early translation of Jacques Dubois (see No. 103).

Durling 3145; Osler 3401 (1561 ed.); Waller 6520 (1542 ed.); Wellcome 4279 (1548 ed.).

48. ALBERTUS MAGNUS (ca. 1200–1280). *De secretis mulierum.* Lyons: Apud Anthonium de Harsy, 1598. 381 [9] pp. 11.7 cm. Vellum.

It was through the immense scholarly labors of Albertus Magnus that the medieval Christian world came to know Greek and Arabian science and philosophy. A German scholastic theologian and scholar of the Dominican order, he taught in Cologne and Paris, his most noted pupil being Thomas Aquinas. In addition to his theological works, he also engaged in scientific research.

This little book on obstetrics and the diseases of women is one of scores of editions and translations which were published from the fifteenth into the eighteenth centuries, so great was its popularity, although it is largely superstitious and astrological.

Durling 90; Wellcome 137 (1553 ed.).

*49. BRUNO DA LONGOBURGO (ca. 1200–1286). *La cyrogia di Maistro Bruno.* [Venice: Per Simone de Luere, 1510]. 40 *ll.* 20.8 cm. Modern boards.

Since Bruno was born in Longoburgo in Calabria, it is thought that he probably studied at Salerno. He later practiced and taught at Padua where he gained a wide reputation as a surgeon. The present work is the first Italian translation of his *Chirurgia magna* which he completed in 1252. In it he mentions not only Greek authorities but such Arabian medical authorities as Avicenna, Abulcasis, and Haly Abbas. Bruno discusses a wide variety of surgical matters in this work including hernia, erysipelas, fractures, ear diseases, cancers, dislocations, and nerve wounds. In his view, goiters are best cured by surgical removal and he suggests using ants to suture intestinal wounds.

Durling 738.

*50. *Codex Granatensis.* Edición facsimil del Codice-67 de la Biblioteca universitaria de Granada. Cuidó de la edición L. García Ballester. 2 vols. [Granada: Universidad de Granada] 1973–1974. Vol. I: 116 *ll.*; Vol. II: 330 pp., col. illus. 44.9 cm. A facsimile.

This is a facsimile edition of an early fifteenth century illustrated codex which was brought to Spain from Austria during the eighteenth century. The codex comprises nineteen manuscripts and includes Books 4 through 12 of *De natura rerum,* the *Tacuinum sanitatis,* and the anonymous treatise, *De avibus nobilibus.* Research at the University of Granada has shown that the author of *De natura rerum* was Thomas de Cantimpré (ca. 1201–ca. 1276) and not Albertus Magnus to whom the work has been ascribed. The *Tacuinum sanitatis* is a set of tables of general medical and dietetic information, originally written in the eleventh century by Ibn Butlān (see No. 41). *De avibus nobilibus,* written in the form of a letter near the end of the twelfth century, deals with falcons, their diseases, and the remedies for treating them. The second volume of the set contains an account of the studies made on the codex as well as a transcription of the Latin text and translations into Spanish and English.

ARNALDUS DE VILLANOVA (ca. 1240–1311). *Sententiarum medicinalium morborum curationibus.*

See No. 111.

*51. PIETRO D'ABANO (1250–1315?). *Conciliator differentiarum philosophorum et medicorum.* Venice: Gabriele di Pietro, for Thomas de Tarvisio, 1476. [280] *ll.* (lacking first preliminary leaf). 39.3 cm. Modern vellum, in slipcase.

Pietro d'Abano was one of the most illustrious and influential men of his time. A Paduan physician, he was consulted by such men as Pope Honorius IV and was in great demand for lectures, consultation, and teaching. Dante was among his pupils. A defender of Italian Averroism, Pietro disputed much of the church dogma and scholastic philosophy. For his heretical and outspoken views he ran afoul of the Inquisition and was condemned, but he died before he could be executed.

Conciliator is Pietro's greatest work and one which made a great impression on his age. In fact, its influence was such that its method of dialectics became the fashion for student dissertations and disputations at Padua through the seventeenth century. Pietro d'Abano presents the scattered medical knowledge, particularly from the Arabic and Grecian schools, in a series of questions with answers from both schools of thought, in true scholastic fashion, with the hope that the truth would emerge and the contradictions be resolved. Among important and novel views that Pietro expresses are that air has weight, that the heart is the source of veins and arteries, and that the brain is the source of nerves which convey sensation.

This handsome copy is decorated with two fine gilt and colored initials and is rubricated throughout with initials in red and blue.

Cushing, Incunabula 113 (1472 ed.); Goff P 432; Hain-Copinger 2; Klebs 773.2; Osler 7470 (1472 ed.); Waller 111; Wellcome 4940 (1483 ed.).

*52. ———. *Expositio problematum Aristotelis.* [Venice]: Johannes Herbort, de Seligenstadts, 1482. [314] *ll.* 30.5 cm. Eighteenth century mottled calf with gilt tooled arms of Pope Pius VI on front and back covers.

This scarce incunable is Pietro's commentary on the Alexandrian pseudo-Aristotelian *Problemata,* an anonymous compilation of medical problems. A Latin translation of the *Problemata* accompanies the commentary.

Goff P 437; Hain-Copinger 17; Klebs 776.2; Osler 245 (1475 ed.); Wellcome 4939.

*53. HENRI DE MONDEVILLE (ca. 1260–ca. 1320). *Chirurgie.* Paris: Félix Alcan, 1893. lxxxii, 903 pp., front., diagrs. 27.6 cm. Original wrappers.

De Mondeville was a French physician, chief surgeon to King Philip the Fair of France, and taught at the University of Paris. His surgery is said to have been in advance of his time, although he relied chiefly on Avicenna.

Like many other encyclopedic texts on surgery until about 1700, de Mondeville's work is a combination of surgery, anatomy, physiology, pharmacology, and

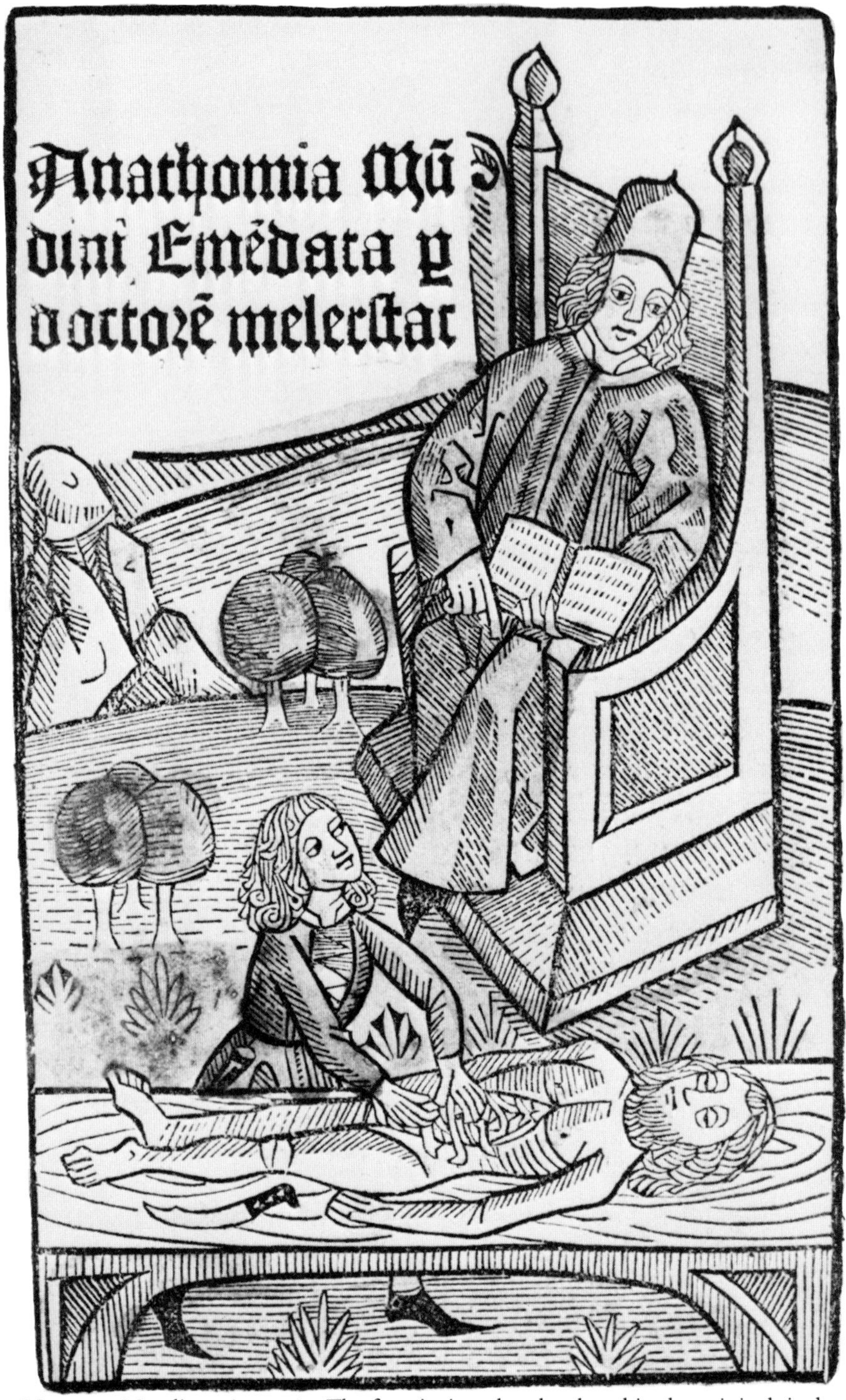

No. 54. Mondino. *Anatomia.* The frontispiece, hand-colored in the original, is the book's only illustration.

philosophy. It was not published until 1892, after discovery of manuscripts in the libraries in Berlin, Erfurt, and Paris. This French translation was done by Jules Édouard Nicaise (1838–1896) from a codex in the Bibliothèque Nationale in Paris.

Choulant-Frank, p. 45; Osler 3433; Waller 6619.

*54. MONDINO DEI LUZZI (d. 1326). *Anatomia*. [Leipzig: Martin Landsberg, 1493?]. [40] *ll.*, woodcut. 20.8 cm. Full maroon levant by Rivière.

Mondino, son of a Bolognese pharmacist, enjoyed a great reputation as an anatomist and also as a noted statesman, serving as Ambassador to Bologna for a number of years. He was probably the first to introduce the systematic teaching of anatomy into medicine and it is from his era that the body began to be dissected in an orderly fashion, one part after another. Written in 1316, his *Anothomia* was copied, expanded, altered, and republished for almost two centuries and was one of the most influential of all pre-Vesalian works devoted strictly to anatomy.

This early edition, published some fifteen years after the first printing, was edited by Martin Pollich of Mellerstadt (d. 1513) who was a professor at Leipzig until 1502 and then at Wittenberg where he assisted in founding the university. On the title page is a hand-colored illustration of a familiar teaching scene of the time.

Choulant-Frank, p. 93; Cushing, Incunabula 103; Garrison-Morton 361 (1487 ed.); Goff M 874; Hain 11633; Waller 105; Wellcome 4484.

*55. ———. *Anatomia Mundini*. Marburg: In officina Christiani Egenolphi [1541]. [4] 67 *ll.*, 41 plates. 19.7 cm.

This edition of Mondino's anatomy was prepared by Johannes Dryander, called Eichmann, who is generally regarded as one of the first anatomists to make illustrations from his own dissections. This important and rare book is especially interesting for its woodcuts. Nearly half of the plates were copied from Berengario da Carpi's commentary on Mondino's *Anothomia* published in 1521 and most of the remaining plates are Dryander's. Many of them were taken from Dryander's *Anatomiae* first issued in 1537 (see No. 139) and at least six of his plates are believed to have been taken from Vesalius' *Tabulae anatomicae sex*. Only forty-one of the original forty-six plates are present in this copy.

Choulant-Frank, pp. 88–96; Cushing M452; Durling 3233; Osler 3439; Waller 6746; Wellcome 4486.

*56. ———. *Anatomia Mundini per Carpum castigata, & postmodum cum apostillis ornata, ac noviter impressa*. Venice: [Melchiorre Sessa, 1540?]. 76 *ll.* 10.7 cm. Contemporary limp vellum. Bound with No. 154.

This tiny book contains one of the many editions of Mondino's *Anothomia*. The exact date of publication is not given in the book and some authorities feel that it may have been published as late as 1575. The work is here edited by Jacopo Berengario da Carpi (see No. 92) and is without illustrations.

Cushing M453; Osler 3440; Wellcome 4487.

MVNDINI.

In hac figura uidentur formæ, ſitus, & uerus numerus omni-
um oſſium corporis humani: exceptis oſſibus capitis, & dorſi,
quorum iuncturæ omnes non poſſunt uideri, niſi in corporib.
decoctis, uel exiccatis in cimiterijs.

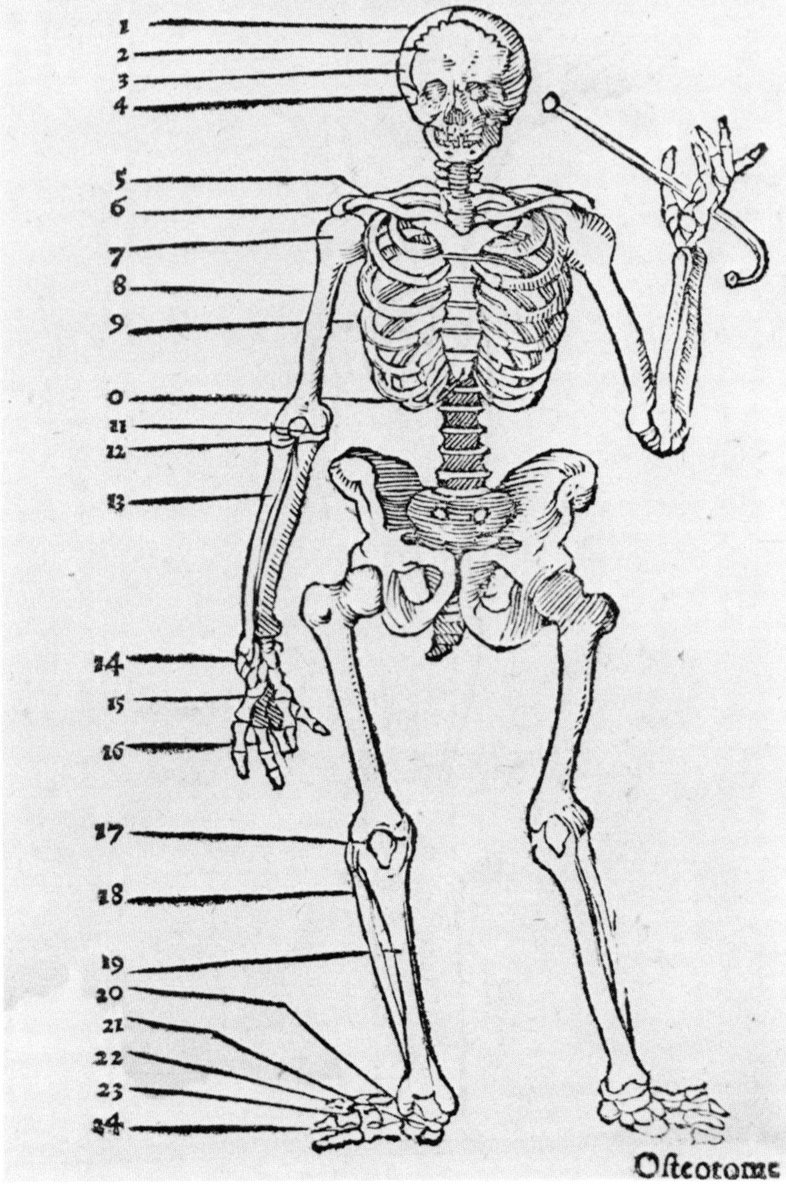

No. 55. Mondino. *Anatomia Mundini.*

*57. ———. *Anatomies de Mondino dei Luzzi et de Guido de Vigevano.* Paris: E. Droz [ca 1926]. 91 pp., illus., 16 plates (part col.). 33 cm. A facsimile: No. 239 of 340 copies.

Mondino's *Anothomia* was not published until 1478 at Pavia, Italy, and did not contain illustrations as did many of the later editions. This compilation by medical librarian and historian, Ernest Wickersheimer (1880–1965), contains a facsimile of the 1478 edition of Mondino's *Anothomia* as well as the text and eighteen plates from Guido de Vigevano's (fl. 14th century) *Anathomia*. Vigevano's manuscript was completed in 1345 and is MS. 569 in the collection of the Musée Condé at the Bibliothèque de Château de Chantilly. In his *Anathomia,* Vigevano discusses the usefulness of using drawings for the demonstration of anatomy and also the church's attitude toward dissection of the human body. According to Wickersheimer, the Papal Bull of Boniface VIII in 1300 was not aimed at curtailing dissection but was intended to halt the practice of boiling and dismembering the bodies of crusaders who had died away from home for easier transportation back to Europe. The plates are among the earliest anatomical drawings of the time and are intended to show the techniques of dissection and a limited number of diagnostic techniques.

Cushing M455.

DINO DEL GARBO (d. 1327). *Expositio . . . de generatione embrionis cum questionibus eiusdem.*

See No. 84.

———. *Scriptum . . . super libro de natura fetus Hypo[cratis].*

See No. 84.

*58. GUILIELMUS VARIGNANA (ca. 1270–1339). *Secreta sublimia ad varios curados morbos verissimis autoritatibus illustrata additionibus nonnullis flosculis.* [Lyons: Impressum per Jo. de Cambrey, 1522]. [iv] lvi (misnumbered xli) *ll.* 20 cm.

Professor of medicine at the University of Bologna, Varignana was one of the most important members of a well-known Jewish family of Bologna physicians. His sons, Pietro and Matteo, were also teachers at the University of Bologna, following in the footsteps of their father. Fielding H. Garrison notes that Guilielmus' father, Bartolomeo, conducted the first recorded postmortem examination on a case of suspected poisoning at Bologna in 1302.

This rare book is divided into five sermones or sections: the first contains nineteen tracts on pathology, the second deals with fevers, the third with abscesses and wounds, the fourth with toxicology, and the fifth discusses leprosy, plague, and various skin diseases.

Durling 2199; Wellcome 6494 (1519 ed.).

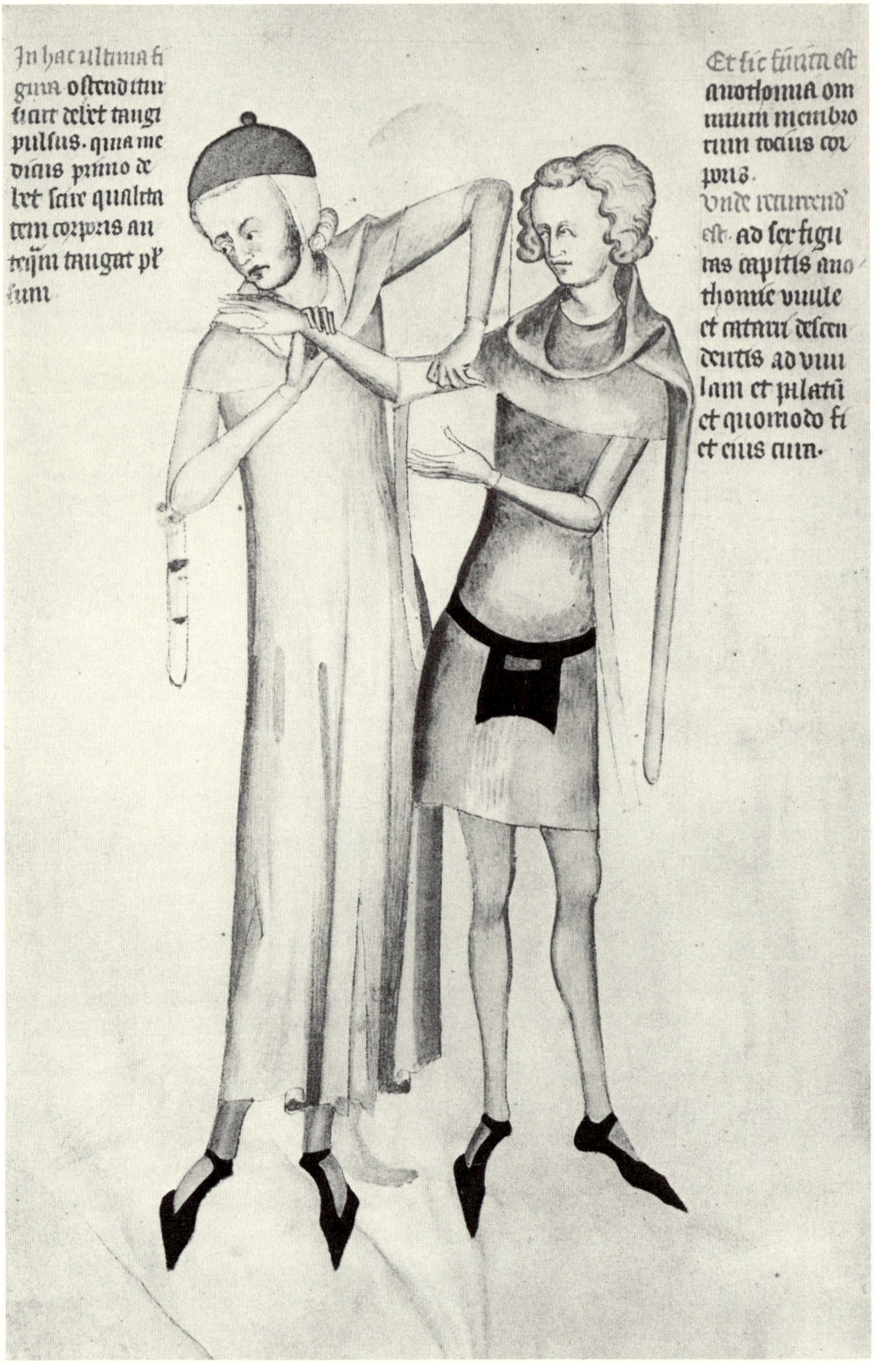

No. 57. Guido de Vigevano. *Anatomies de Mondino dei Luzzi et de Guido de Vigevano.* One of the earliest depictions of palpation of radial and brachial pulses.

*59. MATTHAEUS SILVATICUS (d. ca. 1342). *Liber pandectarum medicinae.* [Venice: Octaviani Scoti per Bonetum Locatellum, 1498]. 181 [1] *ll.* 29 cm. Antique calf.

As medicine began to emerge from the dark ages, the medieval student was confronted with an amazing variety of new words. Many of these words were of Greek, Arabic, Hebrew, or Syriac origin and the medical student was especially interested in mastering the meaning and composition of the new drugs whose uses were important in his practice. Thus it is not surprising to find that dictionaries were among the first books to be printed.

Silvaticus, a Mantuan physician, lived during the fourteenth century and prepared this dictionary which first appeared in printed form in the early 1470's. Arranged in alphabetical order, his dictionary is mainly a treatise on Arabic drugs. Special sections, sometimes covering several pages, are devoted to the more important drugs. In the longer entries, the Latinized form of the Arabic word is followed by its Latin and Greek equivalents. A description of the drug is given and its uses by such authorities as Avicenna, Mesuë, Serapion, Galen, and Dioscorides are provided. Freind, in his *History of physick,* Vol. 2, p. 265 (see No. 490) says "either through the fault of the original Writer or the Transcribers, that there is scarce any understanding it; there being hardly one line, where there is not a barbarous or unintelligible expression: so that there wants another Dictionary to explain his meaning." Nevertheless, the work was popular and by 1498 had already gone through eight editions.

In the present edition, for the first time, the editor, Georgius de Ferrariis, has incorporated the *Synonyma medicinae* of Simon Genuensis (fl. 1285). Genuensis (or Simon of Genoa) was physician to Pope Nicholas IV and prepared his dictionary of the materia medica after many years of travel and study in the late thirteenth century.

Durling 4205 (1507 ed.); Goff S 517; Hain 15202; Klebs 919.9; Waller 143 (1580 ed.); Wellcome 5970 (1480 ed.).

*60. JOHN OF GADDESDEN (1280?–1361). *Rosa anglica practica medicine a capite ad pedes noviter impressa & per que diligentissime emendata.* [Venice: Impressa mandato & expensis heredum Octaviani Scoti, per Bonetum Locatellum, 1502]. 135 *ll.* 28.1 cm.

John studied at Merton College, Oxford, then practiced first at Oxford and later in London, where he was highly esteemed among his contemporaries. He was the first Englishman to be appointed çourt physician to an English king, Edward II, and is said to have been Chaucer's model for the "Doctour of Phisik" in the *Canterbury tales.* His famous treatise, *Rosa anglica,* appearing around 1314, was first printed at Pavia in 1492. It was the first printed medical book written by an Englishman and this is a copy of the very scarce second edition. It is not noted for its scientific approach to medicine and is not much more than a medical advisor for the layman. However, John covered his subject quite thoroughly and the book is typical of other medical works of the period.

Durling 2607; Garrison-Morton 2191 (1492 ed.); Osler 7447 (1492 ed.); Wellcome 2486.

GUIDO DE VIGEVANO (fl. 14th century). *Anathomia.*

See No. 57.

*61. GUY DE CHAULIAC (ca. 1300–ca. 1368). *Guidon in cirugia.* [Venice: Per Cesaro Arrivabeno, 1521]. [4] cxxxviii (misnumbered cxl) [1] *ll.* 2 copies. Copy 1: 31.1 cm. Modern vellum. Copy 2: 29.6 cm. Modern vellum, in slipcase.

Guy de Chauliac was undoubtedly the most famous surgeon of the later Middle Ages. He studied at Montpellier, Paris, and Bologna, receiving his Magister in 1325. During the great plague he was physician to Pope Clement VI and later to the popes at Avignon, where he became acquainted with Petrarch.

His *Chirurgia magna* was the standard surgical text during the later Middle Ages and was frequently found in manuscript form before its first printed publication in 1478. It was still being reprinted and translated two centuries later, so great was its influence. The present edition is representative of the scores of editions of the work.

Guy was a reactionary, however, not following some of the reasonable principles of several of his predecessors, and his persistence in the meddlesome surgery of cautery, salves, and plasters, retarded surgery for at least two centuries because of his great authority.

This exhaustive treatise tells the personal and educational requirements of a physician; discusses pathology, medical treatment, surgery, and drug therapeutics; and altogether shows a spirit of aggressiveness which made Guy de Chauliac respected but not particularly loved.

Durling 2245; Waller 3820.

*62. ———. *La grande chirurgie.* Rouen: Chez Romain de Beauvais, 1615. [32] 711 [24] pp., front. (port.). 16.1 cm. Bound with No. 220.

Another typical edition of Guy's famous work, this time edited by Laurent Joubert. Joubert was one of the most celebrated members of the medical faculty at Montpellier and served as chancellor of the faculty for many years. His best known works were his Latin edition of Guy's surgery and his very popular *De vulgi erroribus* (1579). Joubert's annotations on the work were published as a separate volume and are here bound together with his edition of Guy (see No. 220).

Cushing G488; Waller 3827.

63. ———. *Le maistre en chirurgie, ou l'abregé complet de la chirurgie de Guy de Chauliac.* Paris: De l'Imprimerie de la Veuve d'Houry, 1740. [12] 560 pp. 16.4 cm. Calf.

This edition of Guy's surgery was first published at Paris in 1691 by Laurent Verduc (d. 1703) of the noted family of French surgeons. Although the work was originally published under the name of Verduc's father, Laurent (d. 1695), the younger Verduc actually edited the book. Written chiefly in the form of questions and answers, this edition—most likely the sixth—also contains an etymological dictionary of Greek words found in the text.

Cushing G492; Waller 9874 (1731 ed.); Wellcome III, p. 184.

*64. ———. *La grande chirurgie*. Paris: Félix Alcan, 1890. cxci, 747 pp., illus., 4 plates. 25.4 cm.

Guy de Chauliac's *Chirurgie* was first written in manuscript form in 1363 and is presented here in a modern French edition by the well-known French surgeon, essayist, and medical historian, Jules Édouard Nicaise. The book was published on the sixth centenary of the University of Montpellier where Guy studied and taught.

Cushing G489; Osler 2855; Waller 3830.

*65. FRANCESCO PETRARCA (1304–1374). *De remediis utriusque fortunae*. Cremona: Bernardinus de Misintis and Caesar Parmensis, 1492. 166 *ll.*, woodcuts: 1 initial, printer's device. 31.3 cm.

Although remembered chiefly as a poet, Petrarch also wrote philosophical essays and engaged in extensive correspondence with leaders of the Church and of Italian political life. He was trained in civil law at Montpellier and Bologna and never received any formal medical education. Petrarch experienced three major injuries during his lifetime and also suffered from fevers for at least three decades so he had many occasions to be ministered to by physicians of his day. It was perhaps from this close contact with the medical profession that he developed his great animosity toward physicians, directed more against their professional ethics than their therapeutics. He had little faith in their ability to benefit the patient and believed that they sold their services under false pretences. *De remediis utriusque fortunae* is his longest prose work; it became very popular after the invention of printing and was published in at least seven languages during the sixteenth century. A lengthy and repetitious exposition of Petrarch's moral philosophy, the book is concerned with attitudes toward good fortune as well as reactions to various misfortunes including such illnesses as gout, scabies, plague, toothache, pains in the legs, blindness, speech and hearing loss, agues, stomach pains, madness, and poisons.

Goff P 409; Hain-Copinger 12793; Wellcome 4928.

TOMMASO DEL GARBO (d. 1370). *Expositio . . . de generatione embrionis*.

See No. 84.

*66. JACOBUS Forliviensis (d. 1413). *Expositio . . . in primum Avicenne Canonem cum questionibus eiusdem . . . castigata . . . per Hieronymum Bompillum de Oleariis*. [Venice: Per Jacobum Pentium de Leucho, 1508]. [8] 214 *ll.* 31.7 cm. Modern quarter vellum.

Jacobus (also known as Giacomo della Torre) taught philosophy and medicine at Bologna and, from 1407 until his death, at Padua. He was a celebrated teacher and his well-known commentaries on Hippocrates, Galen, and Avicenna were used as standard textbooks for many years.

The present work is his commentary on the theoretical portion of Avicenna, edited by Hieronymus Bompilus de Oleariis (fl. 1508), a Veronese physician, who appends further commentaries on Avicenna by Jacques Desparts (ca. 1380–1458), the chief French representative of the Arabist school. Avicenna's text is included.

Durling 2561.

———. *Expositio cum questionibus aureum capitulum de generatione embrionis.*

See No. 84.

ANTONIO CERMISONE (d. 1441). *Consilia.*

See No. 70.

*67. VALASCUS DE TARENTA (ca. 1382–ca. 1418). *Practica, sive Philonium.* Lyons: Mathias Huss, 1490. [2] cclxvii (misnumbered cclxxii) [1] *ll.* 31.5 cm.

Valascus, a Portuguese by birth, received his education at Montpellier and was one of the foremost teachers and practitioners in Europe near the end of the fourteenth and beginning of the fifteenth centuries. In the *Philonium,* first published in 1488, he presents a general textbook of medicine intended to cover all of medicine except surgery. In keeping with the traditional arrangement, *a capite ad calcem,* he discusses diseases of the head, respiratory system, intestinal tract, liver, spleen, kidneys and bladder, sex organs, fevers, and epidemic diseases.

Goff V 7; Hain-Copinger 15251; Klebs 1010.3; Osler 7501; Wellcome 6420 (printed by J. Trechsel).

*68. SANTE ARDUINO (fl. 1430). *Opus de venenis.* Basel: [Per Henricum Petri, et Petrum Pernam, 1562]. [16] 569 (misnumbered 573) [14] pp. 30.9 cm. Contemporary limp vellum.

Arduino, a physician of Venice, was an active student of drugs and their actions and first prepared this work on poisons early in the fifteenth century. Although the book is primarily a compilation based on the work of earlier authors, Arduino often refers to his own personal experiences.

Also included with Arduino's *Opus* is Ferdinando Ponzetti's (d. 1528) *De venenis.* Ponzetti was a physician who later became Apostolic Secretary and then Cardinal. According to the dedicatory letter by the editor, Theodor Zwinger (1533–1588), this first collected edition was published at the suggestion of Konrad Gesner.

Durling 254; Wellcome 389.

*69. GIOVANNI ARCOLANI (ca. 1390–1458). *Opera, quibus . . . omnium morborum & symptomatum . . . causas & remediorum praesidia exponit, partium quoque situ*

& constitutione demonstratis. In quibus sunt & commentarii in Razis Arabis nonum lib. ad regem Almansorem . . . Sunt autem ad optimorum exemplarium fidem castigata. Basel: Per Henricum Petrum, 1540. [12] 747 pp., illus. 30.9 cm. Eighteenth century boards, rebacked in calf.

Arcolani, professor of medicine and surgery at Bologna and later at Padua, was one of a number of individuals who led in the struggle to break away from the rigid scholasticism of his time. This work, first published in 1480 under the title *Practica,* is chiefly a commentary on the ninth book of Rhaze's *Almansorem* (see No. 36). It was long used as a text in medical schools during the late fifteenth and sixteenth centuries and is of special interest in the history of dentistry because it contains the first description of the use of gold leaf in filling teeth. There are also several chapters on diseases of the teeth in which he treats his subject fully and with considerable accuracy. Arcolani also included material on the anatomy and physiology of the teeth but his information is largely incomplete and inaccurate. This has been attributed to the fact that he obtained most of his material from books and did not take time to verify it by direct observation. The single page of illustrations at the beginning of the book depicts a curved forceps used for extracting teeth, another forceps called a "stork's bill" used for removing tooth fragments and roots, two cautery irons, and a catheter.

Durling 249.

*70. BARTHOLOMAEUS MONTAGNANA (d. 1460). *Consilia . . . cum tribus tractatibus de balneis Patavinis et de compositione et dosi medicinarum ac antidotario.* [Venice: Per Simonem de Luere, 15,14]. [6] 413 *ll.* 30.8 cm.

Montagnana was first in a long line of famous professors of the same name who taught at Padua for nearly two hundred years. In the *Consilia,* Montagnana presents over three hundred case histories complete with physical condition, diagnosis, and treatment. This, the first edition published in the sixteenth century, was edited by Jacobus de Vitalibus (fl. 1510). Apart from the *Consilia,* the volume also contains three other works of Montagnana: his book on balneology, and two treatises on drugs and antidotes. Also included are the *Consilia* of Antonio Cermisone (d. 1441) and a monograph on the antidote theriac by Francesco Cavallo (d. 1540), both contemporaries of Montagnana at Padua.

Durling 3234; Osler 7464 (1497 ed.); Waller 102 (1476 ed.); Wellcome 4400 (1476 ed.).

71. BERNARDUS TREVISANUS (1406–1490). *Traicté de la nature de l'oeuf des philosophes.* Paris: [Chez Pierre Moët] 1659. 64 pp. 16.4 cm.

Nothing is known with certainty about the life and career of Bernardus Trevisanus, and some authorities feel that perhaps two or even three individuals wrote the works attributed to him. An alchemist, his writings reveal that he was well-acquainted with the writings of Avicenna, Geber, Albertus Magnus, Arnaldus de Villanova, and Thomas Aquinas. His works remained popular and were reprinted as late as the eighteenth century.

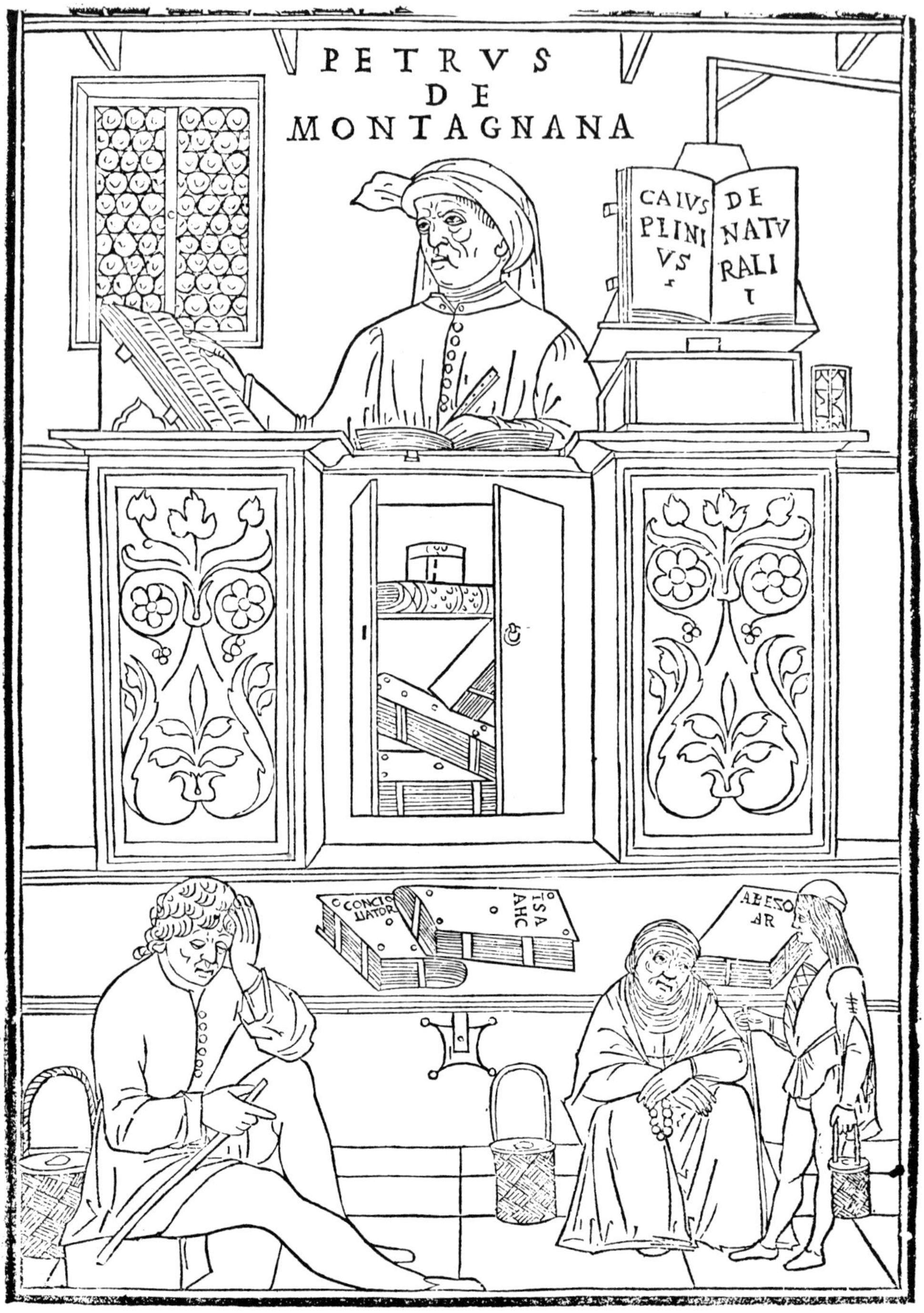

No. 72. Ketham. *Fasciculus Medicinae.* Montagnana teaching from the works of Pliny, Pietro d'Abano, Isaac Judaeus, and Avenzoar.

In this work on the nature of the philosophers' stone, he reiterated the alchemical doctrine that the philosophers' stone is composed of mercury alone. He asserted that the mysterious elixir which would transmute base metals and prolong life was made of pure mercury and contained within itself the entire *magisterium.*

Osler 2023 (1624 ed.); Wellcome 808 (1624 ed.).

*72. JOHANNES DE KETHAM (fl. 1460). *Fasciculus medicine.* [Venice: Per Cesarem Arrivabenum, 1522]. [63] *ll.,* illus., charts, diagrs. 29.2 cm. Nineteenth century quarter calf.

Little is known of Johannes de Ketham. He was born in Swabia and was practicing medicine in Vienna in 1460. Even his connection with this book is tenuous; it is possible that his only association with it was that he was the owner of the manuscript from which the first edition of Venice, 1491, was printed, though he may also have edited the text. His name does not appear in the Italian translation of 1493/94 or the Spanish translation of 1495, which form the second and third editions respectively. Indeed, the name "de Ketham" is probably a corruption, by the Italian printers, of "von Kirchheim."

The work is a collection of medical texts then current among students and practitioners, some of which had been in use for centuries, others more recent. Among the most important is the *Anothomia* of Mondino, which is the first modern treatise on anatomy, but which did not appear until the second edition of the *Fasciculus medicinae.*

But the texts themselves, while not unimportant, pale alongside the illustrations which accompany the volume. Those appearing in the first edition were the first realistic illustrations to a medical book and are among the best woodcuts of the fifteenth and early sixteenth centuries. Among them are Zodiac Man, the Bloodletting Man, the Planet Man, the dissection scene, the Female Figure with Uterus, and, of special interest, the full-page woodcut showing Petrus de Montagnana teaching.

The work was popular for a generation from the time of its first appearance in 1491, but after 1523 it was not much used. But during this twenty-four-year period it went through fourteen known editions and translations. In this 1522 edition, the thirteenth in the line of editions, the ten woodcuts had been altered or redrawn and recut over the years and even the older plates had suffered from wear over the years. But, despite this, they remain here of more than usual interest and beauty.

"This edition [1522], as its title-page tells us, is drawn from the 1500 edition. . . . We meet now, however, with a number of additions . . . and the Ketham myth has reached its final form, for the volume opens with the phrase 'Here begins the *Fasciculus medicinae* composed by that most consummate Master of the Arts and of Medicine Dominus Johannes de Ketham the Alemanian. . . .'" (Charles Singer in his introduction to *The fascicula di medicina, Venice, 1493,* Florence, 1925. Part I, p. 40).

Choulant-Frank, pp. 115–122; Cushing K58; Durling 2660; Waller 5174; Wellcome 3549 (Italian ed.).

*73. NICCOLÒ LEONICENO (1428–1524). *De epidemia quam Itali morbum gallicum, Galli vero Neapolitanum vocant.*

ULRICH VON HUTTEN (1488–1523). *De admiranda guaiaci medicina & morbi Galeni* [sic, i.e. gallici] *curatione.*

PIETRO ANDREA MATTIOLI (1500–1577). *Morbi gallici novum . . . opusculum quo vera . . . eius cura percipi potest.*

LORENZ FRIES (ca. 1490–1531). *Epitome opusculi de curandis pustulis, ulceribus, & doloribus mali Frantzoss.*

SCRIBONIUS LARGUS (fl. ca. 40 A.D.). *De compositione medicamentorum* [Selections].

JUAN ALMENAR (fl. 1500). *Libellus de morbo gallico.*

ANGELO BOLOGNINI (fl. 1517). *Liber de cura ulcerum exteriorum. Et De unguentis.* Venice: [Per Joannem Patavinum & Venturinum de Ruffinellis] 1535. 192 *ll.* 14.9 cm. Bound with No. 95.

Once the venereal origin of syphilis had been established, no country wanted to take responsibility for its having developed within its own borders. As a result, each country blamed its neighbor and during the fifteenth and sixteenth centuries syphilis was known among Italian physicians as *morbus gallicus* (the French disease). This small book contains seven works, all but one of which deal with syphilis which first appeared in Italy late in the fifteenth century and quickly spread throughout Europe. Niccolò Leoniceno's description of syphilis was one of the first to appear, having initially been published in 1497. Juan Almenar, a Spanish physician, published another early description of syphilis in 1502 in which he advocated the use of mercury and a variety of vegetable substances for its treatment. Ulrich von Hutten, a German poet and man of letters, described his personal experiences with syphilis and its treatment with guaiacum in a book that gained wide popularity. Pietro Andrea Mattioli (see No. 141), an Italian botanist, published a classic commentary on Dioscorides and also wrote this small treatise on syphilis in which he reported extensively on syphilis of the newborn and specified mercury for treating the disease. The book also contains works on syphilis by Lorenz Fries, a Dutch physician, and Angelo Bolognini, an Italian military surgeon. Twenty prescriptions and remedies from Scribonius Largus' popular *De compositione medicamentorum* (see No. 14) are also included in this work.

Cushing L213; Durling 2812; Osler 3231; Wellcome 3780.

*74. [GIROLAMO MANFREDI] (ca. 1430–1492). *Opera nova intitulata Il perchè.* Ancona: [Per Bernardino Guerralda Vercelleso, 1514]. [8] 75 *ll.* 20.3 cm. Limp vellum.

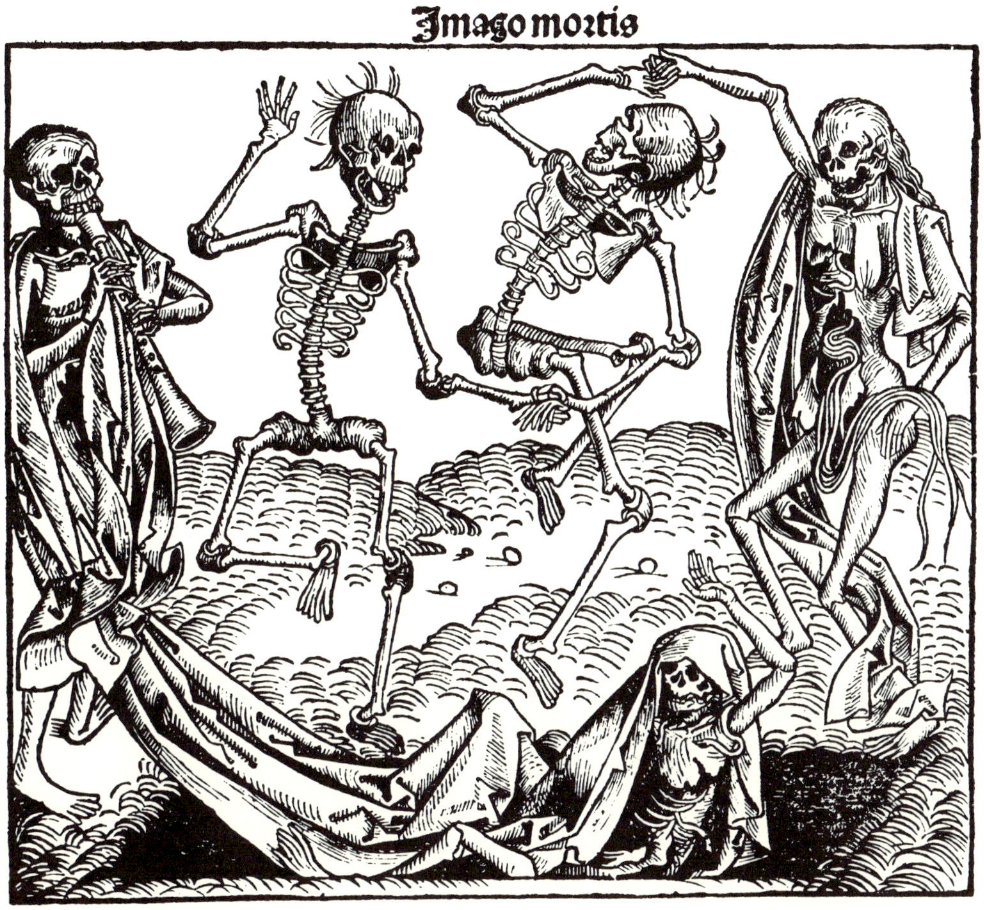

No. 78. Hartmann Schedel. *Liber Cronicarum* (Nuremberg Chronicle). Perhaps because of its bold animation, this woodcut of the Dance of Death is as impressive as the later Hogarth prints.

Manfredi was an astrologer, philosopher, and general scientist, as well as professor of medicine at Bologna.

The present work, first printed in 1474 under the title *Liber de homine*, passed through many editions until late in the seventeenth century. It contains chapters on diet, sex, evacuation, leprosy, the effects of wine, castrati, and other medical observations, many of which are quite curious.

Durling 2926 (1512 ed.); Waller 6211 (1523 ed.).

75. ———. ———. [Venice: Benedetto di Bendoni, 1532]. [16] 128 *ll.* 14.6 cm. Vellum.

Durling 2929.

76. ———. ———. Venice: Per Alessandro de Viano, 1567. [16] 143 (misnumbered 134) *ll.* 14.9 cm. Vellum.

Other editions of Manfredi's popular and often reprinted work.

Durling 2932.

*77. MARSILIO FICINO (1433–1499). *De vita libri tres, recens iam a mendis situque vindicati, ac summa castigati diligentia. . . . His accessit Epidemiarum antidotus.* Venice: Subsigno diui Giorgii, 1548. 144 *ll.* 14.9 cm. Vellum.

Ficino, leading thinker of the Neoplatonic Academy founded by Cosimo de' Medici in Florence, is probably the most important representative of humanism in later fifteenth-century Italy. His translation of Plato was a best seller by fifteenth-century standards and, in addition, he translated other ancient philosophers and wrote numerous treatises in which he sought to harmonize Platonism with Christianity.

Ficino was a physician as well as a philosopher, and the present work, a late edition of a work originally titled *De triplici vita* and first published in 1489, contains essays on medicine, astrology, and philosophy. Of interest to the medical historian are his chapters on headaches, diseases of the stomach, dietetics, and, in an addition to the main work, a Latin translation of his treatise on combating the plague.

Durling 1547; Osler 2584 (1532 ed.); Wellcome 2256 (1489 ed.).

*78. HARTMANN SCHEDEL (1440–1514). *Liber cronicarum.* Nuremberg: Anton Koberger, 1493. [20] cclxvi [6] cclxvii–ccxcix [1] *ll.*, woodcuts: illus., maps. 43.7 cm.

The Nuremberg Chronicle is one of the most renowned illustrated books of all times and its woodcuts are of great importance in furthering the study and knowledge of art. It is among the earliest illustrated books of the incunable period and has been the subject of many critical studies. The book contains nearly two thousand woodcuts done by Michael Wohlgemuth (1434–1519) and Wilhelm Pleydenwurff (d. 1494). Albrecht Dürer (1471–1528) was an apprentice of the two

Auicenna

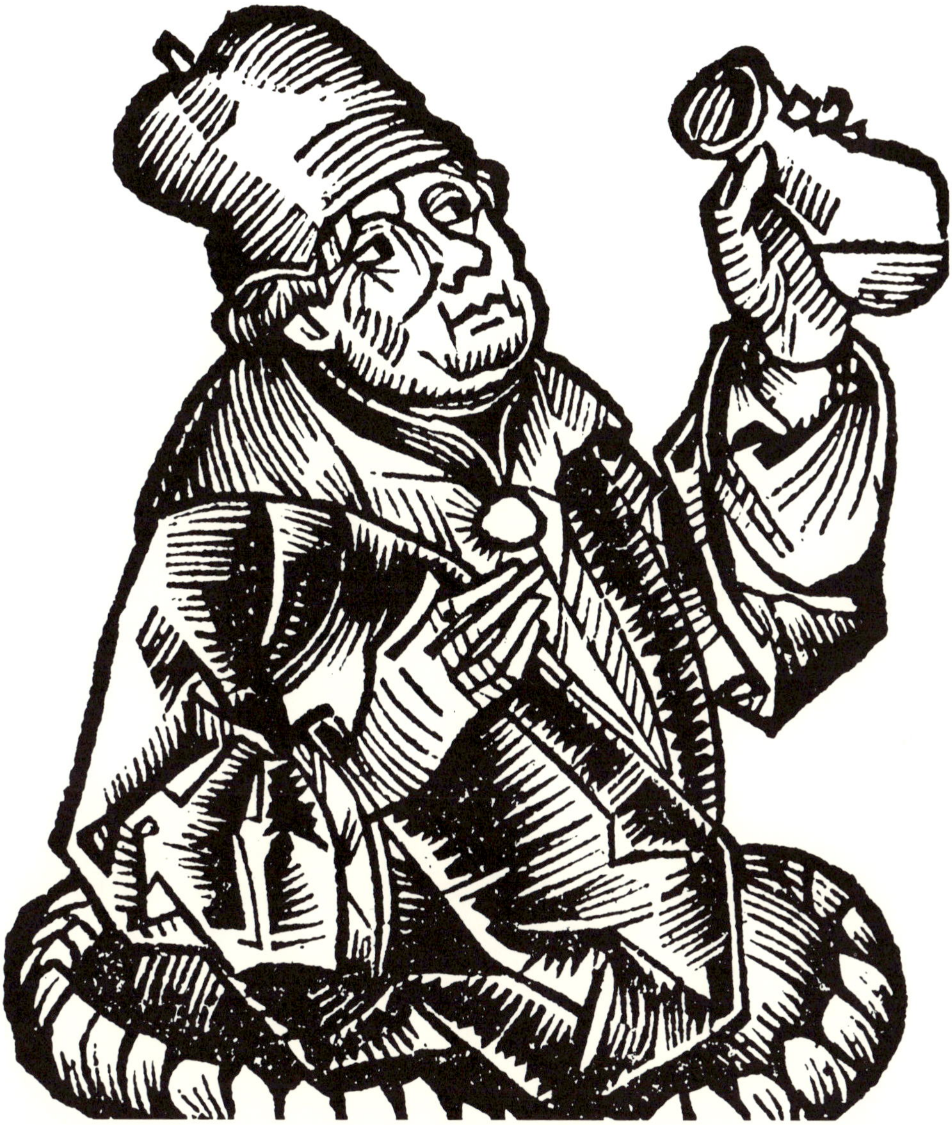

No. 78. Hartmann Schedel. *Liber Cronicarum* (Nuremberg Chronicle). This woodcut was used for the portraits of Galen, Avicenna, Isaac Judaeus, and other notable medical figures.

painters at the time and it is highly probable that he aided in producing the illustrations. Although the *Chronicle* is wide-ranging in scope, its author was a prominent member of the medical community in Nuremberg and was ably assisted in his task by another Nuremberg physician Hyeronimus Muenzer (d. 1508). The book contains numerous biographies. Those of medical significance include Galen, Isaac Judaeus, Rhazes, Serapion the Elder, Avicenna, Avenzoar, and Averroës. There are also reports on epidemics and plagues and the widespread mental affections, such as the sects of flagellants and wandering dancers, as well as material about hospital construction and public sanitation.

Goff S 307; Hain-Copinger 14508; Klebs 889.1; Waller 141 (German ed.); Wellcome 5822.

*79. ANTONIO BENIVIENI (1443–1502). *Di alcune ammirabili ed occulte cause di morbi e loro guarigioni*. Florence: Giovanni Ricordi e Stefano Jouhaud, 1843. 167 pp. 21.2 cm.

Benivieni, a contemporary of Leonardo da Vinci and Savonarola, was born in Florence and studied medicine in his native city as well as in Pisa and Siena. He spent his professional life in Florence where he was among the first physicians to study syphilis. However, he is best known for writing the first book on pathological anatomy—*De abditis nonnullis ac mirandis morborum et sanationum causis*—which was published by his brother in 1507. Here, in 111 observations covering some twenty postmortem examinations, Benivieni has deliberately attempted to determine the precise cause of death. Among his many observations are descriptions of vesical calculus, carcinoma of the stomach, gall stones, and syphilitic periostitis. Neither before Benivieni nor until the work of Bonet in his *Sepulchretum* (1679) (see No. 335) and later by Morgagni in his *De sedibus* (1761) (see No. 498) was there any existing work so important in the development of gross pathology.

The present work is the first translation of this classic in pathology into a modern language. The translator, Carlo Burci (fl. 1840), was professor of pathological anatomy at Arcispedale di S. M. Nuova—a Florence hospital.

Durling 528 (1st Latin ed., 1507); Garrison-Morton 2270 (1st Latin ed.); Waller 894 (1st Latin ed.).

———. *De abditis nonnullis ac mirandis morborum & sanationum causis*.

See No. 14.

GABRIELE DE ZERBIS (1445–1505). *Anatomia infantis*.

See No. 139.

GIORGIO VALLA (1447–1500). *De humani corporis partibus*.

See No. 154.

ALESSANDRO BENEDETTI (ca. 1450–1512). *Sententiae medicinales*.

See No. 111.

80. LEONARDO DA VINCI (1452–1519). *I manoscritti di Leonardo da Vinci della Reale biblioteca di Windsor: Dell'anatomia, fogli A*[–*B*]. 2 vols. Parigi and Torino: Edoardo Rouveyre and Roux e Viarengo, 1898–1901. Vol. I: 202 pp., 34 plates (part fold.); Vol II: 271 pp., 79 plates. Plates have guard sheets with descriptive letterpress and numbered outlines of the figures on the accompanying plate. 35.9 cm. Each volume in slipcase. A facsimile: No. 142 of 400 copies.

It is well known that Leonardo was one of the greatest artists and scientists of the Italian Renaissance. His contributions to science are numerous and include significant accomplishments in mechanics, physics, hydraulics, astronomy, anatomy, architecture, and civil engineering.

As a result of his anatomical studies, he is considered to be the founder of physiological anatomy. After his death, his writings and drawings were forgotten for over two centuries and became scattered among private collectors, libraries, and archives throughout Europe. Thus very little remains of the anatomical drawings that Leonardo had intended eventually to become a treatise on anatomy. The greater part of his extant writings and drawings on anatomy were found at the Royal Library of Windsor Castle in the early 1700's; however, no drawings from the collection were published until 1796. The first effort to make the collection available to the public in facsimile was not made until 1898 when the first volume of this set, containing a transcription of Leonardo's text together with a French translation, was issued. The second volume was published in 1901; unfortunately both volumes contained numerous mistakes due to misunderstandings, ignorance of the subject, and the difficulty of interpreting Leonardo's very fine mirror handwriting.

Choulant-Frank, pp. 99–105; Cushing L158; Garrison-Morton 364; Osler 514; Waller 9986.

81. ———. *Quaderni d'anatomia*. 6 vols. Christiania: Jacob Dybwad, 1911–1916. Col. plates. 41.2 cm. A facsimile: No. 187 of 248 copies.

This work contains the remainder of the drawings not included in *Dell'anatomia* as well as an Italian transcription of the text with translations into English and German. The facsimiles are of excellent quality, but the volumes are not properly annotated and the translations frequently suffer from error.

Choulant-Frank, pp. 99–105; Cushing L162; Garrison-Morton 365; Osler 517; Waller 9987.

82. ———. *Corpus of the anatomical studies in the collection of Her Majesty the Queen at Windsor Castle.* Edited by Kenneth D. Keele and Carlo Pedretti. 2 vols. and atlas: 176 col. plates. New York: Harcourt Brace Jovanovich, 1979. 45 cm. Royal blue Nigerian goatskin. A facsimile: No. 23 of 998 copies.

The editors of this modern edition, Kenneth D. Keele (b. 1930?) and Carlo Pedretti (b. 1928), are acknowledged scholars of Leonardo's work and have carefully

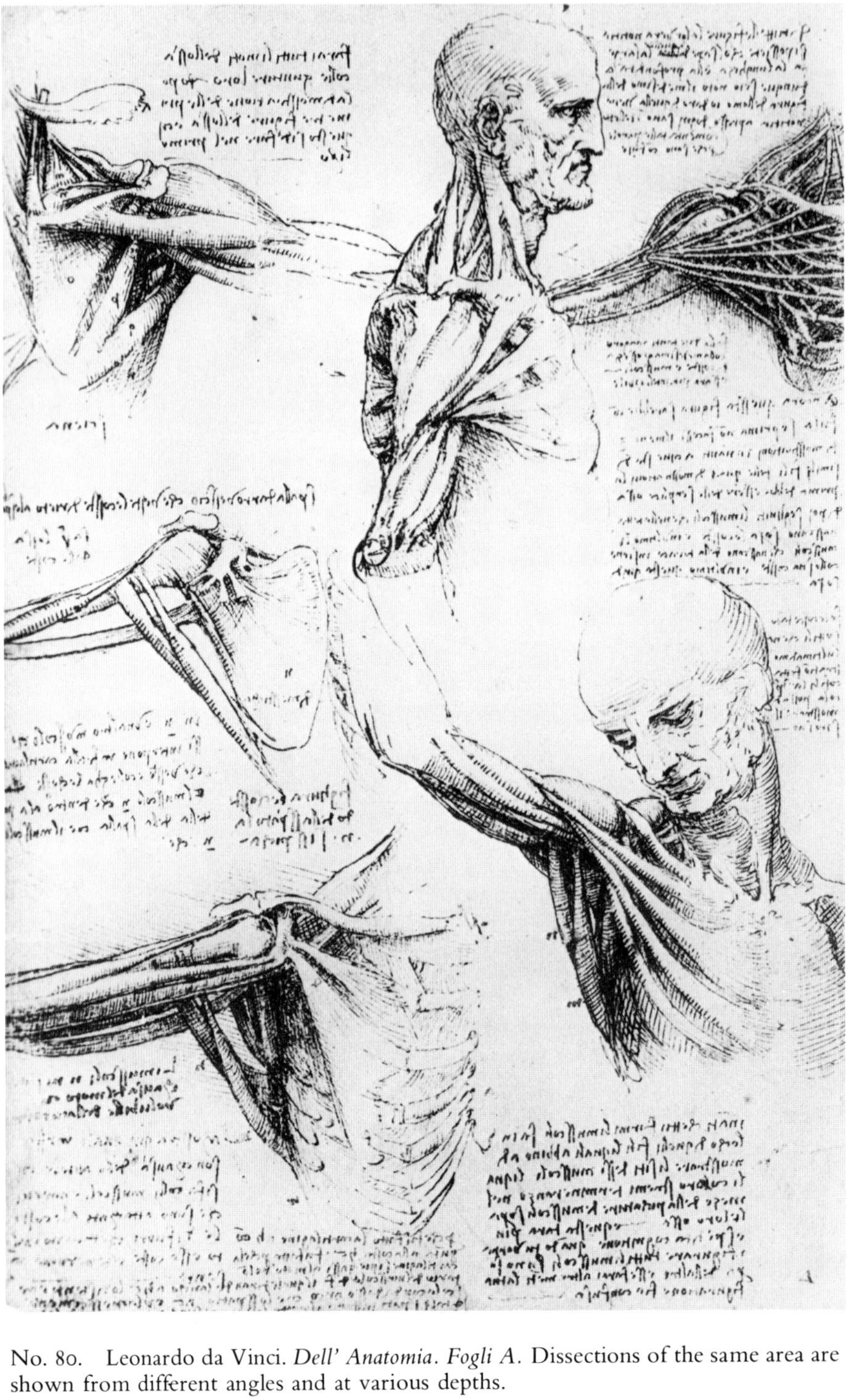

No. 80. Leonardo da Vinci. *Dell' Anatomia. Fogli A.* Dissections of the same area are shown from different angles and at various depths.

studied and reconstructed the chronology of Leonardo's drawings. As a result, many puzzling aspects of Leonardo's notes have now been clarified and our understanding of his manner of collecting and interpreting anatomical information has been greatly increased.

The text volumes contain monochrome reproductions of each drawing along with transliterations of Leonardo's original Italian notes and translations of the notes into English. The editors have also included detailed commentaries and indices. The 201 drawings have also been expertly reproduced in color using modern photographic techniques and have been arranged in chronological order.

*83. ———. *Tabula anatomica Leonardi da Vinci.* Lüneberg: Sumtibus Heroldi et Wahlstabii, 1830. [5] pp., 1 plate. 32.8 cm. A facsimile.

This tall, slender volume contains but one plate, representing a male and female engaged in sexual intercourse. Both individuals are cut in a plane through the median line from front to back and from the shoulders down to the lower end of the abdominal cavity. There are also three other anatomical figures on the plate: one pictures the digestive organs, another the male genitalia, and the third a male torso. All are accompanied by notes in Leonardo's nearly indecipherable mirror writing. The drawing is believed to have been done around 1493 and is among the very few anatomical studies Leonardo did during this period. It is one of the earliest of his drawings to be reproduced in facsimile and was engraved by Francesco Bartolozzi (fl. 1800) for John Chamberlaine (1745–1812) who included it in his *Imitations of original designs by Leonardo da Vinci* in 1796.

Cushing L164; Osler 513; Waller 9988.

JUAN ALMENAR (fl. 1500). *Libellus de morbo gallico.*

See No. 73.

*84. BASSIANUS POLITUS, compiler (fl. 1500). . . . *De generatione embrionis. . . . De natura fetus.* [Venice: Impresse mandato & expensis heredum Octaviani Scoti, per Bonetum Locatellum, 1502]. 90 *ll.* 28.9 cm. Modern vellum.

In this rare little volume are included four works on the embryo and fetus:

JACOBUS Forliviensis (d. 1413). *Expositio cum questionibus aureum capitulum de generatione embrionis.* Commentary on a text of Avicenna concerning reproduction, by Jacobus (also known as Giacomo della Torre), who was a leading exponent of Arabian medicine in the early days of the school at Padua. Contains the text of Avicenna translated into Latin (see also No. 66).

DINO DEL GARBO (d. 1327). *Expositio . . . de generatione embrionis cum questionibus eiusdem.* Garbo was a famous Florentine and Bolognese physician who comments here on the same text of Avicenna.

TOMMASO DEL GARBO (d. 1370). *Expositio . . . de generatione embrionis.* Tommaso, the son of Dino del Garbo, was a Florentine physician and a friend of

Petrarch, with whom he kept up an interesting correspondence. This is another commentary on the Avicennian text.

DINO DEL GARBO. *Scriptum . . . super libro de natura fetus Hypo*[*cratis*]. The text of Hippocrates' treatise on the fetus is given in Latin translation followed by Garbo's commentary.

Cushing J17; Durling 2562.

*85. GIOVANNI DE VIGO (1460?–1520?). *Practi[ca] . . . copiosa in arte chirurgica.* [Venice: Impressum ere ac sollerti cura heredum Octaviani Scotis, & sociorum, 1520]. 113 *ll.* 29.4 cm. Modern full vellum. Bound with No. 86.

Vigo was born near Genoa and came to Rome in 1503 as physician to Pope Julius II. The present work, first published in 1514, immediately met with great success, and in less than thirty years it went through twenty-one editions and was translated into Italian, English, Spanish, French, German, and Portuguese. It is mostly a compilation from other authors blended with Vigo's own experience, showing little originality. Nevertheless, this was the chief surgical textbook until the time of Paré. Part of its great popularity was no doubt due to Vigo's discussion of the two major problems of his time: gunshot wounds and syphilis. He recommended cautery and boiling oil for treating gunshot wounds and mercury-based ointments and inunctions for syphilis. Vigo was also interested in dentistry and was one of the first to use gold leaf to fill cavities of the teeth. In spite of the fact that his works were widely published, early editions, such as the present work, are rare.

Cushing V144 (1514 ed.); Durling 4609; Garrison-Morton 5559.1 (1514 ed.); Waller 9976 (1514 ed.); Wellcome 6610 (1516 ed.).

*86. ———. *Practica compendiosa . . . quam post suam copiosam in chirurgia compilavit.* [Venice: Impensa heredum quondam Octaviani Scoti Modoetiensis, ac sociorum, 1520]. 21 *ll.* 29.4 cm. Modern full vellum. Bound with No. 85.

Vigo first published this popular compendium or epitome of his surgery in 1517. It condenses the nine books of his surgery into five books dealing primarily with wounds and fractures, abscesses, ulcers, and remedies and cures for a variety of ailments.

Durling 4605; Wellcome 6612.

87. ———. *Opera in chyrurgia. Additur chyrurgia Mariani sancti Barolitani.* 2 vols. in 1. [Lyons: Excusa per Anthonium du Ry, impensis Jacobi. q. Francisci de Giuncta Florentini ac sociorum, 1525]. Vol. I: cclxxix [5] *ll.;* Vol. II: [3] lxxxvi [3] *ll.* 15.8 cm. Vellum.

It has been estimated by medical historians that more than fifty editions of Vigo's popular surgery were published. The present work is one of the early editions which, in addition to Vigo's surgery and compendium, contains a surgical treatise by Mariano Santo (ca. 1488–ca. 1550). Santo was a Neapolitan student of Vigo

Magnus Alexander Achillinus.

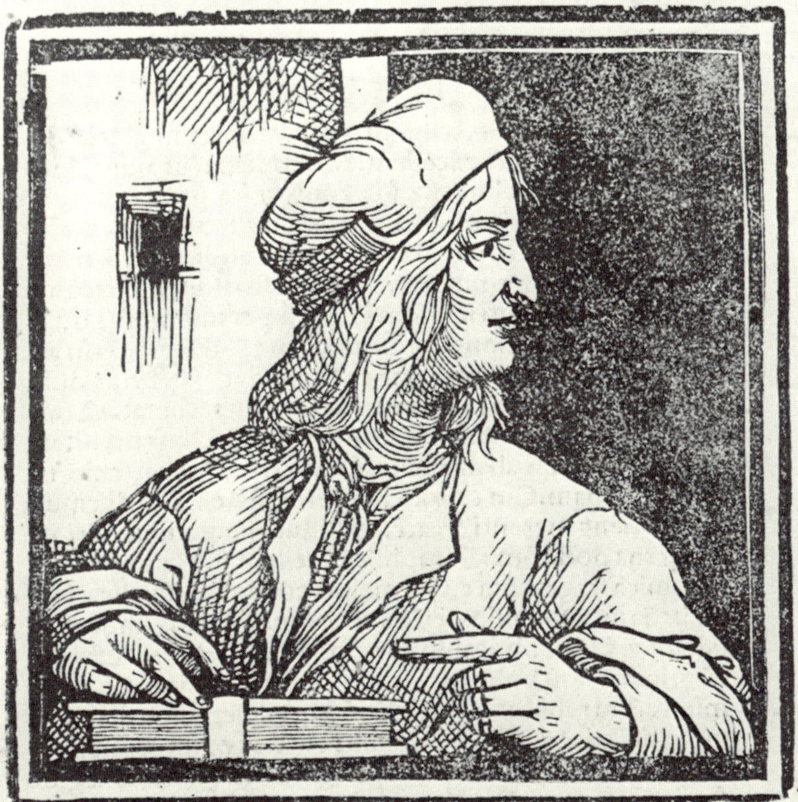

Hannibal Camillus Corrigienſis artium & Medicinæ diſcipulus
Lectori. S. D.

Congeriem ſtudioſa cohors fabricantia noſce
Corporis humani ſemina ſi qua uelit.
Verſet Achilleum nocteſq; dieſq; uolumen.
Quod nimis exiguum ne tamen eſſe putet.
Quicquid enim eximii toto deus orbe creauit
Paruulus in parua molle recondit homo.

Eiuſdem Hannibalis Diſticum.

Omniparens hominem fabrefecit uernula ſummi
Patris. Alexander conſcius illa docet.

No. 89. Achillini. *Anotomicae* [sic] *Annotationes*. The only known portrait of the author.

who achieved great fame through his introduction of the so-called "Marian operation" of lithotomy.

Durling 4610; Osler 4173 (1534 ed.); Wellcome 6614 (1531 ed.).

Purchased from the James Emmett Conn Memorial Book Fund.

*88. GIOVANNI MANARDO (1462–1536). *Epistolarum medicinalium libri duodeviginti*. Basel: [J. Bebelius] 1535. [28] 467 pp. 31.7 cm. Bound in leaf of vellum manuscript.

Manardo, a native of Ferrara and physician to King Ladislaus of Hungary, was one of the first Italians to rebel against Galen's dogmas and was an early supporter of Paracelsus.

Although the first edition of this work appeared in 1521, this edition of 1535 is essentially a new work, as the earlier edition contained only six books while the later contains eighteen. "The letters illustrate in an interesting way—and this is their value—the transition from Arabian to Greek dominion. The opinions of Avicenna, Hippocrates and Galen are quoted on every page" (Osler 3316). There are several chapters on syphilis, one mentioning that it is believed that the disease was brought by Spanish sailors "ex insula quadam antiqua incognita" ("from an island unknown to the ancients"), usually taken to refer to America.

Durling 2914; Wellcome 4000 (1521 ed.).

*89. ALESSANDRO ACHILLINI (1463–1512). *Anotomicae* [sic] *annotationes*. Bologna: Impressae per Hieronymum de Benedictis, 1520. xviii *ll.*, port. 21.2 cm. Contemporary blind-stamped calf.

Achillini was one of the leading pre-Vesalian anatomists and one of the few physicians who had the audacity to dissect human bodies during the fifteenth century. His works are rare; this one, perhaps his most important and best-known work, was published posthumously by his brother, Giovanni Filoteo (1466–1538). He was actually better known as a teacher of logic and philosophy during his lifetime but today is remembered for his study of the human body. The only illustration in this small, modest volume is a woodcut portrait of the author and a woodcut initial letter A, containing an armorial crest.

Durling 31; Waller 178.

*90. GREGOR REISCH (ca. 1467–1525). *Margarita philosophica*. 2nd ed. [Freiburg? Johannes Schottus, 1504]. [330] *ll.*, illus., fold. map, diagrs. (2 fold.). 20.4 cm. Bound in page of sixteenth century manuscript mounted on boards.

Reisch was a Carthusian prior at Freiburg and confessor to Emperor Maximilian I, as well as assistant to Erasmus. His famous book, *Margarita philosophica*, might be called the first modern encyclopedia. Its twelve divisions cover the trivium, the quadrivium, and the natural and moral sciences. Its numerous illustrations are fine examples of the art of wood-block cutting, and include woodcuts of music, a large

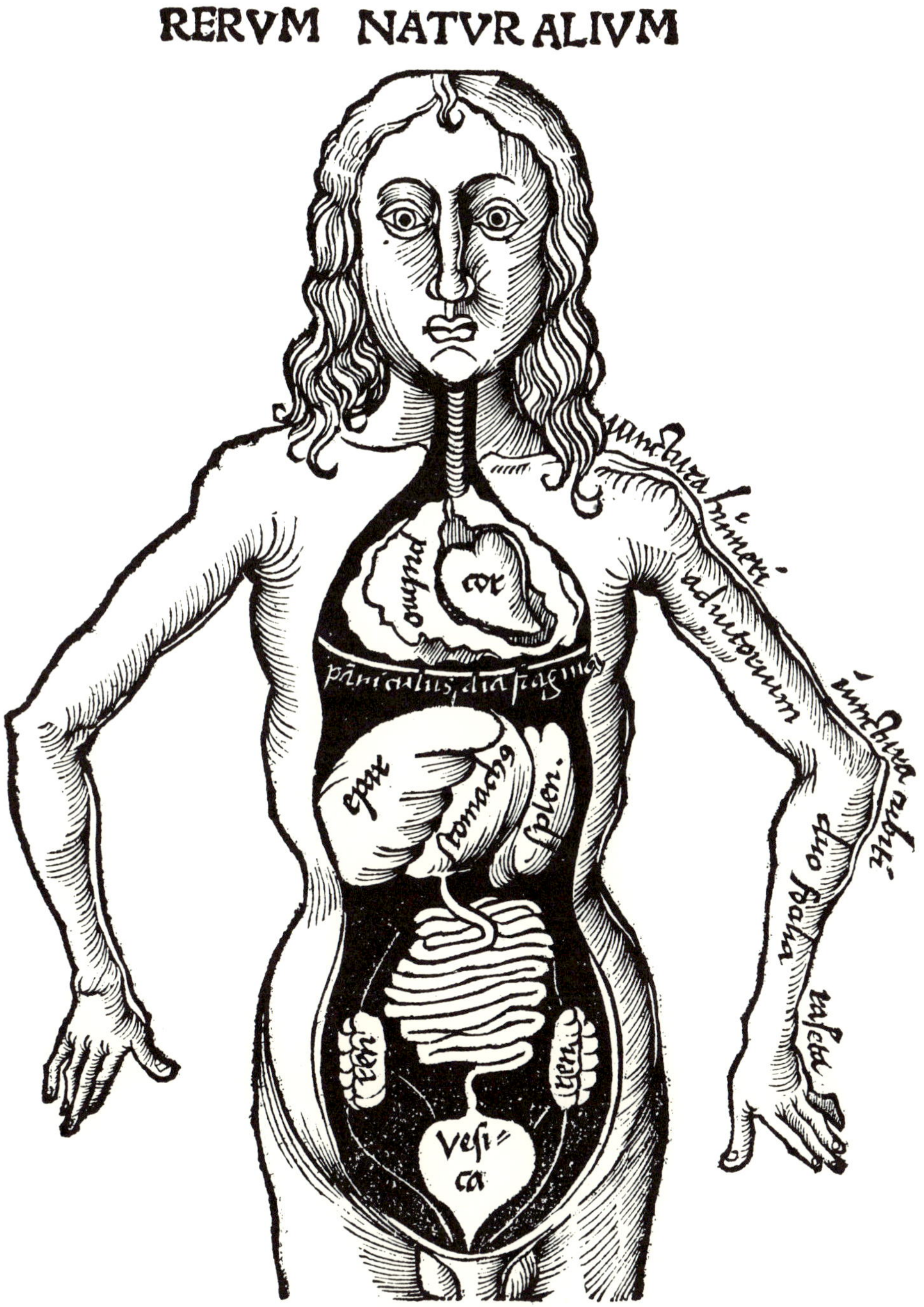

No. 90. Reisch. *Margarita Philosophica.* One of the earliest printed illustrations of the internal organs.

folding map of the Eurasian continent and parts of Africa, and astronomical, astrological, and zoological figures. Four of the plates are of great interest to the history of anatomical illustration, and several others are of medical interest: a man with dissected thoracic and abdominal cavities; two figures of the eye (these did not appear in the first edition and are the earliest printed figures of the anatomy of the eye); a phrenological head showing the brain; a lying-in room showing a woman in childbed, with infant and midwife; and a mineral spring bath. Both the eye and visceral manikin are crude in concept, but are often reproduced for their historial importance in the history of anatomical illustration.

Much more could be said of this immensely fascinating book; the music and the map (often missing from copies of all editions) make extremely interesting studies in themselves. The book was very popular, as attested to by its sixteen editions in the seventeenth century. This edition, the second authorized edition, was preceded by the first edition of 1503 and a "pirated" reprinting of the first edition which appeared the month before this second edition.

Choulant-Frank, pp. 126–129; Cushing R90 (1st ed., 1503); Durling 3847.

FERDINANDO PONZETTI (d. 1528). *De venenis.*

See No. 68.

91. PIETRO BAIRO (1468–1558). *De medendis humani corporis malis enchiridion, quod vulgò Veni mecum vocant.* Basel: Apud Petrum Perna, 1578. [32] 665 [20] pp. 15.5 cm. Vellum.

The year after Bairo received his medical degree at the University of Turin in 1493, he became professor of medicine at Turin and began a long and successful career. At least one of the five known works of Bairo, a highly successful author, remained in print until the early eighteenth century.

The present work, first published in 1512, is a comprehensive treatise on medicine containing numerous recommendations for therapeutic remedies complete with instructions for compounding the remedy. Also included with this work is his *De peste*, a detailed discussion of the plague including his suggestions for curing those afflicted with the disease.

Durling 445; Wellcome 641 (Lyons ed.).

*92. JACOPO BERENGARIO DA CARPI (1470–1530). *Tractatus de fractura calvae sive cranei.* [Bologna: Impressum per Hieronymum de Benedictis, 1518]. cv *ll.*, illus. (woodcuts). 19.1 cm. Limp vellum with ties.

Berengario (or da Carpi, as he is often called) was the great anatomist of the period immediately before the flowering of medicine in the Renaissance. A native of Ferrara, professor of anatomy at Bologna from 1502 to 1522, and one-time professor at Padua, he may be thought of as the immediate predecessor of Vesalius. This work on skull fracture was occasioned by a controversy which had arisen among Berengario and other physicians regarding the post-operative treatment of a head wound suffered by Lorenzo de' Medici. It is especially interesting for the woodcuts of cranial instruments.

Cushing B302; Durling 531; Waller 911; Wellcome 778.

*93. ———. *Isagoge breves, perlucide ac uberime, in anatomia humani corporis.* [Bologna: Impressum per Benedictum Hectoris, 1522]. 72 *ll.*, illus. (woodcuts), including 4 plates. 21.1 cm.

Berengario was an adherent and serious student of Mondino and followed him in all matters pertaining to anatomy. He wrote *Commentaria* on Mondino's *Anothomia* (see No. 54) in 1521 and, because he was such a discerning observer, was able to correct many of Mondino's shortcomings and add many of his own observations. He then decided to write his own anatomical compendium and produced this work in 1522. Although his illustrations are inadequate and lacking in detail, his woodcuts are believed to be the first taken directly from human dissections. The full-length figures are always shown in action poses and his muscle figures and skeletons are drawn against landscape backgrounds in the same fashion used later by Estienne and Vesalius. Although Leonardo da Vinci's anatomical drawings (see No. 80 ff.) received limited circulation, it appears that Berengario was acquainted with them since the influence of Leonardo's artistic techniques is evident in a number of Berengario's woodcuts. The book is of unusual rarity and is an important example of anatomical illustration in the pre-Vesalian period.

Choulant-Frank, pp. 136–142; Cushing B298; Durling 534 (1523 ed.); Garrison-Morton 368; Waller 907; Wellcome 782.

*94. ———. *Anatomia Carpi. Isagoge breves, perlucide ac uberime, in anatomiam humani corporis.* Venice: [Impressum per Bernardinum De Vitalibus] 1535. 63 (misnumbered 61) *ll.*, illus. 18.4 cm. Vellum.

This anatomical compendium, first issued in 1522 and designed to replace the anatomy of Mondino which was still current, shows many innovations, one of which is a distinct break from Galen's influence. Clinician as well as anatomist, Berengario was among the first to use mercury in the treatment of the "French disease"; Benvenuto Cellini received such treatment from him. He gave the first descriptions of the sphenoid sinuses, the pineal gland, the tympanum, the valves of the heart, the lateral ventricles, and chorioid plexuses of the brain. He also noted the difference between the male and female pelvis and chest.

Choulant-Frank, pp. 136–142; Cushing B301; Durling 536; Garrison-Morton 368 (1522 ed.); Osler 2018; Waller 910.

*95. NICOLAUS POL (ca. 1470–1532). *De cura morbi Gallici per lignum guaycanum, libellus.* [Venice? Per Joannem Patavinum & Venturinum de Ruffinellis?] 1535. [8] *ll.* 14.9 cm. Bound with No. 73.

In this short work of nine chapters, Pol sets forth a regimen of treatment for syphilis with guaiacum, a resin extracted from the tree which is native to tropical

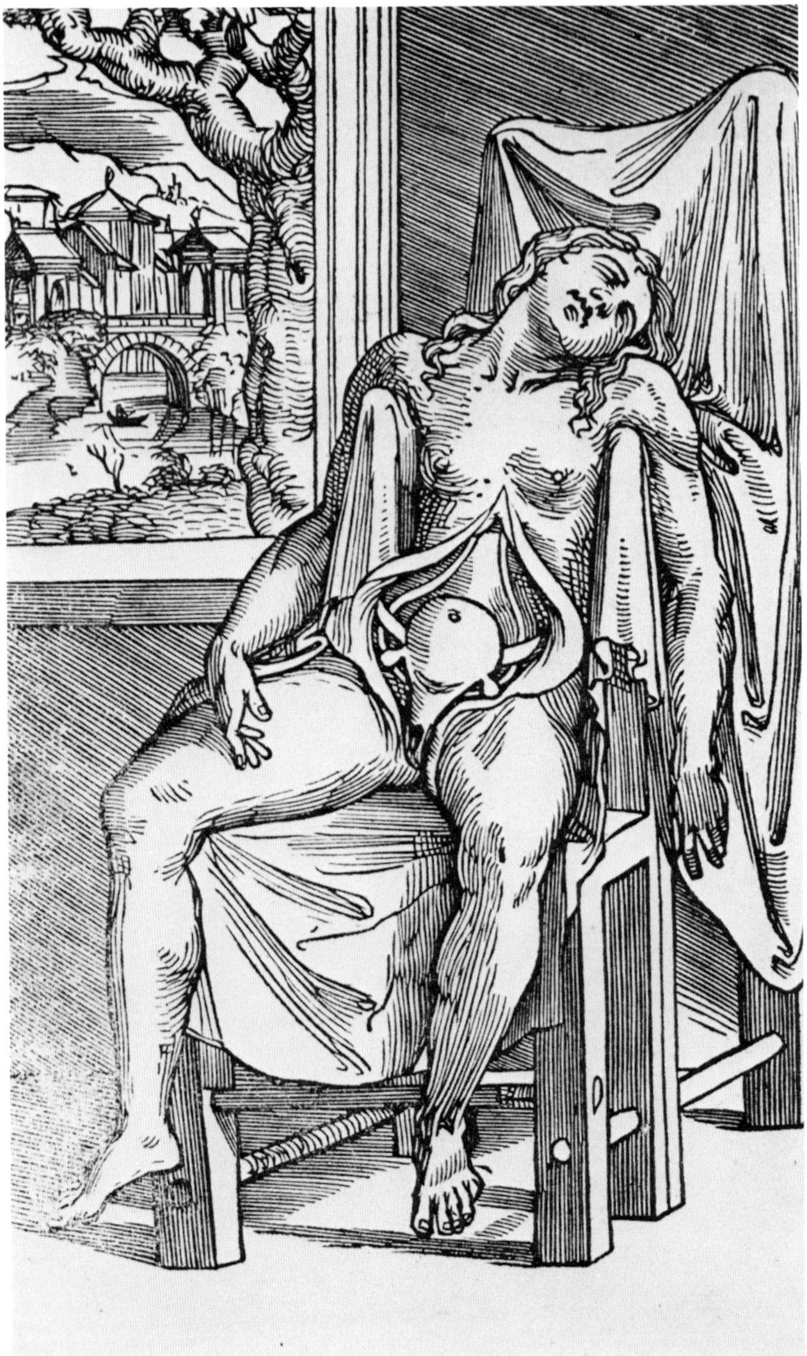

No. 93. Berengario. *Isagoge Breves*. Berengario's illustrations were among the first to be made directly from actual dissections.

America. He states that three thousand Spaniards had been cured of morbus gallicus (the "French disease") by means of guaiacum after many of them had tried other remedies without success. According to Pol, most were cured by a decoction of the wood in fifteen days although some patients required as long as sixty days. Anyone who suffered from the disease, even those who had had it for a decade or longer, could expect to be cured by taking the decoction and following the prescribed regimen.

Cushing P331; Durling 2812; Wellcome 5141.

*96. ALBRECHT DÜRER (1471–1528). *Della simmetria de i corpi humani, libri quattro*. Venice: Presso Domenico Nicolini, 1591. [6] 143 [1] *ll.*, illus., 3 fold. plates. 31.4 cm.

Albrecht Dürer was one of the greatest painters and engravers of the German Renaissance and authored many scientific treatises on such subjects as mathematics, chemistry, engineering, anatomy, and hydraulics. However, painting and engraving were his chief pursuits. His contributions to the techniques of these fields opened up new vistas for graphic artists everywhere. He believed that the beauty of the human body could not be captured completely without a thorough knowledge of its proportions and anatomy.

Dürer's important work on the proportions and symmetry of the human body was first published in German in 1528 and is filled with diagrams and figures. A Latin translation of the book appeared in two parts during the years 1532–1534, and this Italian translation of the Latin edition was published in 1591. The work is divided into four parts as the title indicates. The first two books discuss the proper proportions of the human form and its individual members; the third book gives examples of the human figure after mathematical formulae of proportions are applied to various body parts; and the fourth shows geometric representations of the human figure in motion. A fifth book without illustrations has been added by the translator, Giovanni Paolo Gallucci (1538–ca. 1621).

Choulant-Frank pp. 143–147; Durling 1299; Garrison-Morton 149 (1528 ed.); Wellcome 1920.

LUIGI CORNARO (1475–1566). *L'art de conserver la santé des religieuses, et Les avantages de la vie sobre.*

See No. 386.

*97. LUCA GAURICO (1476–1558). *Super diebus decretoriis (quos etiam criticos vocitant) axiomata.* [Rome: In aedibus Valerii Dorici, & Ludovici fratris Brixianorum] 1546. 138 (misnumbered 136) [1] pp., illus., diagrs. 28.5 cm.

This little-known treatise on astrological medicine is dedicated to Pope Paul III, who was greatly interested in the medical-astrological arguments of the century.

Durling 2027; Wellcome 2705.

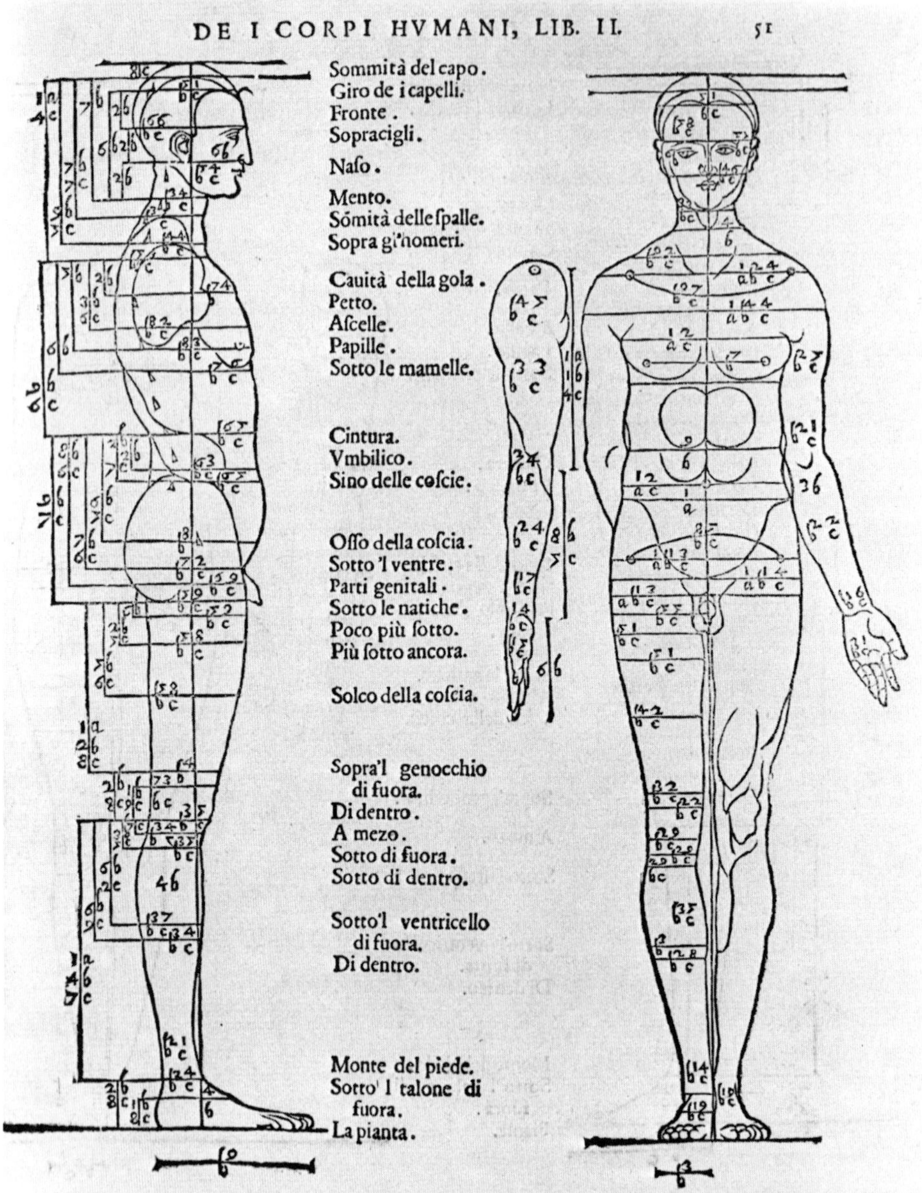

No. 96. Dürer. *Della Simmetria de i Corpi Humani.*

ANGELO BOLOGNINI (fl. 1517). *Liber de cura ulcerum exteriorum. Et De unguentis.*

See No. 73.

*98. GIROLAMO FRACASTORO (ca. 1478–1553). *Syphilis, sive Morbus Gallicus.* Verona: [Stefano dei Nicolini da Sabbio] 1530. [36] *ll.* 20.3 cm. Vellum.

Born of a patrician family in Verona, Fracastoro was the archetypical scholar of the Renaissance—astronomer, biologist, geographer, geologist, mathematician, musician, physician, poet.

Written at a time when syphilis was a terrible scourge in all of Europe, this most famous of all medical poems has given the name to the disease, probably the only poem for which a disease has been named. In it, the shepherd boy, Syphilis, is afflicted with the disease as a result of insulting Apollo. Fracastoro, through the course of the poem, speculates on the origin of the disease, treats of its causes and manifestations, and suggests remedies, especially mercury. There are several references to America, mentioning the curative powers of guaiacum wood and the theory of the American origin of syphilis, which Fracastoro rejects.

The first edition of *Syphilis* is a book of considerable rarity, and this particular copy is inscribed on the flyleaf, "Huius libri possessor est Scribonius," in a sixteenth century autograph, probably that of the philologist and poet, Cornelius Scribonius of Antwerp.

Cushing F284; Durling 1641; Garrison-Morton 2364; Osler 4817; Waller 3173; Wellcome 2391.

*99. ———. *La sifilide.* [Bologna: A. S. Tommaso d'Acquino, 1738]. viii, 137 pp. 27.3 cm. Original pasteboard covers.

More than one hundred editions of Fracastoro's poem have been traced, including translations into six languages. The second Italian translation, with the text in Latin and Italian on facing pages, is of considerable interest for the glossaries of medical terms.

Waller 3190; Wellcome III, p. 51.

*100. ———. *Syphilis, ou, Le mal vénérien.* Paris: C. Lucet, 1796. xiv, 162 [4] pp., front. (port.) 13.4 cm.

The second French edition of this celebrated poem, with Latin and French on facing pages and with notes by the translator.

Waller 3185; Wellcome III, p. 51.

*101. ———. *De sympathia et antipathia rerum liber unus. De contagione et contagiosis morbis et curatione libri III.* Venice: [Apud heredes Lucaeantonii Juntae Florentini] 1546. [4] 76 [3] *ll.* 19.2 cm. New green morocco.

Although his medical poem on syphilis is perhaps more widely known, the present work is a far more important contribution to science, establishes Fracastoro as one of the foremost scientists of all time, and earns him the title of founder of modern epidemiology. *De contagione* contains the first scientifically reasoned statement of the true nature of infection, contagion, and the germ theory of disease and is the foundation of all modern views on the nature of infectious diseases. The influence of Fracastoro's ideas was evident during the seventeenth and eighteenth centuries in the work of Francesco Redi, Giovanni Maria Lancisi, and Antonio Vallisnieri as they contributed to a greater understanding of the nature of infection. Fracastoro's influence is also clearly reflected in the work of such modern scientists as Louis Pasteur, Joseph Lister, and Robert Koch as they broadened and furthered man's knowledge of infectious diseases.

De contagione consists of three books. In the first book Fracastoro presents his germ theory of disease and discusses the three ways that infectious diseases are transmitted: 1) by simple contact, 2) by indirect contact with what he calls fomites—objects that are not in themselves harmful but are able to harbor pathogenic micro-organisms and spread infection and, 3) by transmission from a distance or through the air. In book two he explains the clinical signs of a wide variety of diseases that were prevalent at that time. He gives an early description of typhus and differentiates it from other fevers. He writes of congenital syphilis, recognizes the venereal source of syphilis, and describes its three stages. Fracastoro also discusses the contagiousness of smallpox, measles, tuberculosis, rabies, leprosy, and scabies. In the final book he concentrates on the treatment of contagious diseases and sets forth his general philosophy of therapeutics as well as his specific recommendations for such diseases as measles, smallpox, fevers, typhus, rabies, syphilis, and elephantiasis.

Cushing F275; Durling 1636; Garrison-Morton 2528; Osler 2652; Waller 3163; Wellcome 2393.

*102. ———. *Opera omnia*. Venice: Apud Juntas, 1555. [6] 281 (misnumbered 285), 32 *ll*., illus., ports., diagrs. 22.8 cm. Modern boards.

This first collected edition of Fracastoro's works contains his principal astronomical, philosophical, poetic, and medical treatises, including *Syphilis, sive morbus gallicus* and *De contagione et contagiosis morbis*.

Cushing F280; Durling 1631; Osler 2650; Waller 3168; Wellcome 2396.

*103. JACQUES DUBOIS (1478–1555). *De febribus commentarius ex libris aliquot Hippocratis & Galeni*. Paris: Apud Petrum Drouart, 1554. 91 pp. 27.7 cm.

A most able anatomist and one often quoted both by contemporaries and by medical men for many years to follow, Dubois (also known as Jacobus Sylvius) was Vesalius' teacher at the University of Paris. He was a staunch Galenist and, when Vesalius cast open doubt on much of Galenic "law", Dubois turned on his former pupil, denounced him, and thus caused Vesalius some of the unhappiness which was later to accumulate to such a great degree.

This commentary on Hippocrates' and Galen's teachings concerning fevers was one of the author's better known and most frequently printed works.

Durling 1237; Osler 203 (1556 ed.); Waller 2582 (1555 ed.); Wellcome 6177 (1555 ed.).

*104. ———. ———. Venice: Apud Balthassarem Constantinum, 1555. 64 *ll.* 14.8 cm.

History has not treated Sylvius kindly, chiefly because of his bitter quarrel with Vesalius, and he was, in fact, a rather unpleasant individual. Nevertheless, he made many contributions to scientific knowledge and his name does not deserve all of the abuse to which it has been subjected. Despite his intense allegiance to Galenic medicine, he made a number of improvements in medical nomenclature, giving us the terms jugular, subclavian, phrenic, axillary, and renal vessels. He described the sphenoid bone for the first time and described the jaw bones and spine far better than any previous writer. He also maintained a herbarium to advance his knowledge of materia medica and published a pharmacopoeia in 1548.

The present work is one of two editions of *De febribus* published in Venice in 1555. The other was published by Andrea Arrivabene.

Durling 1238; Osler 203 (1556 ed.); Waller 2582; Wellcome 6177 (printed by Andrea Arrivabene).

*105. ———. ———. Paris: Apud Aegidium Gorbinum, 1561. 52 *ll.* 16.1 cm.

This appears to be the last printing made of *De febribus*. Other copies were printed in earlier years at Paris, Basel, and Venice.

Durling 1242; Osler 203A; Wellcome 6178.

*106. ———. *De mensibus mulierum, et hominis generatione*. Venice: Apud Jo. Franciscum Camotium, 1556. 94 pp. 14.9 cm. Soft boards.

This work contains two of Sylvius' commentaries on the writings of Hippocrates and Galen. The first concerns diseases of the uterus and menstruation while the second deals with human reproduction.

Cushing D283 (Basel ed., 1556); Durling 1251; Waller 2584 (Basel ed., 1556); Wellcome 6179 (1555 ed.).

———. *De mensibus muliebribus liber.*

See No. 228.

107. ———. *Commentarius in Claudii Galeni duos libros De differentiis febrium*. Paris: Apud Aegidium Gorbinum, 1561. 55 [1] *ll.* 16.3 cm. Modern three-quarter calf.

Sylvius based this commentary on Galen's writings about the differences in fevers. The work had been printed earlier in Paris (1555) and in Venice (1556).

Durling 1234; Osler 420 (1555 ed.); Waller 2581 (1556 ed.); Wellcome 6176.

108. PROSPERO CALANO (b. 1480). *Paraphrasis in librum Galeni de inaequali intemperie.* Lyons: Apud Seb. Gryphium, 1538. 287 pp. 17.5 cm.

This work by the Italian physician, Calano, is chiefly devoted to his commentary on Galen's *De inaequali intemperie*. It also contains six additional tracts on such subjects as black bile, heart tremor, and depression that were published between 1530 and 1537 and are assembled for the first time in this volume.

Durling 796; Wellcome 1201.

LUIGI BONACCIUOLI (d. 1540). *Muliebrium liber.*

See No. 228.

———. *Enneas muliebris.*

See No. 239.

FRANCESCO CAVALLO (d. 1540). *Tractatus de animali theria.*

See No. 70.

*109. JEAN TAGAULT (d. 1545). *Institutione di cirugia . . . libri cinque. Aggiuntovi il sesto libro . . . di Giacomo Hollerio.* Venice: Presso Nicolò Moretti, 1596. [20] 421 *ll.*, illus. 14.6 cm. Vellum.

Appearing originally in Latin in 1543, this widely used book by a French surgeon who based his text largely on Guy de Chauliac (see No. 61) was translated into Italian, French, and German. It treats of the nature and cure of wounds, tumors, hernias, ulcers, fractures, and dislocations. A sixth book by Jacques Houllier (see No. 152) describes the tools of surgery. Several interesting woodcuts appear to be reduced copies of plates from Vesalius' *Tabulae anatomicae sex*.

Cushing (other editions); Durling 4308; Waller (other editions); Wellcome (other editions).

*110. EURICIUS CORDUS (1486–1535). *Ain Regiment: wie man sich vor der newen Plage, der Englische Schwaiss genannt, bewaren.* [Augsburg?: n. publ., 1529]. [8] *ll.* 19.2 cm. Bound in vellum leaf of manuscript.

The *sudor anglicus*, or English sickness, is here given one of its earliest descriptions by Cordus (also known as Heinrich Urban), first professor of medicine at the University of Marburg. This disease probably appeared for the first time in 1485, in England, and several severe epidemics during the next century claimed thousands of lives. It was probably, according to clinical descriptions, a virulent form of influenza.

Cushing C407; Durling 1024; Garrison-Morton 5520; Waller 2127; Wellcome 1588.

———. *Ein gemenn Regiment und Diet fuer den Steyn.*

See No. 140.

OTTMAR LUSCINIUS (1487–1537). *Joci ac sales mire festivi.*

See No. 309.

ULRICH VON HUTTEN (1488–1523). *De admiranda guaiaci medicina & morbi Galeni* [sic, i.e. gallici] *curatione.*

See No. 73.

MARIANO SANTO (ca. 1488–ca. 1550). *Compendium in chyrurgia utilissimum volentibus ipsam exercere.*

See No. 87.

*111. OTTO BRUNFELS (1489–1534). *Theses seu communes loci, totius rei medicae.* Strasbourg: Excudebat Georgius Ulricher, 1532. [10] 232 *ll.* 14.4 cm. Modern half vellum.

Brunfels, a German botanist, became a Carthusian monk in his early twenties, a short time after completing his education at Mainz. He abandoned the monastery in 1521 when he became a convert to the Protestant faith and spent several years at various towns in southwest Germany as an evangelical minister and theological writer. Brunfels returned to Strasbourg in 1524 where he established a school and directed his interests to the study of botany and medicine. He is most often remembered for his classic work in botany, *Herbarum vivae icones* (1530–1536), a work which marked the beginning of modern taxonomy. He received a medical degree at Basel in 1532 or 1533 and, after a short period in private practice in Strasbourg, was appointed town physician at Bern in 1533. He died only a year later, probably of diphtheria.

This little-known work of Brunfels, edited by Johannes Munterus (fl. 1513–1532), is a treatise on the pharmacological approach to a wide variety of diseases. Included with it are Alessandro Benedetti's (ca. 1450–1512) *Sententiae medicinales* and Arnaldus de Villanova's *Sententiarum medicinalium morborum curationibus* as well as several other short tracts by Villanova.

Durling, Suppl. I, 29; Wellcome 1105.

*112. ALBAN THORER, editor (1489–1550). *De re medica.* [Basel: In aedibus Andreae Cratandri, 1528]. [12] 125 [1] *ll.* 30.1 cm. Vellum, in slipcase.

This rare volume contains one of the earliest collections of those medical writers and physicians whose works bridged the period between the early Greeks and the Middle Ages. Soranus of Ephesus (ca. 98–ca.138), *In artem medendi isagoge,* is here in its first edition. Oribasius' tract, *De victus ratione*, is presented in its only edition.

The treatise *De re medica*, ascribed to Pliny the Elder (23–79), differs from the only other printed version, published in 1509; Apuleius' (fl. 2nd century) *De herbarum virtutibus* appears in second edition. Two fine woodcut borders and many initials add unusual interest to this work which is seemingly little known to the collectors, bibliographers, and historians of medical works.

Durling 4351; Wellcome 5353.

*113. NICCOLÒ MASSA (1489–1569). *Liber de morbo Gallico*. [Venice: In aedibus Francisci Bindoni, ac Maphei Pasini socii impressus] 1532. [40] *ll.* 21.7 cm. Old vellum, uncut.

Massa, a graduate of Padua, taught and practiced in Venice. His book, *Liber introductorius anatomiae* (1536), is one of the well-known pre-Vesalian anatomies and, although it contained errors, was one of the foremost accounts of anatomical structure of its time. Perhaps Massa's best-known work is the present treatise, of which this is an extremely rare first edition. Divided into six sections, the work, which remained popular throughout the author's lifetime, is a comprehensive description of the symptoms and effects of syphilis. Massa taught that syphilis was usually contracted by sexual intercourse, and he believed that it could also arise spontaneously without contact. In addition, he discusses the role of diet, sleep, and exercise together with the use of drugs, bloodletting, leeches, and guaiac in the treatment of syphilis.

Cushing M178 (1536 ed.); Garrison-Morton 2365; Osler 3341 (1536 ed.); Waller 6300 (1536 ed.); Wellcome 4102.

*114. EUCHARIUS ROESLIN (ca. 1490–1526). *De partu hominis, et quae circa ipsum accidunt, adeoque, de parturientum & infantium morbis atque cura*. Frankfurt: Apud Chr. Egenolphum [1551]. 62 [2] *ll.*, illus. 14.1 cm.

When Roeslin published *Der swangern Frauwen und hebammen Rosegarten* in 1513, he had just become town physician and supervisor of midwives at Worms. Prior to that time he had lived in Freiburg and had been town physician at Frankfurt for several years. Roeslin remained at Worms until 1517 when he returned to Frankfurt and served there as town physician until his death. His son, also named Eucharius, succeeded him as town physician at Frankfurt. Because they had the same name and occupation, they have often been confused with each other or have been thought to be one and the same person.

The "Rosengarten" was the first book written especially for midwives and it was written in the vernacular because those for whom it was intended were not conversant with Latin. The book is essentially a survey of the Greek and Roman literature and contains excerpts from such authors as Hippocrates, Galen, Aëtius, Albertus Magnus, and many others. In addition to obstetrics, Roeslin covers infant care, nursing, and the diseases of infancy. Illustrations of the birth chair, the lying-in chamber, and various positions of the fetus *in utero* are seen for the first time and are the earliest obstetrical illustrations printed from wood blocks. In this edition, the large woodcuts found in earlier editions are absent and many new figures have been added. Four woodcuts of the egg membranes and the placenta are from Vesalius' *Fabrica* (see No. 171).

The book was first translated into Latin for Roeslin's son in 1532. An extremely popular and widely circulated book, it was translated into many languages and appeared in numerous editions until the late 1700's.

Durling 3902; Garrison-Morton 6138 (1513 ed.); Osler 3818 (1513 ed.); Waller 8091 (1513 ed.); Wellcome 5507 (1536 ed.).

*115. ———. *The birth of mankinde, otherwise named the woman's booke*. Set foorth in English by Thomas Raynalde. London: Thomas Adams [1604]. [8] 208 pp. (misnumbered 204), 9 plates. 17.7 cm. Nineteenth century half calf.

An English translation of the "Rosengarten" first appeared in 1540. Based on the Latin version, *De partu hominis*, it was translated and published by Richard Jonas (fl. 1540). The next English edition to appear was published by Thomas Raynalde (fl. 1546) in 1545. Unlike Jonas who had produced a literal translation, Raynalde gave a free translation with many original additions. Raynalde borrowed freely from other authors and included several anatomical plates and descriptive text from Vesalius' *Fabrica*. Extremely popular, there were over ten subsequent editions of Raynalde's translation.

English midwives and physicians were largely dependent on this book for guidance in the practice of obstetrics until the eighteenth century when Smellie and Hunter published their scientific treatises.

Cushing R204 (1540 ed.); Garrison-Morton 6139 (1540 ed.); Russell 720; Waller 8114; Wellcome 5516.

LORENZ FRIES (ca. 1490–1531). *Epitome opusculi de curandis pustulis, ulceribus, & doloribus mali Frantzoss*.

See No. 73.

*116. PARACELSUS (1493–1541). *Von der frantzösischen Kranckheit drey Bücher*. [Nuremberg: Durch Friderich Peypus, 1530]. [54] *ll*. 18.4 cm. Vellum.

Philippus Theophrastus Bombastus von Hohenheim is universally known merely as Paracelsus, a name invented by friends who apparently saw in him a genius "surpassing Celsus." He was born in Switzerland and educated at Basel, where he was appointed town physician and professor at the University. But his unorthodox ideas and teachings put him at loggerheads with the orthodox establishment of his revolutionary time and he spent most of his life wandering through Europe as an itinerant physician, chemist, theologian, and philosopher. Although his ideas were still bound up in alchemy and astrology, and his writings imbued with a mysticism which makes them difficult to interpret, in the field of practical medicine he was usually in advance of his time and attracted many followers. "First, he applied chemical techniques to pharmacy and therapeutics. . . . Secondly, in his medical teaching he abandoned the ruling system of 'humours'; and the beginnings of modern pathology can be seen in his work. . . . His influence on the sixteenth and seventeenth centuries was profound . . . and the work of Helmont . . . is unthinkable without him." (John Carter and Percy H. Muir, *Printing and the mind of man*. London, 1967. p. 66.) Paracelsus was a prolific writer, but few of his works were published during his lifetime. In the century after his death, however, his works came tumbling from the press by the hundreds.

The present rare work is one of the few published during his lifetime and, despite the title, is his famous blast at "quacks" and "false physicians" who preyed on superstition and who treated with useless and sometimes harmful remedies.

Durling 3450 (1553 ed.); Garrison-Morton 2369 (1553 ed.); Sudhoff 7.

*117. ———. *De medicamentorum simplicium gradibus et compositionibus*. Zurich: Excudebat Froschouerus, 1572. [6] 34 (misnumbered 26) *ll.* 15.5 cm. Modern half vellum.

A small handbook of therapeutics, first published in 1562, and containing many recipes for medications.

Durling 3493; Sudhoff 139.

*118. ———. *Opus chyrurgicum*. Strasbourg: Gedruckt bey Paulo Messerschmidt, 1564. [20] cccccxv pp. 31.4 cm. Original half pigskin, blind-tooled, over wooden boards, with two metal clasps.

This first of the larger collected editions of Paracelsus' works on surgery and medicine was edited by one of his pupils, Adam von Bodenstein (1528–1577). To it are added two tracts on syphilis, for which disease Paracelsus is credited with introducing mercury treatment.

Durling 3464; Sudhoff 62.

*119. ———. *Drey Bücher*. Cologne: Gedruckt durch die Erben Arnoldi Byrckmanni, 1564. [16] 292 pp. 19.3 cm. Contemporary blind-stamped vellum over wooden boards, with metal clasps. Bound with No. 120 and No. 121.

This volume contains the first printing of one of Paracelsus' most important works, a defense against the charges of the Carinthian physicians who were protesting his aim to settle in Carinthia. He follows this with an attack, "Von dem Irrgang und Labyrinth der Artzney," or "The labyrinth of physicians," in which he summarizes his doctrines and states his case against the academic doctors. To this he added a third book, on the origin and cure of arthritis.

Durling 3466; Sudhoff 64.

*120. ———. *Phi[lo]sophiae ad Athenienses, drey Bücher. Von Ursachen und Cur Epilepsiae. . . . Vom Ursprung, Cur oder Heilung der contracten Glidern*. Cologne: Gedruckt durch die Erben Arnoldi Byrckmanni, 1564. [206] pp. 19.3 cm. Bound with No. 119 and No. 121.

The first of these three works is a treatise on natural philosophy, which may not be by Paracelsus. The second is the first printing of his treatise on the cause and cure of epilepsy, while the third is on the contractions of paralysis.

Durling 3467; Sudhoff 65; Waller 7121; Wellcome 4754.

*121. ———. *Astronomica et astrologica*. Cologne: Getruckt bey Arnoldi Byrckmans Erben, 1567. [20] 235 [3] pp., 2 ports. 19.3 cm. Bound with No. 119 and No. 120.

Few beliefs were as popular in the sixteenth century as astrology, and references to the stars are to be found throughout Paracelsus' writings. According to his thinking, astrology along with philosophy, alchemy, and virtue were the four cornerstones of medicine. Paracelsus based his astrology on the age-old theory of the interaction of man (microcosm) with the universe (macrocosm) and he considered astral influences to be one of the five causes of disease which also included poisonous and impure substances, psychological, spiritual, and divine causes.

This is the first collected edition of Paracelsus' writings on astrology and astronomy and contains an extensive introduction by the editor, Balthasar Flöter (fl. 1567). A notable aspect of this work is two full-page portraits of Paracelsus.

Durling 3474; Sudhoff 85.

*122. ———. *Von der Bergsucht oder Bergkranckheiten drey Bücher*. [Dillingen: Durch Sebaldum Mayer] 1567. [7] 62 [2] *ll*. 20 cm. Modern half cloth.

This rare first edition of the first monograph devoted to the occupational diseases of miners and metallurgical workers appeared eleven years after Agricola's well-known treatise on mining, *De re metallica,* and was the result of Paracelsus' own observations while studying metallurgical operations at the Fugger mines in the Tirol.

Durling 3476; Sudhoff 88; Wellcome 4762.

123. ———. *Chirurgische Bücher und Schrifften*. Strasbourg: In Verlegung L. Zetzners, 1605. [13] 680 [40] 115 [7] pp. (lacking title page), port. 30.1 cm. Vellum, worn.

This large selection of Paracelsus' works was edited by Johannes Huser (fl. 1589), a Basel publisher who issued Paracelsus' complete medical and philosophical works in 1589 and continued publishing the collected works or portions thereof for a number of years. An appendix to the present edition contains Paracelsus' alchemical works which did not appear in Huser's original edition.

Durling 3516 (1st ed., 1591); Sudhoff 267; Wellcome 4811.

Gift of Edna Dieman and Julia Bennett.

124. ———. *Opera, Bücher und Schrifften*. Vol. I only of 2 vols. Strasbourg: In Verlegung L. Zetzners seligen Erben, 1616. Vol. I: [12] 1127 [53] pp. 31.7 cm. Calf,

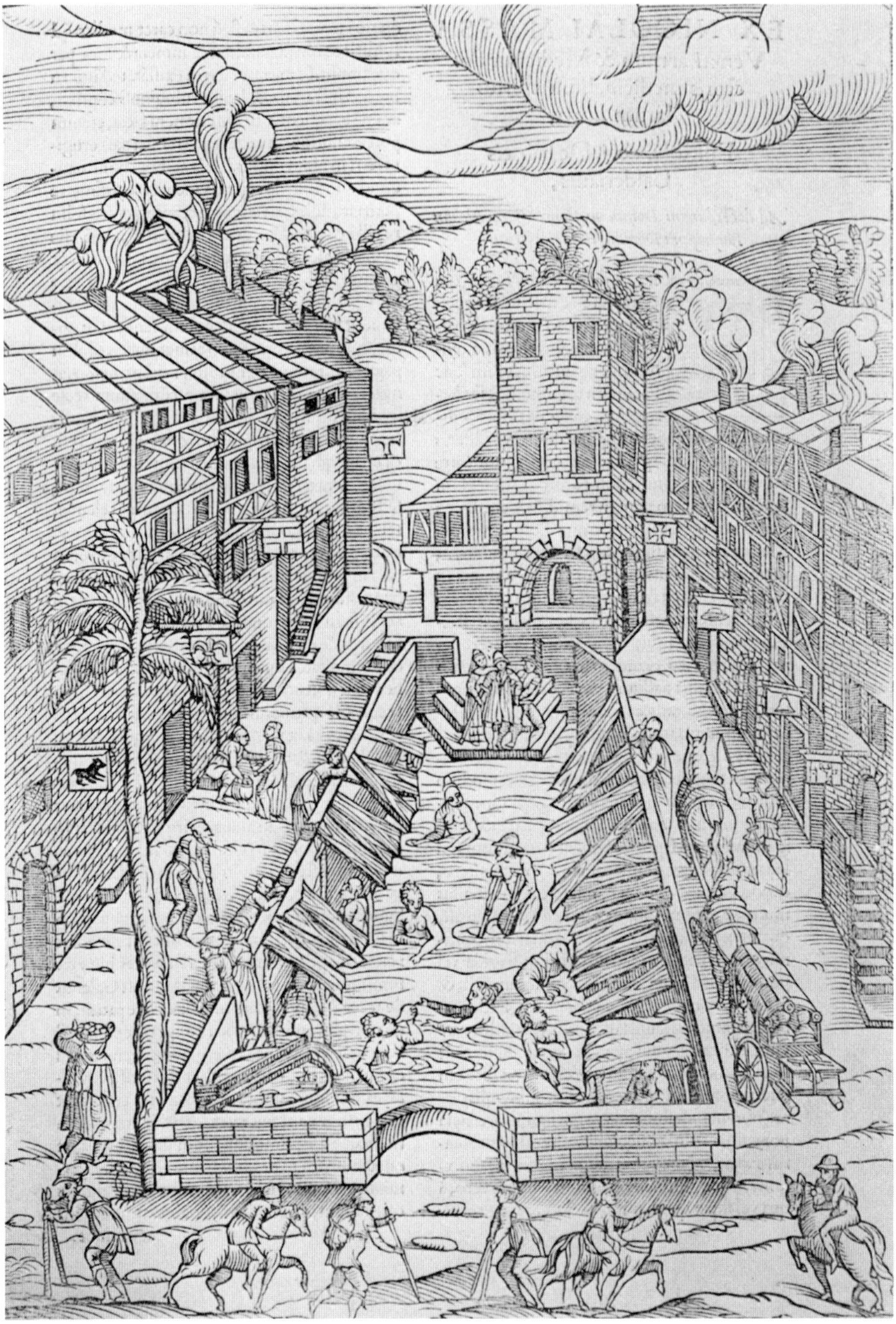

No. 126. Giunta. *De Balneis.* The medieval public bath—practical but unsanitary.

badly worn; unidentified seventeenth century German medical manuscript bound in at end.

So popular were the works of Paracelsus that, for a hundred years after his death, it would be difficult to find a year in which some new edition of one or more of his works was not printed. During the first quarter of the seventeenth century, collections of his works were extremely popular, and this is another edition by the indefatigable Huser.

Durling 3516 (1st ed., 1591); Sudhoff 300; Wellcome 4809.

Gift of Edna Dieman and Julia Bennett.

*125. ———. *Opera omnia medico-chemico-chirurgica. . . . Edidit Fridericus Bitiskius.* 3 vols. in 1. Geneva: Sumptibus Joan. Antonii, & Samuelis De Tournes, 1658. Vol. I: [36] 828 [40] pp.; Vol. II: [24] 718 [30] pp.; Vol. III: [12] 212 [32] 119 [7] 18 pp., front. (port.), illus. 33.6 cm. Old calf, spine restored.

According to Sudhoff, bibliographer of Paracelsus' works, this compendium of the works of Paracelsus, edited by Friedrich Bitiskius, is the most complete of the Latin collected editions. It contains virtually all of Paracelsus' medical and philosophical writings, as well as Tintoretto's beautiful portrait of Paracelsus, which is often missing.

Osler 528; Sudhoff 381–383; Waller 7144.

*126. TOMASO GIUNTA, editor (1494–1566). *De balneis omnia quae extant apud Graecos, Latinos, et Arabas.* Venice: Apud Juntas, 1553. 14, 497 *ll.*, illus. 30.4 cm. Seventeenth century calf.

This work is one of the most complete collections on baths and bathing compiled during the sixteenth century, containing texts by more than seventy authors among whom are Hippocrates, Avicenna, Averroës, Galen, Gesner, Cardano, Savonarola, Fuchs, D'Abano, and Maimonides. Many of these works are printed here for the first and only time so that this volume provides a comprehensive picture of the state of balneology, then at the height of its popularity. The five woodcuts in the work show the plan of a spa, part of the baths at Pfeffers in Switzerland, the baths of Plombière, a map of the baths around Venice and Trieste, and a view of the interior of a Roman bath.

Cushing D88; Durling 1101; Garrison-Morton 1986; Osler 1902; Wellcome 652.

*127. JEAN FERNEL (1497–1558). *Les VII livres de la physiologie.* Paris: Chez J. Guignard, 1655. [24] 384 [8] 385–773 pp. 17.1 cm. Vellum.

Fernel was professor of medicine at the University of Paris where he had a strong influence in breaking down the old hidebound rules of Galen in France. His insistence that physicians should study the human body and not rely on tradition may well have inspired his pupil, Vesalius, to the latter's great anatomical studies.

Fernel's *Physiologiae*, first published in 1542, was later incorporated into his

Medicina (1554), which was used as a standard text throughout Europe for many years, as is shown by this French translation of well over one hundred years after its first publication in Latin. Among several of Fernel's discoveries and descriptions, perhaps his description of "iliac passion" as the first clinical account of appendicitis, with autopsy, stands out as one of the most important.

*128. ———. *De abditis rerem causis libri duo*. Frankfurt: Apud Andream Wechelum, 1581. 272 [23] pp., port. 16.8 cm. Vellum. Bound with No. 130.

In this work Fernel attacks astrology and magic as being superstitious and utterly without foundation. As applied to treatment of sickness, he finds such practices dangerous and states that medicine is to be approached rationally and within the laws of nature.

Durling 1478 (1550 ed.); Waller 2988 (1644 ed.); Wellcome 2199.

*129. ———. *Consiliorum liber. Cui accesserunt responsa quaedam clarorum medicorum Parisiensium*. Lyons: Apud Thomam Soubron, & Moysen des Prez, 1597. 174 pp. 17.7 cm. Vellum. Bound with No. 131.

This separate edition of part of Book II of Fernel's *Universa medicina* (originally titled just *Medicina*) contains his suggestion that aneurysms had their origin in syphilis.

It appears that the publisher of this edition also issued it as part of a complete edition of the *Universa medicina* published in the same year. Thus his customers could purchase the entire work or individual sections, as they preferred. Apparently the original purchaser of this volume wanted only this section and one other (see No. 131), which he then had bound together.

Wellcome 2217.

*130. ———. *Therapeutices universalis, seu medendi rationis, libri septem*. Frankfurt: Apud Andream Wechelum, 1581. 562 [45] pp., port. 16.8 cm. Vellum. Bound with No. 128.

First published in three books and forming part of Fernel's *Medicina*, this work was later enlarged to seven books and included as Part Three of his *Universa medicina* (1557). It included his well-known work on fevers, on the cure of syphilis, and on epilepsy.

Durling 1489 (1569 ed.); Waller 2995 (1555 ed.); Wellcome 2208 (1571 ed.).

*131. ———. ———. Lyons: Apud Thoman Soubron, & Moysen des Prez, 1597. 552 [30] pp. 17.7 cm. Vellum, Bound with No. 129.

The authority and popularity of Fernel's works continued long after their original publication and well into the seventeenth century.

Durling 1489 (1569 ed.); Wellcome 2211.

132. GIOVANNI BATTISTA DA MONTE (1498–1551). *In libros Galeni de arte curandi ad Glauconem explanationes.* Venice: Apud Baltassarem Constantinum, 1554. [8] 562 *ll.* 15.2 cm. Vellum, badly worn; marginal manuscript notes throughout.

Da Monte, better known by his Latin cognomen, Montanus, was not only a very successful physician and teacher, but a noted poet as well. A fellow-student of Vesalius at Padua, he later taught at Padua, and his practical instructions to students mark the beginning of clinical instruction in which he instituted bedside teaching, one of his most notable achievements. Called "the second Galen," he was one of a group of medical humanists who were instrumental in reviving the Greek medical classics and eclipsing the influence and teachings of the Arabist school.

In the present work, Montanus offers his interpretations of Galen's medical works.

Durling 3269; Wellcome 4423.

133. ———. *Lectiones . . . in secundam fen primi canonis Avicennae.* Venice: Ex officina Erasmiana Vincentii Valgrisii, & Balthesaris Constantini, 1557. [39] 832 pp. 15.2 cm. Half vellum.

Montanus' discussions and criticisms of a portion of Avicenna's work.

Durling 3274.

HIERONYMUS BOCK (1498–1554). *Regiment und Arznei für das grausam Hauptwee unnd Bieune.*

See No. 140.

134. ANTONIO MUSA BRASAVOLA (1500–1555). *Examen omnium simplicium medicamentorum, quorum in officinis usus est.* Lyons: Apud Joannem et Franciscum Frellaeos, 1537. [24] 542 (misnumbered 544) [15] pp. 15.5 cm.

Brasavola, like many physicians of his era, also held doctorates in law and theology and taught these subjects as well as medicine. He was a pupil of Niccolò Leoniceno (Leonicenus), a famous Italian medical humanist who also made an important translation of Hippocrates' *Aphorisms.* Brasavola served as personal physician to the Popes Paul III, Leo X, Clement VII, and Julius III; to Emperor Charles V, King Francis I, and King Henry VIII. He wrote some seventy books and articles, is said to have performed a large number of tracheotomies, and described over two hundred different kinds of syphilis.

Among his many works were an authoritative concordance of Galen and this popular work on herbal medicine, first published in 1536, in which he introduced several new drugs into the pharmacopoeia. The work is in the form of a dialogue among Brasavola, an old apothecary, and an herbalist. It is a lengthy treatise and shows that, while he had made significant advances in presenting his material and in his methods, he had not entirely succeeded in freeing himself from the traditional lore and superstitions of the past.

Durling 680; Garrison-Morton 1804 (1536 ed.); Waller 1420a (1544 ed.); Wellcome 1045.

*135. ———. *Examen omnium syruporum, quorum publicus usus est.* Venice: Apud Cominum de Tridino, 1545. 231 [6] pp. 15.9 cm. Limp vellum. Bound with No. 136 and No. 137.

Brasavola's work on herbal remedies was so popular that he wrote a series of similar dialogues about nearly every type of medicine sold in the drugstores of his native city, Ferrara. In this tract, he discusses many of the syrups then in common use and provides numerous recipes from other recognized authorities.

Durling 686; Osler 2119 (1538 ed.); Wellcome 1052.

*136. ———. *Examen omnium electuariorum, pulverum, et confectionum, catharcticorum.* Venice: Ex officina Erasmiana, Vincentii Valgrisii, 1548. 140 [2] pp. 15.9 cm. Bound with No. 135 and No. 137.

Another of Brasavola's many tracts written after his successful *Examen omnium simplicium medicamentorum quorum in officinis usus est,* this one concerned with electuaries, powdered drugs, confections, and cathartics. Electuaries and confections were nearly identical classes of preparations and were prepared from powdered drugs that had been mixed with honey or the syrup of sugared fruit juices.

Durling 677; Wellcome 1056 (1549 ed.).

*137. ———. *Examen omnium catapotiorum, vel pilularum, quarum apud pharmacopolas usus est.* Venice: Ex officina Erasmiana, Vincentii Valgrisii, 1549. 205 [1] pp. 15.9 cm. Bound with No. 135 and No. 136.

The final work in this volume concerned pills and potions and showed a tendency merely to repeat recipes from other authorities rather than to record new discoveries and the results of Brasavola's own personal experiences.

Included at the end of this work is one of the earliest medical writings of Konrad Gesner (see No. 186), *Enumeratio medicamentorum purgantium, vomitoriorum, & aluum bonam facientium,* first published in 1543. It is a short alphabetical index of purgatives.

Brasavola: Durling 676; Osler 2122 (1544 ed.); Waller 1419 (1544 ed.); Wellcome 1054 (1544 ed.).

Gesner: Garrison-Morton 1809; Osler 633.

138. ———. *In libros de ratione victus in morbis acutis Hippocratis & Galeni commentaria & annotationes.* 4 vols. in 1. Venice: Apud Hieronymum Scotum, 1546. 31.4 cm.

This is perhaps the author's scarcest book and is dedicated to Francis I, King of France. It includes Jean Vassès' (1486–1550) Latin translations of Galen's commen-

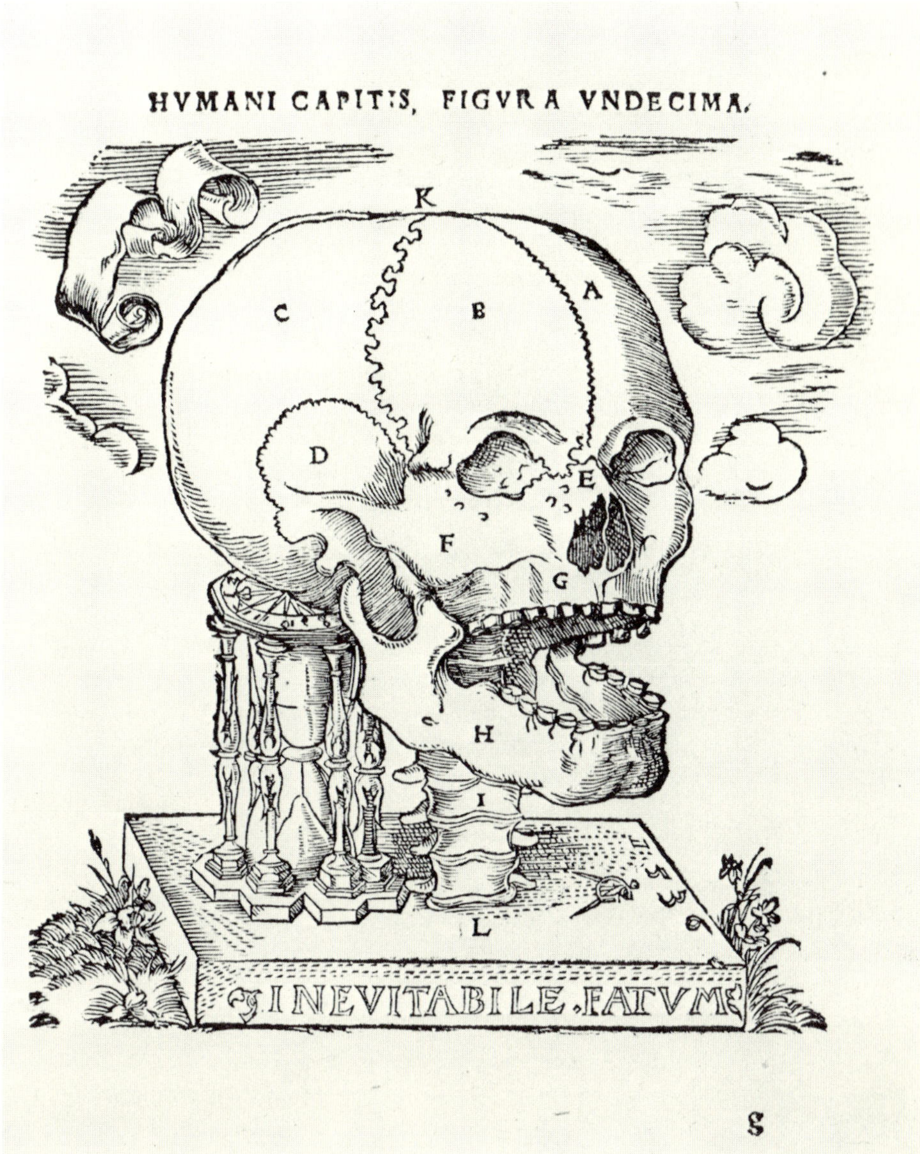

No. 139. Dryander. *Anatomiae.*

tary on Hippocrates' *De victus ratione in morbis acutis* [The regimen in acute diseases], the Latin text of Hippocrates' work, and Brasavola's comments and analysis.

Durling 692; Osler 182.

*139. JOHANNES DRYANDER (ca. 1500–1560). *Anatomiae.* Marburg: Apud Eucharium Ceruicornum, 1537. [72] pp., illus. (woodcuts), fold. table. 20 cm. Full antique calf.

Dryander (also known as Eichmann), professor of surgery at Marburg, was a friend of Vesalius and was "among the first anatomists who made illustrations after their own dissections" (Choulant-Frank, p. 148). His *Anatomiae* appeared six years before Vesalius' great work (see No. 171).

This was the first significant book on the anatomy of the head and contains twenty full-page woodcuts made from Dryander's own dissections. Sixteen of the plates are of the head and brain and were done to show successive stages of dissection. The first eleven plates appeared earlier in his *Anatomia capitis humani* (1536) and the remaining four plates of the chest and lungs were added as an appendix, possibly as models for a second book which was never published. A folding chart containing an explanation of the parts of the head, included here in facsimile, is not present in most copies.

This work also contains a brief tract on the anatomy of the pig traditionally attributed to Copho (ca. 1110), an early teacher at Salerno, and a short essay by Gabriele de Zerbis (1445–1505), professor at Padua, on the anatomy of the fetus.

Choulant-Frank, p. 148; Cushing D275; Durling 1215; Garrison-Morton 371; Waller 2576; Wellcome 1869.

*140. ———. *New Artznei unnd Practicierbüchlein zu allen Leibs gebrechen und Kranckheyten.* Frankfurt: Christian Egenolff, 1551. [8] 140 *ll.*, illus. 15.2 cm. Contemporary blind-stamped pigskin over wooden boards; two clasps and catches.

The present work is a very rare and little-known compendium of practical medicine and contains, as well, tracts by Euricius Cordus and Hieronymus Bock (1498–1554). The colored vignette on the title page and quaint woodcut illustrations through the text go to make this an interesting and charming little handbook.

Durling 1218 (1557 ed.); Waller 2579 (1557 ed.); Wellcome 1871 (1572 ed.).

141. PIETRO ANDREA MATTIOLI (1500–1577). *Kreutterbuch . . . jetzt widerumb mit vielen schönen newen Figuren, auch nützlichen Artzneyen . . . gemehret, und verfertiget durch Joachimum Camerarium.* Frankfurt: Jacob Fischer, 1626. [70] 460 [54] pp., col. illus. 36.8 cm.

Mattioli of Siena studied medicine at Padua where he was graduated in 1523. During his busy and active career, he practiced at Siena, Perugia, Rome, Trent, and Gorizia and was physician to Ferdinand I and later Maximilian II. He wrote

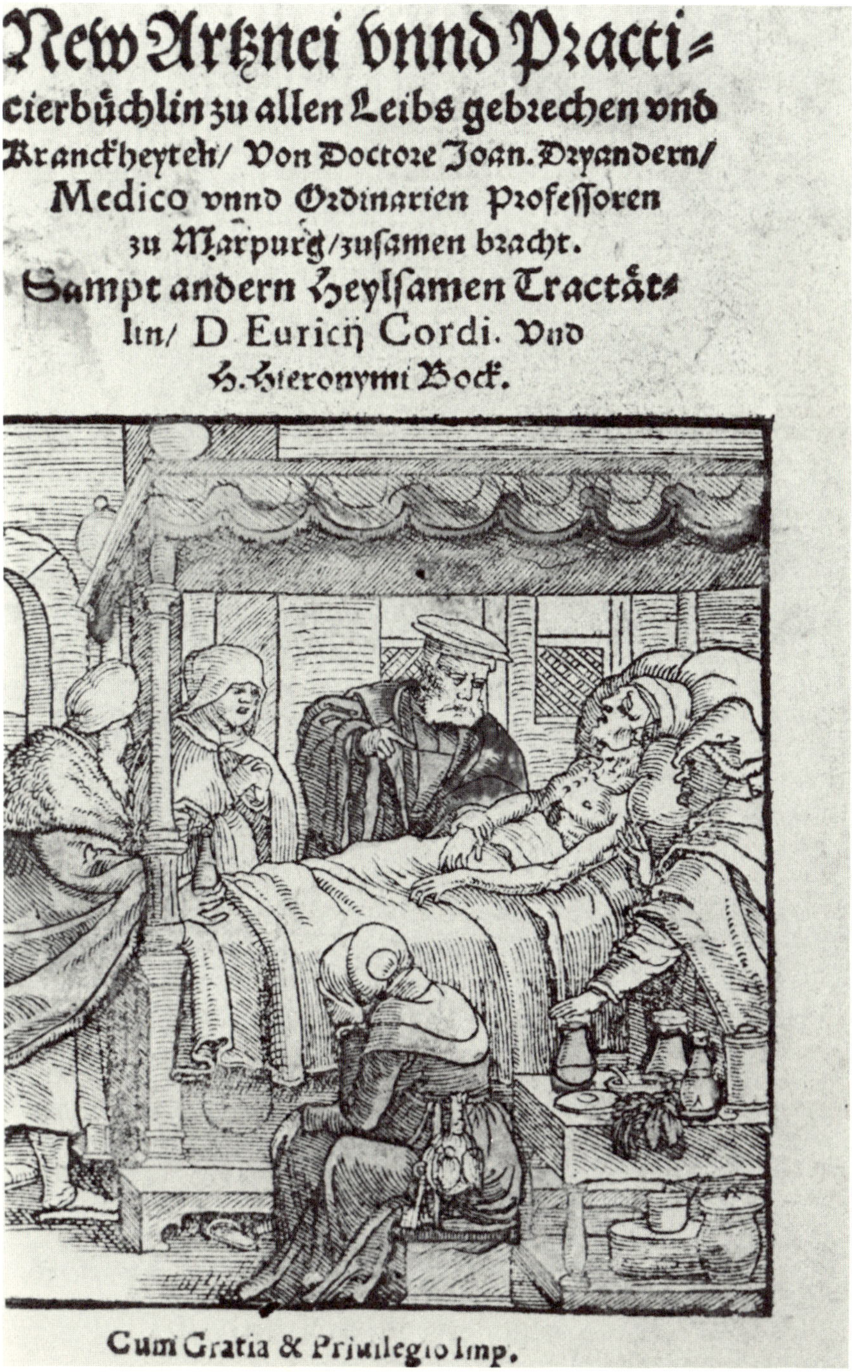

New Artznei vnnd Practi-
cierbůchlin zu allen Leibs gebrechen vnd
Kranckheyten/ Von Doctore Joan. Dryandern/
Medico vnnd Ordinarien Professoren
zu Marpurg/zusamen bracht.
Sampt andern heylsamen Tractät-
lin/ D Eurici Cordi. Vnd
H. Hieronymi Bock.

Cum Gratia & Priuilegio Imp.

No. 140. Dryander. *New Artznei unnd Practicierbüchlein.* Title page vignette of a sixteenth century sickroom scene.

books on syphilis (see No. 73), the practice of medicine, and therapeutics, but his best-known and most popular work was the present book. In this commentary on Dioscorides, Mattioli prepared what many authorities now regard as the encyclopedia of Renaissance pharmacology. He studied hundreds of plants, examined and described them fully, added many new species, and provided excellent illustrations which were far superior to those of any previous work in the field. His commentary, first published in Venice in 1544, went through numerous Latin, French, German, Czech, and Italian editions. The first German edition was published in 1562 and the work continued to be published well into the eighteenth century.

Durling 3019 (1586 ed.); Wellcome 4159 (1590 ed.).

———. *Morbi gallici novum . . . opusculum quo vera . . . eius cura percipi potest.*

See No. 73.

*142. LEONHART FUCHS (1501–1566). *De medendis singularum humani corporis partium a summo capite ad imos usque pedes passionibus ac febribus libri quatuor.* Basel: [In officina Roberti Winter, 1539]. [8] 314 [6] pp. 22.2 cm. Contemporary limp vellum.

Fuchs was a German physician, professor of medicine at Tübingen, a practicing pharmacologist, a fervid Hippocratist, and writer of numerous works, the most famous of which is his herbal, *De historia stirpium* (see No. 143).

The little-known medical text, *De medendis*, first published in 1538, is a handbook of therapeutics covering most diseases of most parts of the body.

Cushing F355; Durling 1686; Wellcome 2434 (Paris ed.).

*143. ———. *De historia stirpium commentarii insignes.* Basel: In officina Isingriniana, 1542. [28] 896 [2] pp., 512 col. plates. 38.1 cm. Full calf.

Prior to the sixteenth century, very little had been done in the field of medical botany and, although numerous herbals in both manuscript and printed form had been produced, they were poor in text and illustration, primarily derived from classical sources. But in the sixteenth century the same spirit which inspired Vesalius and others in the field of anatomy served also as the inspiration for the study of flora from actual specimens, culminating in what is certainly the most celebrated and probably the most beautiful herbal ever published, that of Leonhart Fuchs. He described 400 German plants as well as 100 foreign ones. The 512 woodcut illustrations are neatly colored by hand in pleasing tones and include a full-page hand-colored woodcut of Fuchs as well as portraits of the three illustrators, one of the first instances of such a tribute being paid to artists in a printed book.

This first edition of this lavish herbal is characterized by spacious design and layout, by fine printing, and by the sheer number of illustrations. Its popularity

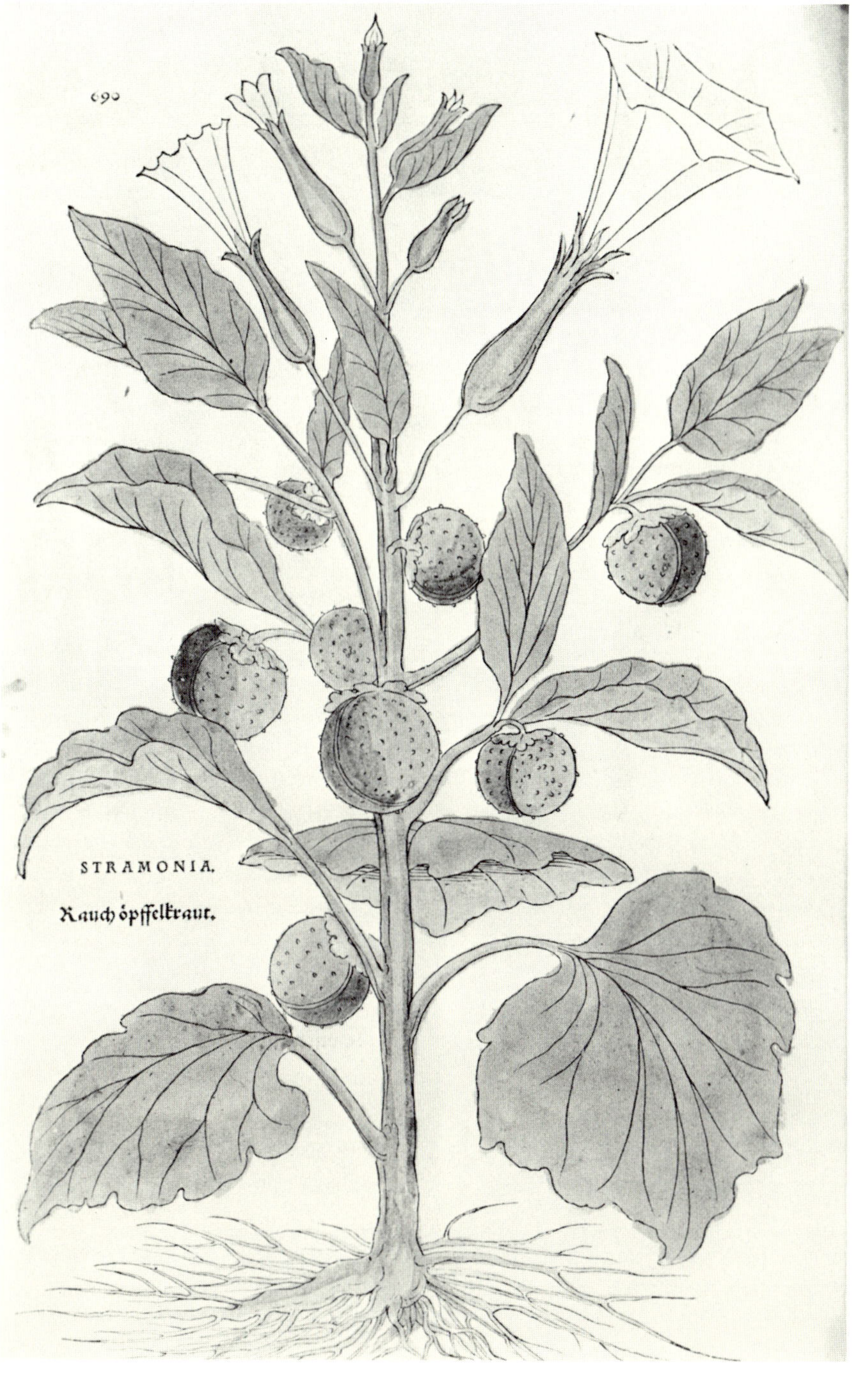

No. 143. Fuchs. *De Historia Stirpium.* The stramonium plant (jimson weed).

was immediate and it was issued in many subsequent editions and translations, but the first edition was never equaled.

Cushing F350; Durling 1675; Garrison-Morton 1808; Wellcome 2438.

144. ———. *De humani corporis fabrica epitomes pars prima, duos, unum de ossibus, alterum de musculis, libros complectens.* Lyons: Apud Antonium Vincentium [excudebat Joannes Frellonius] 1551. 338 [12] pp. (pp. 303–312, 325–336 are lacking from this copy). 16.2 cm. Limp vellum. Bound with No. 191.

This work is Fuchs' "epitome" of Vesalius' text of the *Fabrica* (see No. 172), but it is completely without illustrations. Another edition, carrying Vesalius' name on the title page, appeared the same year in Tübingen. A second volume of this Lyons edition appeared in 1555, but is not present here.

Cushing F354; Cushing Vesalius VI.D.–15; Durling 1685 (Tübingen ed.); Waller 3294.

*145. GARCIA DE ORTA (1501 or 2?–1568). *Aromatum, et simplicium aliquot medicamentorum apud Indos nascentium historia.* 4th ed. Antwerp: Ex officina Plantiniana, apud viduam, & Joannem Moretum, 1593. [1]–224 pp., illus. 16.1 cm. Appears with No. 167 and No. 233.

Orta, a Portuguese clinician and student of materia medica, practiced and taught for a time in Lisbon, then moved to India and settled in Goa where he established a large practice and an extensive medical garden. On the basis of his research into the description, history, clinical uses, and effects of the many herbs and spices in his herbarium, he published, in 1563, *Colóquios dos simples, e drogas e cousas medicinais da India.* In the course of preparing the work, he described the classic symptoms of cholera and he is credited with bringing the disease to the attention of the European world. The initial printing in Portuguese was followed by several editions and translations into French, German, Italian, and Latin. The present fourth Latin edition was translated by Charles de l'Écluse (1526–1609), a noted French botanist.

Cushing O47 (1st Latin ed., 1567); Durling 3417; Osler 2327 (5th Latin ed., 1605); Waller 7006; Wellcome 4658.

*146. GIROLAMO CARDANO (1501–1576). *De utilitate ex adversis capienda, libri IIII.* Basel: [Per Henrichum Petri, 1561]. [72] 1161 pp. 15.8 cm. Contemporary blind-stamped pigskin.

Famous as a philosopher and physician, Cardano was one of the most interesting personalities of the Italian Renaissance and one of the most learned men of his time. He covered almost every branch of knowledge in his writings: philosophy, mathematics, physics, hygiene, medicine, astronomy and astrology, and theology. He was an early follower of Paracelsus and his advanced thinking as well as his disputations and obstinate character made many enemies for him.

This first edition of his work on the uses of adversity contains many autobio-

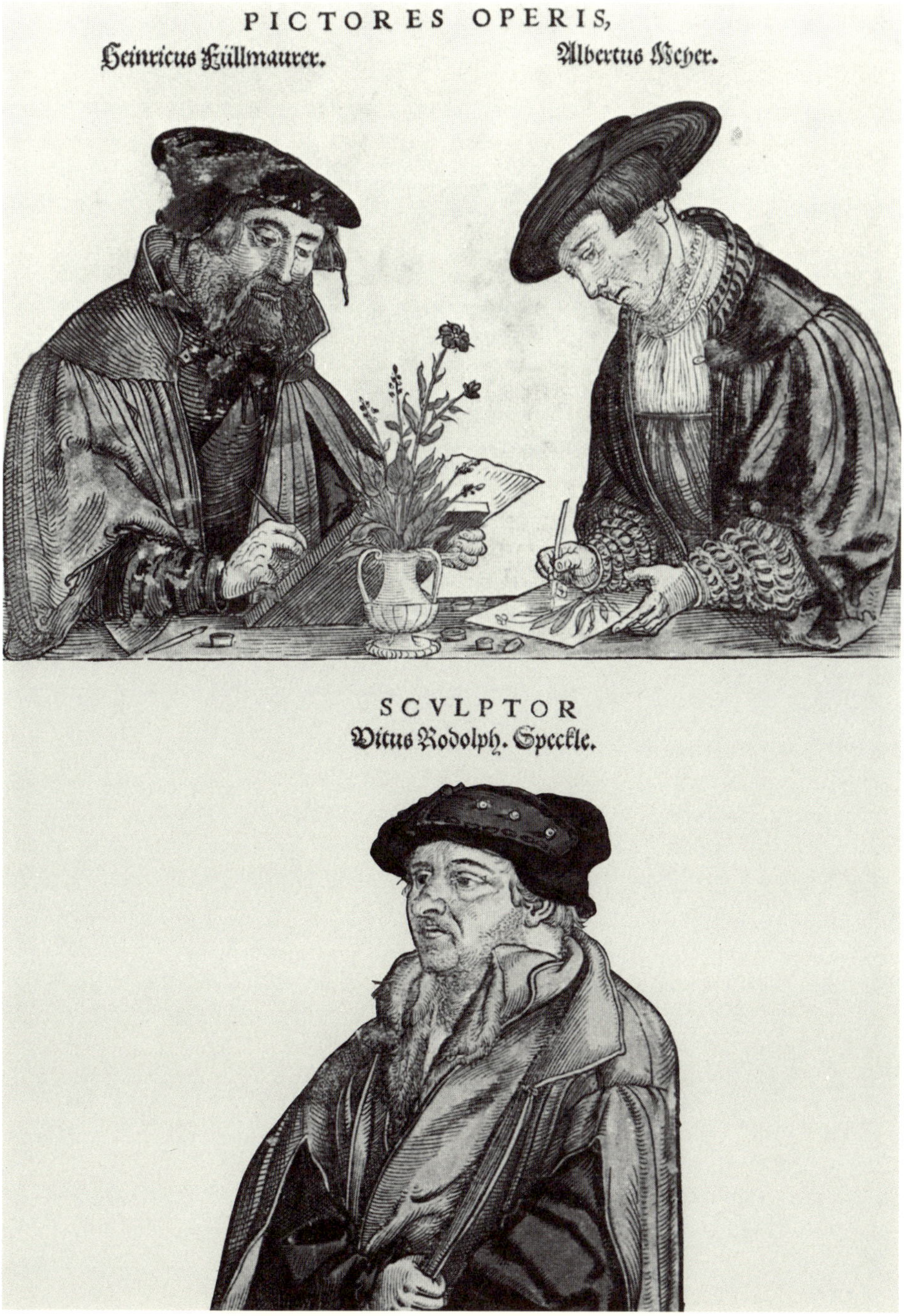

No. 143. Fuchs. *De Historia Stirpium.* The artists, Füllmaurer and Myer, and the engraver, Spreckle.

graphical details and was completed at a time when the author was experiencing a number of misfortunes in his private life. The final chapter is on grief and in it he tells the story of his son who was executed in 1560 for poisoning his wife. The most moving part of the volume is Cardano's defense of his son which is added at the end of the book. The volume also includes a fragment from his son's treatise on fetid foods.

Durling 852; Wellcome II, p. 299 (1648 ed.).

*147. ———. *In septem Aphorismorum Hippocratis particulas commentaria. . . . De venenorum differentiis, viribus, & adversus ea remediorum praesidiis. . . . De providentia temporum liber.* Basel: Per Henrichum Petri, 1564. [8] pp., 1072 columns, [46] pp., illus. 30.1 cm. Modern quarter parchment.

The present work contains a translation into Latin of the *Aphorisms* of Hippocrates with Cardano's extensive commentaries and a treatise on poisons and their antidotes.

Durling 856; Wellcome 1307.

*148. ———. *Contradicentium medicorum libri duo: quorum primus centum & octo: alter verò totidem disputationes continet.* Marburg: Typis Pauli Egenolphi, 1607. [32] 1134 pp. 15.7 cm.

In this work, Cardano examines the question of whether spells and charms have any therapeutic value and concludes that under some circumstances they may be helpful. Facts supporting his conclusion had been recorded earlier by Dioscorides, Aristotle, Avicenna, and others, and Cardano relates several cases to support his viewpoint. He endeavors to present a scientific explanation for these cures and remarks that one should always be aware that there are many enigmas in nature and it is only occasionally that an explanation may be found.

Durling 837 (1564 ed.); Waller 1763; Wellcome 1284 (1564 ed.).

*149. ———. *Opus novum cunctis de sanitate tuenda, ac vita producenda studiosis apprime necessarium.* Rome: [Apud Franciscum Zanettum] 1580. [26] 339 pp., illus. 29.2 cm. Vellum.

This posthumously published work deals largely with hygiene, diet, and geriatrics.

Durling 858; Wellcome 1310.

*150. ———. *De praeceptis ad filios libellus. Ex bibliotheca Gabrielis Naudaei.* Paris: Apud Thomam Blasium, 1635. [8] 30 pp. 17.5 cm. Contemporary calf. Bound with No. 151.

Cardano was a voluminous writer whose collected works, published in 1624, fill ten large volumes. They cover a wide range of knowledge and include this little-known work in which Cardano sets forth his maxims for a successful life. This rare first edition was prepared by Gabriel Naudé (1600–1653).

*151. ———. *De propria vita liber.* Paris: Apud Jacobum Villery, 1643. [96] 374 pp. 17.5 cm. Contemporary calf. Bound with No. 150.

This rare first edition of Cardano's autobiography was edited by Gabriel Naudé who also prepared an extensive introduction containing a great deal of bibliographical information. It is considered by some to be one of the greatest human documents of all times and is most certainly a pioneering work in clinical psychology.

Cushing C76; Wellcome II, p. 300 (1654 ed.).

NICOLAS DE LA ROCHE (fl. 1542). *De morbis mulierum curandis.*

See No. 228.

152. JACQUES HOULLIER (1504?–1562). *De morbis internis, lib. II. . . . De febribus. De peste. De remediis. . . . De materia chirurgica.* Lyons: Expensis Petri Landry, 1578. [24] 296, 83, 68, 132 *ll.* 16.5 cm.

This work, published posthumously, is a general text, without illustrations, of internal medicine, with added treatises on the plague, pharmaceuticals, and surgery. All are commented upon and extended by remarks of the editors, Antoine Valet (d. 1607) and Louis Duret (1527–1586). Houllier, a celebrated French physician, was a leader in France of the reaction against Galen and the return to Hippocratic principles.

Durling 2485; Wellcome 3280 (1611 ed.).

———. *Aggiuntovi il sesto libro della materia di cirugia.*

See No. 109.

*153. CHARLES ESTIENNE (1504–1564). *De dissectione partium corporis humani libri tres.* Paris: Apud Simonem Colinaeum, 1545. [23] 379 (misnumbered 375) pp., illus., plates. 33.7 cm. Vellum.

Estienne was a member of the famous family of printers bearing the same name. He received his medical degree from the University of Paris in 1542, but had apparently been at work on this anatomical *magnum opus* for many years, as some of the plates are dated 1530 and 1531.

This magnificent folio volume is one of the finest of all anatomical treatises. Certainly it was the finest printed in France in its century, and the sixty-two full-page woodcuts, artistically presenting the anatomical subjects in special poses before unusual background settings, are unusually sumptuous and imaginative. The anatomy itself is pre-Vesalian in conception and far from being as accurate as that of Vesalius. Some of the plates show diseased as well as normal anatomy.

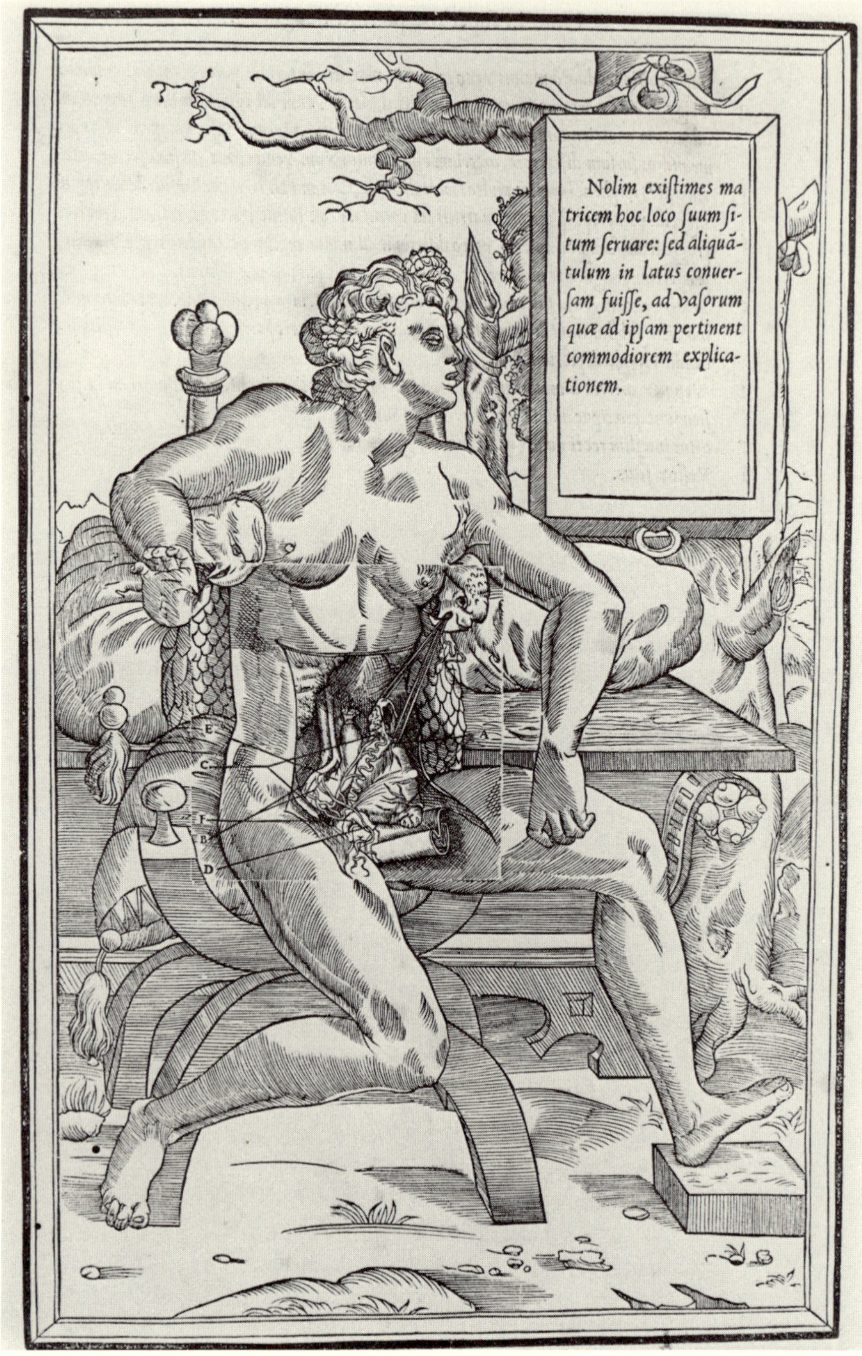
Nolim exiſtimes ma
tricem hoc loco ſuum ſi-
tum ſeruare: ſed aliquã-
tulum in latus conuer-
ſam fuiſſe, ad vaſorum
quæ ad ipſam pertinent
commodiorem explica-
tionem.

No. 153. Charles Estienne. *De Dissectione Partium Corporis Humani.* Good artistry but inaccurate anatomy. Note the parrots supporting the axillae.

Choulant-Frank, pp. 152–155; Durling 1391; Garrison-Morton 378; Osler 2541; Waller 2819; Wellcome 6076.

*154. JOANNES GUINTERIUS Andernacus (ca. 1505–1574). *Institutionum anatomicarum secundum Galeni sententia ad candidatos medicine libri quatuor. . . . Ab Andrea Vesalio . . . auctiores & emendatiores redditi.* Venice: [Melchiorre Sessa, 1540?]. [16] 101 [3] *ll.* 10.7 cm. Contemporary limp vellum. Bound with No. 56.

Guinterius, a German physician, was far better known as a teacher, scholar, and humanist. One of Vesalius' teachers at Padua, he was always more active at scholarly pursuits than at the practice of medicine and practical anatomy.

He first published this work in 1536 as a manual for medical students, and, although the book exerted considerable influence at the time, it was essentially Galenic in tradition and provided little new anatomical knowledge. Vesalius made a number of changes with the publication of this second edition, and it is evident that Vesalius was beginning to suspect the errors in Galen, which he later exposed.

Also included with this work is Giorgio Valla's (1447–1500) *De humani corporis partibus*. Valla was an Italian mathematician and physician who practiced in Milan and Venice. Later in his career he taught at Padua and occupied the chair of rhetoric at Venice. In addition to his several medical and mathematical works, he translated a number of Greek scientific texts into Latin including selections from Aristotle, Hippocrates, Galen, Rhazes, and Averroës.

Cushing G434; Cushing Vesalius III.–2; Durling 2227 (1536 ed.); Osler 582 (1538 ed.); Waller 3791; Wellcome 2968 (1538 ed.).

*155. ———. *Commentarius de balneis, & aquis medicatis in tres dialogos distinctus*. Strasbourg: [Excudebat Theodosius Rihelius, 1565]. [16] 206 pp. 15.3 cm. Half vellum.

In this small book on thermal springs, Guinterius gives many interesting details on the waters of Baden near Vienna, Gastein, Baden-Baden, Ems, Karlsbad, and many other springs throughout Europe.

Durling 2222; Waller 3786.

ANTONIO FRACANZANO (d. 1567). *De morbo Gallico.*

See Nos. 210 and 211.

*156. GUILLAUME RONDELET (1507–1566). *Methodus curandorum omnium morborum corporis humani.* Paris: Apud Jacobum Maceum [ca. 1567]. [702] *ll.* 16.6 cm. Contemporary blind-stamped pigskin over boards.

Rondelet was an active and successful physician and teacher on the faculty of the University of Montpellier where he also served as chancellor during the last ten years of his life. He is perhaps best known for his *De piscibus marinis* (1554), a noteworthy contribution to modern biology and expression of Rondelet's great interest in ichthyology. The majority of his published medical works were on

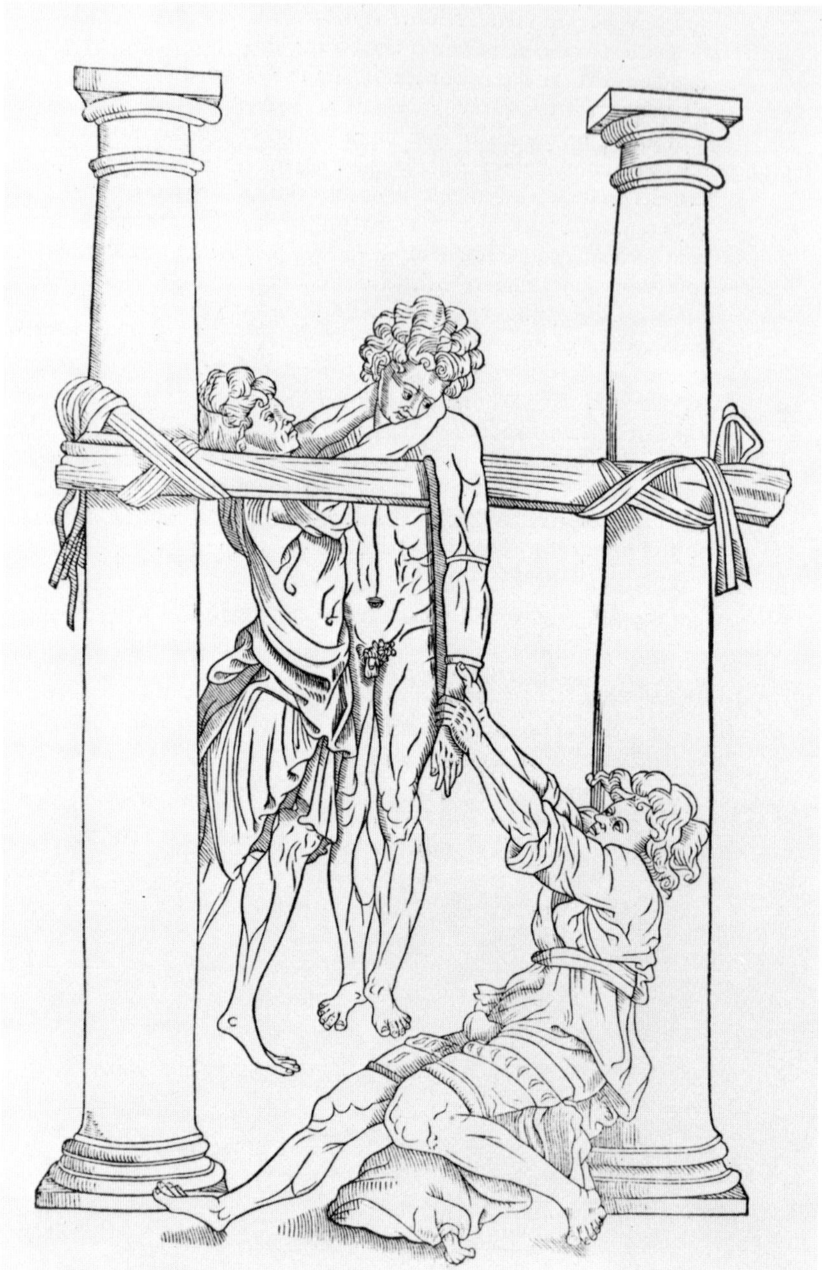

No. 158. Guidi. *Chirurgia*. The reduction of a dislocated shoulder.

therapeutics and the materia medica. However, the bulk of his scientific and anatomical works were never published because his friend and biographer, Laurent Joubert (see No. 220), was unable to find a publisher willing to undertake the expense of publishing Rondelet's considerable writings.

The present work is a lengthy treatise on numerous diseases, injuries, and fevers, and includes instructions for compounding suitable remedies. Rondelet infrequently refers to other authors so it is highly likely that this is an original work. As is so often found in works of this period, considerable attention is given to the diagnosis and treatment of worms, which were common because of the poor sanitary conditions of that day.

Cushing R230 (1575 ed.); Durling 3927; Osler 3832 (1576 ed.); Waller 8157 (1570 ed.); Wellcome 5552 (1570 ed.).

*157. BALDASAR HESELER (1508 or 9–1567). *Andreas Vesalius' first public anatomy at Bologna, 1540; an eyewitness report, by Baldasar Heseler, together with his notes on Matthaeus Curtius' lectures on Anatomia Mundini*. Uppsala: Almqvist & Wiksells Boktryckeri Aktiebolag [1959]. 343 pp., illus., port., fold. map. 25.2 cm.

Heseler, a German physician, was a medical student at Bologna when he made these notes from lectures on Mondino dei Luzzi's *Anatomia corporis humani* (see No. 54), given by Matthaeus Curtius (1475–1542), a noted Italian physician and teacher, and demonstrated by none other than Andreas Vesalius. Heseler's notes, found in a manuscript in the Royal Library in Stockholm, cover twenty-five lectures and twenty-six demonstrations and are of great interest and importance because they provide a contemporary and intimate insight into attitudes and opinions toward Curtius' lectures and Vesalius' demonstrations.

*158. GUIDO GUIDI (1508–1569). *Chirurgia è Graeco in Latinum conversa*. Paris: Excudebat Petrus Galterius, 1544. [35] 533 pp., illus. 35.9 cm. Contemporary blind-tooled calf, rebacked and restored.

Guidi, a successful Florentine surgeon, was invited to Paris in 1542 to help the French King Francis I apply the medical advances of the Italian Renaissance to French medicine. Francis appointed Guidi as his personal physician and to the chair of surgery at the newly founded Collège de France. Upon the death of Francis I in 1547, Guidi was recalled to Italy by Cosimo I, ruler of Tuscany, and became his personal physician and professor of philosophy and medicine at Pisa. Most of Guidi's works were published by his nephew, and in his *De anatomia corporis humani* (1611) is the first published figure of the sympathetic nervous system as well as descriptions of the anatomical structures in the pterygoid bone that bear his name: the Vidian canal, Vidian nerve, and Vidian artery.

When Guidi came to Paris, he brought with him a copy of a tenth-century Greek surgical manuscript as a gift for the French monarch. Under the patronage of the King, Guidi was able to complete his Latin translation and commentary on the manuscript and published the present work. In large part, the book is a compilation of what was then known about treating wounds and fractures, particularly

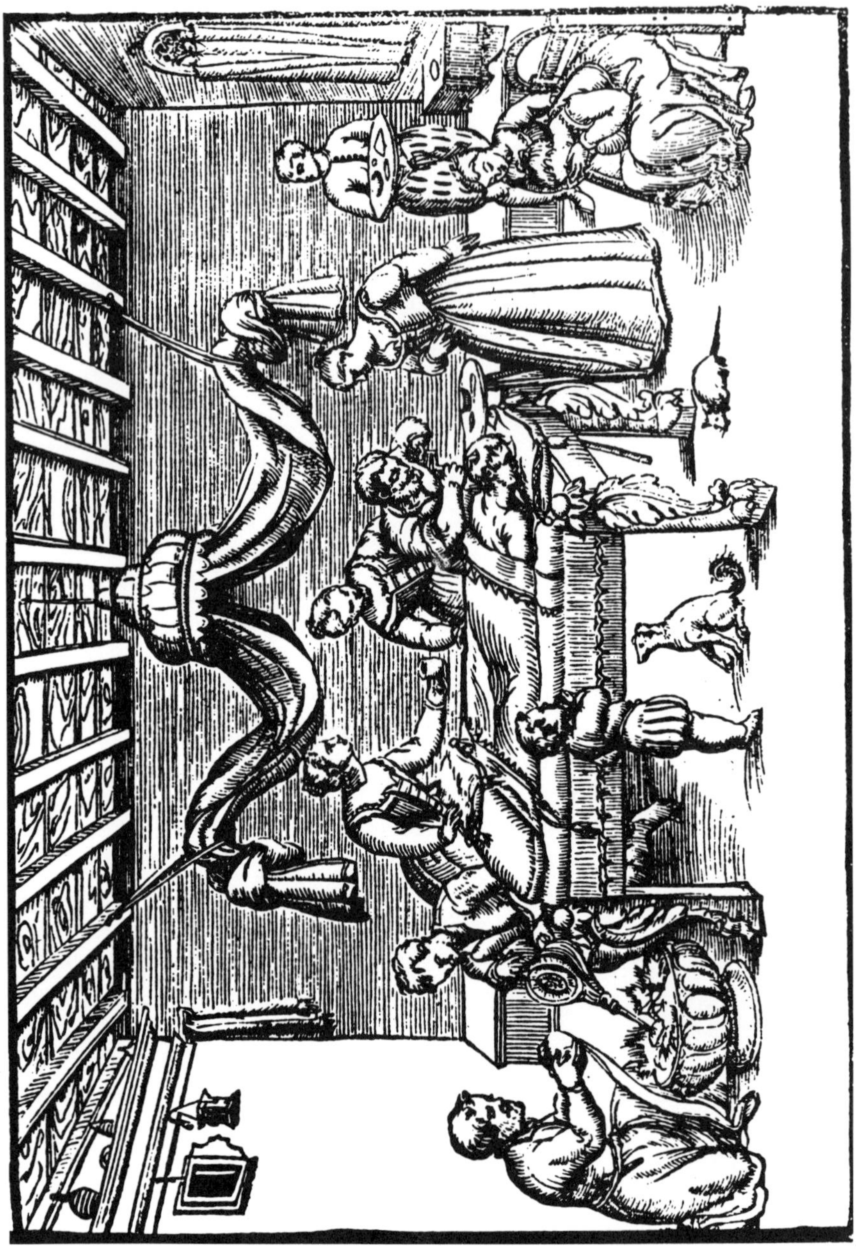

No. 159. Croce. *Chirurgiae.* A sixteenth century neurosurgical scene.

those conditions resulting from war wounds. Most of the book is devoted to Hippocrates' writings on ulcers, fistulas, and head wounds with Guidi's commentaries and observations, and Galen's commentaries on Hippocrates' works on fractures and joints. Also included are Galen's work on bandages as well as Oribasius' *De laqueis* (see No. 25) and *De machinamentis* (see No. 25). It is thought that many of the sketches for the more than 200 woodcuts in the book came from the drawings of the Italian mannerist Francesco Primaticcio (1504–1570) who copied and partially redrew the Greek manuscript. This book is often considered to be the finest textbook of surgery to be printed in the sixteenth century, and the various instruments, bandages, orthopedic machinery, and surgical procedures are beautifully illustrated.

Choulant-Frank, pp. 211–212; Cushing G445; Durling 2204; Osler 155; Waller 1960; Wellcome 6596.

*159. GIOVANNI ANDREA DALLA CROCE (1509?–1580). *Chirurgiae . . . libri septem*. Venice: Apud Jordanum Zilettum, 1573. [4] 142 [7] *ll.*, illus., plates. 29.8 cm. Vellum.

Not a great deal is known of Croce's life. He was born at Venice, is known to have been a member of the College of Surgeons there, and about 1560 is mentioned as being one of the city's most successful surgeons.

The present work is Croce's major contribution and is chiefly an historical compilation of the writings of the important authorities from Hippocrates to Abulcasis. Croce's recommendations for wound management are surprisingly modern and are similar to some of those used during the early years of this century. Noteworthy in his *Chirurgiae* are the many excellent illustrations that appear throughout the text. Nearly all of the best known and most frequently used surgical instruments are depicted in historical sequence. The various types of arrows, spears, and bullets used in the warfare of his day are also illustrated as well as several scenes of the typical operating room of the sixteenth century. Croce's work went through several editions and was also translated into German and Italian.

Cushing C477; Durling 1082; Wellcome 1666.

160. PAMPHILO FIORIMBENE (fl. 1550). *Collectanea de febribus*. [Venice: Impressum per Nicholaum Bascarinum] 1550. [4] 119 *ll.* 15.2 cm.

This collection of writings on the nature of fevers and their cure was prepared by the Italian physician, Fiorimbene. The author has drawn chiefly upon the works of Galen although he also includes material from Avicenna, Paul of Aegina, and Cletius.

Durling 1580.

161. CHRISTÓBAL DE VEGA (1510–1573). *Commentaria in librum Galeni De differentia febrium*. Alcalá de Henares: Typis Joannis Mey, 1553. 301 [6] *ll.*, fold. plate. 14.9 cm. Old vellum.

Vega, a Spanish physician, was an active teacher and professor at the university in his native city of Alcalá de Henares. He is perhaps best known for his commentaries on the works of Hippocrates and Galen. He published a number of commentaries on their works and also wrote his own treatise on medicine—*De arte medendi* (1564). The present work is his commentary on Galen's work on fevers. A Latin translation of the original Greek work is also included in the volume.

Durling 4560.

*162. GIOVANNI FILIPPO INGRASSIA (1510–1580). *Quaestio de purgatione per medicamentum. . . . Illustrissimi ducis Terraenovae casus enarratio. . . . Quaestio utrum victus.* 4 pts. in 1 vol. Venice: Sumptibus Angeli Patessii, 1568. Part I: [8] 112 pp.; Part II: 68 pp.; Part III: 101 pp.; Part IV: 50 pp. (the 4 pts. bound in different order from that given on title page). 18.7 cm. Newly rebound in vellum.

"Ingrassia, 'the Sicilian Hippocrates', a graduate of Padua, was a celebrated teacher of anatomy and medicine at Naples. . . . He discovered the stapes, and the lesser wings of the sphenoid are still called the processes of Ingrassias [sic]" (Osler 3052). He also gave the first descriptions of scarlet fever and chicken pox.

In this collection of lesser works of Ingrassia appears the transcript of a letter from Vesalius to Ingrassia, a rare and little-known piece of Vesaliana which indicates that Vesalius was ahead of his time in surgical as well as in anatomical knowledge. During the spring of 1562, John, Duke of Terranova, suffered a penetrating wound of the left chest during a tournament. Under the care of Ingrassia, he failed to respond to treatment and developed a fistula with empyema. Ingrassia sought help and about eight months later Vesalius wrote a long letter of advice ("Consilium pro fistula"), in itself a treatise on his manner of therapy in empyema. In this letter, dated from Madrid, Christmas, 1562, he gives in detail the steps in the procedure, using surgical drainage instead of the usual cauterization. The patient recovered.

Cushing I13; Cushing Vesalius VIII.–C; Durling 2549; Garrison-Morton 3164; Waller 5070.

*163. AMBROISE PARÉ (1510?–1590). *Opera.* Paris: Apud Jacobum Du-Puys, 1582. [12] 884 [22] pp., illus., plates (port.). 34.3 cm. Vellum, new calf back.

Paré, of humble Huguenot beginnings and poorly educated, became the sixteenth century's outstanding surgeon and the greatest military surgeon before his fellow countryman, Larrey (see No. 736), more than two hundred years later. He began his studies as a barber-surgeon and at age nineteen, while working as a surgical dresser and assistant in a Paris hospital, he began to acquire the fund of practical knowledge for which he became a legend in his own time. Probably his best known innovations were his discarding the use of boiling oil in gunshot wounds and the reintroduction of simple ligature instead of red hot cautery after amputation. He invented many surgical and dental instruments and was especially adept at devising ingenious artificial limbs. Beyond his technical skill and imagination, he was a man of utmost honesty, courage, and great modesty.

Although he wrote widely—always in French, as he knew no Latin—his original works are very rare. The first edition of his collected works in French was published in 1579. The present work is the first Latin edition, edited by Paré's pupil, Jacques Guillemeau (1550–1613), who succeeded Paré as surgeon to King Charles IX. It contains a wealth of interesting illustrations showing surgical techniques and instruments, as well as a portrait of the author.

Cushing P88; Durling 3531; Osler 661; Waller 7175; Wellcome 4824.

164. ———. *Opera chirurgica*. Frankfurt: Apud Joannem Feyrabend, impensis Petri Fischeri, 1594. [12] 851 [25] pp., illus., port. 34.3 cm. Blind-tooled vellum, extremely worn and broken.

A re-issue of the 1582 Latin translation (No. 163).

Cushing P89; Durling 3532; Waller 7176.

Gift of Dr. Everett D. Plass.

*165. ———. *Oeuvres complètes d'Ambroise Paré . . . par J.-F. Malgaigne*. 3 vols. Paris: Chez J.-B. Baillière, 1840–1841. Vol. I: cccli [1] 459 pp.; Vol. II: [4] 811 pp.; Vol. III: [4] xxxii, 878 pp., illus. 25.4 cm.

Edited by Joseph François Malgaigne (see No. 933), this three-volume set is the definitive edition of Paré's works. A comprehensive work, it contains a lengthy historical introduction to the development and state of surgery between the sixth and sixteenth centuries, an extensive biography and bibliography of Paré, as well as his collected writings. Malgaigne was an accomplished French surgeon and author and was described by John Shaw Billings as "the greatest surgical historian and critic whom the world has yet seen" (Fielding H. Garrison, *An introduction to the history of medicine*. 4th ed. Philadelphia, 1929. p. 491).

Cushing P87; Garrison-Morton 59; Osler 660; Waller 7174.

*166. MARCO ANTONIO MONTAGNANA (d. 1572). *De herpete, phagedaena, gangraena, sphacelo, & cancro; tum cognoscendis, tum curandis, tractatis accuratissima*. Venice: Apud Paulum Meiettum, 1589. [8] 107 *ll*. 19.2 cm. Marbled boards.

Marco Antonio, another member of the distinguished Montagnana family whose male descendants taught at Padua for over two centuries (see No. 70), was professor of surgery at Padua from 1545 to 1570.

In this early work on ulcers, tumors, gangrene, and cancer, he discusses the etiology, diagnosis, prognosis, and therapy of these diseases in considerable detail. Montagnana relied heavily on ancient authorities and frequently cites Galen, Rhazes, Avicenna, and Celsus.

Durling 3237.

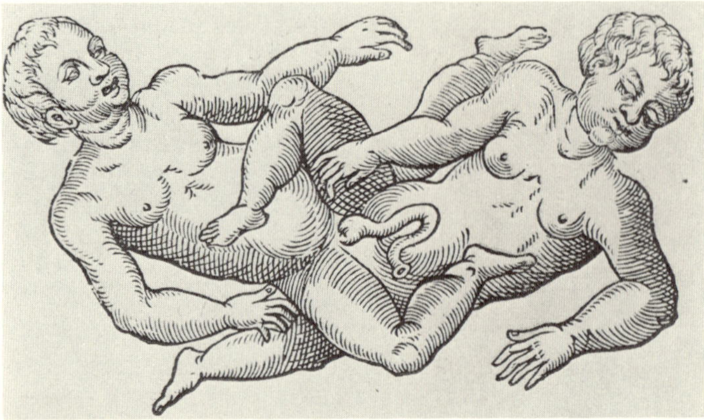

No. 163. Paré. *Opera*. Conjoined twins, born alive and eventually baptized.

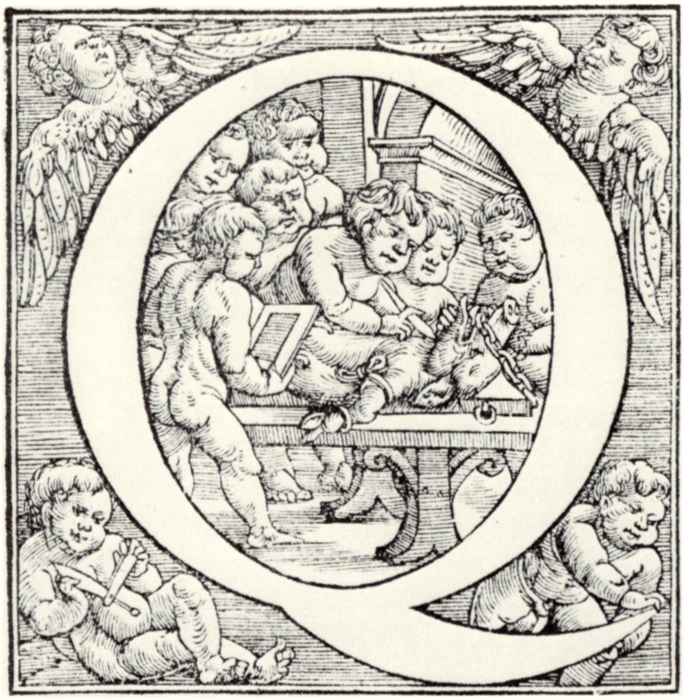

No. 172. Vesalius. *De Humani Corporis Fabrica*. An initial capital letter.

*167. NICOLÁS MONARDES (ca. 1512–1588). *Simplicium medicamentorum ex Novo orbe delatorum, quorum in medicina usus est, historia*. 3rd ed. Antwerp: Ex officina Plantiniana, apud viduam, & Joannem Moretum, 1593. [313]–456 pp. (pp. 449–454 are lacking from this copy), illus. 16.1 cm. Old calf. Appears with No. 145 and No. 233.

Monardes, a Spanish physician, was very much interested in the plants of the New World and established a botanical garden devoted exclusively to American flora. Although he never visited the Americas, he studied their flora and tested the medicinal properties of many plants on his patients. He first published his findings and observations in Spanish at Seville in 1565. This was followed in 1574 by a Latin edition and in 1577 by an English translation with the title *Joyfull newes out of the newe founde worlde*. The work was translated also into Italian, French, Flemish, and German. The present work, translated into Latin by Charles de l'Écluse, is the third Latin edition and contains accounts of such New World plants and drugs as tobacco, curare, guaiac, and chinaroot (sarsaparilla), as well as many other medicinal herbs.

Cushing M445 (1st Latin ed., 1574); Durling 3417; Osler 2327 (4th Latin ed., 1605); Waller 7006; Wellcome 4658.

*168. GIOVANNI ARGENTERIO (1513–1572). *De morbis, libri XIIII*. 2nd ed. Florence: [Excudebat Laurentius Torrentinus] 1556. 19, 358 [26] pp. 29.5 cm.

Argenterio, a native of Piedmont, practiced (though not too successfully) in Lyons and Antwerp before returning to Italy where he taught at several universities. His fame as a teacher was great although (and perhaps because) he ventured to attack Galen and was almost Paracelsian in his attitudes.

The present work, first published in 1550 under the title *Varia opera de re medica*, is a quasi-clinical, quasi-philosophical discussion of the nature of various illnesses, general diagnostic methods, and especially the causes of diseases.

Durling 264; Wellcome 402 (1558 ed.).

169. ———. *In artem medicinalem Galeni*. 2 vols. in 1. Paris: Apud Joannem Poupy, 1578. Vol. I: [16] 762 pp.; Vol. II: [4] 356 [51] pp. 16.5 cm. Quarter vellum.

A lengthy and closely-printed text of commentary on and critique of Galen.

Durling 268 (1566 ed.); Wellcome 405.

170. ———. *Opera nunquam excusa, iamdiu desiderata, ac è tenebris in lucem prodita. In duas partes distincta*. 2 pts. in 1. Venice: Apud Juntas, 1606. Pt. I: [32] 288 pp.; Pt. II: [28] 179 pp. 28.9 cm. Vellum.

Issued first in 1555, this work contains extensive commentaries on the aphorisms of Hippocrates and a treatise on fevers.

Wellcome 407.

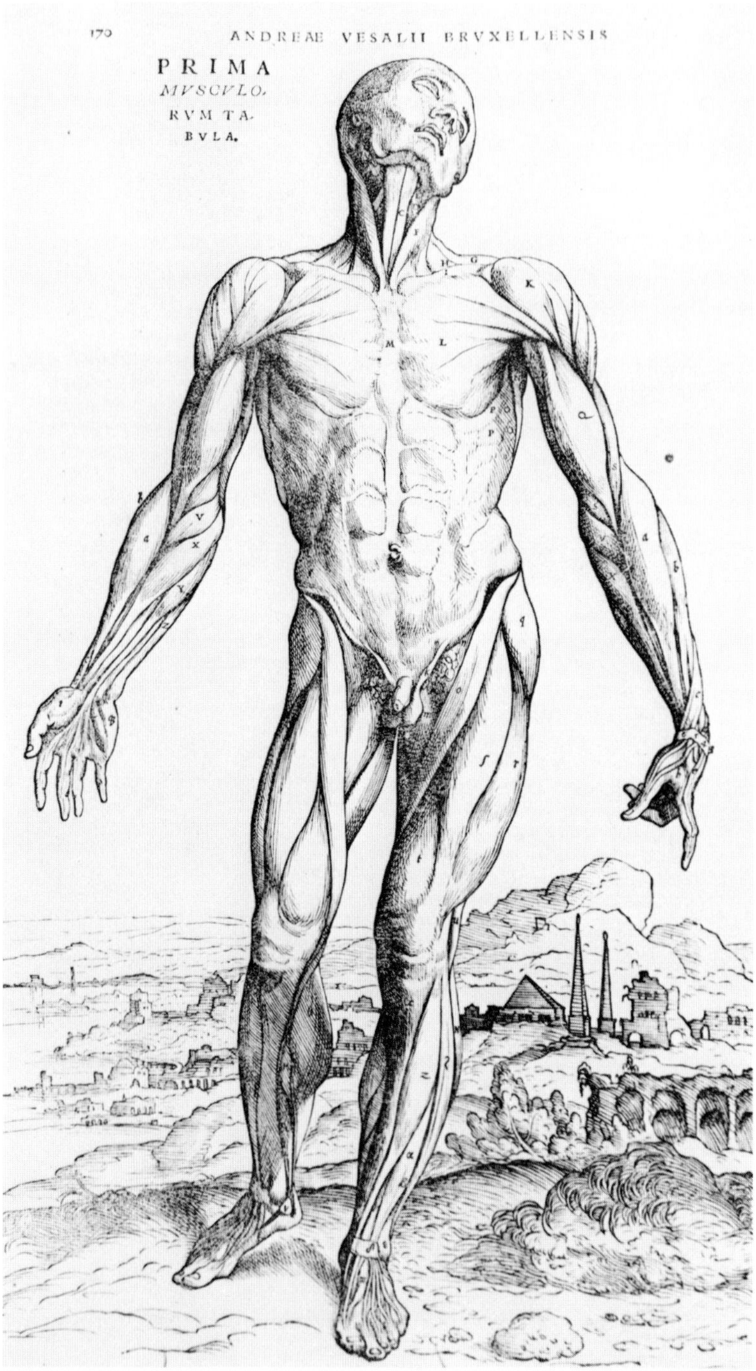

No. 172. Vesalius. *De Humani Corporis Fabrica.* The plate of the first muscleman from the 1543 edition.

*171. ANDREAS VESALIUS (1514–1564). *Paraphrasis in nonum librum Rhazae . . . de affectuum singularum corporis partium curatione*. Lyons: Apud Joan. Tornaesium & Gulielmum Gazeium, 1551. 212 [28] pp. 11.6 cm. Modern three-quarter vellum.

Vesalius is a name known and revered by all students of medicine. In his short lifetime, this Brussels-born Fleming came to occupy one of the foremost places in the history of medicine, not only as the inaugurator of a real science of anatomy, but also as a founder, with Harvey later, of medical science based on fact rather than tradition. To have completed before his twenty-ninth year a task of the magnitude of the *Fabrica* (see No. 172), at a time when bodies for dissection were most difficult to obtain and legal authority difficult to resist, is a feat to which the literary history of the profession offers no parallel. Mainly because he questioned (and actually proved erroneous) many old Galenic "laws," he had a far from tranquil life and, after his studies at Louvain, Montpellier, Paris, and Padua, he was at the center of a great scientific uproar at the last university because of his daring anatomical demonstrations and his strongly-phrased doubts of some old masters. Fortunately he had the backing of the royal court, so, eventually sickened by the continuous sniping of his contemporaries, he discontinued the pursuit of anatomy to become court physician to Emperor Charles V, and in 1556 to his successor, Philip II, at Madrid. In 1563 Vesalius undertook a trip to Jerusalem and, on the return trip in 1564 (the story of which is somewhat hazy), the ship is said to have been wrecked near the island of Zante in the Ionian Sea. Vesalius supposedly died of typhoid fever and was buried in a plain crypt in the little Church of the Virgin at Zante.

Vesalius had been pursuing his medical studies in Paris for three years when he was forced to return to Louvain in 1536 upon the outbreak of hostilities between France and Belgium. He resumed his medical studies at Louvain later that year and, from what is known, prepared the present work as his thesis for the degree of bachelor of medicine. Vesalius undertook this paraphrase of the ninth book of Rhazes (see No. 36) primarily to compare the therapeutics of the Arabs with those of the Greeks. It is likely that he selected Rhazes because he was advised to do so by his mentor, Nicolas Florenas (fl. 1530), and also because Rhazes was held in high repute by Jacques Dubois (see No. 103) under whom he had studied in Paris. Vesalius also wanted to edit and correct the poorly translated text so that the book might be more readily understandable to those who wished to use it. He did improve the text stylistically, provided better identification of many of the drugs, and added numerous marginal notes that called attention to prevailing views or cast doubt on Rhazes' observations.

The book was first published at Louvain in 1537, was reprinted later that year at Basel, appeared in a 1544 edition of Rhazes' *Opera omnia* published at Basel, and was reissued in 1551, 1586, and 1592.

Cushing V65; Cushing Vesalius I.–4; Durling 4592; Waller 9895.

*172. ———. *De humani corporis fabrica libri septem*. Basel: [Ex officina Joannis Oporini, 1543]. [12] 663 (misnumbered 659) [36] pp., illus., 171 plates (2 fold.), port.

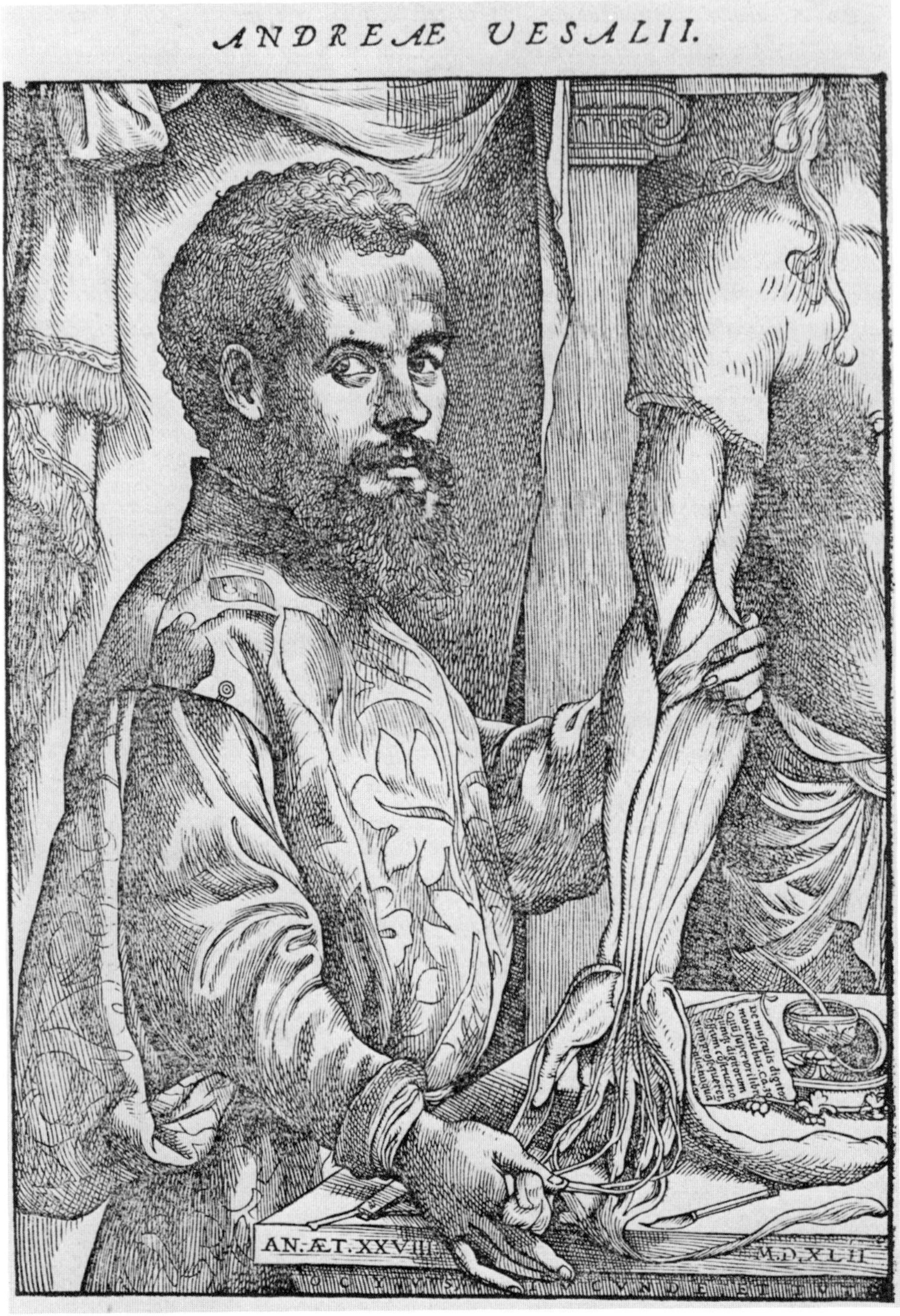

No. 173. Vesalius. *De Humani Corporis Fabrica.* Portrait of Vesalius at age 28 from the 1555 edition.

(facsimile). 41.6 cm. Half vellum. Lacking portrait, replaced in facsimile. With folded leaf m³, sometimes lacking.

It is often a matter of friendly contention among medical historians as to which is the "more important" book, Vesalius' *De humani corporis fabrica* or Harvey's *De motu cordis*. It cannot be denied that the *Fabrica* is the most famous anatomical work ever published, to this day one of the most beautiful in existence, and the milestone in all medical history which definitely showed a break from old traditions.

It cannot be emphasized too often that this was an epochal book. The beautiful woodcuts, executed under the supervision of Vesalius by the artist Jan Stephan van Calcar (1499–1546?), student of Titian, are famous for their beauty, accuracy, and lavishness of detail and number. It was E. Jackschath of Tilsit who pointed out that the background scenes of the "muscle men" illustrations are, when collected into a continuum, a dioramic replica of the Paduan countryside of the time of Vesalius. The often-copied frontispiece dissecting scene, a portrait of Vesalius dissecting the arm, and the innumerable capital letters (depicting grave robbing, naked little boys urinating with abandon, operation for the stone, childbirth, cranial operations, etc.) are as fascinating a study as are the 171 anatomical plates.

Throughout this copy there are many interesting marginal notes, written in Latin in fine, careful script, sometimes revealing the critical opinions of a former owner of this book.

This first edition of the *Fabrica* is the heart of any library of medical history.

Choulant-Frank, pp. 178–180; Cushing V76; Cushing Vesalius VI.A.–1; Durling 4577; Garrison-Morton 375; Osler 567; Waller 9899; Wellcome 6560.

*173. ———. ———. [2nd folio ed.]. Basel: Per Joannem Oporinum [1555]. [12] 824 [48] pp., illus., 171 plates (2 fold.), port. 41.3 cm. Vellum.

In 1552, a small "pocket" edition of the *Fabrica* was pirated in Lyons but, as it had no illustrations, it was neither popular nor profitable. For that matter, neither the first nor the second splendid folio edition was profitable, either, and the printer, Oporinus, suffered losses on both.

By the time of this second folio edition, the plates from the first edition had been copied in England and throughout Europe, and the prospect for sale of a new edition must have been considerably lessened. Even so, the new edition was even more lavish than the first, with heavier paper and larger type, necessitating an entire recutting of the initial letters. Corrections were made in the text by Vesalius with some rearrangement of both the text and the illustrations.

The woodcut title page has always created much interest. It carries considerable dramatic impact and probably fairly represents, with some theatrical touches, an "anatomy" of the sixteenth century. The block for the second edition was entirely recut and, although it closely resembles that of the first edition, there are a few changes. The unclothed man of the first edition, observing from his perch at the left, is clothed in the second edition, "for no other reason that one can see,"

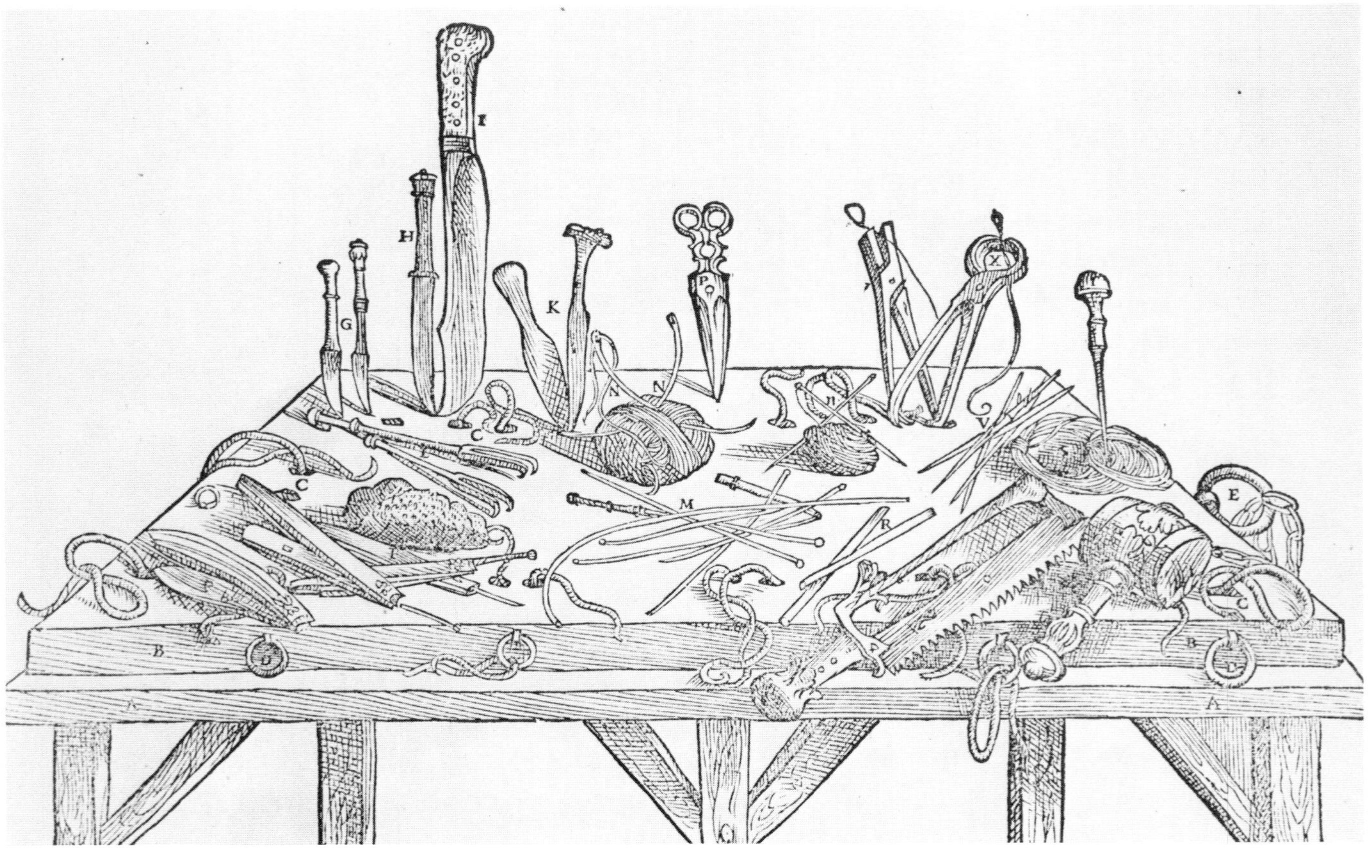

No. 173. Vesalius. *De Humani Corporis Fabrica*. Vesalius' dissection tools.

comments Cushing, "unless to save the nun's embarrassment by clothing the naked figure." (Cushing Vesalius, p. 90). The wood blocks were cut in Venice and transported by mule across the Alps to Basel, where Oporinus—artist, printer, and friend of Vesalius—received them with detailed instructions from the author.

Choulant-Frank, pp. 181–182; Cushing V78; Cushing Vesalius VI.A.–3; Durling 4579; Garrison-Morton 377; Osler 568; Waller 9901; Wellcome 6562.

*174. ———. ———. [3rd folio ed.]. Venice: Apud Franciscum Franciscium Senensem, & Joannem Criegher, 1568. [12] 510 [45] pp., illus. 31.8 cm. Modern parchment.

This posthumous edition of the *Fabrica*, printed without license by Senense in Venice, is set up much like the 1555 edition, but the woodcuts, redrawn by the artist Johann Criegher (or Krüger), are slightly reduced copies of the originals, and entirely new capital initials were used in this edition. The fact that publishers for many years found it profitable to put out new editions of Vesalius' work indicates that the solid truths set forth in the 1543 edition were quickly accepted by all but a few diehards, and Vesalius, instead of Galen, became the medical bible.

Choulant-Frank, p. 182; Cushing V79; Cushing Vesalius VI.A.–4; Durling 4580; Osler 569; Waller 9902.

*175. ———. *Anatomia.* [4th folio ed.]. Venice: Apud Joannem Antonium et Jacobum de Franciscis [1604]. [6] 510 [45] [19] pp., illus. 31.1 cm. Soft boards.

This fourth folio edition of the *Fabrica* shows considerable loss of identity with the 1543 original. The title has changed and some new plates were added by Criegher, the artist, but the text is essentially unchanged. This edition, published by the sons of the publisher of the third folio edition of 1568, was a purely business adventure, and a successful one. The book was widely distributed and is said to have been the text used by the anatomist Fabricius ab Aquapendente. The over-all tone of the book is sadly cheapened; yet even in this plagiarized, "commercialized" form it is a beautiful book and better done than many anatomy texts which succeeded it. The original Calcar woodblocks were never used in their entirety other than for the authorized first two editions.

Choulant-Frank, pp. 182–183; Cushing V80; Cushing Vesalius VI.A.–5; Osler 570; Waller 9903; Wellcome 6563.

*176. ———. *Opera omnia anatomica & chirurgica, cura Hermanni Boerhaave & Bernhardi Siegfried Albini.* 2 vols. Leiden: Apud Joannem du Vivie, et Joannem & Hermannem Verbeek, 1725. Vol. I: [42] 572 pp.; Vol. II: [8] 577–1156 [52] pp., plates, port. 44.4 cm. Contemporary paneled calf, rebacked.

Edited by Hermann Boerhaave (see No. 474 ff.) and Bernhard Siegfried Albinus (see No. 525 ff.), this is the first collected edition of Vesalius' works. Although it is not complete, no expense was spared in producing the two-volume set, which contains superbly engraved copperplates by Jan Wandelaer (1690–1759). The

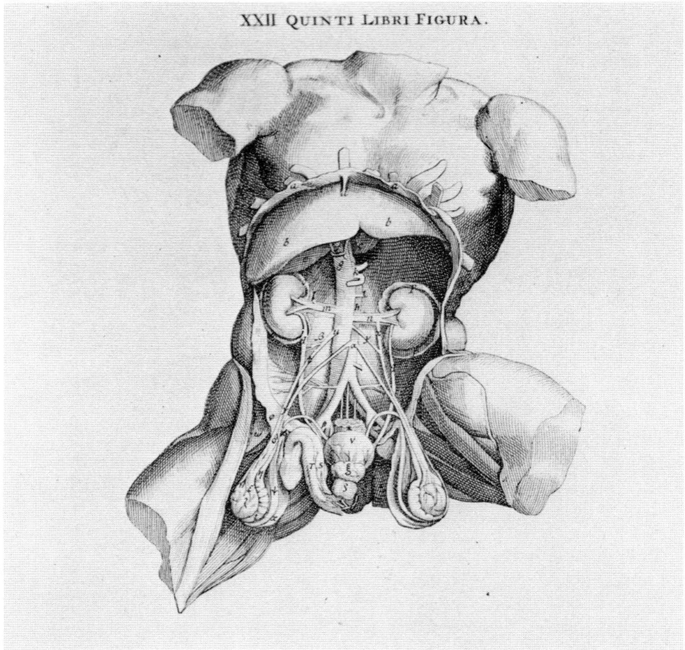

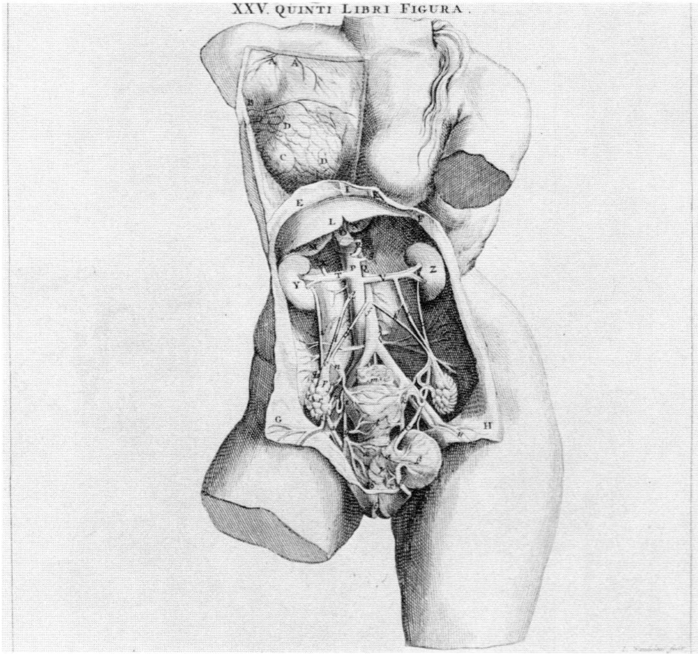

No. 176. Vesalius. *Opera Omnia Anatomica & Chirurgica.* The artist Wandelaer's accurate plates from the collected edition of Vesalius' works by Boerhaave and Albinus. (Figures XXII and XXV.)

editors, famous physicians in their own right, have done a magnificent job in clearly showing the astonishing achievements of Vesalius.

Choulant-Frank, p. 183; Cushing V108; Cushing Vesalius VI.D.–8; Lindeboom 554; Osler 579; Waller 9917.

177. ———. *Icones anatomicae.* [Munich]: Academia Medicinae Nova-Eboracensis et Bibliotheca Universitatis Monacensis, 1934. [10] 130, xiii [3] pp., with folio leaf "To the reader" laid in, plates (part fold.), port. 54.6 cm.

The publication of this large and beautiful volume of original wood blocks from Vesalius' *Fabrica, Epitome*, and *Tabulae anatomicae sex* was a joint project of the New York Academy of Medicine and the Library of the University of Munich where the wood blocks had been preserved. Of the 277 illustrations reproduced in the work, 227 are from the original blocks with the remaining fifty being reproduced photographically. No changes or improvements were made in any of the blocks, and they were reproduced just as they were and printed on paper "specially made from the best hempen fibres." The only exception was a block from the *Epitome* which had to be restored to supply a hand which had been damaged on the original block. Vesalius' letter to the printer is included and it explains the order and arrangement of the wood blocks. In addition, that part of the text explaining the symbols used in the figures and illustrations has also been reprinted. This was the last time that these wood blocks—which had been preserved for nearly four hundred years—were ever used; they were destroyed during World War II as a result of Allied bombing raids.

Cushing V110; Cushing Vesalius VI.A.–16; Waller 9907.

*178. ———. О СТРОЕНИИ ЧЕЛОВЕЧЕСКОГО ТЕЛА. 2 vols. [Moscow]: Akademiî nauk SSSR, 1950–1954. Vol. I: 1055 pp.; Vol. II: 960 pp., illus. 22 cm. Modern cloth.

This Russian translation of Vesalius' *De humani corporis fabrica*, by V. N. Ternovskii and S. P. Shestakov, is the only complete translation of this famous work into a modern language. An epilogue by the noted Russian physiologist, Ivan Petrovich Pavlov (see No. 1105), is appended.

*179. ———. *De humani corporis fabrica librorum epitome.* Basel: [Ex officina Joannis Oporini, 1543]. [27] pp., illus., port. 52.3 cm. Vellum.

Vesalius was fully convinced of the importance of using anatomical diagrams for teaching purposes and prepared the *Epitome* to meet that end. In actuality, the *Epitome* is an illustrated compendium of all that was contained in the *Fabrica* and it represents an extremely skillful condensation of the immense amount of detail in the *Fabrica*. Almost all of the wood blocks used in the *Epitome* were prepared especially for it and do not appear in the *Fabrica*. The figures are some six centimeters taller than those of the *Fabrica* in order to provide as much detail as possible and to make them easier to follow. Vesalius also included two plates of various anatomical features which were supposed to be cut out and pasted upon human figures elsewhere in the book.

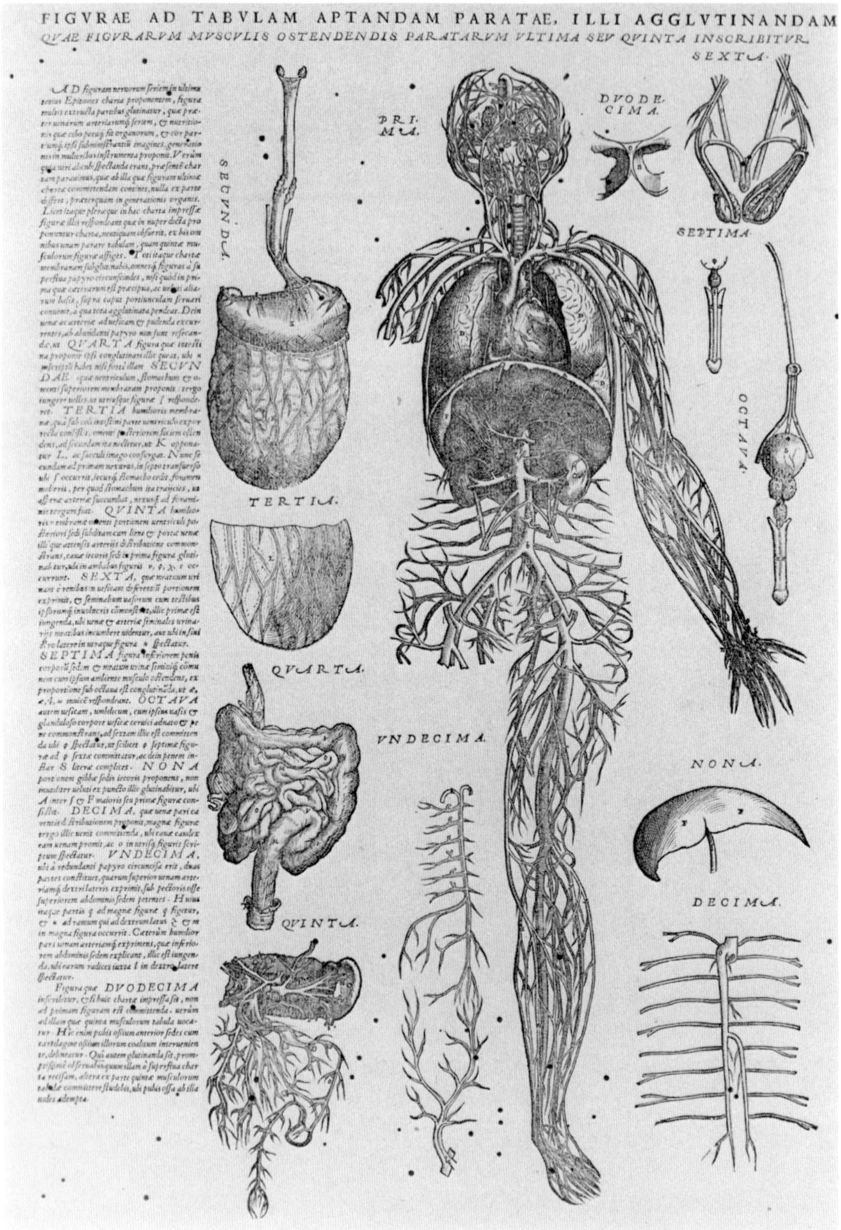

No. 179. Vesalius. *Epitome*. The vascular system and parts of the abdominal viscera intended to be cut out and pasted on other figures in the book. (The numerous black dots are worm holes.)

Apparently the work was never intended to be bound together but rather was for use in separate sheets. As a result, it is a very rare work and is incomplete in most of the existing copies. This is reflected in the library's complete copy which appears to have been assembled from at least four other copies. Cushing lists only eleven copies in the United States and seven in Europe.

Choulant-Frank, p. 180; Cushing V85; Cushing Vesalius VI.B.–1; Durling 4581; Garrison-Morton 376; Osler 571; Waller 9908; Wellcome 6565.

*180 ———. *Epitome anatomica. Opus redivivum, cui accessere, notae ac commentaria P. Paaw*. Leiden: Ex officina Justià Colster, 1616. [8] 226 pp., illus., fold. plate. 19.9 cm. Old calf.

This is basically a reprint of the *Epitome* with commentary and notes after each chapter by Pieter Pauw (see No. 251). The text is taken largely from the *Epitome* and Pauw has added a chapter on the names of the parts of the human body. The beautiful woodcuts of the *Epitome* have been replaced by thirteen small copper engravings from the *Fabrica* which are scattered through the text. Pauw, a pupil of Fabricius at Padua, was professor of anatomy at Leiden and wrote a number of anatomical works which reflected the new anatomical concepts set forth by Vesalius. He was also successful in having an anatomical theater constructed at Leiden while he was there.

Choulant-Frank, p. 181; Cushing V105; Cushing Vesalius VI.D.–19; Osler 578; Waller 9921; Wellcome 6567 (1633 ed.).

*181. ———. *The epitome of Andreas Vesalius*. New York: Macmillan Co., 1949. xxxvi, 103 [27] pp., illus., port. 25.2 cm.

This scholarly work was translated from the Latin by Levi R. Lind (b. 1906) so that the very rare *Epitome* would be more readily available to modern readers. It more than fulfills that role, containing, in addition to the translation, facsimiles of the Latin text and figures, a very helpful introduction to the life and work of Vesalius, and a most useful table of Vesalius' Greek marginal notes which gives the Greek, Latin, and modern term for nearly all of the parts of the body.

Waller 9911.

*182. ———. *Epistola, rationem modumque propinandi radicis Chynae decocti*. Basel: [Ex officina Joannis Oporini, 1546]. 204 (misnumbered 404) [16] pp., port. 26.7 cm. Half morocco.

This very rare work is actually a monograph in the form of a long letter to a physician friend, Joachim Roelants (fl. 1546). Commonly called the "China-root epistle," it was copied by Vesalius' brother, Franciscus, who felt that it was so important that it should be published and, appreciating the quality of printing in the *Fabrica*, took it to Oporinus for publication. The China root (*Smilax china*), a plant of the sarsaparilla family, had recently been brought from the West Indies and had come into vogue as a medication in decoction form for various ailments. Vesalius describes his use of it (probably of doubtful value in his own mind) in the treatment of Emperor Charles V, to whom Vesalius was personal physician at the time. But the great importance and value of this book lies in the intimate, often sad, experiences which Vesalius relates concerning the creation of the *Fabrica*, his defense against his critics (especially Sylvius, his old teacher in Paris) for his denial of much of the Galenic tradition, and in his seeing his works plagiarized, badly copied, and misquoted. On page 196 he tells of his rash act, later regretted, of burning many of his own works, translations and original manuscripts, and other books which he valued greatly. This book, therefore, has great biographical value. It is Vesalius in person revealing much of his life and thought.

Cushing V111; Cushing Vesalius VII.–1; Durling 4587; Waller 9923; Wellcome 6570.

*183. ———. *Anatomicarum Gabrielis Falloppii observationum examen*. Venice: Apud Franciscum de Franciscis, Senensem, 1564. [4] 171 pp. 21.6 cm. Limp vellum.

Fallopius, Vesalius' pupil and a later occupant of the chair of anatomy at Padua, had published his *Observationes anatomicae* in 1561 (see No. 207). In it he pointed out certain errors of his teacher. Three days after receiving a copy of Fallopius' work, Vesalius began a letter to his devoted pupil, and it is that letter which prefaces this work of Vesalius in which he discusses the differences in their anatomical findings. Fallopius was never harshly critical of Vesalius and, indeed, was always most respectful in his corrections of the man whom he called "the prince of anatomists . . . and divine teacher." Vesalius' reply was written in kind: he acknowledges the preeminence of Fallopius as an anatomist, praises his discoveries, and defends or admits graciously his own errors and lapses. He says of Fallopius' work, "It might almost be called an appendix to my *De humani corporis fabrica*."

By the time Vesalius' reply was published, both he and Fallopius were dead. This first edition of his last work is very rare, few copies being known in the United States or abroad, and it almost never appears for sale.

Cushing V114; Cushing Vesalius IX.–1; Durling 4575; Wellcome 6564 (1609 ed.).

*184. ———. *The bloodletting letter of 1539, an annotated translation and study of the evolution of Vesalius's scientific development, by John B. de C. M. Saunders and Charles Donald O'Malley*. New York: Schuman [1947]. 94 pp., illus. 23.2 cm.

Vesalius wrote this letter to Nicolas Florenas, a friend and professor of medicine at Louvain, in response to Florenas' request for additional information concerning the marginal notes printed with the vena cava table of the *Tabulae anatomicae sex*. The particular note that interested Florenas was the one concerning the azygos vein and its relation to the question of bloodletting in cases of pleurisy. Vesalius responded by giving his views, methods, and treatment regimen and continued with a long discussion in answer to Florenas' query as to where and how one should draw blood from the hemorrhoidal vessels. Translated and heavily annotated by John B. de C. M. Saunders (b. 1903) and Charles O'Malley (1907–1970), this was the first time a complete work of Vesalius had appeared in English translation.

Waller 9927.

*185. KONRAD GESNER (1515–1565). *Der erste [-ander] Theil, dess köstlichen unnd theuren Schatzes Euonymi Philiatri, darinn behalten sind vil heimlicher guter Stuck der Artzney.* 2 vols. in 1. [Zurich: In Verlegung J. Gessners] 1583. Vol. I: [7 (lacking 1 preliminary leaf)] 368 [18] pp.; Vol. II: [8] 307 (misnumbered 305) [12] pp., illus. 19.4 cm. Vellum.

"A striking figure, typically Renaissance in his universality, was the Swiss Konrad Gesner, whose attainments in botany, zoology, medicine and surgery, philology and general scholarship brought him the name of the 'German Pliny'" (Arturo Castiglioni, *A history of medicine*. New York, 1946. p. 487). In addition, his *Bibliotheca universalis* in twenty volumes remained the best general bibliography until Albrecht von Haller's bibliographies appeared more than two hundred years later.

The present work, the first edition of which was published in Latin in 1552 under the pseudonym Euonymus Philiater, treats of chemistry and distilling processes for the purposes of medical treatment. It was a frequently published and frequently translated work. The woodcuts illustrating distilling apparatus are of special interest.

Wellcome 2789.

*186. ———. *Epistolarum medicinalium . . . libri III.* Zurich: Excudebat Christoph. Frosch., 1577. [8] 140 [28] *ll.*, illus. 20.3 cm. Modern quarter leather and marbled paper.

These 226 letters on a wide variety of medical topics, edited by Caspar Wolf (see No. 228), Gesner's literary executor, and published posthumously, indicate the wide interests and scientific insights of this great Renaissance scholar. The book contains two botanical tracts and three fine woodcuts of plants from Gesner's huge collection of drawings and woodcuts of plants which were to form the illustrative portion of his projected history of plants. Only a handful were published in the sixteenth century, and the plates passed from one botanist or publisher to another until, in the eighteenth century, they came into the hands of the botanist and bibliographer, Christopher Trew (1695–1769), who published them in *Opera botanica* (1754–1771), using such wood blocks as were still usable or having copperplates engraved from the drawings. The original drawings and blocks then were lost to view until 1929, when they were discovered in the attic of the library of the University of Erlangen. In 1973 appeared the first fascicule of a large project to publish the facsimile the corpus of the works of Gesner found at Erlangen.

Inscribed on the title page of this copy of the *Epistolarum* is the signature of

Johannes Gesner, eighteenth century descendant of Konrad and an important naturalist of his time.

Durling 2067; Osler 647; Waller 3521; Wellcome 2805.

———. *Enumeratio medicamentorum purgantium, vomitoriorum, & aluum bonam facientium.*

See No. 137.

*187. GIOVANNI BATTISTA CANANI (1515–1579). *Musculorum humani corporis picturata disectio (Ferrara 1541?). Facsimile edition, annotated by Harvey Cushing & Edward C. Streeter.* Florence: R. Lier, 1925. 98 pp., illus., facsims. 21 cm. A facsimile.

A native of Ferrara, Canani came from a distinguished medical family and developed into an anatomist at an early age. He was trained by Marcantonio della Torre, an associate of Leonardo da Vinci, and was Pope Julius III's personal physician until his death in 1555, after which he became chief physician at the University of Ferrara. He discovered the palmaris brevis muscle in the hand and was the first to describe the valves in the veins, a fact which he communicated to his contemporary, Vesalius.

In 1541, he published a small volume of twenty leaves on the muscles of the arm and forearm. This was to be the initial book of a seven-book series on the musculature of the bones that he planned to produce; however, it was the only book that was completed. It is thought that he felt his work was so overshadowed by Vesalius' *Fabrica* that he destroyed as many copies as he could recover. Nevertheless, as far as we know today, his illustrations are the first copperplate engravings to be used in medical illustration. Unfortunately, the engraver, Girolamo da Carpi (1501–1556), failed to solve many of the technical problems, and the plates leave much to be desired. Nonetheless, Canani's technique of picturing each muscle separately and showing its relationship to the bones was a new and unique approach to teaching anatomy. At the time this facsimile copy was printed, there were only eleven copies of the original known to be extant. This facsimile was made from Dr. Harvey Cushing's copy.

Choulant-Frank, pp. 150–151 (1541 ed.); Cushing C56; Garrison-Morton 373 (1541 ed.); Waller 1746.

*188. REALDO COLOMBO (1516?–1559). *De re anatomica libri XV.* Venice: Ex typographia Nicolai Beuilacquae, 1559. [8] 269 (misnumbered 169) pp. 33.3 cm. Contemporary vellum.

Colombo was a pupil of Vesalius at Padua and in 1544 succeeded him in the chair of anatomy, a position which he held for only a year before moving to Pisa and eventually to Rome, where he was professor of anatomy.

In this first edition of an important work in the history of anatomy, Colombo introduced a description of pulmonary circulation and denied that the blood went through the ventricular septum. He probably had no clear idea of the greater circulation, but this historic breakthrough in his demonstration of the lesser circulation through the lungs secures his place of importance in the line culminating in Harvey's demonstration of the circulation of the blood sixty-nine years later.

Colombo was particularly strong in regional anatomy, but the book is weakened by a total lack of illustration except for the very fine full-page woodcut on the title page depicting a dissecting scene.

Cushing C339; Durling 992; Osler 897; Waller 2076; Wellcome 1546.

*189. ———. ———. [2nd ed.]. Paris: In officina Joannis Foucherii, 1562. [8] 495 pp. 16.5 cm. Contemporary calf.

The second edition, following in Paris three years after the first edition, attests to the widespread contemporary use and recognized importance of Colombo's work.

Durling 993.

*190. ———. *De re anatomica libri XV. Hisce iam accesserunt Joannis Posthii. . . . Observationes anatomicae*. [4th ed.]. Frankfurt: Apud Joannem Wechelum, 1590. [8] 517 pp. 17.1 cm. Contemporary limp vellum.

This fourth edition has added to it the anatomical observations of Johannes Posthius (1537–1597) in an attempt to expand and update the work of Colombo.

Wellcome 1548 (incomplete).

191. GUGLIELMO GRATAROLI (1516–1568). *De literatorum & eorum qui magistratibus funguntur conservanda praeservandaque valetudine*. Basel: [Per Henrichum Petri, 1555]. 101 [3] pp. 16.2 cm. Limp vellum. Bound with No. 144.

Grataroli, a native of Bergamo, took his degree at Padua and later taught at Basel. He wrote one of the earliest histories of medicine and botany. The present work on hygiene is one of several works ranging widely over the fields of medicine, mnemonics, botany, and epidemiology.

Durling 2156; Waller 3709 (1562 ed.); Wellcome 2917.

192. LEONARDO FIORAVANTI (1517–1588). *Del compendio de' secreti rationali . . . libri cinque*. Venice: Appresso Marc' Antonio Bonibelli, 1597. [22] 187 [1] *ll.*, port. 14.7 cm. Vellum.

Fioravanti, a celebrated physician and alchemist of Bologna, was primarily a compiler of the opinions, techniques, "recipes," etc., of other physicians, and many of his works deal with the "secrets" and "mysteries" of medicine, alchemy, and the more esoteric and occult philosophies of his time. Still, enough of his medical and surgical work is of sufficient interest and importance to warrant his mention in the history of these subjects. In the cloudy picture, the question whether Vesalius, Berengario, Fallopius, and others may have performed human vivisection, the name of Fioravanti stands out sharply, since he calmly allowed that he had performed living dissection on a Saracen—his infidelity apparently being sufficient justification.

The present work is probably the sixth edition of a highly regarded handbook of medicine which contains five books devoted to various aspects of medicine, surgery, alchemy, and cosmetics. First published in 1564, this popular book remained in publication until the mid-seventeenth century.

Durling 1559 (1564 ed.); Wellcome 2293 (1566 ed.).

*193. ———. *La cirugia . . . distinta in tre libri*. Venice: Gli Heredi di Melchior Sessa, 1570. [24] 200 *ll.* 15.2 cm. Limp vellum.

Although sometimes accused of charlatanry, Fioravanti was actually a very observant and clever, though sometimes unorthodox, clinician. In this work he presents a collection of remarkable surgical cures brought about by means of his balsams, syrups, and other concoctions.

Durling 1556; Waller 3052 (1669 ed.); Wellcome 2302 (1582 ed.).

*194. ———. *Il tesoro della vita humana*. Venice: Appresso gli heredi di Melchior Sessa, 1570. 327 pp., port. 15.2 cm. Contemporary limp vellum.

This is the first known edition of the present work and is an important source for the early history of plastic surgery. The book is written mainly in the form of letters from Fioravanti to his colleagues; in one letter he describes a splenectomy performed by a stonecutter at Palermo in the spring of 1549.

Durling 1578; Waller 3051 (1582 ed.); Wellcome 2305 (1582 ed.).

*195. ANDREA CESALPINO (1519–1603). *Quaestionum peripateticarum lib. V*. 2nd ed. Venice: Apud Juntas, 1593. [20] 291 *ll.* 22.2 cm. Calf with marbled boards.

Cesalpino, a contemporary of Vesalius, was a noted botanist, physiologist, and philosopher of the Italian Renaissance. One of his teachers was Realdo Colombo (see No. 188), the anatomist who succeeded Vesalius at Padua. This important work, first published in 1571, shows that Cesalpino was aware that the blood circulated, but his discussions were largely philosophical in nature and were not readily accepted by the medical community. Although William Harvey was undoubtedly familiar with Cesalpino's work, it is not known with certainty what influence Cesalpino had on Harvey's experiments.

Cushing C155; Durling 925; Garrison-Morton 756; Osler 901; Waller 1878; Wellcome 1182.

GIOVANNI MARINELLI (fl. 1560). *Le medicine partenenti alle infermità delle donne*.

See No. 234.

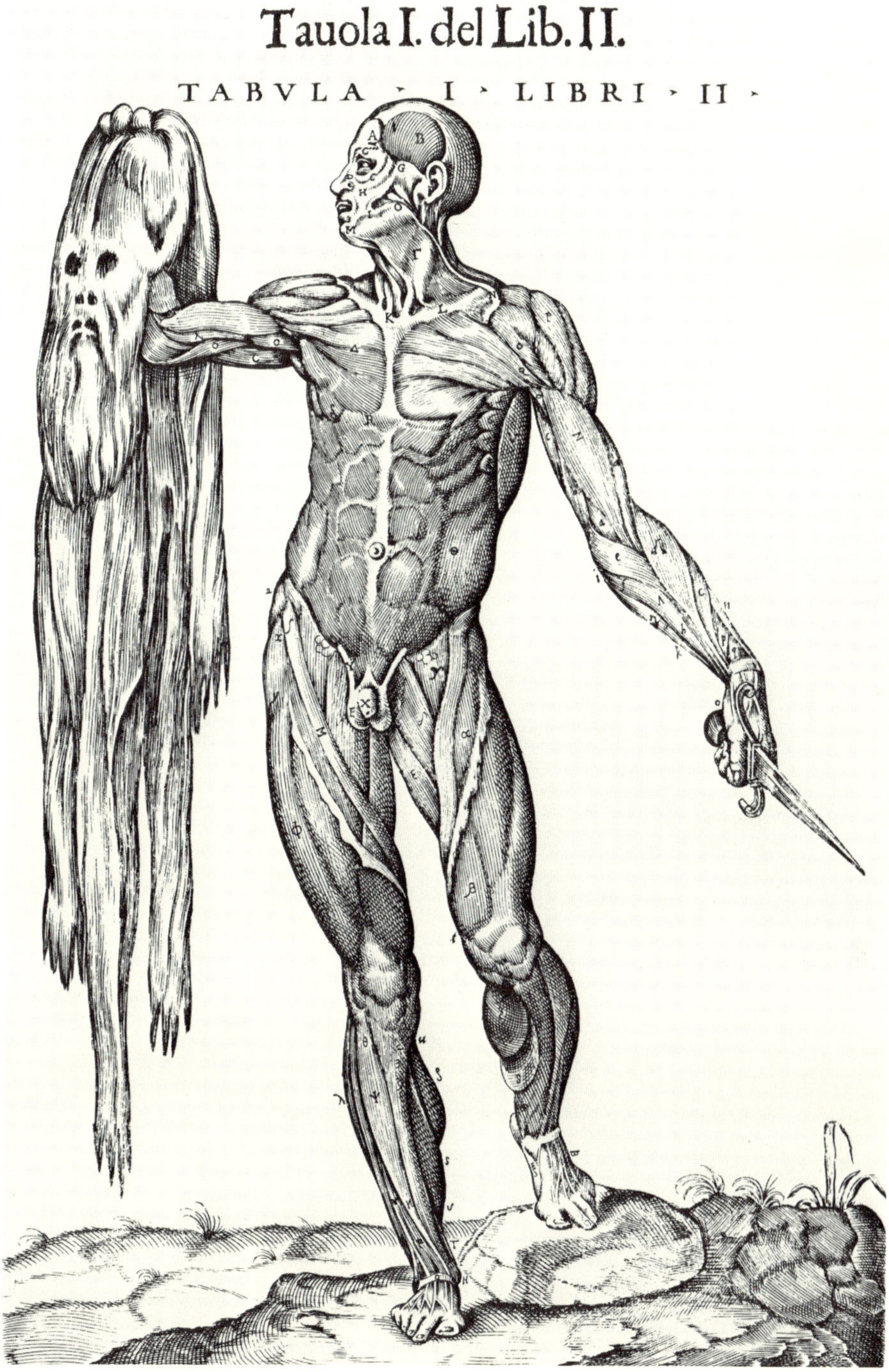

No. 196. Valverde. *La Anatomia del Corpo Umano.* One of many dramatic figures, this muscleman is holding his own skin.

*196. JUAN DE VALVERDE (fl. 1560). *Vivae imagines partium corporis humani, aereis formis expressae*. Antwerp: Ex officina Christophori Plantini, 1572. 171 (misnumbered 172) [4] pp., 42 plates. 27.9 cm. Vellum.

Valverde studied at Padua as a pupil of Realdo Colombo (see No. 188) and became the leading Spanish anatomist of his time. His anatomical atlas was first published in 1556 in Spanish and was widely used, reprinted, and translated for the next hundred years. "Nearly all the plates are copied from Vesalius and Valverde's text is plagiarized from the *Fabrica*" (Osler 576). Even so, the plates have some distinctive features of their own and the engraved title page depicting Adam and Eve on either side of the imprint is attractive. This Latin edition, with the forty-two plates, was published by the Plantin press and is unusual in that, although the title page dates it as 1572, the colophon indicates 1579.

Cushing Vesalius VI.D.–45; Durling 4536; Waller 9808; Wellcome 6481.

*197. ———. *La anatomia del corpo umano*. Venice: Nella stamperia de Giunti, 1586. [18] 82 [4] 83–154 *ll.*, illus., 46 plates, port. 30.2 cm. Limp vellum, in slipcase.

This Italian edition of Valverde's anatomical work contains, for the first time, four additional plates of "muscle men."

Choulant-Frank, p. 206; Cushing V16; Cushing Vesalius VI.D.–37; Durling 4533; Osler 576; Waller 9806; Wellcome 6478.

198. ———. *Anatomia del corpo humano*. Venice: Nella stamperia de Giunti, 1608 (colophon dated 1606). [18] 154 *ll.*, plates, port. 28.9 cm.

Another of the many editions and reprints of Valverde's anatomy, this one is nearly identical to the 1606 edition with the exception of the 1608 date on the title page. Although many of the plates have been reversed and re-engraved, the setting of type is unchanged.

Cushing V20; Cushing Vesalius VI.D.–40; Osler 576 (1586 ed.); Waller 9806 (1586 ed.).

*199. BARTOLOMEO EUSTACHI (1520?–1574). *Opuscula anatomica*. Venice: Vincentius Luchinus excudebat, 1564. [12] 323 [7] 95 [204] pp., 8 plates. 19.4 cm. Early nineteenth century quarter morocco, in quarter morocco box.

At first a Galenist in his teaching in Rome but later an adherent to the "new school," Eustachi was the first to describe the Eustachian tube, the adrenal glands, the thoracic duct, and many of the finer structures of the teeth.

This rare volume is the first compilation of his works on the teeth, kidney, ear, and venous system. Eustachi was among the first to study the teeth in any detail, and his treatise contains an early description of the first and second dentitions as well as the tooth's basic composition of enamel and dentin. He also attempted to explain why the tooth was sensitive to various stimuli. His treatise on the kidney shows that he possessed knowledge of the organ that surpassed that of his prede-

TABULÆ ANATOMICÆ

CLARISSIMI VIRI

BARTHOLOMÆI EUSTACHII

Quas è tenebris tandem vindicatas

ET

Sanctissimi Domini

CLEMENTIS XI.

PONT. MAX.

Munificentiâ dono acceptas

Præfatione, Notisque illustravit, ac ipso suæ Bibliothecæ dedicationis die publici juris fecit

JO. MARIA LANCISIUS

Intimus Cubicularius, & Archiater Pontificius.

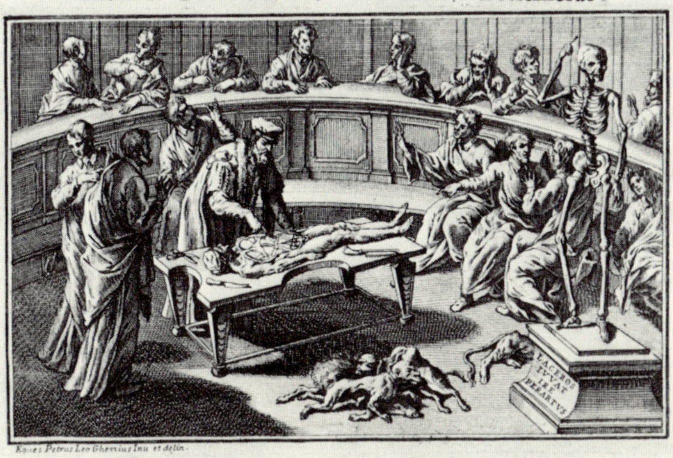

ROMÆ MDCCXIV.

Ex Officina Typographica FRANCISCI GONZAGÆ in Via lata.

PRÆSIDUM PERMISSU.

No. 201. Eustachi. *Tabulae Anatomicae.*

cessors, and it also contains the first account of the adrenal gland. His work on the ear includes descriptions of the tube that bears his name as well as the tensor tympani and stapedius muscles. In his treatise dealing with the venous system, he described the thoracic duct and the Eustachian valve—the valvula venae cavae inferioris in the right ventricle of the heart. The eight plates mentioned in No. 201 were first published in this work.

Choulant-Frank, p. 200; Cushing E111; Durling 1408; Garrison-Morton 801, 1093, 1139, 1228, 1538, 3668; Wellcome 2091.

*200. ———. ———. Delphis: Apud Adrianum Beman, 1726. [12] 358 [6] 98 [11] 47 pp., 10 plates (2 fold.). 18.1 cm. Half vellum.

This edition of *Opuscula anatomica*, containing Eustachi's four major treatises on the teeth, kidney, ear, and venous system, is a reprint of the second edition which was published at Leiden in 1707. Like the second edition, it contains an introduction by Hermann Boerhaave and ten anatomical plates.

Choulant-Frank, p. 200.

*201. ———. *Tabulae anatomicae . . . quas è tenebris tandem vindicitas . . . praefatione, notisque illustravit . . . Jo. Maria Lancisius*. Rome: Ex officina typographica Francisci Gonzagae, 1714. xliv, 115 [13] pp., 47 plates. 34.9 cm. Vellum, in slipcase.

With the intention of publishing an anatomical text, Eustachi had completed the drawings for his work and the plates had been engraved by 1552. The text, however, was never completed and Eustachi's notes to the plates were lost except for the eight which had been published in his lifetime. The plates were inherited by Eustachi's assistant and were eventually deposited in the Vatican Library, where they were uncovered a century and a half later and published by the papal physician, Giovanni Maria Lancisi (see No. 445), who added his elucidations and included the previously published eight plates with Eustachi's commentary. In all, there are forty-seven plates. Although from an artistic standpoint they are not as well done as the anatomical plates of Vesalius, from the point of view of anatomy they are sometimes more accurate than Vesalius'. Had the plates been published at the time they were executed, Eustachi would undoubtedly have ranked with Vesalius as a founder of modern anatomical studies. Indeed, the title page vignette illustrating a dissection, the forty-seven plates themselves, and the large initial capital letters decorated with pastoral and hunting scenes make his a splendid anatomical atlas, with few peers and fewer superiors.

Choulant-Frank, p. 202; Cushing E113; Garrison-Morton 391; Osler 2543; Wellcome II, p. 536.

*202. ———. ———. Geneva: Sumptibus Cramer & Perachon, 1717. [12] xvi, 34 [9] pp., 21 plates. 41.9 cm. Quarter calf and marbled boards.

This is a separate publication of the edition of the *Tabulae anatomicae* which had appeared as a major appendix to Manget's *Theatrum anatomicum* (see No. 443) in

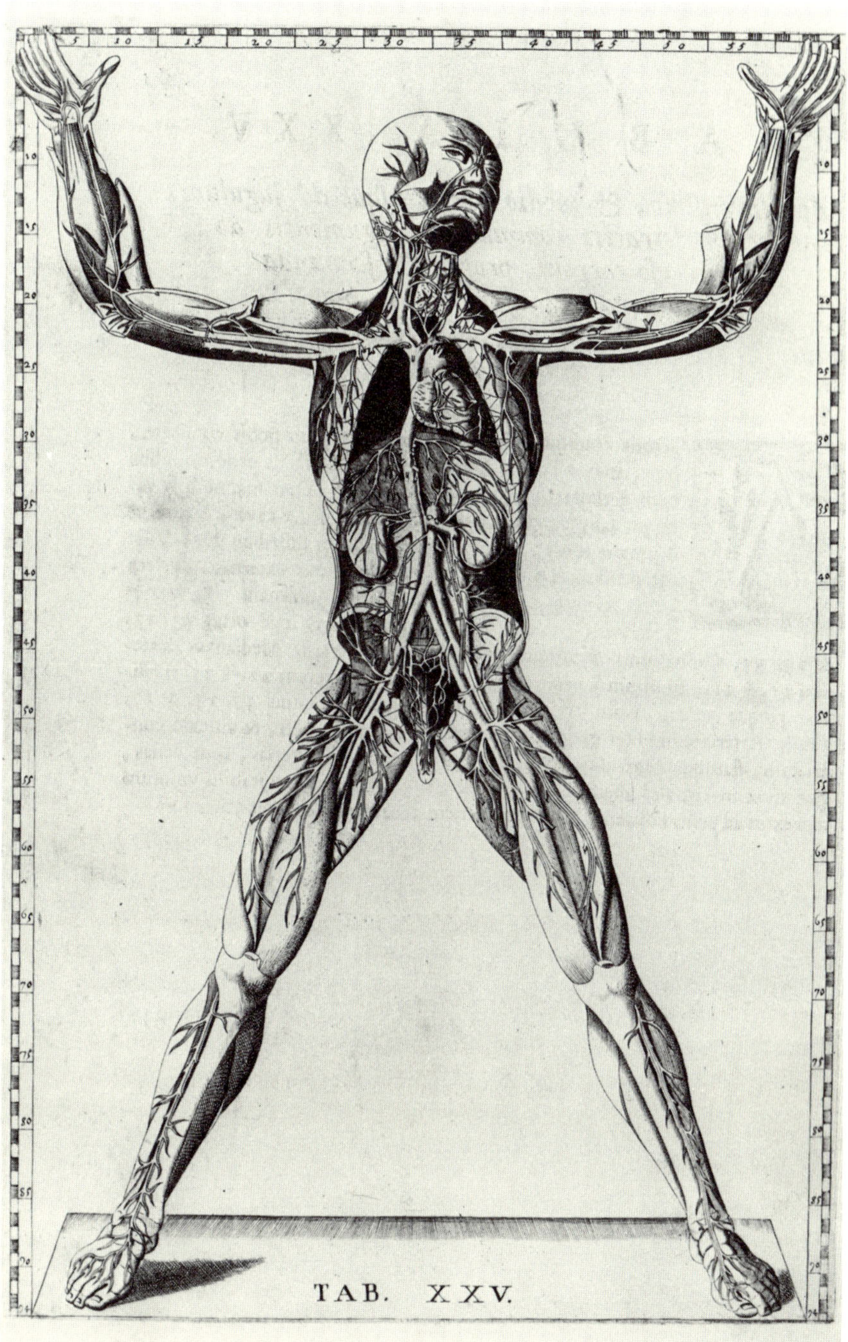

No. 201. Eustachi. *Tabulae Anatomicae.* A composite figure from several dissections.

the same year, the sole difference being the addition of a portrait of Lancisi as a frontispiece. The original plates of the 1714 edition have been re-engraved and slightly reduced, and instead of one figure per plate there are now usually as many as can be crowded in, so that the original forty-seven plates have now been reduced in number to twenty-one.

*203. ———. *Bernardi Siegfried Albini . . . explicatio tabularum anatomicarum*. Leiden: Apud Joannem Arnoldum Langerak, et Joannem & Hermannum Verbeek, 1744. [6] 28, 275 (misnumbered 277) [3] pp., 89 plates. 39.4 cm.

Albinus (see No. 525) not only produced his own outstanding anatomical atlas but, with Boerhaave, he produced an excellent edition of Vesalius (see No. 176) and this edition of Eustachi. The plates are newly engraved by the artist Wandelaer and nearly all are accompanied by outline drawings, making a total of eighty-nine full-page plates. Albinus has added his own extensive descriptions and commentaries.

Choulant-Frank, p. 202; Waller 337 (incomplete).

204. ———. ———. Venice: Typis Bartholomei Locatelli, 1769. [12] xvi, 34 [9] pp., 21 plates. 46.7 cm. Half vellum, uncut.

A reissue of the earlier Roman edition. The title page vignette has been recut and is almost totally without the distinction of the original.

Choulant-Frank, p. 204; Osler 2544; Wellcome II, p. 536.

*205. PIETER VAN FOREEST (1522–1597). *Observationum et curationum medicinalium libri tres*. Leiden: Ex officina Plantiniana, Apud Franciscum Raphelengium, 1590. [24] 90 [6] 323 [21] 919 [7] pp. 16 cm. Contemporary blind-stamped vellum.

Foreest was a Dutch clinician who practiced for many years in Alkmaar and later at Delft. He studied medicine in Italy and was a pupil and colleague of Vesalius. His wide-ranging interests included botany, and he brought a large number of medicinal plants with him when he returned to Holland. He was a prolific writer and began publishing his *Observationes et curationes* series in 1588. At the time of his death, this comprehensive series on diseases numbered thirty-two books. It was his practice to issue three or four books at a time, and the first seven books had already been published before this work, containing the eighth through tenth books, appeared. This work is primarily devoted to diseases of the head, and, in all probability, is the first edition. The tenth book contains a rare consilium (letter of consultation) from Vesalius to Foreest concerning a serious case of nosebleed in a young man. Only six of the many consilia that Vesalius undoubtedly wrote have survived.

Cushing Vesalius VIII.D.–1; Durling 1612; Waller 3125 (1660 ed.); Wellcome 2360 (incomplete).

*206. ULISSE ALDROVANDI (1522–1605). *Monstrorum historia*. 2 vols. in 1. Bologna: Typis Nicolai Tebaldini, 1642–1657 (colophon dated 1658). Vol. I: [8] 748 [28] pp.; Vol. II: 159 [7] pp., illus. 35.4 cm. Half calf with vellum sides.

Aldrovandi and Konrad Gesner (see No. 186) were the most important zoologists of the sixteenth century. Aldrovandi, a native of Bologna, first studied law but eventually changed his field to medicine. Accused of Lutheranism in 1549, he was sent to Rome for trial but was later released by the Inquisition. He returned to Bologna where he studied botany and became professor of natural history and philosophy at the University in 1560. He was successful in persuading the University to start a botanical garden and became its first director. He also established a museum of natural history at Bologna which is still in existence.

He was the author of an enormous thirteen-volume encyclopedia of biology of which only four volumes appeared during his lifetime. The remaining volumes were prepared from his manuscripts by his pupils and published by the university senate. He invested much of his own money in the project and employed many artists and engravers during the thirty years that he worked on it. This work on the history of monsters was part of the encyclopedia and is an exhaustive treatise on the deformities of humans, animals, fishes, insects, and plants. There are several hundred excellent woodcuts in the book and, like a number of other works of the period, many depict abnormalities that are not consistent with the facts.

Osler 1769; Waller 10725; Wellcome 172.

*207. GABRIEL FALLOPIUS (1523–1562). *Observationes anatomicae*. Venice: Apud Marcum Antonium Ulmum, 1561. [8] 222 [1] *ll.* 15.4 cm. Limp vellum.

Though a pupil, friend, local supporter, and successor to Vesalius in the chair of anatomy at Padua, Fallopius did have the temerity to point out, in this modest text on anatomy, some errors in the *Fabrica*. This occasioned Vesalius' answer in the *Anatomicarum Gabrielis Falloppii observationum examen* (1564) (see No. 183).

Fallopius was a poor man and published this book at his own expense. Even a more ardent anti-Galenist than Vesalius, he corrected Vesalius on the course of certain cerebral arteries, described the clitoris and the arteria profunda of the penis, first fully examined the Fallopian tubes, and gave a clear account of the ocular muscles and cranial nerves. *Observationes* was Fallopius' most important work and the only one published in his lifetime. There are no illustrations in the book.

Cushing F27; Durling 1440; Garrison-Morton 1208; Osler 593; Waller 2935; Wellcome 2147 (1562 ed.).

*208. ———. ———. Paris: Apud Bernardum Turrisanum, 1562. 133 *ll.* 16.2 cm.

This Paris edition quickly followed the first and second editions published in Venice in 1561 and 1562 respectively.

Cushing F27 (1st ed., 1561); Durling 1442; Garrison-Morton 1208 (1st ed.); Osler 594; Waller 2935 (1st ed.); Wellcome 2147.

GABRIELIS FALLOPPII
MEDICI MVTINENSIS
OBSERVATIONES
Anatomicæ.

AD PETRVM MANNAM
medicum Cremonensem.

Cum Priuilegio Summi Pontificis, Regis Philippi, Senatusque Veneti.

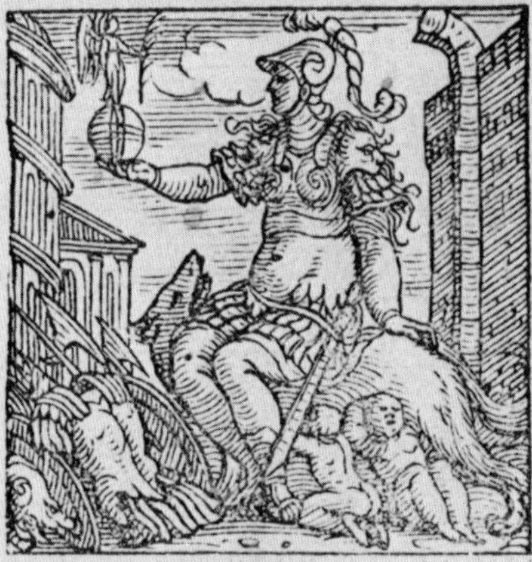

VENETIIS.
Apud Marcum Antonium Vlmum
M D LXI.

No. 207. Fallopius. *Observationes Anatomicae.* This title page vignette is the book's only illustration.

*209. ———. *Libelli duo, alter de ulceribus: alter de tumoribus praeter naturam*. Venice: Apud Donatum Bertellum, 1563. [3] 1, 101 [1] *ll*. 21 cm. Vellum.

Fallopius was a clinician as well as an anatomist, and this treatise on diseases of the skin (ulcers and tumors) is one of the most complete of its kind up to the time of its publication.

An interesting bibliographical point in this copy is the canceling of leaf 1 with a substitute leaf, but the cancelland was not removed, thus leaving both the original leaf and its substitute in place.

Cushing F25; Durling 1438; Waller 2934; Wellcome 2156 (1566 ed.).

*210. ———. *De morbo Galllico* [sic]. . . . *Additus etiam est in calce De morbo Gallico tractatus, Antonii Fracanciani*. Padua: Apud Lucam Bertellum & socios, 1563 (colophon dated 1564). [4] 64, 16 [2] *ll*. 20.3 cm. Bound in a portion of a vellum manuscript leaf.

In this classic work on "the French disease," Fallopius wrote more knowingly of the Europe-wide scourge of syphilis than previous authors on the subject and was one of the first to oppose the use of mercury in its treatment.

Antonio Fracanzano (d. 1567), a teacher of Fallopius at Padua and later his colleague there, contributed a short tract to this work on syphilis published in the year after Fallopius' death.

Durling 1433 (1564 ed.); Garrison-Morton 2370; Waller 2928; Wellcome 2152.

*211. ———. ———. Padua: Apud Lucam Bertellum & socios, 1564. [4] 64, 16 [2] *ll*. 18.7 cm. Vellum.

This slightly variant issue of No. 210 differs from it only in a resetting of the date on the title page. Interestingly, the work by Fallopius has its own colophon dated 1564 and the work by Fracanzano has its own title page dated 1563, although the colophon is dated 1564. Even in resetting the date on the title page, the printer failed to drop the extraneous *l* from *Galllico*.

Fallopius: Durling 1433.
Fracanzano: Durling 1628.

*212. ———. *Opera quae adhuc extant omnia*. Frankfurt: Apud haeredes Andreae Wecheli, 1584. [12] 848 [32] pp. 32.3 cm. Contemporary blind-stamped pigskin.

Many of Fallopius' writings which were no longer available in original or single editions in the late sixteenth century were preserved in this first edition of his collected works. Included here are his treatises on tumors, ulcers, syphilis, and *Observationes anatomicae* from which so many common anatomical terms have been derived. Also among the contents of this volume are commentaries on Galen and Hippocrates, discussions of metals and fossils, notes on pharmacology, and letters to contemporaries.

Durling 1426; Waller 2937.

*213. FRANCISCO DE VALLES (1524–1592). *Controversiarum medicarum et philosophicarum*. Frankfurt: Apud heredes Andreae Wecheli, Claudium Marnium & Joann. Aubrium, 1590. [8] 452 [10] pp. 32.8 cm. Stamped pigskin.

Valles, a native of Covarrubias, Spain, studied medicine at Alcalá de Henares and eventually became a professor on the faculty. He also served as chief physician in the court of the Spanish monarch, King Philip II. This third edition of his text on general medicine covers a variety of subjects and relies heavily upon references and quotations from Galen, Aristotle, Hippocrates, Avicenna, and other early medical authorities. Works such as this continued the long dependence on Galen and his predecessors and contained little original thought or new knowledge.

Durling 4513; Waller 9786 (1606 ed.); Wellcome 6462.

214. ARCANGELO PICCOLOMINI (1525–1586). *In librum Galeni de humoribus, comemtarii* [sic]. Paris: Apud Bernardum Turrisianum, in Aldina biblioteca, 1556. 170 *ll.* 18.1 cm. Vellum.

Piccolomini was primarily an anatomist of Verona. This work, an extensive exposition of, and commentary on, the natural humors of the body as expounded by Galen, is the sort of work which sustained for so long a belief in Galen's anatomy and physiology. The Greek and Latin texts of Galen are followed by the commentary in Latin.

Durling 3624; Waller 7433; Wellcome 5006.

*215. FRANCISCO BRAVO (ca. 1525–ca. 1595). *The opera medicinalia.* [1st ed. reprinted]. With a biographical and bibliographical introduction by Francisco Guerra. 2 vols. Folkestone: Dawsons, 1970. Vol. I: [6] 77 pp., 9 plates; Vol. II: 610 pp., illus., facsims. 16.4 cm. Imitation vellum, in slipcase. A facsimile: No. 108 of 250 copies.

Bravo was born at Osuna, in southern Spain, and received his medical education at the University in the early 1550's. He began to practice medicine in Seville shortly thereafter and came to New Spain sometime in the 1560's where he established a practice in Mexico City. The *Opera medicinalia* was published in Mexico City in 1570, and, as far as is known, is the first medical book to have been published in the New World. The book shows that he possessed great learning and sound judgment and contains many clinical descriptions and medical doctrines on venesection, materia medica, and diet as well as the first description of typhus to appear in the western hemisphere. Only three copies of the original volume are known to exist. This facsimile was made from the 1570 edition of the *Opera*.

216. LUIS DE MERCADO (1525?–1606). *De pulsibus libri duo*. Padua: Apud Paulum Meiettum, 1592. [10] 184 *ll.* 19.7 cm. Vellum.

Mercado was one of the best-known physicians of the sixteenth century, professor of medicine at Valladolid, and physician to Kings Philip II and Philip III. He is best known for his extensive treatise on gynecology and obstetrics. In the present work he shows the pulse, in its variety of forms, to be indicative of many conditions of health and disease.

Durling 3077.

217. LUIGI LUISINI (b. 1526). *Aphrodisiacus; sive, De lue venerea.* 2 vols. in 1. Venice: Apud Baretium Baretium & Socios, 1599. Vol. I: [4] 736 [28] pp.; Vol. II: [24] 196, 216 [2] 96 [6] pp. 29.5 cm.

Luisini, the compiler of this important collection of works on venereal diseases, was born in Udine and practiced medicine in Venice. He first published the anthology in 1566, followed by this edition in 1599. The work contains the writings of such notable men as Fallopius, Fracastoro, Leoniceno, Massa, Hutten, Montanus, Vesalius, and many others through the early sixteenth century. Boerhaave published a revision of this work in 1728, updating it to the mid-1500's.

Cushing L379 (1728 ed.); Durling 1108 (1st ed., 1566); Garrison-Morton 2372 (1st ed.); Waller 6099 (1728 ed.); Wellcome 3892 (1st ed.).

*218. HENRI ESTIENNE, compiler (1528–1598). *Medicae artis principes, post Hippocratem & Galenum.* 5 pts. in 1 vol. [Geneva]: Excudebat Henricus Stephanus, 1567. Part I: [8] pp., 346 columns [8] pp.; Part II: [5] pp., 347–692 (misnumbered 700) columns, 701–[743] (misnumbered 751) columns, 752–760 (misnumbered 768) columns; Part III: 696 (misnumbered 697) columns; Part IV: [4] pp., 866, 856 (misnumbered 846) columns; Part V: 434 columns [107] pp., illus. 34.9 cm. Modern boards.

Henri Estienne, the printer and publisher, brought together in this huge volume of nearly two thousand pages many of the Greek, Roman, and medieval medical writers exclusive of Hippocrates and Galen, from Celsus in the first century to Nicolaus Myrepsus in the thirteenth century. Included are such writers as Scribonius Largus, Rufus of Ephesus, Alexander Trallianus, Paulus Aegineta, Oribasius (with a number of woodcut illustrations), Theophilus, and others. This is one of the earliest compilations of medical works and was much used in its day.

Cushing M257; Durling 3049; Garrison-Morton 55; Waller 6417; Wellcome 4177.

*219. ———. ———. 5 pts. in 2 vols. [Geneva]: Excudebat Henricus Stephanus, 1567. Vol. I: Part I: [8] pp., 346 columns [8] pp.; Part II: [5] pp., 347–692 (misnumbered 700) columns, 701–[743] (misnumbered 751) pp., 752–760 (misnumbered 768) columns; Part III: 696 (misnumbered 697) columns; Vol. II: Part IV: [4] pp., 866, 856 (misnumbered 846) columns; Part V:434 columns [107] pp., illus. 34.8 cm.

Another copy of this widely circulated and much-used compilation of medical works. The writings of many of the authors who are included in this voluminous work were not easily available from any other source at that time.

Cushing M257; Durling 3049; Garrison-Morton 55; Waller 6417; Wellcome 4177.

*220. LAURENT JOUBERT (1529–1583). *Annotations . . . sur toute la chirurgie de M. Guy de Chauliac*. Rouen: Chez Romain de Beauvais, 1615. 32, 403 [11] pp. (Lacking first and last leaves, replaced in manuscript), illus., front. (port.). 16.2 cm. Bound with No. 62.

Annotations on Guy de Chauliac's *La grande chirurgie* in Joubert's edition of 1615, with which it is bound.

Waller 5202; Wellcome II, p. 367 (1641 ed.).

*221. LEONARDO BOTALLO (1530–1590). *De curatione per sanguinis missionem. De incidendae venae, cutis scarificandae, & amplicandarum* [sic] *modo*. Lyons: Apud Joan. Huguetan, 1580. [10] 212 [4] pp., illus. 16.3 cm.

Botallo, a native of Asti in northwestern Italy, studied medicine under Gabriel Fallopius (see No. 207) and Vittore Trincavelli (1496–1548) and graduated from Pavia. He achieved great repute as an anatomist and has long been known for his description of the ductus arteriosus or duct of Botallo. Exactly how his name became associated with the duct is not known, though it was not by the discovery of the duct because its existence was known in Galen's time. In his treatise on gunshot wounds, he advocated a milder treatment than currently in vogue and gave one of the first descriptions of hay fever in his *De catarrho commentarius*, 1564.

This small work on bloodletting is primarily an instruction manual and also discusses the therapeutic results that can be expected. Botallo, like many of his contemporaries, was an enthusiastic advocate of frequent and copious bloodletting. The two illustrations in this work are of instruments used in scarification preparatory to actual bloodletting.

Cushing B525 (1577 ed.); Durling 651; Waller 1332 (1577 ed.); Wellcome 1001 (1577 ed.).

*222. ———. *Opera omnia medica & chirurgica*. Leiden: Ex officina Danielis & Abrahami à Gaasbeeck, 1660. [16] 800 [24] pp., 4 fold. plates. 15.1 cm. Contemporary vellum.

Joannes van Horne (see No. 342) has here edited Botallo's collected works. In this book will be found Botallo's descriptions of the ductus arteriosus, ligamentum arteriosum, and foramen ovale as well as plates illustrating them. Also included are his works on anatomy, gunshot wounds, hay fever, syphilis, and bloodletting. This book was once in the collection of Johann Friedrich Blumenbach (see No. 692).

Garrison-Morton 802.1; Waller 1335; Wellcome II, p. 209.

223. GIROLAMO MERCURIALE (1530–1606). *De arte gymnastica libri sex*. 3rd ed. Venice: Apud Juntas, 1587. 3, 308 [27] pp., illus. 23.6 cm. Limp vellum.

Mercuriale, professor of medicine at Bologna and Pisa, is probably best known to modern students of medical history for the present work, first published in 1569. It was the first complete text on gymnastics and stresses the importance that all forms of exercise have in maintaining good health. Relying heavily on ancient practices, this work is an excellent compendium of the physical therapy of earlier times. Mercuriale describes ancient gymnasia and baths and discusses mild exercises such as dancing as well as more strenuous pursuits such as wrestling and boxing. He also gives full consideration to the health benefits of proper exercise and concludes the book with a section of therapeutic exercises. The book contains many excellent woodblock illustrations of wrestling, boxing, and other sports.

Durling 3090; Garrison-Morton 1986.1 (1st ed., 1569); Osler 3387 (1st ed.); Waller 6480 (1601 ed.); Wellcome 4226.

224. ———. *Variarum lectionum, in medicinae scriptoribus & aliis, libri sex*. Venice: Apud Juntas, 1588. [8] 135 [16] *ll*. 22.9 cm. Quarter vellum.

A critical analysis and commentary on many passages of classical and later authors: Celsus, Plutarch, Galen, Hippocrates, Paracelsus, and others. First published in 1585.

Durling 3114; Osler 3389 (1st ed., 1585); Waller 6493 (1598 ed.).

*225. ———. *De decoratione*. Venice: Apud Paulum Meietum, 1585. [10] 38 *ll*. 23.5 cm. Modern calf with blind-stamped and gilt panel design.

The present work was originally published in 1572 and also appeared as the second part of the author's work on diseases of the skin, *De morbis cutaneis*, in the same year. *De decoratione* inspired the famed Gaspare Tagliacozzi to publish, in 1597, his own classic work on plastic surgery (see No. 236).

Durling 3093 (1587 ed.); Osler 3390; Waller 6481 (1601 ed.); Wellcome 4243 (1587 ed.).

*226. ———. *De morbis puerorum tractatus*. Venice: Apud Paulum Meietum, 1588. [16] 107 *ll*. 20.7 cm.

The present work, first published in 1583, was one of the first books devoted entirely to pediatrics. The dedication indicates that the book is based on the lecture notes of one of Mercuriale's students, Jan Hieronim Chrosciejowski (fl. 1583–1612), also known as Johannes Groscesius. The work is divided into three parts: diseases of children, fevers of children, and worms. Although the book is filled with references to Arabian, Greek, and Roman authors, Mercuriale used his own judgment in interpreting their observations instead of slavishly adhering to their opinions as was common with many writers of the fifteenth and sixteenth centuries.

Durling 3102; Waller 6483 (1583 ed.); Wellcome 4241.

*227. ———. *Praelectiones . . . in Epidemicas Hippocratis historias*. Venice: Apud Juntas, 1597. [xvi] 208, 56 [2] *ll*. 31.4 cm.

This work, a collection of lectures given by Mercuriale at the University of Pisa, is largely devoted to a history of epidemics based on the writings of Hippocrates. It also contains Mercuriale's remarks on the plague as well as three shorter lectures on conception, the baths and mineral waters of Pisa, and the various qualities of wine and water.

Durling 3107; Wellcome 4249.

*228. CASPAR WOLF, compiler (1532–1601). *Gynaeciorum, hoc est, de mulierum tum aliis, tum gravidarum, parientium & puerperarum affectibus & morbis*. Basel: Per Thomam Guarinum, 1566. [20] pp., 868 [42] columns, [8] 63 pp., illus. 21.4 cm.

During the Renaissance there was a great upsurge of interest in the diseases of women, and it was during this period that this first encyclopedia of gynecology was published. Konrad Gesner (see No. 186) assembled a collection of the most important works on the diseases of women and was planning to publish them in a single volume but died before the work could be finished. However, he had asked Wolf, his friend and successor at the University of Zurich, to complete the task. Wolf finished the volume, which turned out to be a compendium on both gynecology and obstetrics. In addition to his own essay on gynecology, which contained excerpts from Theodorus Priscianus, Cleopatra, Moschion, and other sources, Wolf also included the following: excerpts from the works of Abulcasis; a book on diseases of women by Trotula (fl. 1050); a treatise by Nicolas de La Roche (fl. 1542), a French physician; a book on conception, miscarriage, delivery, infant care, and related subjects by Luigi Bonacciuoli (see No. 239); a treatise on menstruation and diseases of women by Jacques Dubois (Sylvius); and Gesner's and Wolf's own verion of Moschion. Caspar Bauhin (see No. 246) revised this work in 1586 and Israel Spach edited a third and final edition in 1597 (see No. 245).

Cushing G501 (1586 ed., incomplete); Durling 2252; Garrison-Morton 6011; Waller 3897; Wellcome 3033.

*229. HIERONYMUS FABRICIUS ab Aquapendente (ca. 1533–1619). *De visione, voce, auditu*. 3 pts. in 1 vol. Venice: Per Franciscum Bolzettam, 1600. Part I: [12] 133 pp.; Part II: [14] 83 pp.; Part III: [8] 38 pp., illus. 36.3 cm. Contemporary vellum.

One of the great Paduan anatomists and teachers, pupil of Fallopius, teacher of Harvey, and friend of Galileo, Fabricius built at his own expense the anatomical theater at Padua, which is still preserved intact. During his long life, he produced a number of important works on anatomy, embryology, and physiology, characterized by numerous large, clear copperplate illustrations which long remained unexcelled.

The major portion of this work on the organs of vision, speech, and hearing is devoted to the eye, and it is clear that Fabricius was one of the first to grasp the true form and proper location of the lens. Although his description of the ear is sound, it contributed no new knowledge about the ear or the sense of hearing. An extremely competent comparative anatomist, he was at his best in dealing with the laryngeal apparatus.

Cushing F7; Durling 1415; Osler 2558; Waller 2888; Wellcome 2118.

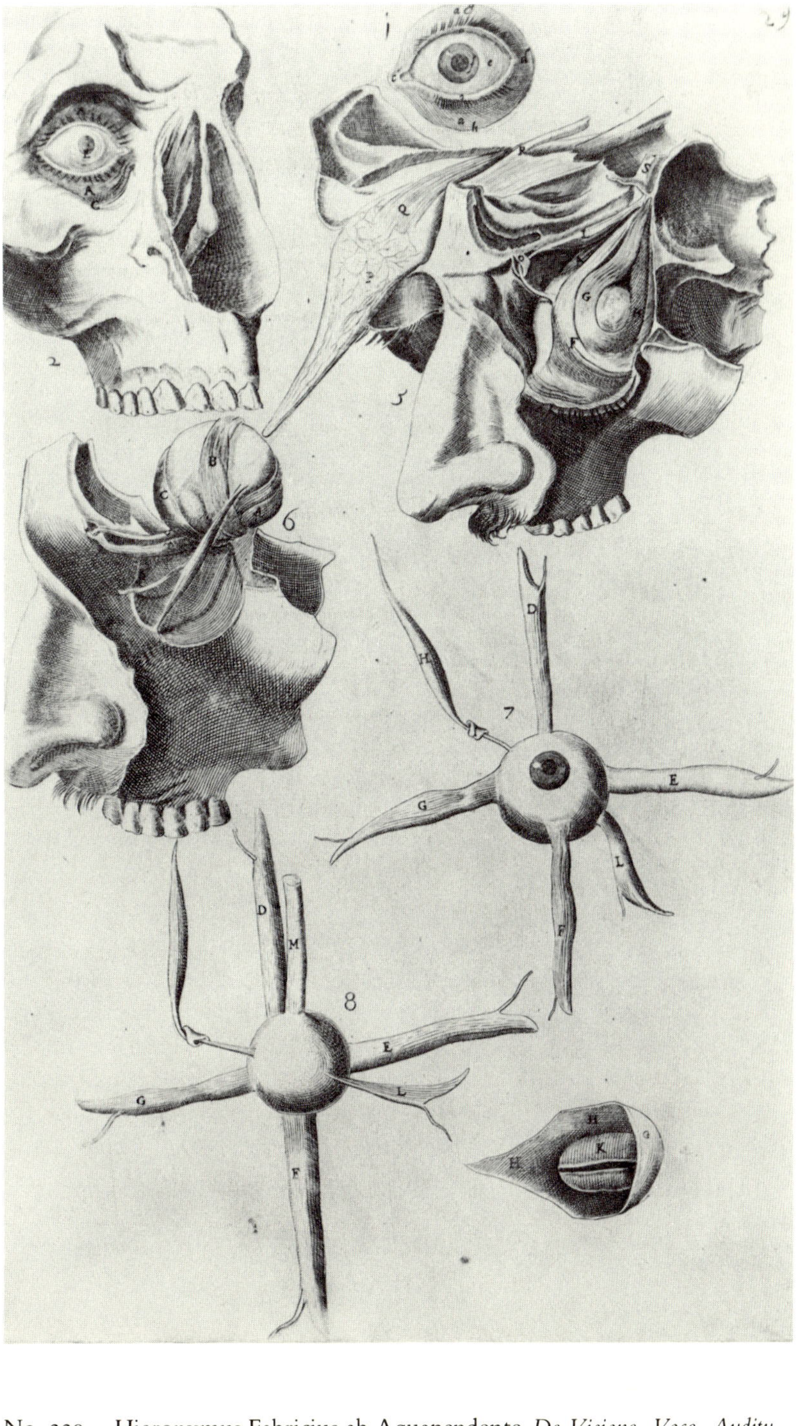

No. 229. Hieronymus Fabricius ab Aquapendente. *De Visione, Voce, Auditu.*

*230. ———. *Opera chirurgica.* 2 pts. in 1 vol. Padua: Apud Franciscum Bolzettam, 1641. Part I: [26] 204 pp.; Part II: [15] 187 pp., 2 plates. 30.8 cm. Old paper over boards, vellum back.

The first edition of this textbook of surgery was published in 1617 and described techniques entirely new for that age. It was reprinted many times, even into the eighteenth century.

Cushing F9 (1647 ed.); Waller 2890 (1647 ed.); Wellcome III, p. 4.

*231. ———. *Opera omnia anatomica et physiologica . . . cum praefatione Bernardi Siegfried Albini.* Leiden: Apud Johannem van Kerckhem, 1738. [50] 452 [22] pp., front. (port.), plates (part fold.), diagrs. 33 cm. Quarter vellum, uncut.

This eighteenth-century volume of collected works of Fabricius, with an introduction by Bernhard Siegfried Albinus (see No. 525), contains a large number of beautiful plates. The plates of the arm veins in Harvey's *De motu cordis* (see No. 256) were apparently redrawn from the original of that shown on page 154 of this work by Fabricius, who was Harvey's teacher at Padua.

Osler 2557 (1687 ed.); Waller 2891 (1687 ed.); Wellcome III, p. 4 (1687 ed.).

VOLCHER COITER (1534–1576). *Tractatus anatomicus, de ossibus foetus abortivi, et infantis, dimidium annum nati.*

See No. 336.

*232. GIOVANNI BATTISTA DELLA PORTA (1535?–1615). *De humana physiognomonia libri IIII.* Naples: Apud Josephum Cacchium, 1586. [4] 272 (misnumbered 265) pp., illus., port. 32 cm.

A Neapolitan natural philosopher and investigator into many fields of science, Porta was also the author of some of the best Italian comedies of his age. His contributions to optics include the camera obscura and a description of the opera glass. As an early ecologist, he was one of the first to group plants according to their geographical location and distribution in his *Phytognomonica* (1583).

The present work, one of the first on physiognomy, contains a series of woodcuts which show facial resemblances between man and animals with an accompanying text that compares various animal traits to their human counterparts.

Cushing P346; Durling 3720; Garrison-Morton 150; Osler 3714; Waller 7566; Wellcome 5196.

FELIX PLATTER (1536–1614). *De origine partium, earumque in utero conformatione.*

See No. 239.

JOHANNES POSTHIUS (1537–1597). *Observationes anatomicae.*

See No. 190.

*233. CHRISTOVAM DA COSTA (ca. 1540–1599). *Aromatum & medicamentorum in Orientali India nascentium liber.* 2nd ed. Antwerp: Ex officina Plantiniana, apud viduam, & Joannem Moretum, 1593. [225]–312 pp., illus. 16.1 cm. Old calf. Appears with No. 145 and No. 167.

Costa was born on the island of Mozambique and practiced as a surgeon at Burgos in northern Spain. He was an active traveler and spent some years in India, chiefly at Goa, where he made the acquaintance of Garcia de Orta (see No. 145).

Costa first published this work in Spanish at Burgos in 1578. Although it contained Costa's commentary, it was largely an illustrated translation of Orta's *Colóquios dos simples, e drogas e cousas medicinais da India.* It was later translated into French, Italian, and Latin and became well known throughout Europe. The present work is the second Latin edition and is here translated by the noted botanist, Charles de l'Écluse.

Cushing A33 (1st Latin ed., 1582); Durling 3417; Osler 2327 (3rd Latin ed., 1605); Waller 7006; Wellcome 4658.

*234. GIROLAMO MERCURIO (1540–1616). *La commare o' raccoglitrice.* Venice: Per Domenico Louisa, 1713. [xxxii] 390 pp., illus. 23.4 cm.

Mercurio, a native of Rome, studied medicine at Bologna and Padua before entering the Dominican monastery at Milan. He studied theology and philosophy for a time but preferred medicine and eventually left the monastery to travel and study in other European countries. After several years, he returned to Venice where he practiced medicine until his death.

First issued in 1596, this was one of the earliest works on obstetrics to be published in Italy. It maintained an authoritative position in Italy and Germany for more than one hundred and twenty-five years, and Mercurio's writings remain as the outstanding contribution to Italian obstetrics during the sixteenth and seventeenth centuries. The work is divided into three parts: the first deals with natural labor and care of the mother and child, the second with abnormal presentations, and the third with diseases that complicate pregnancy and affect the newborn. It is interesting to note that the illustrations are taken from the 1596 edition and have been used again in this edition more than one hundred years later. This work also contains a treatise by Pietro de Castro (1603–ca. 1657) on colostrum and skin diseases of children and a treatise on the diseases of women by Giovanni Marinelli (fl. 1560).

Cushing M297 (1601 ed.); Garrison-Morton 6144 (1596 ed.); Waller 6494 (1618 ed.); Wellcome 4259 (1601 ed.).

*235. PETRUS SEVERINUS (1542–1602). *Idea medicinae philosophicae, fundamenta continens totius doctrinae Paracelsicae, Hippocraticae, & Galenicae.* Basel: Ex officina Sixti Henricpetri, 1571. [14] 416 [12] pp. 20.3 cm. Limp vellum.

Severinus (or Soerensen), a precocious student, was born and received his early education in Denmark and his doctorate in France in 1571. He was devoted to the

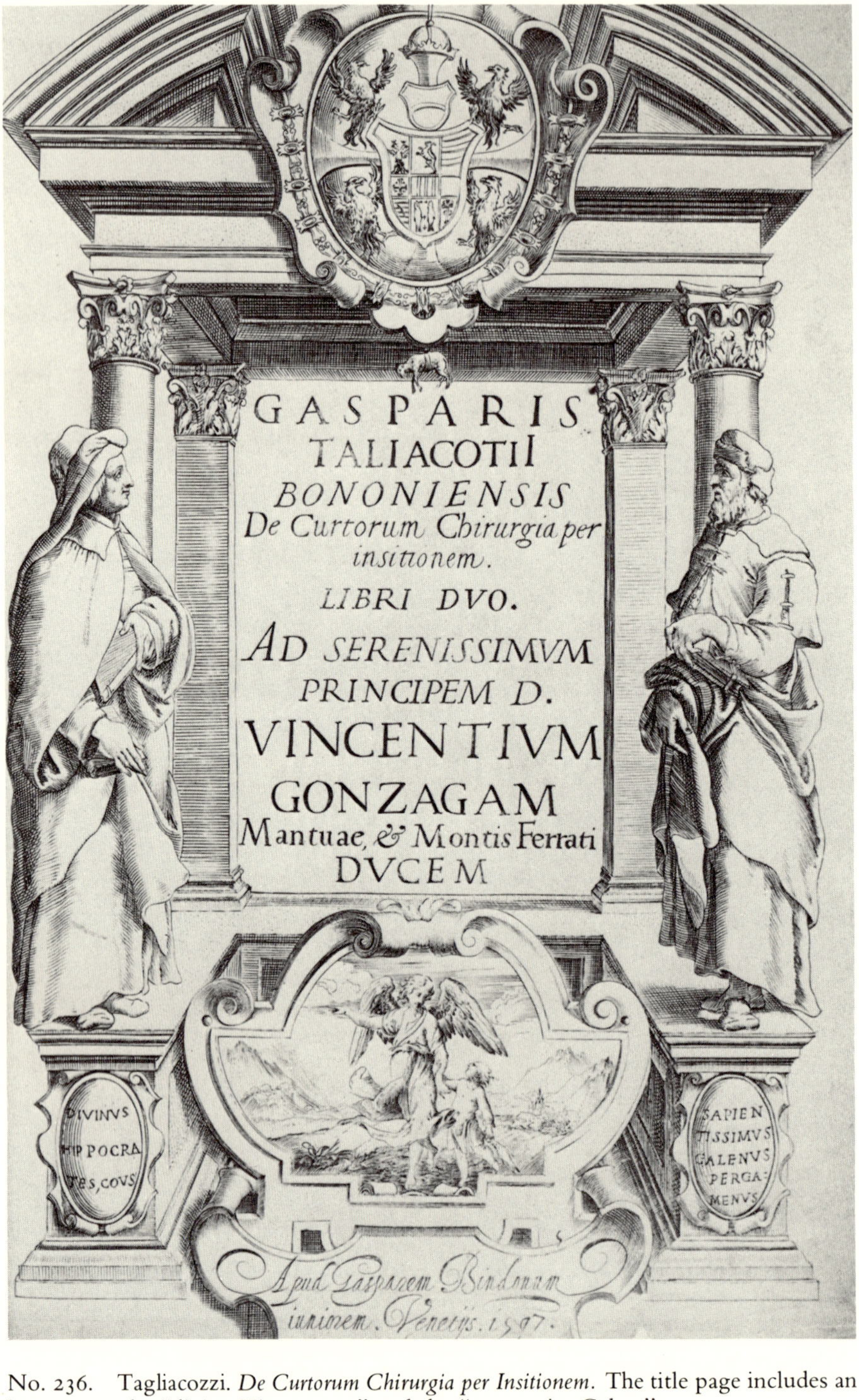

No. 236. Tagliacozzi. *De Curtorum Chirurgia per Insitionem.* The title page includes an homage to the "divine Hippocrates" and the "most wise Galen."

doctrines of Paracelsus, whom he supports in this rare book. Severinus extended Paracelsus' ideas concerning invisible agents of disease in the concept of *pathologia animata*.

Durling 4231; Waller 9059; Wellcome 5954.

*236. GASPARE TAGLIACOZZI (1545–1599). *De curtorum chirurgia per insitionem, libri duo*. Venice: Apud Gasparem Bindonum, juniorem, 1597. [28] 94, 95, 47 [32] pp., illus. 31.4 cm. Vellum.

Tagliacozzi studied under Girolamo Cardano at Bologna and later became professor of surgery and anatomy at that institution. This work, "Concerning the surgery of the mutilated by grafting," is a classic in the history of plastic surgery and is especially noteworthy for its description of rhinoplasty. Rhinoplasty had been practiced in ancient India and, in the thirteenth century, by a family of itinerant Sicilian surgeons who kept the operation a family secret. The volume is divided into two parts: the first, "Theory of the art of plastic surgery," is about the structure, function, and physiology of the nose; and the second part, "Practice of the art," describes and illustrates the instruments and operative procedures for restoration of the nose, lip, and ear. Tagliacozzi also fully discussed the complications, such as hemorrhage and gangrene, that often occurred during these operations. The numerous full-page woodcuts are well-executed and illustrate many of the techniques described in the text. The immediate popularity of the work caused it to be pirated by another Venetian printer, and that is the edition mentioned by Osler.

Cushing T16; Durling 4310; Garrison-Morton 5734; Osler 4079 (Venice, Meietus, 1597); Waller 9451; Wellcome 6210.

237. BARTHOLOMEO CASTELLI (d. 1607). *Lexicon medicum Graeco-Latinum*. Leipzig: Fritsch, 1713. [4] 788 pp. 25.3 cm.

Castelli was professor of theology, philosophy, and medicine at Messina. He first published his lexicon in 1598 at Messina, and it gained wide popularity, being published in many editions through the end of the eighteenth century. The present work was first revised and edited by Jakob Pancraz Bruno (1629–1709) at Nuremberg in 1682.

Durling 884 (1st ed., 1598); Garrison-Morton 6794 (1st ed.); Osler 6963; Waller 1816 (1746 ed.); Wellcome II, p. 311.

238. JOANNES DONATUS SANTORUS (fl. 1590). *Epistolarum medicinalium libri septem*. Naples: Ex typographia Stelliolae, sumptibus Sipionis Ricii, 1596. [12] 607 [2] pp. 20.3 cm. Limp vellum.

Comparatively few medical texts printed in Naples have come down to us. This work by a Neapolitan physician, dedicated to the Cardinal Archbishop of Naples, consists of a series of letters from the author to medical colleagues concerning fevers, purgatives, the humors, malignancy, and a variety of other topics.

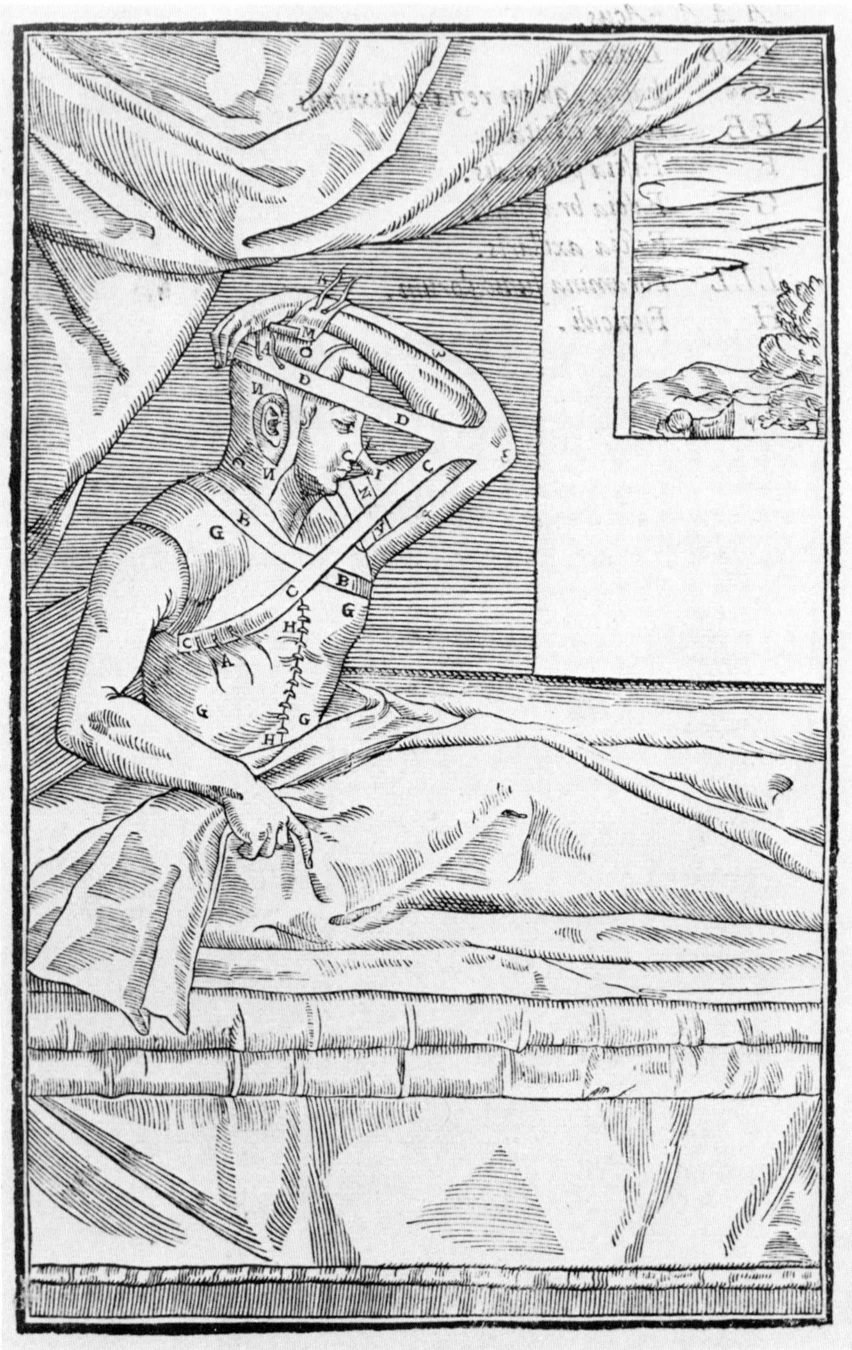

No. 236. Tagliacozzi. *De Curtorum Chirurgia per Insitionem.* Grafting skin to the nose.

*239. SÉVERIN PINEAU (1550?–1619). *De integritatis et corruptionis virginum notis: graviditate item & partu naturali mulierum, opuscula.*

LUIGI BONACCIUOLI (d. 1540). *Enneas muliebris.*

FELIX PLATTER (1536–1614). *De origine partium, earumque in utero conformatione.*

PIERRE GASSENDI (1592–1655). *De septo cordis pervio, observatio.*

MELCHIOR SEBISCH (1578–1674?). *De notis virginitatis.* Leiden: Apud Franciscum Hegerum, 1641. 182, 298 [40] pp., illus., fold. plates. 12.7 cm. Vellum.

Although this curious collection of treatises, chiefly on gynecology and obstetrics, went through several editions, it is not often found, particularly with all of the plates, as some editions were confiscated because of the frank (for those times) discussion of virginity and its method of loss.

Pineau was a Parisian physician and surgeon to the king. The present edition of his work, an unusual treatise on the anatomical signs of virginity, also contains tracts on embryology, gynecology, and obstetrics.

Bonacciuoli, a physician in Ferrara, first published this gynecological work, dedicated to Lucrezia Borgia, early in the sixteenth century.

Platter was an anatomist, the earliest supporter of Vesalius north of the Alps, and professor of medicine at Basel. One of the earliest German anatomists to dissect the human body, he published, in 1583, a well-known book of anatomy illustrated with numerous plates, many of which were copied from Vesalius. The present work is the gynecological portion of his book on anatomy.

A famed French philosopher, astronomer, physicist, and opponent of Harvey, Gassendi here gives the first description of the foramen ovale of the heart and its vestigial nature in the mature organ, thus finally proving the impervious nature of the interventricular septum. This interesting treatise on the heart appears only in this collection; there is no separate edition.

Sebisch, professor of medicine in the university of his native Strasbourg, provides here another curious tract on virginity.

Garrison-Morton 802 (1639 ed.); Osler 3680 (1650 ed.); Waller 7450; Wellcome 5042 (1639 ed.).

*240. PROSPER ALPINI (1553–1617). *De medicina Aegyptiorum.* Paris: Apud viduam Gulielmi Pelé, & Joannem Duval, 1646. [xi] 150 [25] 39 [1] *ll.*, illus. 22.2 cm. Vellum. Bound with No. 241.

Alpini, an Italian physician and botanist, graduated from Padua and traveled through Greece, Crete, and Egypt from 1580 to 1583. Following his travels, he returned to Padua where he remained as professor of botany and director of the botanical garden until his death. This work, first published in 1591, was one of several major books that resulted from his travels and is a comprehensive account of medicine as it was practiced in Egypt.

Following Alpini's work is Jakob de Bondt's (see No. 291) *De medicina Indorum.* The work contains an account of the various tropical diseases Bondt treated and has been regarded as one of the first authoritative works on such diseases. In it are the first modern descriptions of beri-beri and cholera.

Cushing A146 (1645 ed.); Durling 178 (1st ed., 1591); Garrison-Morton 6468 (1st ed.); Osler 1796 (1st ed.); Waller 12509 (1st ed.); Wellcome 232 (1st ed.).

*241. ———. *De plantis Aegypti liber.* Padua: Typis Pauli Frambotti Bipliopolae, 1640. [xvi] 144, 4 [4] 5–54 [12] 80 pp., illus. 22.2 cm. Bound with No. 240.

While in Egypt, Alpini studied its plant life and this work is the result of his findings and observations. In this, the second edition, there are more than seventy full-page illustrations of Egyptian plants, among them the earliest representations of the coffee and cotton plants. This edition is the first to contain the notes and observations of Johann Vesling (see No. 303) who succeeded Alpini as director of the University's botanical garden. Also included in this work is Alpini's *De balsamo* in which are set forth, in the form of a dialogue between an Egyptian and a Hebrew physician, the merits and uses of balsam.

Durling 179 (1st ed., 1592); Osler 1799 (1st ed.); Wellcome 233 (1st ed.).

*242. ANDRÉ DU LAURENS (1558–1609). *Historia anatomica humani corporis et singularum eius partium multis controversys & observationibus novis illustrata.* Frankfurt: Apud Matthaeum Beckerum, impensis Theodorici de Brii viduae & duorum filiorum [1599]. [23] 442 [28] pp., illus. 30.7 cm. Contemporary vellum.

A graduate of Montpellier, Du Laurens succeeded Laurent Joubert as professor in 1586 and later as chancellor of the faculty. He taught at Montpellier until 1598 when he was called to Paris as court physician. In this position he eventually became personal physician to Marie de Medici and King Henry IV. This work became very popular and went through a number of editions. It remains as one of the more important anatomical texts of the late sixteenth century. Although the book contains many illustrations, few of the plates are taken from Du Laurens' own observations as he took most of his figures from Vesalius, Valverde, Coiter, and others.

Choulant-Frank, p. 222; Cushing D311; Durling 1313; Osler 3174; Waller 2629; Wellcome 1935.

*243. ———. *De mirabili strumas sanandi vi solis Galliae regibus christianissimis divinitus concessa liber unus.* Paris: Apud Marcum Orry, 1609. [xv] 307 (misnumbered 293), [18] pp., fold. plate. 17.5 cm. Limp vellum.

During the Middle Ages, tuberculosis of the lymph glands of the neck was very common and was known variously as scrofula, struma, and the "King's Evil." For centuries it was believed that the "royal touch" could cure this disease and many English and French monarchs were in the habit of touching their afflicted subjects during major religious holidays. Du Laurens was a firm believer in the effectiveness of the "royal touch" and, in this work, reports that King Henry IV often touched and healed as many as 1,500 individuals at a time. The work contains a magnificent folding copperplate engraving showing the King touching a number of sufferers who are gathered about him in a circle. The University of Iowa copy has an interesting provenance and can be traced back to Jean Auguste de Thou, its original owner, who died in 1617.

Cushing D308; Garrison-Morton 3806; Waller 2626; Wellcome 1940.

*244. ———. *Toutes les oeuvres de Me. André Du Laurens.* Rouen: Pour Raphael du Petit Val, 1621. [601] *ll.*, illus. (port.) 36.1 cm. Mottled calf.

This is the second edition of the French translation of Du Laurens' collected works. From what is known about his works, it appears that the French translation preceded the publication of the Latin text. In addition to the author's textbook of anatomy and his account of scrofula, the volume contains works on geriatrics, melancholy and other mental afflictions, and an early ophthalmological work which describes the anatomy and diseases of the eye. The volume has an exceptionally well-engraved title page, the author's engraved portrait, and numerous historiated and ornamental woodcut initials.

Cushing D317 (1st ed., 1613); Wellcome 1942.

*245. ISRAEL SPACH, compiler (1560–1610). *Gynaeciorum.* Strasbourg: Sumptibus Lazari Zetzneri, 1597. [36] 28, 1080 [33] pp., illus. 32.1 cm. Contemporary elaborately blind-tooled pigskin.

In the Renaissance there was a growth of interest in diseases of women and encyclopedic works on the subject were issued by Caspar Wolf (see No. 228) and Caspar Bauhin (see No. 246). They constituted compilations of the best that had been written up to their time. Spach, a Strasbourg physician, reprinted most of Wolf's and Bauhin's compilations and added several other treatises. Included in this huge collection are works by Platter, Moschion, Le Boë, Montanus, Paré, and many others. The work is profusely illustrated with woodcuts of anatomical subjects (some taken from Vesalius), as well as of various instruments for medical and surgical treatment.

Durling 2254; Garrison-Morton 6013; Waller 9096; Wellcome 6030.

*246. CASPAR BAUHIN (1560–1624). *Theatrum anatomicum.* Frankfurt am Main: Typis Matthaei Beckeri, 1605. [16] 1314 [8] 197 [46] pp., illus., ports. 19.5 cm. Old vellum.

A native of Basel, Bauhin studied first in his native city, then at Padua and Montpellier, and returned to Basel to complete his medical degree in 1581. He remained at Basel and was appointed professor of Greek in 1582, becoming professor of anatomy and botany in 1589. He was made professor of practical medicine on the death of Felix Platter in 1614 and later served as city physician and rector of the University. Although Bauhin made no major original contributions in anatomy, he did erect an anatomical theater and encouraged the study of anatomy at the University.

Bauhin's *Theatrum anatomicum* became a very popular text because it was systematic, provided adequate coverage of the ancient authorities, did not dwell too much on the controversies, had useful footnotes, mentioned anatomical anomalies, and gave pathological findings. It is well-illustrated but does not contain any original plates, the 131 anatomical engravings being taken from the anatomies of Vesalius, Valverde, Eustachius, Coiter, and other anatomists. Harvey chose this work as the basis for his Lumleian Lectures to London's College of Physicians in 1616.

Choulant-Frank, p. 229; Cushing B177; Garrison-Morton 379; Waller 784; Wellcome 724.

*247. WILHELM FABRICIUS VON HILDEN (1560–1634). *Opera quae extant omnia, partim ante hac excusa, partim nunc recens in lucem edita.*

MARCO AURELIO SEVERINO (1580–1656). *De efficaci medicinae libris tribus.* Frankfurt am Main: Sumptibus Joannis Beyeri, 1646. [24] 1044 [36] 297 [14] pp., illus. 33.6 cm. Contemporary blind-stamped vellum.

Fabricius received an excellent classical education as a boy, but a series of family misfortunes left him without the means to obtain a formal medical education. As a result, he became an apprentice in the less desirable craft of surgery and subsequently received the training which prepared him for a distinguished career. Although he was a bold and accomplished operator, his writings show that he was conservative in theory, yet possessed great capacity for progress in the search for sound surgical operations.

This large folio edition of his collected works includes his separately published monographs on dysentery, burns, lithotomy, and anatomy. Congenital malformations, skull fractures, carcinoma of the eye and penis, hydrocele, gangrene, mineral water baths, the concept of removing some healthy tissue along with the necrotic tissue in amputation, and a special operation for hernia are among the many topics discussed in his writings. Among the numerous instruments and appliances he designed were a bullet extractor, a tourniquet for controlling hemorrhage, a urinal for ambulatory use, and a field-chest of drugs and instruments for use by the army.

Also included with Fabricius' *Opera* is Marco Aurelio Severino's *De efficaci medicinae libris tribus.* Professor of anatomy and surgery at Naples, Severino became well known as a teacher and surgeon. He employed trephination, operated upon harelip, epulis, empyema, and is said to have been the first to perform tracheotomy to relieve suffocation in diphtheria. Among his works is this important contribution in which he discusses surgical anatomy, phlebotomy, paracentesis, and cautery.

Fabricius: Waller 2908; Wellcome III, p. 4.
Severino: Waller 8888.

*248. GIULIO CASSERIO (1561–1616). *De vocis auditusque organis historia anatomica.* 2 pts. in 1 vol. Ferrara: Excudebat Victorius Baldinus, 1600–1601 (pt. 1,

1601). Part I: [56] 191 pp.; Part II: 126 pp., 34 plates, 2 ports. 37.1 cm. Contemporary boards, leather back.

Preceding Spigelius (see No. 281), Casserio was next to the last in the line of great anatomists in the Vesalian tradition at Padua. Medical historians rank the accuracy and artistry of the illustrations in this and other works of Casserio in the same category as those of Vesalius, with Casserio setting the standard in copperplates as Vesalius had done in woodcuts. The thirty-four full-page anatomical copperplates of the vocal organs and of the organs of hearing in man and other animals are accompanied by engraved portraits of Casserio and of the Duke of Parma.

Choulant-Frank, p. 223; Cushing C113; Garrison-Morton 286; Waller 1809; Wellcome 1333.

*249. SANTORIO SANTORIO (1561–1636). *Medicina statica: being the aphorisms of Sanctorius . . . to which is added, Dr. Keil's Medicina statica Britannica.* By John Quincy. 5th ed. London: T. Longman and J. Newton, 1737. viii, 463 [17] pp., front., fold. plate. 19.3 cm.

Santorio (or Sanctorius) was a graduate of Padua and returned there at the age of fifty to take the chair of medicine. He experimented unceasingly, using himself as the subject of his experiments. In his original physiologic studies of weight gain and loss, respiration, pulse, body temperature, and other metabolic processes, he was a leading representative of the new Iatrophysical School. He invented a clinical thermometer and other devices, most of which were forgotten for a hundred years until they were revived and improved upon for more general use. Crude as they were, however, his quantitative experiments opened a new approach in the blossoming field of physiology, which expanded through the studies of such men as Borelli, Malpighi, Le Boë, and Helmont.

The first edition of the present work appeared in 1614 and was an astounding success, going through many editions and translations for a century and a half. The book was first translated into English in 1676 and, in 1712, was translated by John Quincy (see No. 462) in a series of editions that continued into the nineteenth century. It contains the account of his famous balance seat in which he sat in a suspended chair counterbalanced by weights so that he could determine the amount of respiration (or, in his term, "insensible perspiration") which took place through the skin.

Cushing S71 (1723 ed.); Osler 3915 (1st ed., 1712); Waller 8487 (1720 ed.).

*250. ———. *De medicina statica aphorismi. Commentaria, notasque addidit A. C. Lorry.* Paris: Apud P.-G. Cavelier, 1770. [xxxvi] 395 pp., plate. 16.5 cm.

This late Parisian edition is the first to contain the commentary and additions of the French dermatologist, Anne-Charles Lorry (1726–1783), and is an indication of the significance of Santorio's work more than 150 years after its first appearance.

Waller 8482.

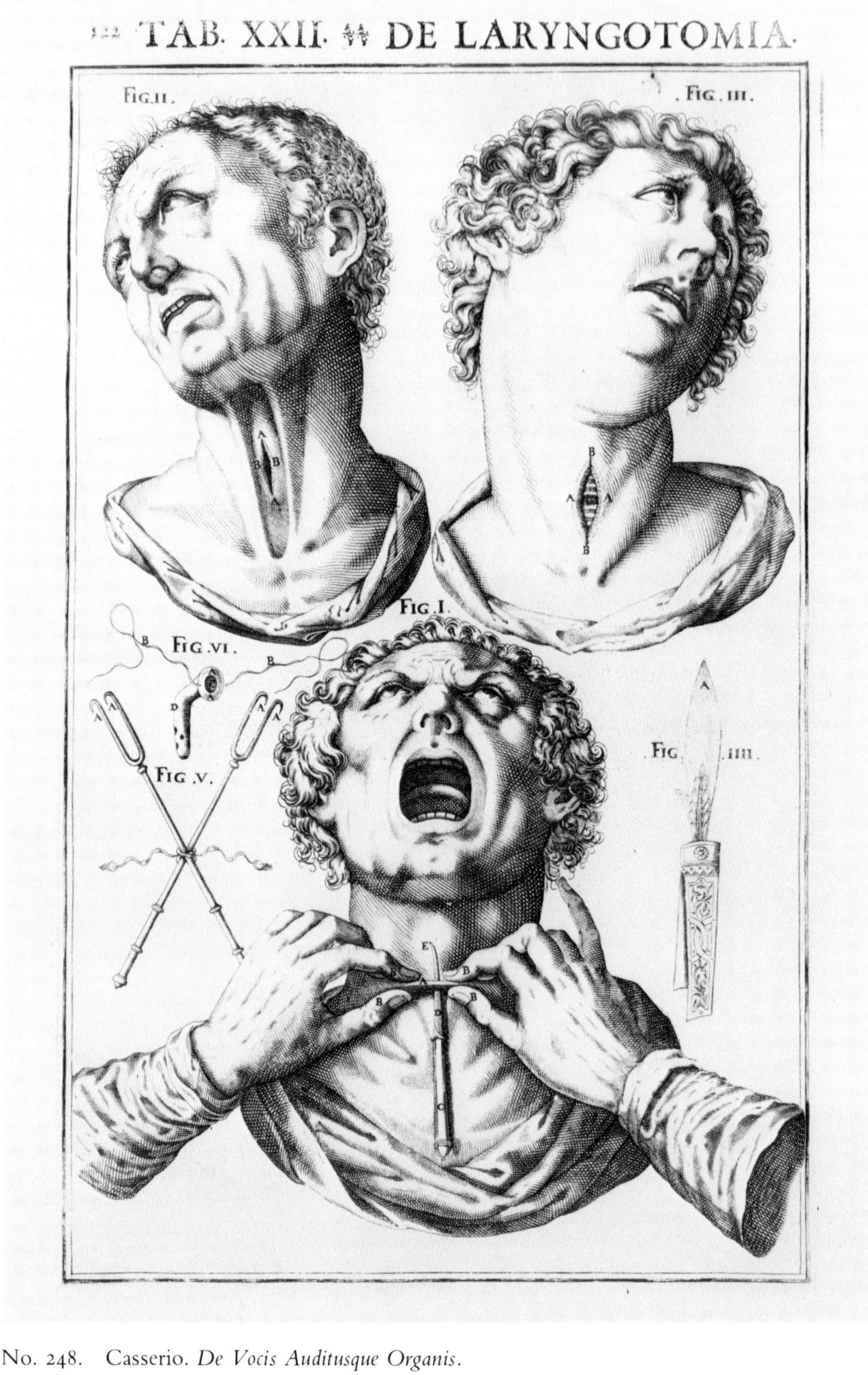

No. 248. Casserio. *De Vocis Auditusque Organis.*

*251. PIETER PAUW (1564–1617). *Primitiae anatomicae. De humani corporis ossibus.* Leiden: Ex officina Justi à Colster, 1615. [xvi] 188 pp., illus., 4 fold. plates. 19.7 cm. Limp vellum.

Pauw studied at Leiden, Paris, and Rostock, and was a pupil of Fabricius at Padua. He was professor of anatomy and botany at Leiden and founded the first anatomical theater there in 1597. A follower of Vesalius, he edited an edition of the *Epitome* in 1616 (see No. 179) and made a number of important contributions to craniology and osteology. Perhaps the first osteological work to be published in the Netherlands, this volume on the skeletal system contains several fine folding plates of the skeleton and skull.

Cushing P161; Waller 7254; Wellcome 4682.

EMILIO PARISANO (1567–1643). *Exercitationes.*

See Nos. 256 and 257.

*252. [ROBERT BURTON] (1577–1640). *The anatomy of melancholy.* 2nd ed. Oxford: Printed by J. Lichfield and J. Short, for H. Cripps, 1624. [4] 64 [4] 557 [7] pp. 28.6 cm.

This deeply serious work by a layman was said by Osler to be "a great medical treatise" (Osler 4621). The author, under the assumed name of Democritus Junior, offers many causes for melancholy, discusses the cure of its many forms and, in his studious discussion, throws much light on the customs and social attitudes of the day. It is a medical work in that, in all its seventy and more editions, it has continued to express the author's understanding of human psychiatric problems. Almost half of the thousand references to other authors are medical. The work was one of Dr. Samuel Johnson's favorites.

Cushing B880; Osler 4622; Wellcome 1161.

*253. JEAN BAPTISTE VAN HELMONT (1577–1644). *Opuscula medica inaudita.* 2nd ed. Amsterdam: Apud Ludovicum Elzevirium, 1648. [8] 110, 115, 88 pp. 19.4 cm. Vellum. Bound with No. 254.

A Belgian mystic, Helmont was nonetheless the most prominent chemist of the first half of the seventeenth century. Originally an alchemist and a follower of Paracelsus in that his outlook was universal, he himself marks the transition from alchemy to the science of chemistry in the modern sense.

This work, first published in 1644 and issued in a corrected second edition in 1648 in conjunction with *Ortus medicinae* (see No. 254), contains a lengthy treatise on the stone, as well as shorter ones on fevers, the humors of Galen, and the plague.

Cushing H239; Osler 2932; Waller 4306; Wellcome III, p. 241.

*254. ———. *Ortus medicinae; id est, Initia physicae inaudita.* Amsterdam: Apud Ludovicum Elzevirium, 1648. [34] 808 (misnumbered 800) pp., front. (ports., coats of arms). 20 cm. Vellum. Bound with No. 253.

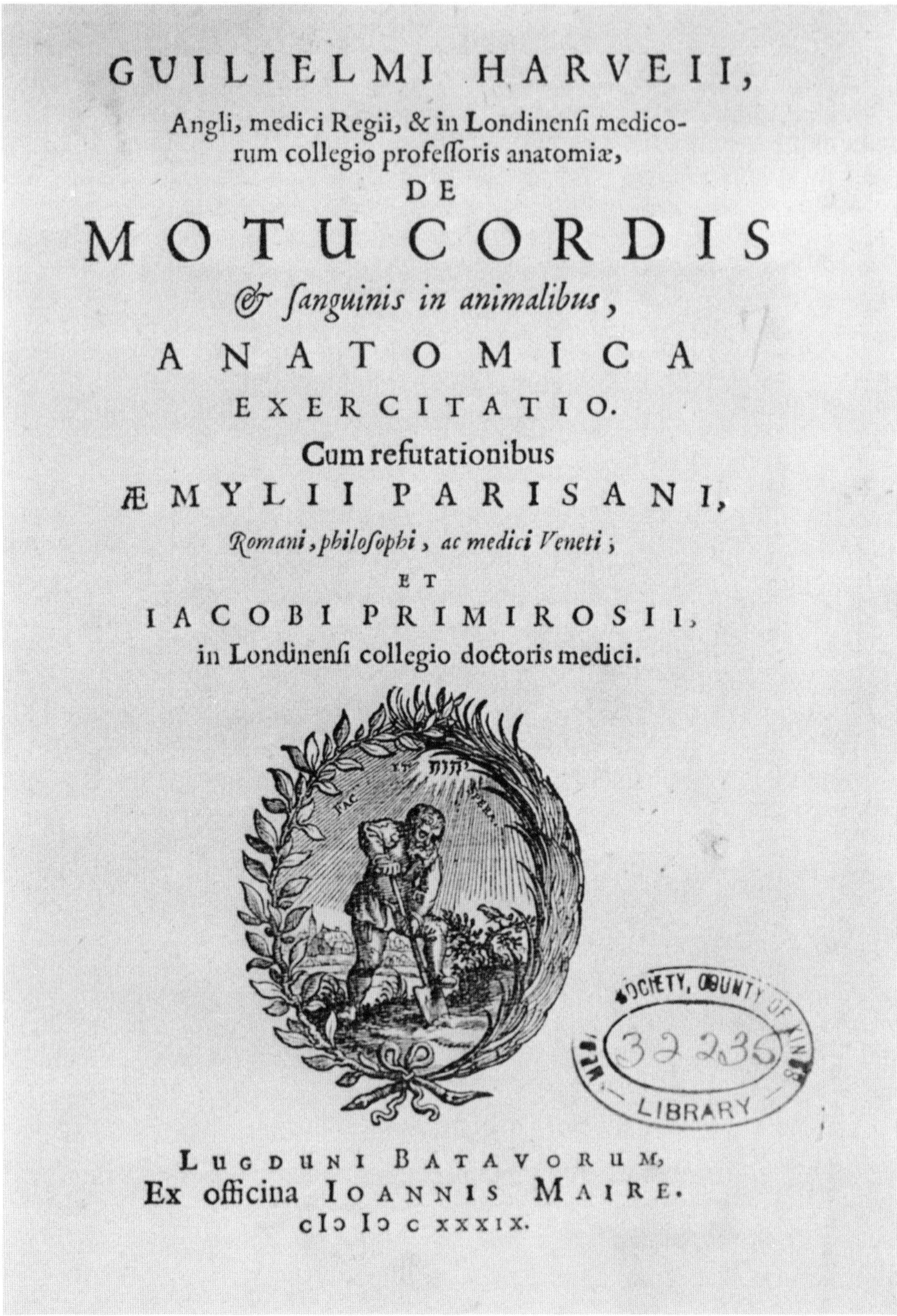

GVILIELMI HARVEII,

Angli, medici Regii, & in Londinensi medicorum collegio professoris anatomiæ,

DE

MOTU CORDIS

& sanguinis in animalibus,

ANATOMICA

EXERCITATIO.

Cum refutationibus

ÆMYLII PARISANI,

Romani, philosophi, ac medici Veneti;

ET

IACOBI PRIMIROSII,

in Londinensi collegio doctoris medici.

LUGDUNI BATAVORUM,

Ex officina IOANNIS MAIRE.

cIↃ IↃ c XXXIX.

No. 256. Harvey. *De Motu Cordis.*

Helmont's most important work, *Ortus medicinae* [Birth of medicine], was published four years after his death by his son. Its publication in Amsterdam, a Protestant country, was thought necessary to avoid the Inquisition, whose disfavor Helmont had earlier incurred because of his mystical and magical tastes not entirely in keeping with Church dogma.

In this work, Helmont established his name as one of the founders of biochemistry, although some authorities believe that he is perhaps overrated because of his vacillations between mysticism and science. In any event, his discovery of digestive juices in the stomach and intestine, and especially his first use of the specific gravity of urine for diagnostic purposes, mark him as a man of no insignificant importance in the history of medicine.

Cushing H241; Garrison-Morton 665; Osler 2929; Waller 4307; Wellcome III, p. 241.

*255. ———. *Deliramenta catarrhi; or, The incongruities, impossibilities, and absurdities couched under the vulgar opinion of defluxions.* London: Printed by E. G. for William Lee, 1650. [12] 75 pp. 18.4 cm. Full calf.

This is the only English edition of Helmont's treatise on catarrhal discharges and phlebotomy and was translated and adapted by Walter Charleton (see No. 333), a British physician. In it, Helmont opposes the popular views of his day regarding the uses of bloodletting, purgatives, and several other therapies then in vogue. He devotes a considerable portion of the book to a discussion of the Galenic theory of phlegm and mucus and presents his own views on these matters while refuting and criticizing the position of his contemporaries.

Cushing H238; Osler 2933; Waller 4304; Wellcome III, p. 242.

*256. WILLIAM HARVEY (1578–1657). *De motu cordis & sanguinis in animalibus, anatomica exercitatio.* Leiden: Ex officina Joannis Maire, 1639. [4] 267, 84 pp., illus., 2 plates. 18.8 cm. Contemporary limp vellum.

There is probably no name better known in the history of medicine than that of William Harvey. An Englishman, educated at Cambridge and then at Padua when Fabricius was in the chair of anatomy, Harvey returned to London and set up in practice. In 1615 he was made professor of anatomy and surgery at the College of Physicians. By 1616 he had perfected his theory of the circulation of the blood, publishing his findings in 1628 in an unimposing little book, *Exercitatio anatomica de motu cordis et sanguinis in animalibus* [An anatomical disquisition concerning the motion of the heart and blood], usually called just *De motu cordis*. It is probably the most important book in the history of medicine. What Vesalius was to anatomy, Harvey was to physiology; the whole scientific outlook on the human body was transformed, and behind almost every important medical advance in modern times lies the work of Harvey. The first edition of Harvey's little book has become one of the greatest rarities. It was printed on poor paper and almost always badly bound. Even the later editions are scarce.

Although this is actually the third edition of *De motu cordis,* it is only the second

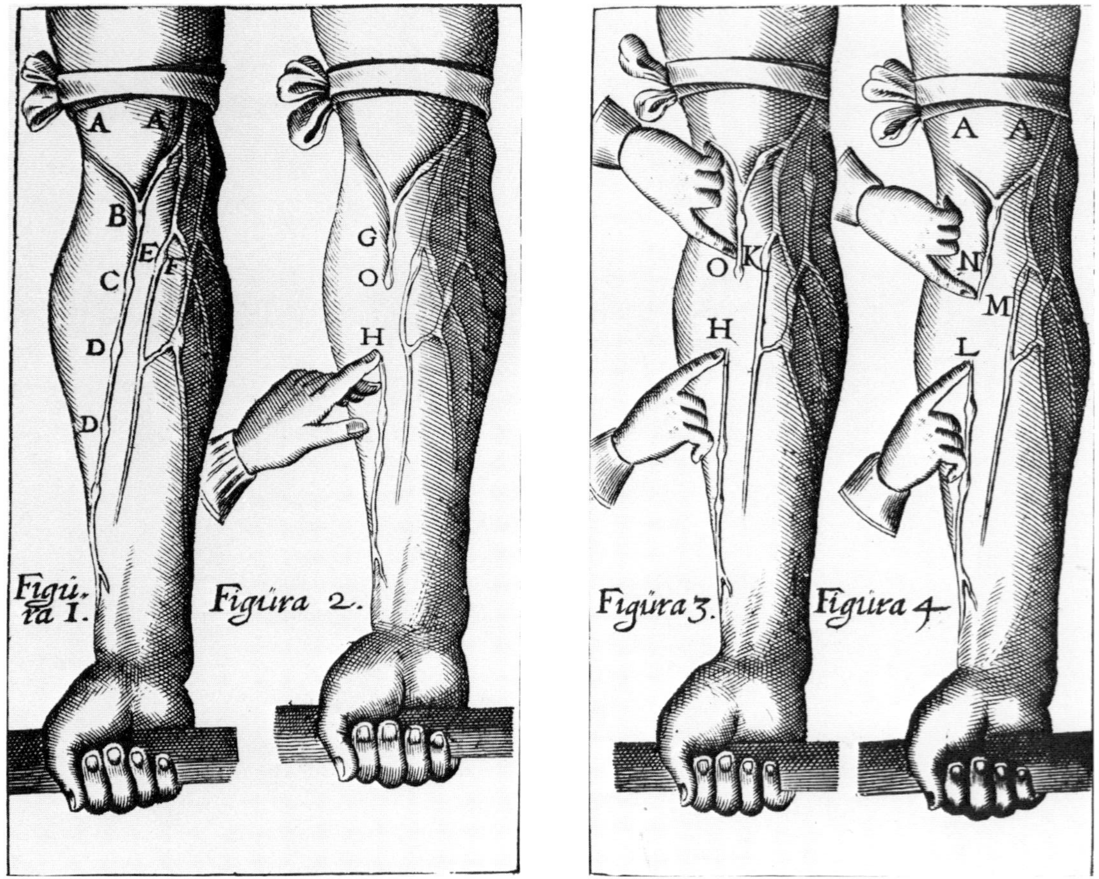

No. 256. Harvey. *De Motu Cordis.* These figures, the only ones in any edition of *De Motu Cordis,* were taken from Fabricius (No. 231).

complete edition. The second edition of 1635 was lacking parts of the introduction, chapters One and Sixteen, and the plates. In this edition, the text of Harvey's treatise is printed passage by passage alternatively with the refutations of Emilio Parisano (1567–1643), one of Harvey's many opponents. The criticism and denials of James Primerose (see No. 287), first published in 1630, are also included as a separate tract at the end of the book.

Cushing H144; Garrison-Morton 759 (1st ed., 1628); Keynes 3; Osler 692 (1st ed.); Russell 352; Waller 4089; Wellcome 3070.

*257. ———. *Recentiorum disceptationes de motu cordis, sanguinis, et chyli, in animalibus.* Leiden: Ex officina Joannis Maire, 1647. 267, 84, 240, 51, 104 pp., plates. 18.3 cm. Contemporary vellum, edges restored.

Although the present work is chronologically the sixth edition of *De motu cordis,* it is actually a reprint of the 1639 edition (see No. 256) with Parisano's refutations printed in the same fashion. Also included with *De motu cordis* are treatises by James Primerose, Johannes Walaeus (1604–1649), Henricus Regius, and Roger Drake (1608–1669) on the pros and cons of Harvey's research and theories.

In addition to these works, the 1640 edition of Gaspare Aselli's (1581–1626) *De lactibus sive lacteis venis* is included in the book. Johann Friedrich Blumenbach (see No. 692), a previous owner of this book, has made several annotations which record his rediscovery of the lacteal vessels which were traced by Aselli to the mesenteric glands but not followed to the thoracic duct.

Keynes 6; Russell 355; Wellcome III, p. 220.

*258. ———. *The anatomical exercises of Dr. William Harvey.* London: Printed by Francis Leach, for Richard Lowndes, 1653. [37] 111 [20] 123, 86 pp. 14.5 cm. Old calf, rehinged.

This is the first of four English editions of *De motu cordis.* It contains a preface by Zachariah Wood as well as Jacobus de Back's (ca. 1594–1658) *Discourse of the heart.*

Cushing H137; Keynes 19; Osler 7698; Russell 368; Waller 4105; Wellcome III, p. 219.

*259. ———. *Exercitationes anatomicae, de motu cordis & sanguinis circulatione. . . . Accessit dissertatio de corde Doct. Jacobi de Back.* Rotterdam: Ex officina Arnoldi Leers, 1654. [32] 285 [19] 252 [24] pp., 2 plates. 12.8 cm. Eighteenth century mottled calf.

This edition of 1654 is the first to contain Harvey's two essays, *Exercitationes duae anatomicae,* delayed responses to his harsh critic, Jean Riolan (see No. 285). And, in addition, a treatise on the heart by Jacobus de Back is included.

Cushing H153; Keynes 8; Osler 696; Russell 357; Waller 4092; Wellcome III, p. 219.

*260. ———. ———. Rotterdam: Ex officina Arnoldi Leers, 1660. [32] 285 [19] 252 [24] pp., 2 plates. 13.6 cm. Vellum.

An almost exact reprint of the 1654 edition (No. 259).

Cushing H153; Keynes 9; Osler 697; Russell 358; Waller 4093; Wellcome III, p. 219.

*261. ———. ———. Rotterdam: Ex officina Arnoldi Leers, 1671. [32] 285 [19] 252 [24] pp., 2 plates. 12.9 cm. Vellum.

Almost exact reprint of the 1654 edition (No. 259).

Cushing H155; Keynes 11; Russell 360; Waller 4095; Wellcome III, p. 219.

*262. ———. *De motu cordis, & sanguinis in animalibus, anatomica exercitatio, cui postrema hac editione accesserunt clarissimi viri Johannis Walaei. . . . Epistolae duae, quibus Harveii doctrina roboratur.* Bologna: Typis Longhi, 1697. [22] 178 [2] pp., illus. 13.7 cm.

The illustrations in this uncommon edition are crudely copied woodcuts of the usual valves in the veins and appear on either side of the final leaf. Also included are two letters of Johannes Walaeus, anatomist of Leiden, in corroboration of Harvey's thesis. These letters had first appeared in the Padua edition of 1643 but had been included in only two other editions between then and this Bologna edition.

Keynes 13; Russell 362; Waller 4097; Wellcome III, p. 219.

*263. ———. ———. Leiden: Apud Johannem van Kerckhem, 1736. [14] 170 pp., 2 plates (on double leaf). 19.9 cm. Blind-stamped white vellum.

This edition, printed by Johann van Kerckhem, contains a preface by Bernard Siegfried Albinus, the famous eighteenth-century anatomist (see No. 525). Keynes states that "this form of van Kerckhem's edition is rare, the sheets of the greater part of the issue having been published in 1737 as Part I of the *Opera*" (Keynes 14).

Cushing H151; Keynes 14; Russell 363; Waller 4098.

*264. ———. *Exercitationes anatomicae, de motu cordis et sanguinis circulatione.* Glasgow: In aedibus R. Urie, Sumptibus D. Baxter, 1751. x [2] 299 pp., 2 plates. 14.7 cm.

An especially well-printed book, containing the replies of Harvey to Riolan, two engraved plates, and a good index.

Cushing H156; Keynes 15; Osler 699; Russell 365; Waller 4100; Wellcome III, p. 219.

*265. ———. *Exercitatio anatomica de motu cordis et sanguinis in animalibus . . . Atque hisce praefactionem addidit Bernardus Siegfried Albinus.* Leiden: Apud Gerardum Potuliet, et Cornelium de Pecker, 1753. [14] 170 pp. 19.8 cm. Vellum.

This edition is a reissue of the 1736 edition (No. 263) with a title page redesigned slightly by the printers, Gerard Potuliet and Cornelius de Pecker.

Laid into this copy is a letter dated 5 November 1954 to Dr. John Martin from Sir Geoffrey Keynes, Harvey's present-day biographer and bibliographer, who states:

> Very many thanks for letting me know that you have acquired a copy of 14a. It is the only copy I have yet heard of besides Dr. Waller's. It is certainly *very* uncommon. Congratulations!

Keynes 14a; Russell 364; Waller 4099.

*266. ———. *Exercitationes de motu cordis et sanguinis*. Edinburgh: Ven. apud Joannem Carfrae et Filium; atque Longman et Socios, London, 1824. xviii, 250 pp., 2 plates. 22.3 cm.

This was the last Latin edition of *De motu cordis*.

Keynes 16; Osler 700; Russell 366; Waller 4101; Wellcome III, p. 219.

*267. ———. *La circulation du sang*. Paris: G. Masson, 1879. [4] iii, 287 pp., illus. 21.6 cm. Morocco-backed marbled boards.

This work was the first translation of *De motu cordis* into French. The translator, Charles R. Richet (1850–1935), also includes a long introduction in which he gives an historical review of the development of man's knowledge of circulation up to Harvey's time. Richet later received the Nobel prize for his work in anaphylaxis.

Cushing H143; Keynes 28; Osler 704; Russell 370 (i); Waller 4112.

*268. ———. *An anatomical dissertation upon the movement of the heart and blood in animals, being a statement of the discovery of the circulation of the blood*. Canterbury: G. Moreton, 1894. x, 72 [2] 91 pp., front. (port.), plates. 21.5 cm. Quarter parchment and cloth. A facsimile.

This work is a facsimile reproduction of the 1628 edition of *De motu cordis*. It contains a photogravure portrait of Harvey from the painting in the National Portrait Gallery and facsimile reproductions of the two plates in the 1628 edition. A short biography of Harvey at the beginning of the book is followed by the facsimile of the original text. An English translation of Harvey's Latin text is included after the original text.

Cushing H136; Keynes 23; Russell 370 (d); Waller 4108.

269. ———. *The anatomical exercises of Dr. William Harvey*. London: Nonesuch Press, 1928. xvi, 202 pp., fold. plate. 20.2 cm. Niger morocco.

This work was issued on the occasion of the tercentenary celebration of the first publication of *De motu cordis*. In it, Geoffrey Keynes has carefully edited and presented the text of the 1653 edition (see No. 258).

Cushing H139; Keynes 25; Osler 7698A; Russell 370 (f); Waller 4110.

270. ———. *Exercitatio anatomica de motu cordis et sanguinis in animalibus.* With an English translation and annotations by Chauncey D. Leake. Springfield, Ill.: C. C. Thomas [1928]. 72, 154 pp., front., plates, ports. 23.5 cm.

This translation of *De motu cordis* was prepared by Chauncey D. Leake, professor of pharmacology at the University of California, on the tercentenary of Harvey's birth. The book contains a facsimile of the 1628 edition as well as Leake's translation and notes. A highly respected work, it is now in the fifth edition (1978).

Cushing H149; Keynes 25a; Russell 370 (g).

*271. ———. *Exercitationes de generatione animalium.* Amsterdam: Apud Ludovicum Elzevirium, 1651. 568 [5] pp. 13 cm. Calf. With added engraved title page carrying London imprint and intended for the English trade.

After the publication of *De motu cordis*, Harvey turned his attention to the study of generation. Even if Harvey had not discovered the circulation of the blood, his remarkable work on embryology would have placed him in the front ranks of biological scientists. Without benefit of the compound microscope, his work was necessarily limited; nevertheless, nothing comparable had been done since Aristotle. He disbelieved the previously-held doctrine of "preformation" of the fetus, maintaining instead that it proceeds from the ovum by gradual building up of its parts. Always slow to publicize his findings, Harvey was only after some years persuaded by his friend, Sir George Ent, to put them into print. The first edition was published in London in 1651, followed by three Amsterdam editions of the same year. This Elzevir edition is believed to be the first of the three Amsterdam editions.

Cushing H158; Keynes 35; Osler 712; Russell 376; Waller 4119; Welcome III, p. 220.

*272. ———. ———. Amsterdam: Apud Joannem Janssonium, 1651. [34] 415 [4] pp. 13.3 cm. Contemporary calf.

This may be the second of the three Amsterdam editions and was published by Joannes Jansson. This copy contains the engraved title page showing Jove seated on a pedestal holding an egg in his hands. He has raised the upper half of the egg with his right hand to reveal animals, insects, and plants springing forth from the lower half. At his side is an eagle clutching thunderbolts in its talons.

Cushing H160; Keynes 37; Osler 711; Russell 378; Waller 4121; Wellcome III, p. 220.

*273. ———. ———. Amsterdam: Apud Joannem Janssonium, 1651. [34] 415 [4] pp. 13.3 cm. Vellum. Lacks extra engraved title page present in some copies.

A variant issue of No. 272 in which the place of publication is altered from Amstelodami to Amstrodami.

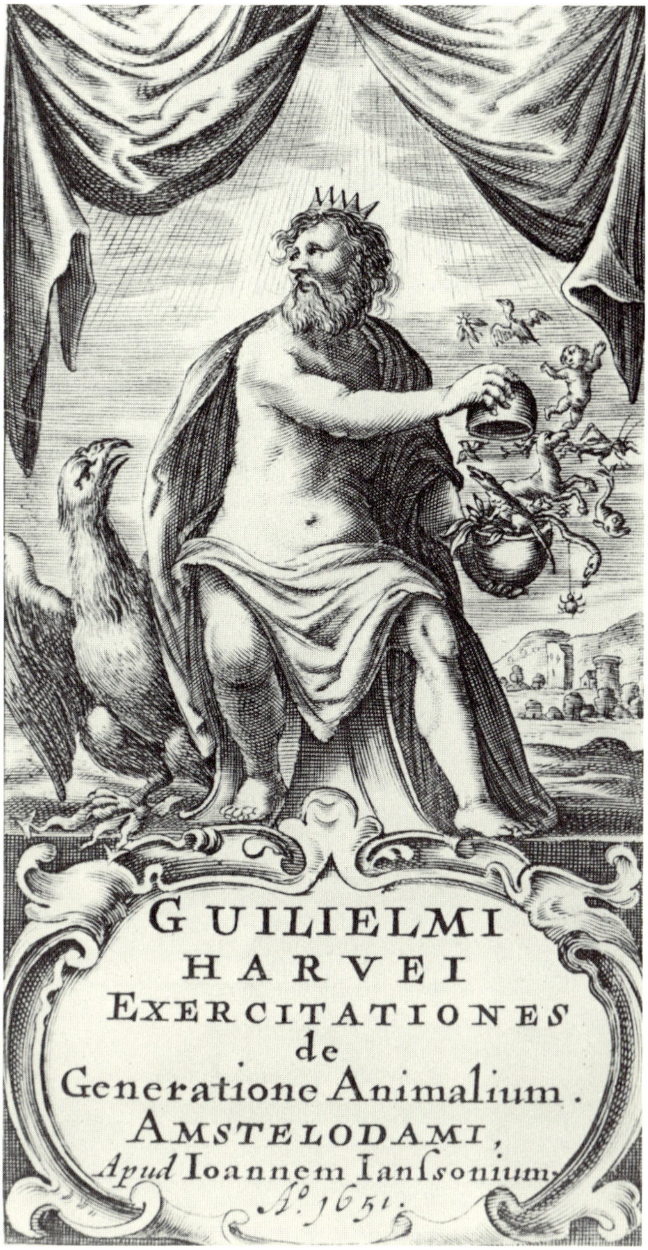

No. 271. Harvey. *Exercitationes de Generatione Animalium.* The engraved allegorical title page.

Cushing H160; Keynes 37; Osler 711; Russell 378; Waller 4121; Wellcome III, p. 220.

*274. ———. *Anatomical exercitations.* London: Printed by James Young for Octavian Pulleyn, 1653. [46] 566 [1] pp., port. 16.8 cm. Antique calf.

This is the first English edition of *De generatione animalium* and contains William Faithorne's original copper engraving of Harvey. According to Keynes "many copies of the book lack the engraving, and many have never contained it" (Keynes, p. 49).

Cushing H140; Keynes 43; Osler 714; Russell 384; Waller 4126; Wellcome III, p. 220.

*275. ———. ———. Padua: Typis heredum Pauli Frambotti, 1666. [36] 604 [5] pp. Two copies. Copy 1: varies between 14.2 and 16.5 cm. Vellum, uncut. Copy 2: 14.2 cm. Vellum.

Keynes 40 mentions a copy on "large paper" for sale in Paris in 1951. Copy 1, above, is that copy, although it is not on large paper but merely untrimmed. There is a similar copy in the Yale Medical Library.

Cushing H163; Keynes 40; Osler 713; Russell 381; Waller 4123; Wellcome III, p. 220.

*276. ———. ———. The Hague: Apud Arnoldum Leers, 1680. [36] 582 [4] pp. 12.9 cm. Vellum.

Cushing H164; Keynes 42; Russell 382; Waller 4125; Wellcome III, p. 220.

*277. ———. *Observationes et historiae omnes & singulae è Guiljelmi Harvei libello De generatione animalium excerptae, & in accuratissimum ordinem redactae.* Amsterdam: Typis Abrahami Wolfgang, 1674. [32] 240 pp., 8 plates. 13.1 cm. Contemporary calf.

This small book, edited by Justus Schrader (b. 1646), contains Wilhelm Langley's (1616–1668) excerpts and comments on Harvey's *De generatione animalium* along with his own observations and experiments. The first six plates, depicting various stages in the development of the chick embryo, are the first illustrations of Harvey's text to be published. The remaining two plates illustrate hernial protrusions and accompany a series of postmortem reports prepared by Joannes van Horne, Franciscus Le Boë (Sylvius), Frederik Ruysch, Jan Swammerdam, and others.

Cushing H168; Keynes 41; Osler 715; Russell 383; Waller 4124; Wellcome III, p. 220.

*278. ———. *Opera omnia.* [London: Excudebat Guilielmus Bowyer] 1766. [8] xxxviii [2] 673 pp. Two copies. Copy 1: 30.3 cm. Vellum-backed boards, uncut. Copy 2: 29.2 cm. Half morocco.

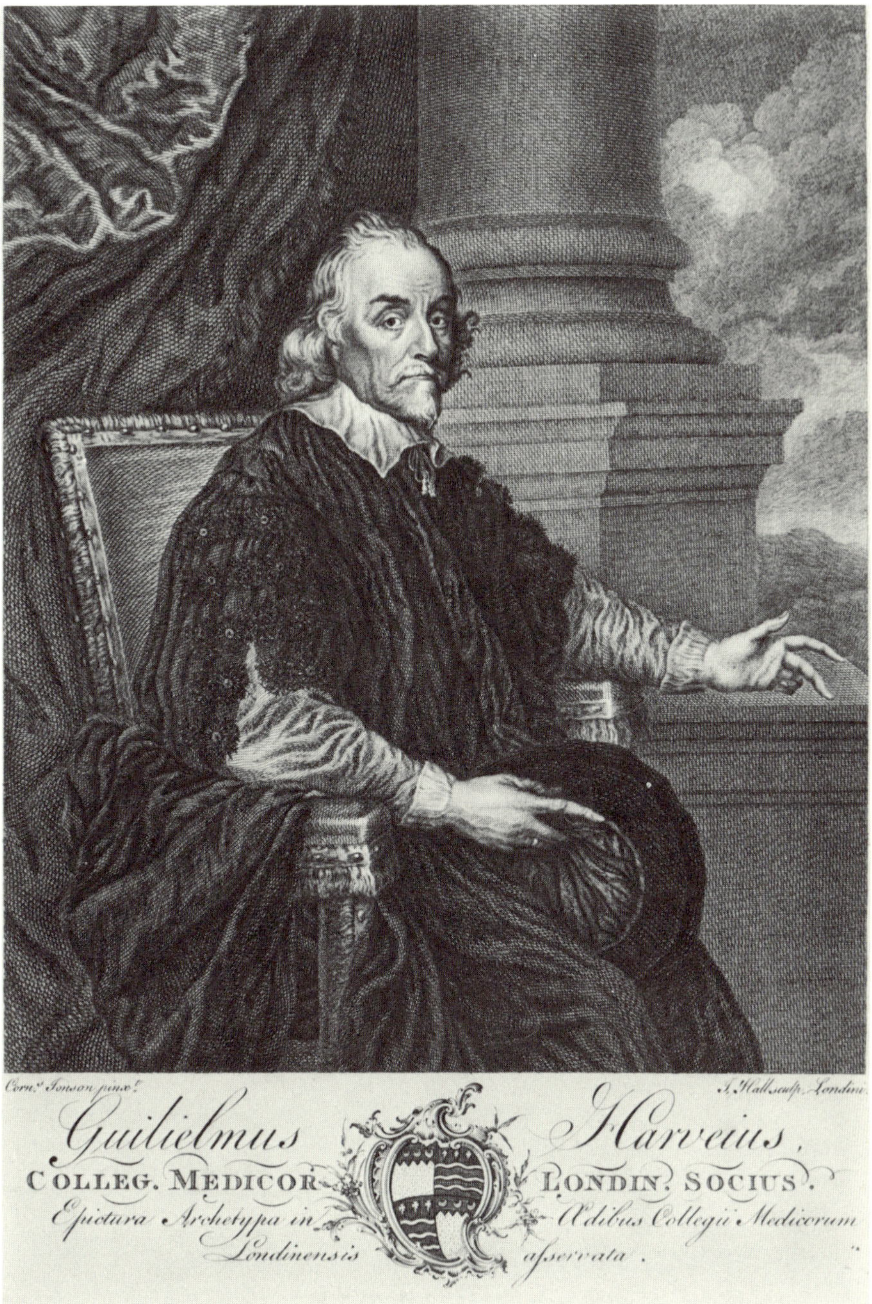
Corn.s Jonson pinx.t
I. Hall sculp. Londini.
Guilielmus Harveius,
COLLEG. MEDICOR. LONDIN. SOCIUS.
Epictura Archetypa in Ædibus Collegii Medicorum
Londinensis asservata.

No. 278. Harvey. *Opera Omnia.* The poorly proportioned hands in this portrait of Harvey have been repainted to repair earlier damage to the painting from which this engraving was copied.

Harvey's major works in Latin have been printed only twice in collected form and this work is perhaps the better of the two. The text of this edition was prepared with extreme care and there is an extensive list of textual corrections following his works on the heart. In addition to his major works, the volume contains Harvey's biography, an autopsy report on Thomas Parr, a number of his letters, and the text of his diploma from Padua. Copy 2 is inscribed "Wm. Morley Fletcher from Wm. Osler. Oxford, March 11/15."

Cushing H172; Keynes 47; Osler 717; Russell 386; Waller 4128; Wellcome III, p. 220.

279. ———. *The works.* London: Printed for the Sydenham Society, 1847. xcvi, 624 pp. 22 cm.

This is the only collected edition of Harvey's works in English. They were translated by Robert Willis (1799–1878), a scholarly and well-educated English country physician, at the request of the Sydenham Society. In addition to Harvey's major works, the book contains Willis's life of Harvey, Harvey's will, the autopsy report on Thomas Parr, and a number of Harvey's letters which are translated here for the first time.

Cushing H176; Keynes 48; Osler 718; Russell 387; Waller 4129; Wellcome III, p. 220.

*280. ———. *Prelectiones anatomiae universalis.* London: J. & A. Churchill, 1886. viii, 195 pp., plates (facsims.). 25 cm. A facsimile.

This work is a facsimile reproduction of the notes Harvey used to prepare the Lumleian Lectures of 1616–1618. It was in these notes that he first recorded his discovery of the circulation. Opposite each page of Harvey's handwritten manuscript is a printed version of the Latin and occasional English that Harvey used to record his thoughts and observations. This is an interesting association copy for it was once owned by the library of the Royal College of Physicians.

Cushing H173; Garrison-Morton 758; Keynes 52; Osler 719; Russell 350 note; Waller 4131.

*281. ADRIAAN VAN DE SPIEGEL (1578–1625). *De semitertiana libri quatuor.* Frankfurt: Apud Jo. Theodori De Bry, 1624. [12] 160 [4] pp. 19.8 cm. Newly rebound in quarter morocco.

Spiegel (or Spigelius) was born in Brussels, studied at Padua as a pupil of Fabricius ab Aquapendente, taught anatomy at Padua from 1618 to 1624, and is considered by historians to be the last of the great Paduan anatomists. Although known primarily as an anatomist, Spiegel was a busy and much-sought clinician, and this account of malaria also contains a description of what is now known as typhoid fever.

Garrison-Morton 5229; Osler 4005.

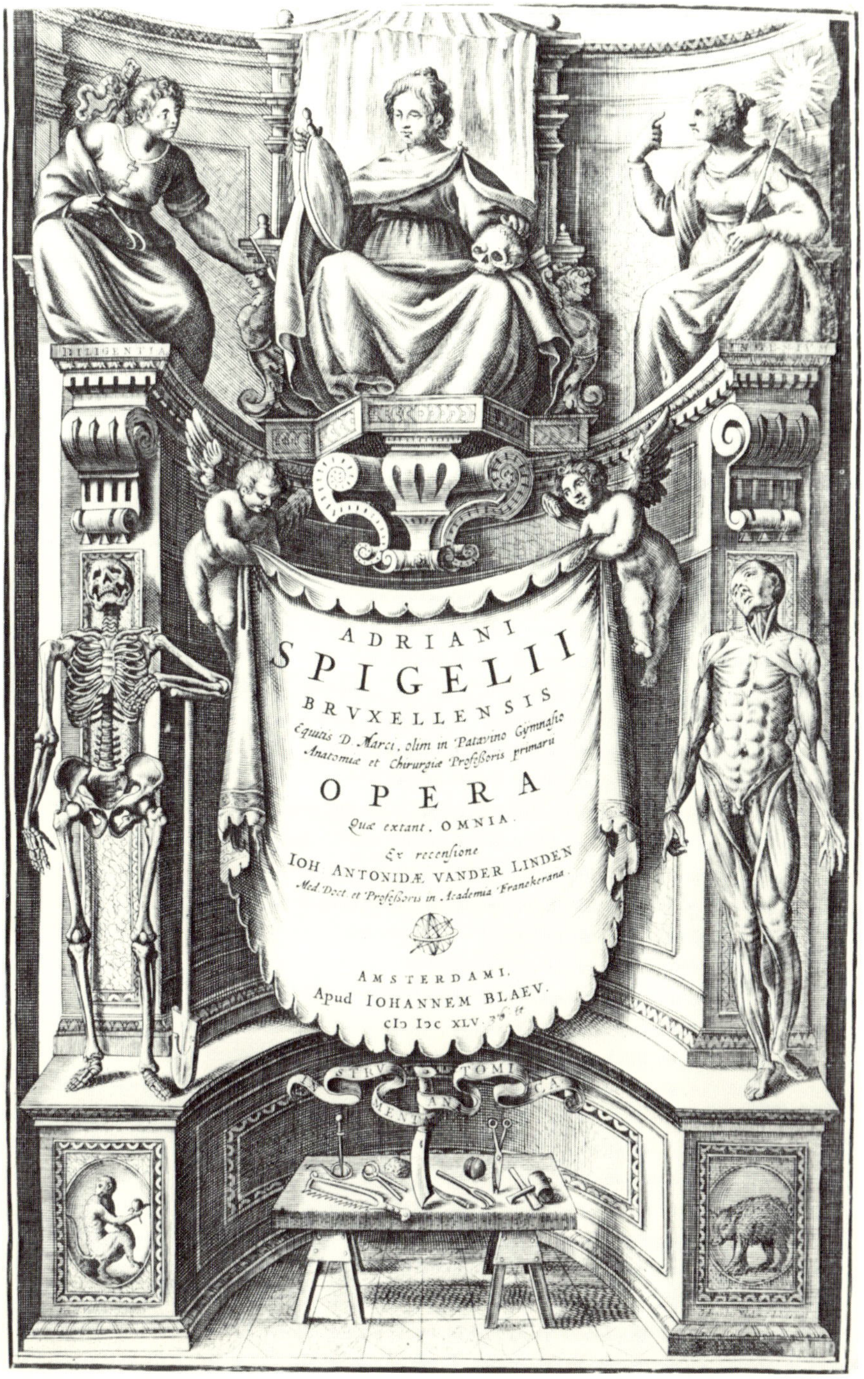

No. 284. Spiegel. *Opera.* The engraved title page from Spiegel's collected works.

*282. ———. *De formato foetu. . . . Epistolae duae anatomicae. Tractatus de arthritide.* Padua: Apud J. B. de Martinis, & L. Pasquatus [1626]. [8] 104 pp., 9 plates. 39.8 cm. Vellum.

"Spigelius' son-in-law, the physician Liberalis Crema of Padua, had bought several. . .copperplates from Casserius' grandson and when in 1626 he wished to publish a few selections from the posthumous works of his father-in-law, he chose nine appropriate plates and added them with his own explanations to these selections. . . .The plates. . .deal with the pregnant uterus, placenta, and the child. They are among Casserius' most beautiful engravings. Four of them represent entire female figures with the abdomen cut open. . . .The work was published at Crema's expense and is rare" (Choulant-Frank, p. 226).

Choulant-Frank, p. 226; Cushing S360; Waller 9119; Wellcome 6038.

283. ——— and GIULIO CASSERIO (1561–1616). *De humani corporis fabrica libri decem, tabulis XCIIX aeri incisis elegantissimis.* Venice: [Apud Evangelistam Deuchinum] 1627. [12] 330 (misnumbered 328) [12] pp., 97 plates. 41 cm. Calf, rebacked.

This lengthy and detailed anatomy text by Spiegel did much to bring order to anatomical nomenclature and to describe accurately certain muscle groups, particularly those of the back. When Spiegel died he asked in his will that a German physician, Daniel Bucretius (1600–1631), publish his unillustrated manuscript. In order to furnish illustrations, Bucretius asked the heirs of Casserio for the plates which Casserio had prepared for an anatomical work which had not been completed at the time of his death in 1616. Of the original seventy-eight, one was destroyed, and Bucretius added twenty plates by the same artists and engravers who had done Casserio's plates. Bucretius published the plates separately as well as with Spiegel's text under the title *Tabulae anatomicae*. They are among the finest produced in the seventeenth century and are remarkable for their accuracy, beauty of execution, and tasteful arrangement.

Choulant-Frank, p. 225; Cushing C114 and S361; Garrison-Morton 381; Waller 1812 and 9121; Wellcome 6040 (1632 ed.).

*284. ———. *Opera quae extant omnia. Ex recensione Joh. Antonidae vander Linden.* 2 vols. in 1. Amsterdam: Apud Johannem Blaeu, 1645. Vol. I: [24] 303 [14] 199 [4] 48 [3] xxxvi [10] xxxvii–lxxxvi [5] pp.; Vol. II: [8] 155 [8] pp., illus., plates, port. 40.8 cm. Newly rebound in full polished calf.

This splendidly produced collection of Spiegel's works edited by Johannes Antonides van der Linden (1609–1664), contains 117 copperplate engravings, many of them of primary importance in the history of medical and anatomic illustration. Of first interest are the plates of Casserio and the twenty plates added by Daniel Bucretius for Spiegel's *De humani corporis fabrica* (see No. 283).

In addition to Spiegel's works, these volumes contain Gaspare Aselli's *De lactibus sive lacteis venis*, with four engravings; William Harvey's *De motu cordis*, with a fine

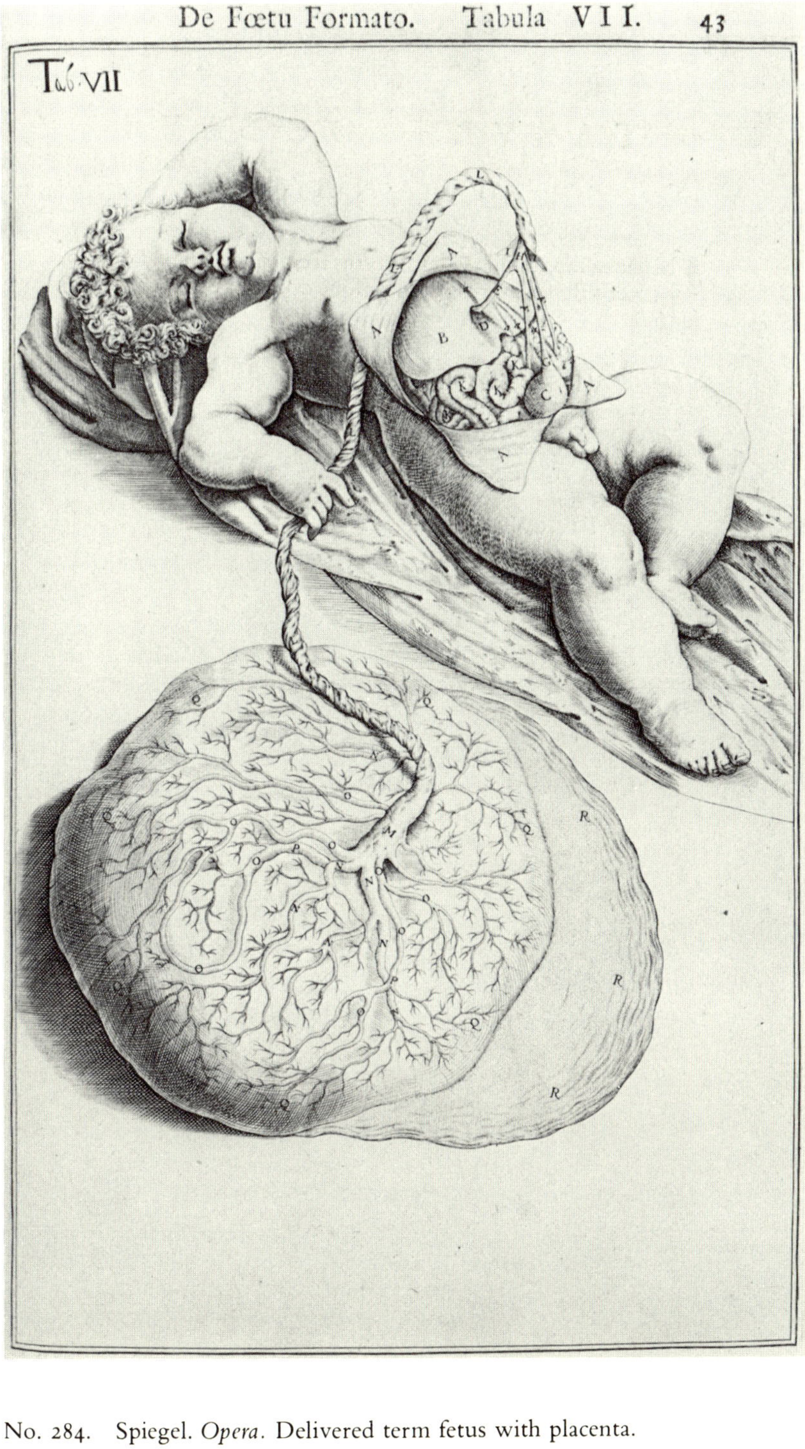

No. 284. Spiegel. *Opera.* Delivered term fetus with placenta.

version of the plate illustrating the valves of the veins; Johannes Walaeus' *Epistolae duae, de motu chyli & sanguinis*; and Linden's *De monstrosis vermibus, observatio rara.*

Choulant-Frank, p. 226; Cushing S363; Keynes 5; Waller 9124.

MELCHIOR SEBISCH (1578–1674?). *De notis virginitatis.*

See No. 239.

MARCO AURELIO SEVERINO (1580–1656). *De efficaci medicinae libris tribus.*

See No. 247.

*285. JEAN RIOLAN (1580–1657). *Opuscula anatomica nova. . . . Instauratio magna physicae & medicinae, per novam doctrinam de motu circulatorio sanguinis in corde.* London: Typis Milonis Flesher, 1649. [4] 536 pp. 18.7 cm. Vellum.

Riolan was a brilliant Parisian anatomist, but he was the leading opponent and most persistent critic of Harvey's teaching on the circulation of the blood. He was the critic whom Harvey took most seriously, but Harvey remained silent for twenty-one years, until the appearance of this book, to which Harvey replied in two essays published together in the same year. (These appeared in later editions of Harvey's *De motu cordis*. See Nos. 256 ff. in this catalogue). Riolan maintained the belief in partial circulation through the lungs and that the chief circulation was through the septum of the heart. Curiously enough, "Riolan maintained that if dissections no longer agreed with the descriptions of Galen, it should be attributed to the fact that nature had changed since Galen's time, but that one should not admit that Galen was wrong" (Arturo Castiglioni, *A history of medicine*. New York, 1946. p. 519). A large portion of this work is on the anatomical works of Spiegel, Bartholin, Du Laurens, Bauhin, Hofmann, Vesling, and Parisano.

Cushing R168: Osler 733; Russell 703; Waller 8000.

*286. ———. *A sure guide; or, The best and nearest way to physick and chyrurgery. . . . Being an anatomical description of the whole body of man, and its parts. . . . Written in Latin. . . . Englished by Nicholas Culpeper.* 3rd ed. London: Printed by John Streater, 1671. [8] 288 [11] pp., 24 plates. 29.7 cm.

First published in 1649, this work was considered the best anatomical textbook of its time. Riolan added greatly to anatomical knowledge, and his textbook was widely used for many years, being translated into several languages. The twenty-four plates are taken from the *Syntagma anatomicum*, an anatomical manual by Johann Vesling (see No. 303).

Cushing R170; Osler 3810; Russell 705.

*287. JAMES PRIMEROSE (1580–1659). *De vulgi erroribus in medicina libri IV.* Rotterdam: Ex officina Arnoldi Leers, 1658. [20] 561 pp. 12.6 cm. Contemporary sheep, spine repaired.

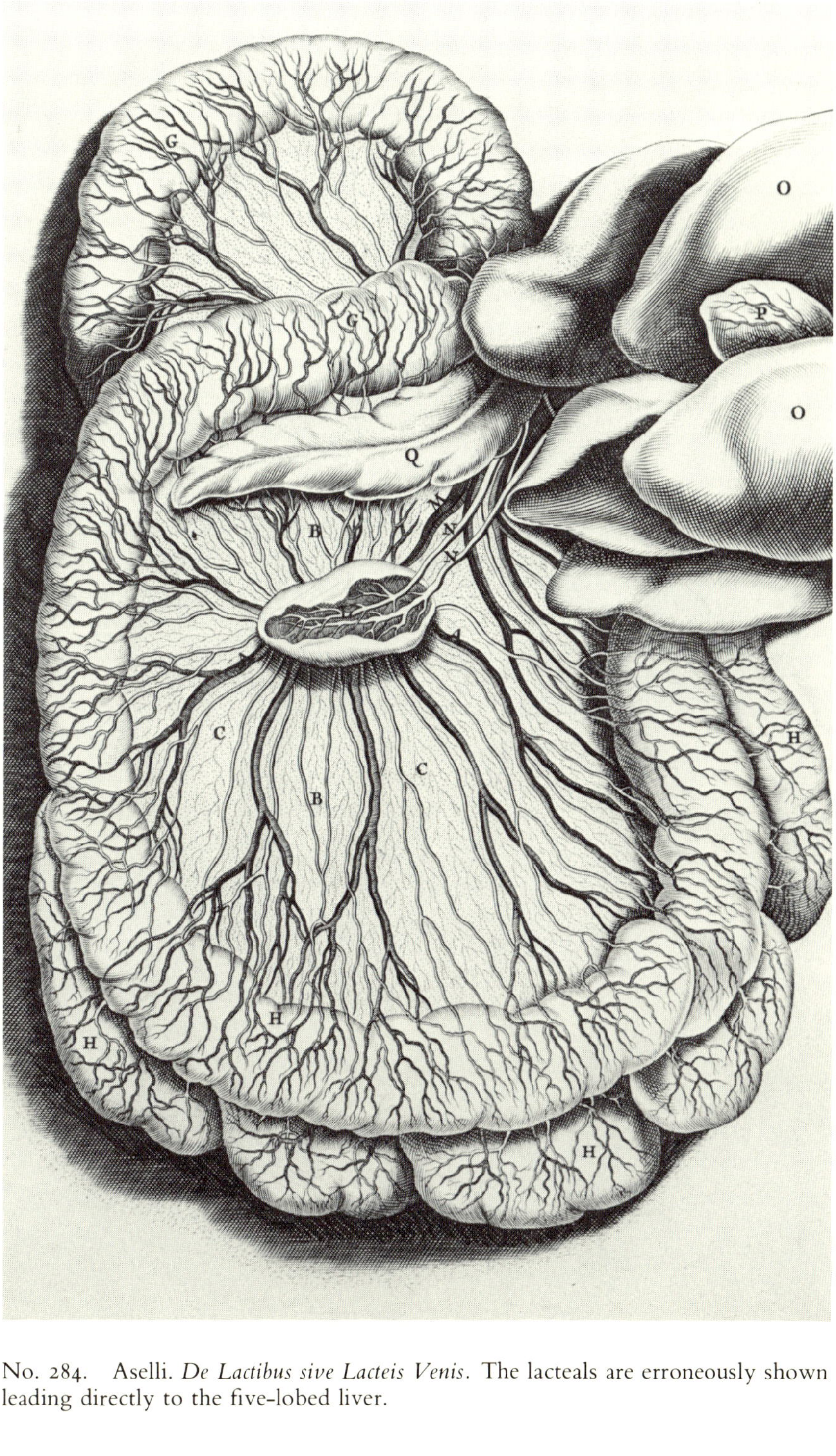

No. 284. Aselli. *De Lactibus sive Lacteis Venis.* The lacteals are erroneously shown leading directly to the five-lobed liver.

Primerose, though of Scottish parentage, was born and educated in France. He went to England, where he became a Fellow of the College of Physicians of London, William Harvey having been on his examining board. In 1630 Primerose issued a violent attack on Harvey's teaching on the circulation of the blood (see No. 256). The present book, first published in London in 1683, is a curious work on a variety of topics, including the choice of physicians and nurses, on taking mercury, on tobacco and opium, and the falsity of astrology and almanac prognosticators, as well as a continued attack on Harvey.

Cushing P395; Osler 3735.

———. *Exercitationes & animadversiones.*

See Nos. 256 and 257.

———. *Animadversiones in theses, quas pro circulatione sanguinis Henricus Le Roy disputandas proposuit.*

See No. 257.

———. *Animadversiones in Johannis Walaei disputationem medicam.*

See No. 257.

———. *De usu lienis sententia.*

See No. 257.

———. *Antidotum adversus Henrici Regii Spongiam.*

See No. 257.

GASPARE ASELLI (1581–1626). *De lactibus, sive lacteis venis.*

See Nos. 257 and 284.

*288. CASPAR BARTHOLIN (1585–1629). *Institutiones anatomicae.* Leiden: Apud Franciscum Hackium, 1641. [xx] 408 [12] 409–496 [44] pp., illus., 8 fold. plates. 18.2 cm. Polished calf.

The Bartholin family—Caspar, Thomas (see No. 324), and Caspar *secundus* (1655–1738)—made many contributions to Danish medicine during the seventeenth century when ducts, glands, and blood vessels were recognized as conduits for body fluids rather than as static tubes or reservoirs. Caspar *secundus* gave the family name to the major sublingual duct and to Bartholin's glands at the vaginal orifice. Thomas is known for his description of the thoracic duct and his work with the lymphatic vessels. Thomas also edited and republished many of Caspar's writings including the present work. It was first published in 1611 and went through four editions as well as several translations. The majority of the book's seventy anatomical engravings and eight folding plates were taken from the work

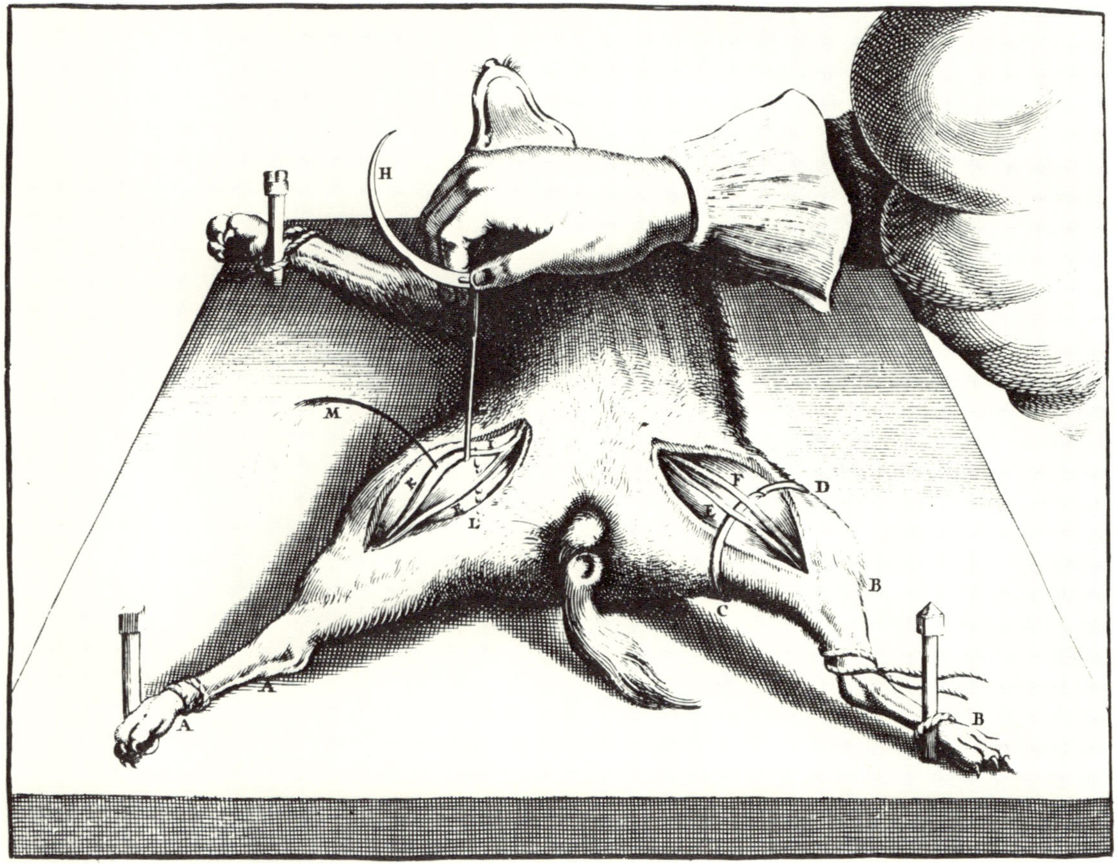

No. 284. Walaeus. *De Motu Chyli & Sanguinis*. Demonstration of centripetal flow of venous blood in the crural vein (K) of the dog.

of other anatomists. Many of the engravings of the brain were drawn by Sylvius and appear in print for the first time in this edition. The work also contains the *Epistolae duae . . . de motu sanguinis* of Johannes Walaeus, an ardent supporter of Harvey.

Cushing B96; Waller 702 (1645 ed.); Wellcome II, p. 106.

*289. [PETER LAUREMBERG] (1585–1639). *Anonymi Introductio anatomica.* Leiden: Apud Philippum Bonk, 1744. xvi, 157 [31] pp., 3 fold. plates. 20.1 cm. Old marbled limp boards.

This introductory work to the study of anatomy is of unknown authorship but has been attributed to the editor of the 1618 edition, Peter Lauremberg. The text, printed with Greek and Latin on opposite pages, borrows freely from ancient authors, particularly Aristotle. The work has been heavily annotated by Daniel Wilhelm Triller and Johann Stephan Bernard (1718–1793). The two full-page engravings of male figures and the folding plate of a head were taken from a Leiden manuscript of indefinite date and are merely linear drawings with rather poor proportions.

Osler 3057 (1618 ed.); Waller 432; Wellcome III, p. 456.

*290. THOMAS REINESIUS (1587–1667). *Ad viros clariss[imos] D. Casp. Hofmannun, Christ. Ad. Rupertum . . . Epistolae.* Leipzig: Sumtibus Johannis Scheibii, 1660. [10] 681 [11] pp., front. (port.), illus., fold. tables. 20 cm.

Reinesius, town physician of Altenburg, Germany, was a scholar of some renown who carried on a considerable correspondence. These seventy-five letters to the physician Caspar Hofmann (1572–1648) and the historian Christoph Adam Rupert (1612–1647), both professors at the University of Altdorf, are mostly on topics outside the sphere of medicine. One of the letters, however, from Reinesius to Hofmann, dated Ascension Day, 1640, is of considerable interest for the early history of the reception of Harvey's theory of the circulation. Hofmann, one of the few contemporaries quoted in Harvey's *De motu cordis*, was visited by Harvey in 1636, when he demonstrated circulation to him. Even so, Hofmann continued to reject Harvey's theory. Reinesius' letter deals at length with Harvey's theory, its attack by Primerose and others, and with earlier theories.

291. JAKOB DE BONDT (1592–1631). *De medicina Indorum.* Leiden: Apud Franciscum Hackium, 1642. [6] 212 [4] pp. 12.3 cm. Modern calf, in slipcase.

A Dutch physician educated at Leiden, Bondt entered the service of the East India Company and was sent to Djakarta, Java, where he spent the last four years of his life, dying at the early age of thirty-nine. His writings were preserved and published posthumously by his brother. This important and rare work is divided into four sections: 1) criticisms of the third book of Garcia de Orta's (see No. 145) treatise on Asian materia medica; 2) the maintenance of a healthy diet; 3) Indian methods of treatment; and 4) obervations from autopsies. Bondt includes the first

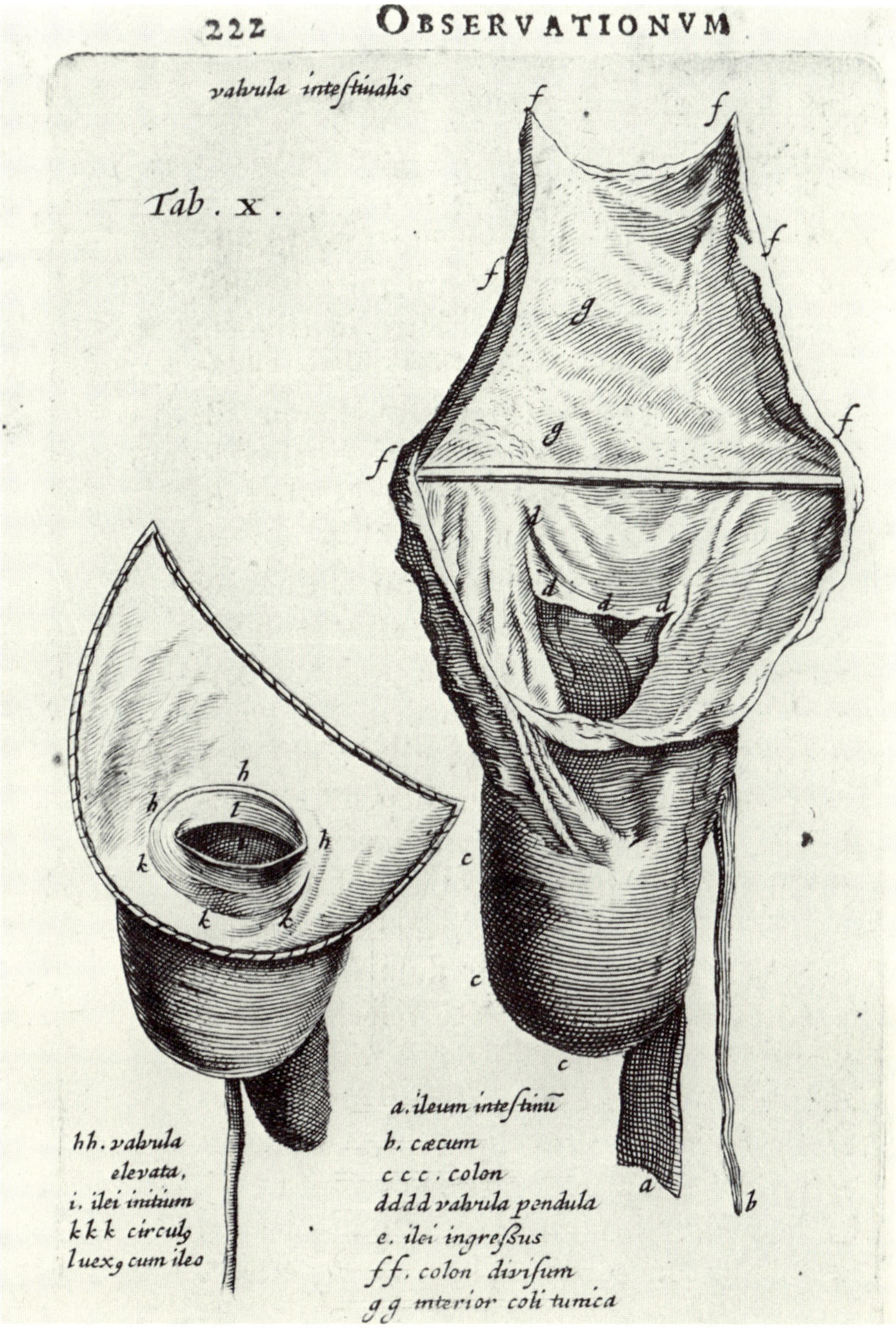

No. 292. Tulp. *Observationes Medicae.* The ileo-cecal valve, "Tulp's valve."

modern descriptions of cholera, tropical dysentery, and yaws in this work, making it a milestone in the history of medicine.

Garrison-Morton 2263; Waller 1297; Wellcome II, p. 201.

PIERRE GASSENDI (1592–1655). *De septo cordis pervio, observatio.*

See No. 239.

*292. NICOLAAS TULP (1593–1674). *Observationes medicae.* Amsterdam: Apud Ludovicum Elzevirium, 1652. [16] 403 pp., illus. 15 cm. Limp vellum.

Along with other distinguished anatomists in Holland, Tulp, a professor of anatomy at Amsterdam, left a rich legacy of anatomical discoveries. His name is current in the eponym "Tulp's valve" (the ileo-cecal valve) and his face is familiar as the central figure in Rembrandt's painting, "Doctor Nicolaas Tulp Demonstrating the Anatomy of the Arm," which hangs in The Hague.

The present work, Tulp's only book, was first published in 1641. This enlarged edition contains the first descriptions of beri-beri and of what is probably diphtheria. Several interesting plates complement the book, including a well-known one showing a most comically bemused chimpanzee, erroneously labeled an "orang-outang."

Cushing T177; Garrison-Morton 3737; Osler 4126 (1672 ed.); Waller 9716.

JACOBUS DE BACK (ca. 1594–1658). *Dissertatio de corde.*

See Nos. 258, 259, 260, and 261.

*293. JOHANNES SCULTETUS (1595–1645). Χειροπλοθῆκη . . . *Armamentarium chirurgicum XLIII.* Ulm: Typis & impensis Balthasari Kühnen, 1655. 10, 132 [3] pp., 43 plates. 36.7 cm. Contemporary vellum.

Scultetus, born at Ulm on the Danube, was a pupil of Hieronymus Fabricius ab Aquapendente and Adriaan van de Spiegel at Padua where he received a doctorate in medicine, surgery, and philosophy. He eventually settled in Ulm as the city physician after having practiced for a time in Padua and Vienna. His "arsenal of surgery" was published a decade after his death by his nephew, Scultetus the Younger, who edited Scultetus' notes and issued them along with the excellent engravings. The work contains accounts of surgical instruments, methods of bandaging and splinting, numerous operative procedures (including amputation of the breast), obstetrical delivery by forceps, and one hundred of his case reports.

Cushing S172 (1665 ed.); Garrison-Morton 5571; Waller 8792.

*294. RENÉ DESCARTES (1596–1650). *Passiones animae.* Amsterdam: Apud Ludovicum Elzevirium, 1650. [23] 98 [5] pp. 20.2 cm. Modern decorated boards.

Cartesian physiology and philosophy had a powerful influence on the thinking of such men as Robert Hook, Giovanni Borelli, Jan Swammerdam, and Thomas

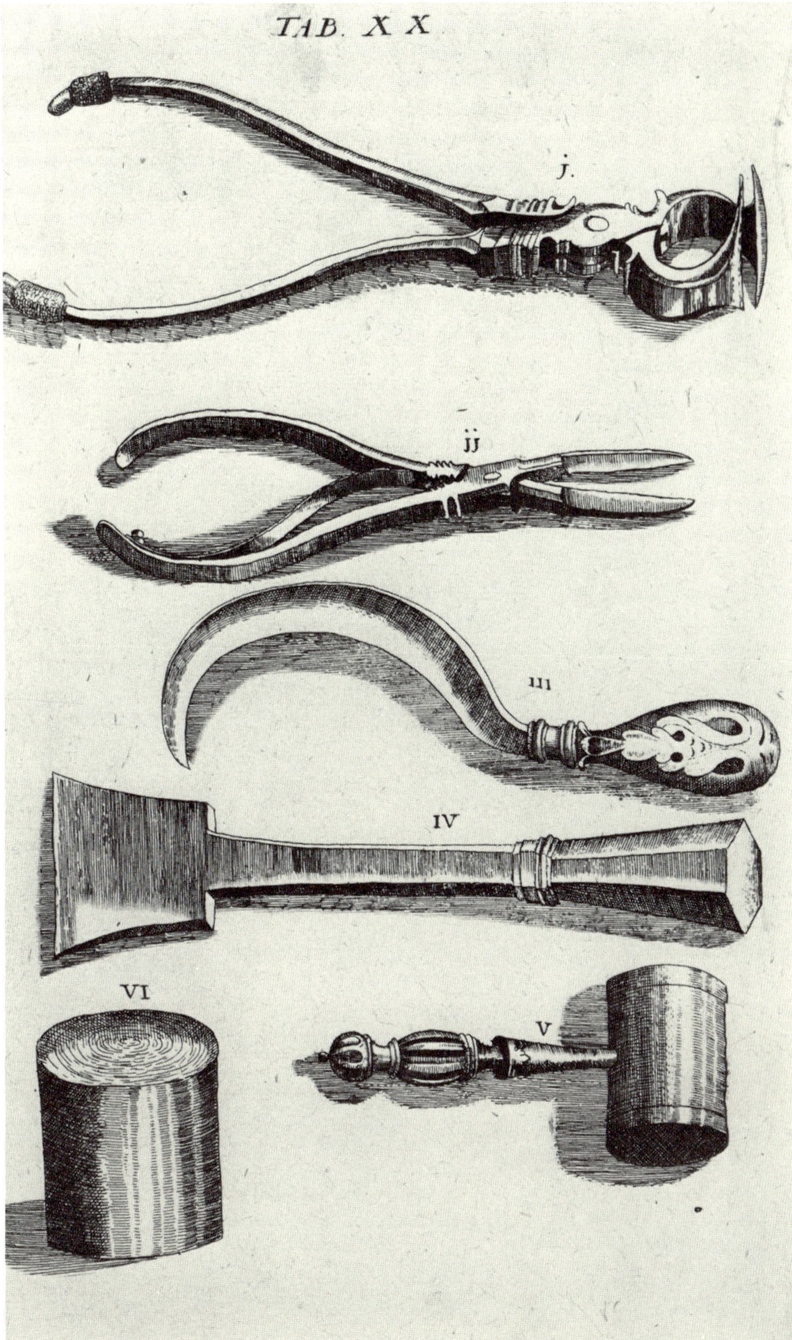

No. 293. Scultetus. *Armamentarium Chirurgicum.* Seventeenth-century instruments used in orthopedic surgery.

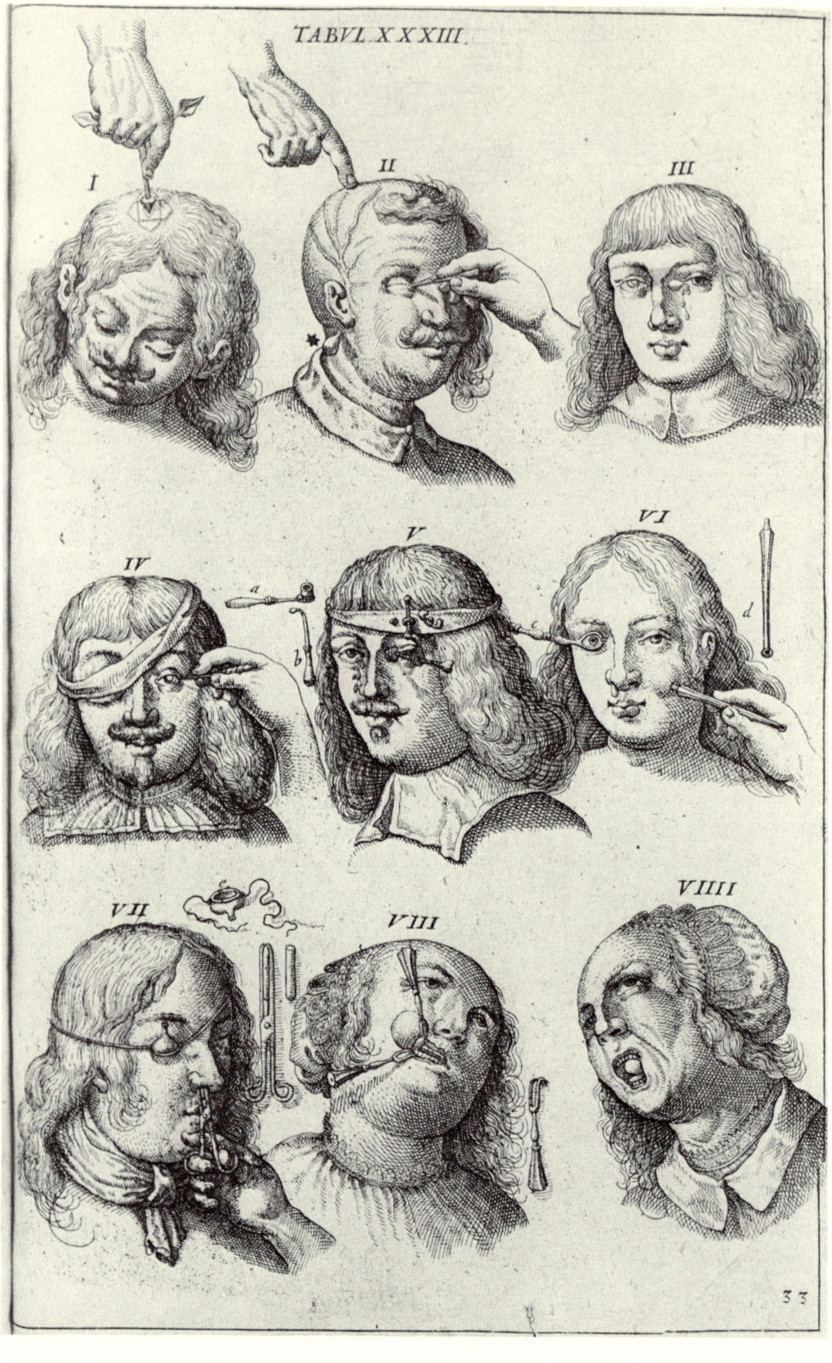

No. 293. Scultetus. *Armamentarium Chirurgicum.* Cranial, ophthalmic, and maxillofacial surgery.

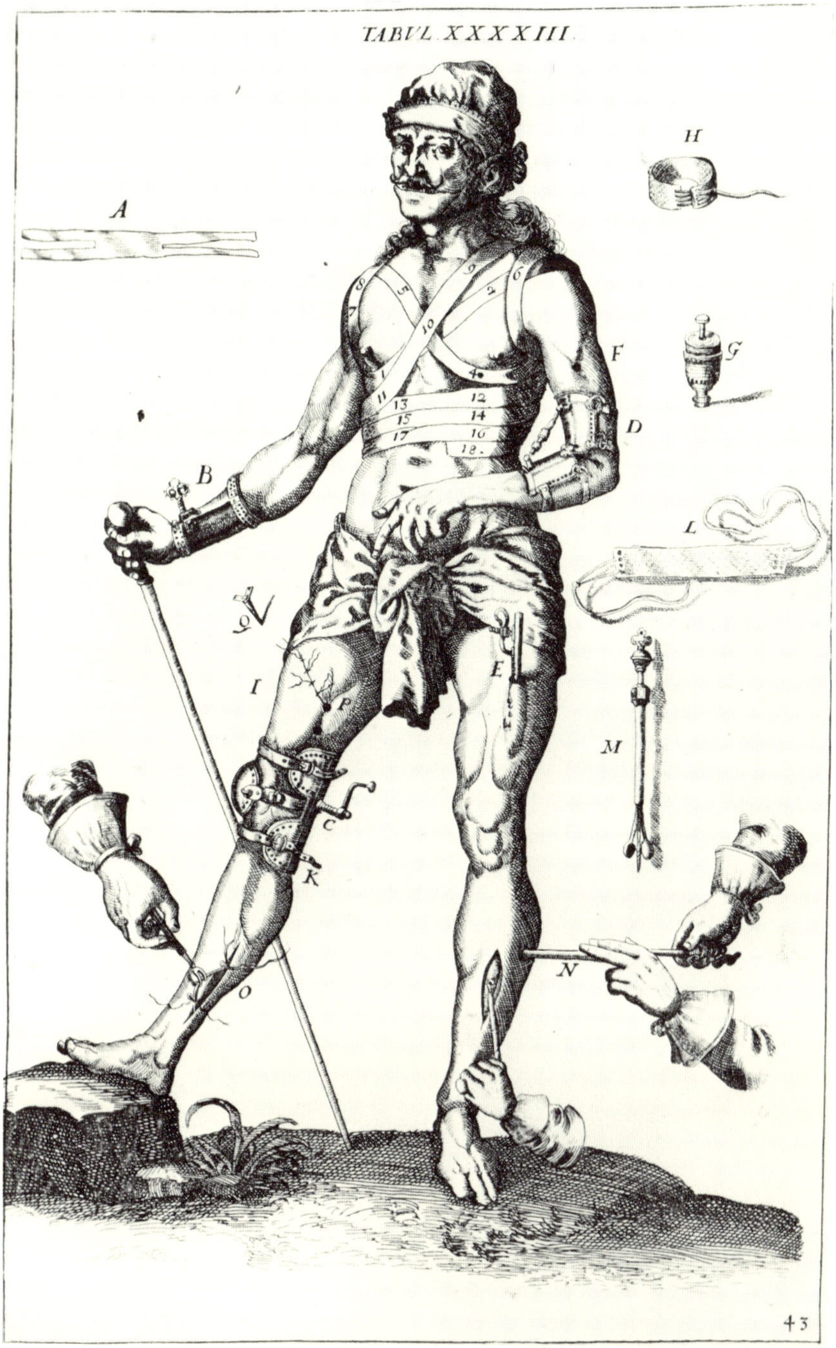

No. 293. Scultetus. *Armamentarium Chirurgicum.* Scultetus bandage (1–18), surgical appliances, instruments, and surgical exposures.

Willis. Descartes' theories helped to explain in understandable mechanistic terms the more puzzling problems of human physiology during a time when scientific research was expanding rapidly. This work, written for Queen Christina of Sweden, was first published in French a year before this Latin edition appeared. It was the last book that Descartes wrote, and in it he discusses psychology, ethics, and the relationship between mind and body.

Garrison-Morton 4965 (French ed., 1649); Wellcome II, p. 453.

*295. ———. *De homine. Figuris et latinitate donatus a Florentio Schuyl*. Leiden: Ex officina Hackiana, 1664. [36] 123 (misnumbered 121) [4] pp., illus., fold. plates. 20 cm. Quarter calf, newly rebound.

Descartes was prepared to publish this book in 1633 but decided to withhold it when he learned of Galileo's condemnation by the Church. As a result, the first edition was not published until 1662, twelve years after Descartes' death. The Latin translation preceded the French edition by two years, the present second Latin edition appearing the same year as the first French edition. It is sometimes called the first book on physiology, and that could be argued, but there is no doubt that the Cartesian philosophy exerted a tremendous effect on the evolution of medicine. This book could only have been written by a man who was basically a mathematician; it is step-by-step reasoning. Unfortunately, Descartes had little practical knowledge of the subject with which he was dealing and, when later investigation failed to confirm his theoretical structure, his work passed into oblivion. The many interesting illustrations have frequently been copied by other authors.

Cushing D118; Garrison-Morton 574 (1st ed., 1662); Osler 931 (1st ed.); Waller 2376; Wellcome II, p. 453.

*296. ———. *L'homme*. Paris: Charles Angot, 1664. [70] 448 [8] pp., illus. 23 cm. Contemporary calf.

This first French edition is the original text as composed by Descartes and edited by his good friend, Claude Clerselier (1614–1684). This edition also contains the first printing of his treatise *De la formation du foetus*, completed just before his death. The fine woodcuts in this edition were partly based on Descartes' drawings from the manuscript and partly prepared by the co-editors, Louis de la Forge (1632–1666?) and Gérard van Gutschoven (fl. 1660).

Cushing D121; Osler 933 (1677 ed.); Wellcome II, p. 453.

*297. PIETRO DA CORTONA (1596–1669). *Tabulae anatomicae*. Rome: Impensis Fausti Amidei, Ex typographia Antonii de Rubeis, 1741. [4] 84 pp., 27 plates. 43.4 cm. Contemporary vellum.

Cortona was an Italian painter and architect, and this rare volume containing twenty-seven large anatomical plates has been attributed to him. Begun in 1618, the plates were engraved by Luca Ciamberlano, but it is not known why they lay unpublished for more than a century. They were edited, in this first edition, by

DE RENE' DESCARTES. 81

perficie interieure du cerueau, ſe raporte à chacun des autres membres; & chacun des autres points de la ſuperficie de la glande H à chacun des coſtez vers leſquels ces membres peuuent eſtre tournez : En ſorte que les mouuemens de ces membres, & leurs idées, peuuent eſtre cauſez reciproquement l'vn par l'autre.

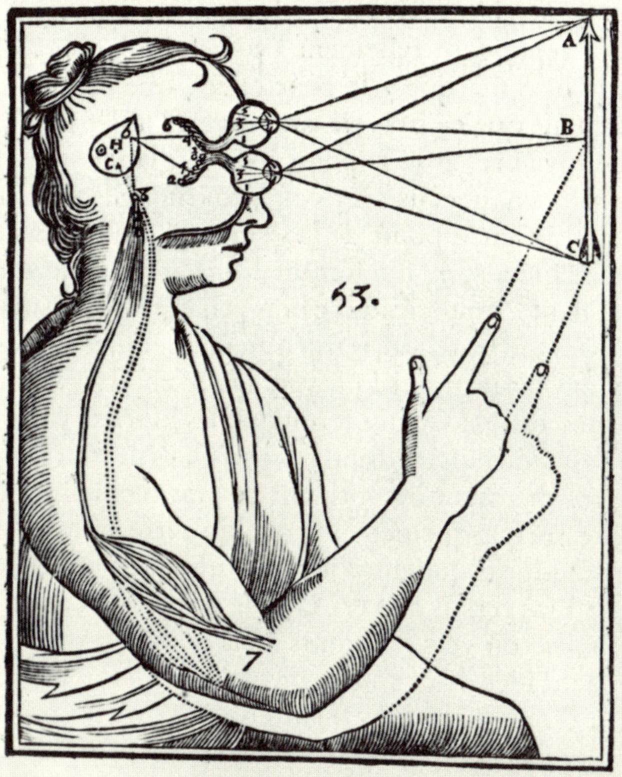

Et de plus, pour entendre icy par occaſion, comment, lors que les deux yeux de cette machine, & les organes LXXVIII. Comment vne idée

L

No. 296. Descartes. *L'homme*. Light rays strike the retinas, nerve forces are then directed through the pineal gland, the "seat of the soul," and vital spirit activates the muscles.

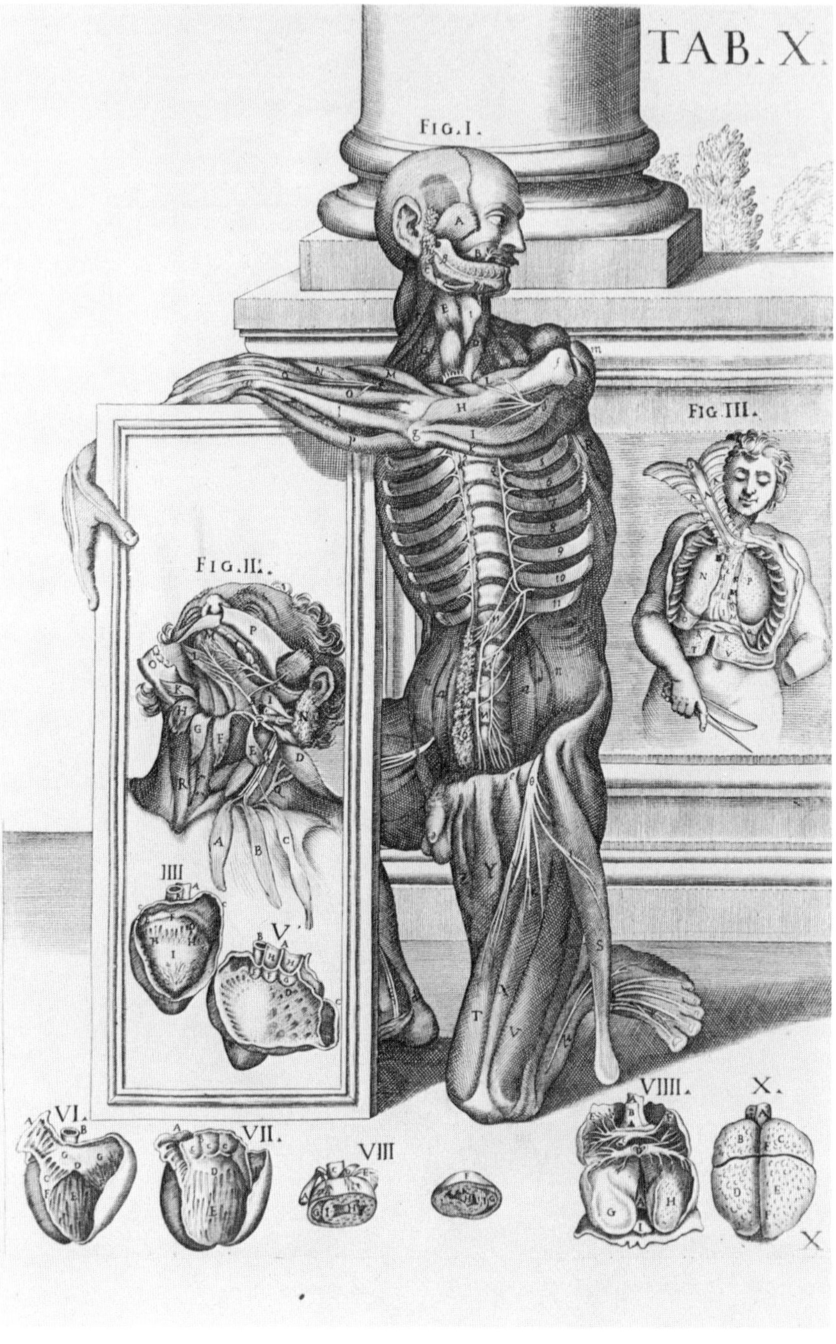

No. 297. Pietro da Cortona. *Tabulae Anatomicae.*

Gaetano Petrioli (fl. 1740) and it is likely that either he or a previous owner of the plates added the numerous torsos and other anatomical parts that surround each main figure. The anatomical additions were taken from the works of Vesalius, Casserius, and others by a different artist and engraver. The figures were removed from the plates in the second and last edition. Cortona's figures are, for the most part, representations of entire bodies in action or in some active attitude and were intended for use by physicians.

Choulant-Frank, p. 235–239; Cushing B334; Waller 983 (1788 ed.); Wellcome II, p. 146.

*298. GIOVANNI IMPERIALI (1596?–1670). *Musaeum historicum et physicum*. 2 pts. in 1 vol. Venice: Apud Juntas, 1640. Pt. I: [16] 122 pp.; Pt. II: [8] 219 [22] pp., ports. 22.2 cm. Old vellum.

The first part of this work is a collection of engraved full-page portraits and short biographical sketches of famous men of science, medicine, and religion. Among the nearly sixty portraits are those of Arnoldus de Villanova, Ulisse Aldrovandi, Jean Fernel, Girolamo Fracastoro, Giovanni Argenterio, Jean Riolan, Giovanni Battista della Porta, and Andreas Vesalius. The second part is an interesting study of memory and the nature of genius based in part on the lives of the men whose portraits appear in the first section of the book.

Cushing I3; Osler 6686; Waller 16011; Wellcome 3394.

THOMAS BRIAN (fl. 1637). *Der englische Wahrsager*.

See No. 465.

*299. FRANCIS GLISSON (1597–1677). *Anatomia hepatis*. London: Typis Du-Gardianis, 1654. [48] 458 [13] pp., illus., 2 fold. plates. 16.5 cm. Calf.

Glisson was a graduate of Cambridge and Regius professor of physic there for more than forty years, although he was almost never in residence, as he carried on a busy medical practice in London. He was a founder of the Royal Society and one-time president of the Royal College of Physicians. In this book he gives the first description of the capsule of the liver and describes its blood supply. Here, too, is the description of the sphincter of the bile duct. In its time, the *Anatomia hepatis* was the most important treatise thus far on the physiology of the digestive system.

Cushing G288; Garrison-Morton 972; Russell 322; Wellcome III, p. 126.

*300. ———. ———. The Hague: Apud Arnoldum Leers, 1681. [50] 552 [12] pp., front. (port.), illus., plates (diagrs., part fold.). 13 cm. Vellum.

A later edition of the work which assured Glisson's fame. This copy has the famous frontispiece, the ornamental title page, and a full-page portrait of the author.

Osler 2760; Waller 3585; Wellcome III, p. 126.

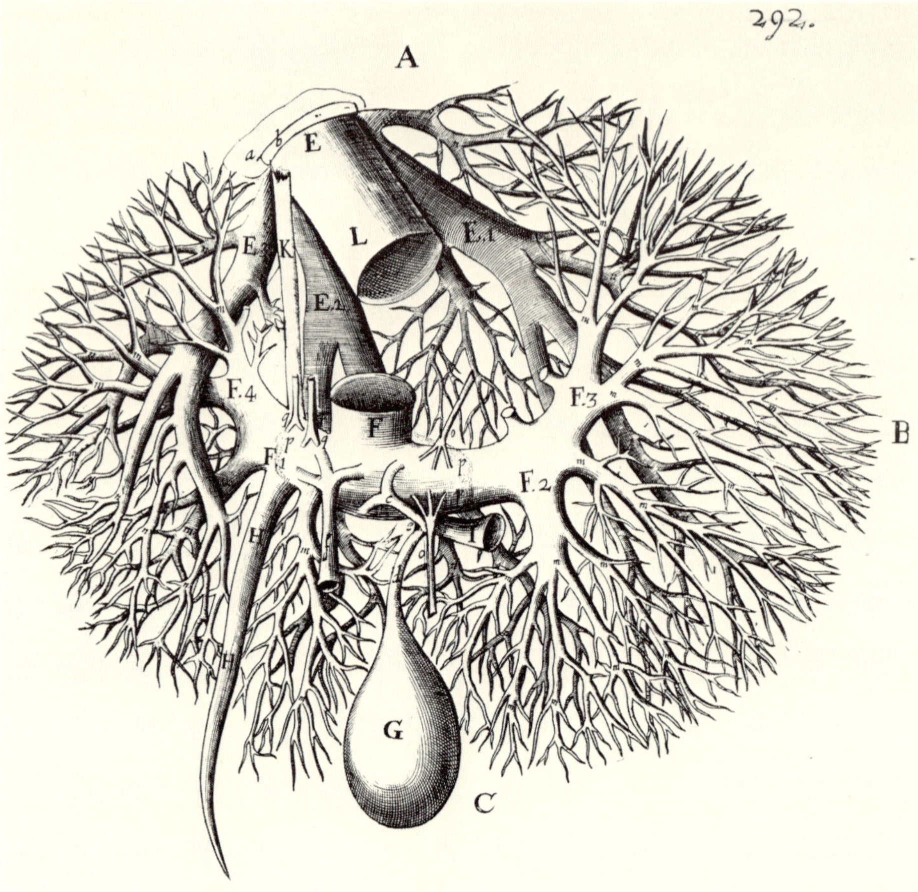

No. 299. Glisson. *Anatomia Hepatis.* A schematic portrayal of the biliary and vascular systems of the liver.

*301. ———. *Tractatus de rachitide sive morbo puerili.* The Hague: Apud Arnoldum Leers, 1682. [18] 412 pp., illus. 12.7 cm.

Glisson was a most able clinician as well as anatomist, physiologist, and pathologist, and the present work, first published in London in 1650, gave the first clinical description of rickets with an early note on Barlow's disease (infantile scurvy).

Garrison-Morton 3729 (1650 ed.); Osler 2757 (1650 ed.); Waller 3589 (1650 ed.); Wellcome III, p. 126.

*302. ———. *Tractatus de ventriculo et intestinis. Cui praemittitur alius, De partibus continentibus in genere; & in specie de iis abdominis.* Leiden: Apud Petrum vander Aa, 1691. [32] 591 pp., front. (port.), plates. 13 cm. Vellum.

First published in 1677, this important work on the stomach and intestines contains Glisson's original concept of "irritability" not only as the prime cause of muscular contraction but as a property of all human tissues. The view was materialistic and mechanistic and, like all of Glisson's hypotheses, shows an attempt by an able thinker to explain important physiological phenomena. This edition also contains Glisson's treatise on the abdomen.

Cushing G292 (1st ed., 1677); Garrison-Morton 579 (1st ed.); Osler 2762 (1st ed.); Wellcome III, p. 126 (1st ed).

*303. JOHANN VESLING (1598–1649). *Syntagma anatomicum, locis plurimis auctum, emendatum, novisque iconibus diligenter exornatum.* 2nd ed. Padua: Typis Pauli Frambotti, 1651. [14] 274 [10] pp., 24 plates, port. 24.8 cm. Limp vellum.

A native Westphalian, Vesling lived for a time in Egypt and Palestine before becoming professor of anatomy at Padua in 1632. He was also director of the botanical gardens and made scientific journeys to Canada and the Orient to study botany. He published the first edition of his anatomical manual in 1641 without illustrations. This second edition contained twenty-four copperplates and a finely engraved title page depicting the anatomical theater at Padua. The work proved to be very popular and was translated into German, Dutch, and English.

Choulant-Frank, p. 243; Cushing V119; Osler 4166; Waller 9932.

*304. ———. *The anatomy of the body of man.* London: Printed by Peter Cole, 1653. [15] 192 pp., 24 plates, port. 28 cm. Contemporary calf.

This is the first English edition of Vesling's *Syntagma anatomicum*, translated by Nicholas Culpeper, the English physician and herbalist.

Choulant-Frank, p. 243; Cushing V116; Russell 834.

*305. HENRICUS REGIUS (1598–1679). *Fundamenta physices.* Amsterdam: Apud Ludovicum Elzevirium, 1646. [16] 306 pp., illus., diagrs. 19.9 cm.

Regius was professor of botany, theoretical medicine, and anatomy at Utrecht and a pupil, friend, and ardent follower of Descartes. This book on physical philosophy created something of a sensation when it appeared because the author departed from his adherence to Cartesian doctrine and, as a result, was denounced by Descartes. The book contains numerous scientific and anatomical woodcuts, with those of the magnet being of special interest. The book is very rare and is not found in the major medical bibliographies.

———. *Spongia*.

See No. 257.

*306. GUY PATIN (1601–1672). *Lettres choisies*. 2nd ed. Paris: Chez Jean Petit, 1688. [20] 432 pp., front. (port.). 14.9 cm. Vellum.

"Guy Patin, an eminent member of the Faculty of Paris, declared Harvey's theory 'paradoxical, useless, false, impossible, absurd and harmful.' This statement is characteristic of Patin. . . . He carried on violent quarrels in the name of the faculty with all innovators, against the physicians of Montpellier, against Renaudot, van Helmont, and many others. His letters . . . give a vivid and bold picture of the condition of physicians and of the Paris Faculty at that time" (Arturo Castiglioni, *A history of medicine*. New York, 1946. pp. 519–520). Although Patin was dean of the faculty at Paris and was a brilliant lecturer, "he contributed little or nothing to the literature of the profession" but his letters "remain as a permanent contribution to literature" (Osler 5277). This edition contains 196 letters, many of them treating of medical topics in Patin's typical vein.

*307. ———. ———. 3rd ed. 2 vols. Paris: Chez Jean Petit, 1692. Vol. I: [22] 573 pp.; Vol. II: 583 pp. 15.2 cm. Calf.

A reissue of what appears to be a third edition of Patin's letters with the addition of three hundred letters above what appeared in the second edition. Altogether there have been some fifteen editions or printings of portions of the correspondence.

Osler 5277; Waller 17548.

*308. ATHANASIUS KIRCHER (1602–1680). *Scrutinium physico-medicum contagiosae luis, quae pestis dicitur*. Rome: Typis Mascardi, 1658. [16] 252 [15] pp. 22.4 cm. Contemporary vellum.

Kircher was one of the earliest scientists to use the microscope to investigate the causes of disease. A very learned individual, Kircher was a mathematician, physicist, optician, Orientalist, musician, and physician. In this work, he details seven experiments on the nature of putrefaction, showing how maggots and other living creatures are developed in living matter. He also describes his finding that the blood of plague patients is filled with countless "worms" that are invisible to the naked eye but visible through the microscope. He was one of the earliest to suggest the germ theory of disease.

Cushing K94; Garrison-Morton 5118; Osler 3120 (1659 ed.); Waller 5295; Wellcome III, p. 395.

309. MENSA PHILOSOPHICA. Leipzig: Imprimebant haeredes Francisci Scnelboltzii, typis haeredum Beyeri, 1603. [24] 526 pp. 12.6 cm.

This popular and well-known book has been attributed to Michael Scott (1175?–1234?) and Theobaldus Anguilbertus (fl. 1500), but the authorship is not certain. First published at Cologne in 1480, it appeared in eight more editions before 1500 and several more during the sixteenth century. Its medical importance lies in the fact that much of the book is devoted to matters concerning various foods, wine, and the diet as well as hygiene. The book also contains Ottmar Luscinius' (1487–1537) *Joci ac sales mire festivi* [Wondrously festive jokes and witticisms].

Cushing, Incunabula 99 (1485 ed.); Durling 3066 (1500 ed.); Goff M 491 (1480 ed.); Hain-Copinger 3984 (1480 ed.); Klebs 676.1 (1480 ed.); Osler 7491 (1589 ed.); Waller 19988 (1514 ed.); Wellcome 5888 (1514 ed.).

PIETRO DE CASTRO (1603–ca. 1657). *Il colostro.*

See No. 234.

JOHANNES WALAEUS (1604–1649). *Epistola prima de motu chyli et sanguinis.*

See No. 257.

———. *Epistola secunda de motu sanguinis.*

See No. 257.

———. *Epistolae duae, quibus Harveii doctrina roboratur.*

See No. 262.

———. *Epistolae duae, de motu chyli & sanguinis.*

See Nos. 284 and 288.

———. *De motu chyli et sanguinis.*

See No. 325.

*310. JOHANN RUDOLPH GLAUBER (1604?–1668?). *Pharmacopoea spagyrica.* 3 pts. in 1 vol. Amsterdam: Apud Joannem Janssonium, 1654–1657. Pt. I: 76 pp.; Pt. II: 128 pp.; Pt. III: 48 pp. 15.2 cm. Vellum.

Glauber, a German chemist, is probably best remembered for the salt named after him (Glauber's salt). His chemical and pharmaceutical philosophy was much like that of Paracelsus, a blending of the animal, vegetable, and mineral kingdoms. But he was a keen observer and experimenter, keeping reliable records, which assured him a place among the pioneers of technical chemistry.

This work is one of his many pharmaceutical works. Waller records a total of seven parts of this work.

Osler 2745 (Pts. I and II only); Waller 3577; Wellcome III, p. 123.

GEORGE ENT (1604–1689). *Mantissa anatomica.*

See No. 333.

*311. Sir THOMAS BROWNE (1605–1682). *Pseudodoxia epidemica; or, Enquiries into very many received tenents and commonly presumed truths.* London: Printed by T.H. for E. Dod, 1646. 386 pp. 26.5 cm.

Browne, a noted physician, was also one of the great English writers of the seventeenth century. He is perhaps best known for his popular and often translated *Religio medici* which expounds his personal religious philosophy and the tenets by which he lived. The present work, often called "Vulgar errors," is an unusual and interesting work in which Browne attacks falsely-held traditions, superstitions, and folklore relating to the nature of plants, animals, and man. This copy has been extensively annotated by someone with an excellent classical education and scholarly background.

Cushing B774; Osler 4488; Waller 19462; Wellcome II, p. 253.

*312. ———. *The works.* 4 pts. in 1 vol. London: Printed for Tho. Basset, Ric. Chiswell, Tho. Sawbridge, Charles Mearn, and Charles Brome, 1686. Part I: [18] 316 [11] pp.; Part II: [12] 102 pp.; Part III: [8] 52 pp.; Part IV: [5] 103 [3] pp., front., illus. 32.4 cm.

This first collected edition of Browne's works contains a full-page portrait by the sculptor R. White. In addition to *Pseudodoxia epidemica,* it contains his popular *Religio medici, Hydriotaphia or urn-burial, The Garden of Cyrus,* and other miscellaneous tracts. It does not contain two of his popular philosophically oriented works: *A letter to a friend* and *Christian morals.*

Osler 4522; Waller 1539; Wellcome II, p. 253.

*313. HONORÉ FABRI (1606–1688). *Tractatus duo: quorum prior est de plantis, et de generatione animalium; posterior de homine.* Paris: Apud Franciscum Muguet, 1666. [28] 440, 142 pp., fold. diagr. 23.9 cm. Contemporary calf.

The author of this work, a Jesuit priest and scientist of some renown, here presents the anatomy, physiology, and reproduction of man and plants. He also claims to have taught the principles of the circulation of the blood without having knowledge of Harvey's work. The sole illustration is a line drawing which demonstrates the role of light rays in the eye.

Wellcome III, p. 3.

314. GEORGE BATE (1608–1669). *Pharmacopoeia Bateana; or, Bates' dispensatory.* 4th ed. London: Printed for W. Innys, 1713. [16] 744 [12] pp. 18.3 cm. Blind-stamped calf.

Bate was physician-in-ordinary to the English Kings Charles I and Charles II, and to Oliver Cromwell. Bate's formulas and recipes were first published in 1688 by James Shipton (fl. 1710), a London apothecary. In 1694, William Salmon (see No. 429) translated the work from Latin and issued it under the present title. Salmon combined Bate's work with Jonathan Goddard's (1617?–1675) *Arcana Goddardiana.* Goddard, a London physician, was well known for a preparation called "Goddard's Drops" which he is reputed to have sold to Charles II for £1,500 and which he prepared from "Human bones, or rather Skulls well dry'd" (p. 136). Salmon's edition of the *Pharmacopoeia* was well received, went through several editions, and was translated into a number of European languages.

Cushing B157 (1694 ed.); Wellcome II, p. 113 (1694 ed.).

ROGER DRAKE (1608–1669). *Contra animadversiones Jac. Primirosii.*

See No. 257.

*315. GIOVANNI ALFONSO BORELLI (1608–1679). *De motu animalium.* 2 vols. Rome: Ex typographia Angeli Bernabò, 1680–1681. Vol. I: [12] 376 [12] pp., 14 plates; Vol. II: [4] 520 pp., 4 plates. 20.3 cm. Quarter calf.

Pupil of Galileo and teacher of Malpighi, Borelli's lasting fame is his dominating influence in the establishment of the Iatrophysical, or Iatromechanical, School of thought. The flourishing school of anatomy at Padua had given place to a new breed of scientists who wanted to know the *function* of anatomy. A Neapolitan mathematician, Borelli set up a laboratory in his home in Pisa in order to make application of mechanical laws to all physical phenomena. He regarded the human body essentially as a machine, its functions explained by the laws of physics. Though he carried this principle beyond the actual fact, he did make some original discoveries pertaining to the mechanics of respiration and circulation. He particularly investigated the action of muscles, and *De motu animalium* includes extensive calculations on the motor forces of muscles. The illustrations showing human beings and animals in various positions of muscle exertion could only have been conceived by one who was primarily a physicist and not an anatomist.

Cushing B499; Garrison-Morton 762; Osler 2087; Wellcome II, p. 204 (1685 ed.).

JOHANNES ANTONIDES VAN DER LINDEN (1609–1664). *De monstrosis vermibus, observatio rara.*

See No. 284.

*316. IJSBRAND VAN DIEMERBROECK (1609–1674). *Anatome corporis humani.* Lyons: Sumpt. Joan. Antonii Huguetan, 1679. [14] 606 [6] pp., 13 fold. plates. 24.3 cm. Old calf.

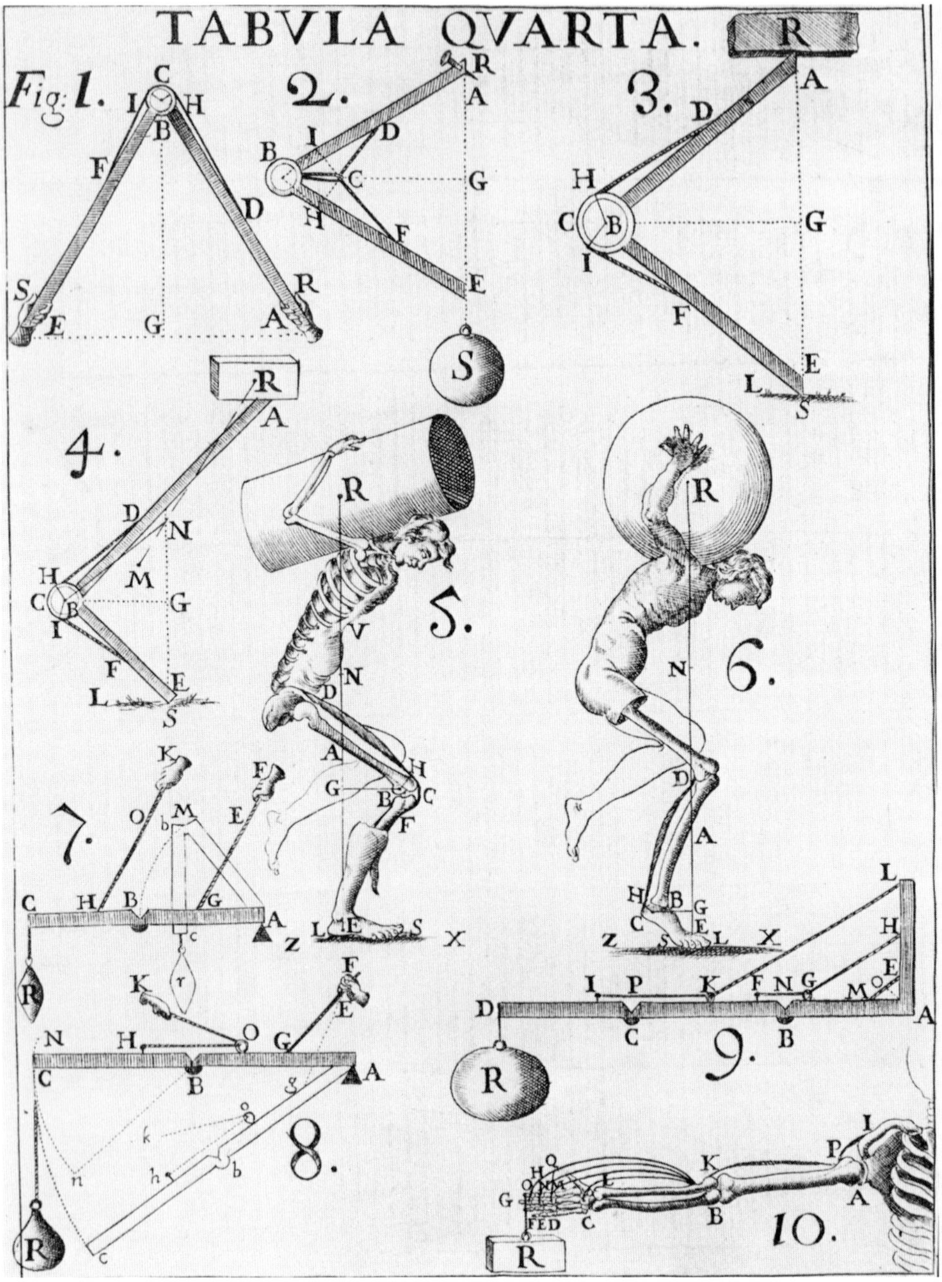

No. 315. Borelli. *De Motu Animalium.* The effects of muscular contraction, muscular tension, and weight bearing.

Diemerbroeck, professor of anatomy and medicine at Utrecht, is remembered not only for his studies of the plague but more especially for this work on anatomy. The first edition was published in 1672; it quickly became popular throughout Europe and was widely used through all of its later editions. The thirteen folding plates are finely etched and their simplicity makes them highly effective and instructive.

Cushing D149; Waller 2451 (Geneva, 1679 ed.); Wellcome II, p. 467.

*317. NATHANIEL HIGHMORE (1613–1685). *Exercitationes duae, quarum prior de passione hysterica: altere de affectione hypochondriaca.* Oxford: Excudebat A. Lichfield, impensis R. Davis, 1660. [11] 184 pp. 13.7 cm. Contemporary calf.

A contemporary and friend of William Harvey, Highmore, in his major work—*Corporis humani disquisitio anatomica* (1651)—presented several new anatomical findings including Highmore's antrum (sinus maxillaris) and Highmore's body in the testes. Highmore was among the many prominent scientists and physicians who founded the Royal Society in 1660. In his *History of generation* (1651), he disagreed with Harvey and continued to espouse the old doctrine of the preformation of the embryo as did other notable investigators such as Marcello Malpighi, Jan Swammerdam, and Théophile Bonet. In this work, Highmore concluded that hysteria was caused by a congestion of the blood in the heart and lungs. He was soon corrected, however, by Thomas Willis (see No. 343) who correctly surmised that it was a nervous disorder.

Osler 7713 (2nd ed., 1660); Waller 4457 (1677 ed.); Wellcome III, p. 263.

*318. FRANS LE BOË (1614–1672). *Idea praxeos medicae.* Venice: Typis Combi, & La Noù, 1672. [14] 655 [20] pp. 14.6 cm.

Le Boë, or Sylvius as he is usually called, was, if not the founder, certainly the outstanding proponent and most influential of the Iatrochemists who explained and treated all disease chemically, basing their treatment on a supposed chemical relationship between the disease and the drug. A Dutch scientist, he was graduated from Basel and returned to Leiden where he became one of the greatest teachers of his time. He was keenly interested in the new developments of his day and was a strong supporter of Harvey. He was a pioneer of bedside teaching, and in the present work an engraved title page shows the interior of a sickroom with a patient lying in a canopied bed and a physician, a nurse, and several others in attendance.

This little volume is the second edition of a general handbook on medical practice for the use of students and physicians, following Le Boë's principles.

Waller 9431.

*319. THOMAS WHARTON (1614–1673). *Adenographia; sive, Glandularum totius corporis descriptio.* Amsterdam: Sumptibus Joannis Ravesteinii, 1659. [24] 261 pp., fold. plate. 12.9 cm.

A successful London physician, Wharton also carried out many anatomical investigations. He studied the entire glandular system and, after discovering that the submaxillary gland had a duct (Wharton's duct), hypothesized that all glands have a secretory duct. In this treatise, he describes the glands of the body including some, such as the choroid plexuses of the cerebral ventricles, which are actually not glands. The single folding plate in this volume illustrates the submaxillary gland, kidney, pancreas, and the thymus gland.

Cushing W146; Garrison-Morton 1116 (1st ed., 1656); Osler 4221; Russell 855; Waller 10264.

*320. NICHOLAS CULPEPER (1616–1654). *Pharmacopoeia Londinensis; or, The London dispensatory*. London: Printed by J. Streater, 1672. [24] 305 [37] pp. 17 cm.

Culpeper, son of an English clergyman, studied at Cambridge and acquired an extensive medical background by reading and serving apprenticeships under two different apothecaries. He began active practice in 1640 as a physician-astrologer—a not unusual practice for doctors of his day. He soon achieved great fame and developed quite a large practice. Although in essence Culpeper was a quack without sound scientific training, he was aware that science must be based upon study and careful observation. It was in this spirit that he translated many notable scientific works including such authors as Galen, Sennert, Rivière, Riolan, Vesling, and Glisson.

The English medical profession was shocked and angered in 1649 when Culpeper published an English translation of the Latin pharmacopoeia. This unauthorized translation outraged the College of Physicians, and they declared that Culpeper had infringed upon their rights because they held a monopoly on the official dispensatory. The fact that all their secret remedies were now easily read in the vernacular was a matter of great concern, and Culpeper was subjected to many bitter attacks by the medical profession. Nevertheless, his pharmacopoeia became quite popular and had already been printed eleven times when this 1672 edition was published.

Cushing C621; Wellcome II, p. 414.

321. ———. ———. London: Printed for H. Sawbridge, 1683. [24] 305 (misnumbered 269) [37] pp. 17 cm.

By 1683, Culpeper's *Pharmacopoeia* had been printed at least thirteen or fourteen times. The last English edition was printed in 1718 and an American edition was printed in Boston in 1720. The Wellcome *Catalogue of printed books* lists some seventeen different printings of this work and Cushing lists nineteen.

Cushing C624; Wellcome II, p. 414.

322. ———. *English physician; and complete herbal*. 2 vols. in 1. London: Lewis and Hamblin, 1807. Vol. I: [2] xvi, 400 pp.; Vol. II: [4] 256 [58] pp., port., col. plates. 26.5 cm.

In 1653, Culpeper again trespassed on the monopoly claimed by the recognized medical writers when he published this work. It, like its predecessors, had enormous success and continued to be issued until the mid-nineteenth century. In it, Culpeper argues that every physician should be an astrologer and sets forth the reasons why medicinal plants and herbs are dependent on the movement of the stars. E. Silby, another physician-astrologer, began editing the work in 1789, and it continued under his name until the early 1800's. This particular edition has a number of tinted anatomical plates as well as twenty-nine colored plates of various medicinal herbs and plants.

Wellcome II, p. 416.

323. ———. *School of physick.* London: Printed for N. Brook, 1659. 461 (misnumbered 361) pp., front. (port.). 16 cm.

Culpeper was an extremely prolific writer and, in addition to his translations, prepared numerous texts on therapeutics. Because of his great fame, many of his therapeutically oriented works were more popular in the home than as reference works for the physician. Culpeper left many unpublished works at his death, and his wife ensured that they were published. This work appeared just a few years after his death and is devoted to the various herbal remedies that may be used to treat a variety of diseases. The book also contains a short introductory testimony by Culpeper's wife and Culpeper's horoscope done by John Gadbury, a close friend.

Cushing C632; Wellcome II, p. 417.

WILHELM LANGLEY (1616–1668). *De generatione animalium observationes quaedam.*

See No. 277.

*324. THOMAS BARTHOLIN (1616–1680). *Historiarum anatomicarum rariorum centuria I et II.* Amsterdam: Apud Joannem Henrici, 1654. [16] 326 [9] pp., illus., plates (2 fold.). 15.2 cm. Old morocco, rebacked.

Bartholin, a Danish physician, naturalist, physiologist, and anatomist, was one of several seventeenth century researchers who greatly expanded the knowledge of the working anatomy of various glands and their ducts, the biliary system, and the lymphatic system. Bartholin is commonly credited with the first description of the thoracic duct in man and Jean Pecquet (see No. 349) with recognizing it in animals a few years earlier.

Bartholin was a prolific writer and this little volume, the first edition of which was published in 1641, was one of several of his collections containing descriptions and illustrations of anatomical anomalies (including a superb illustration of a horseshoe kidney), monsters (i.e., human freaks), and normal structures, together with some brief case histories of unusual anatomical and clinical structures.

Cushing B118; Osler 1927 (Copenhagen, 1654 ed.); Waller 737 (Copenhagen, 1654 ed.); Wellcome II, p. 107 (different eds. of same year).

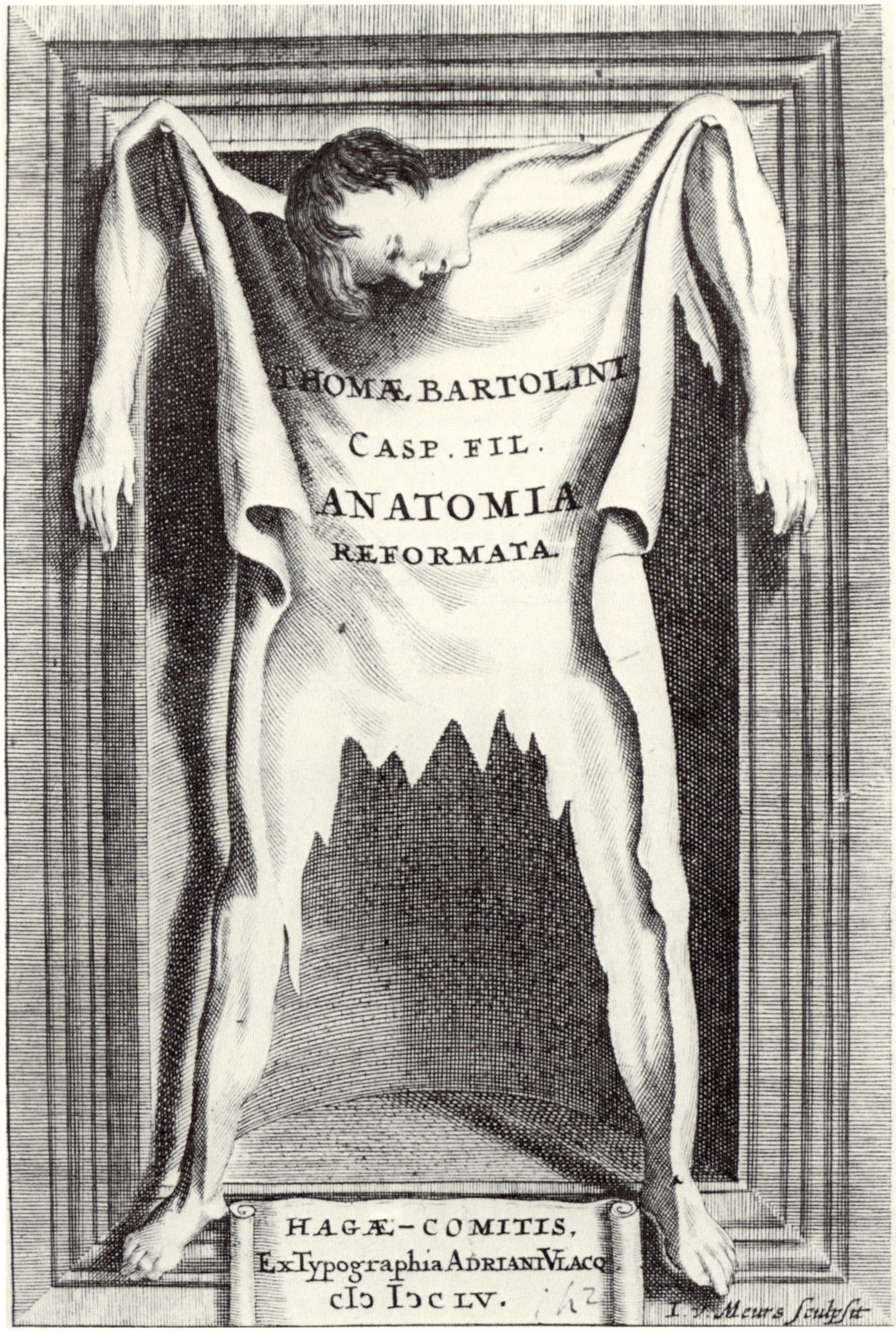

No. 325. Bartholin. *Anatomia.*

*325. ———. *Anatomia*. The Hague: Ex typographia Adriani Vlacq, 1655. [16] 592 [13] pp., illus., plates (part fold.), port. 18.8 cm. Half calf, marbled boards.

Like his father, Caspar Bartholin (see No. 288), the equally famous Danish anatomist, Thomas wrote several anatomical treatises which became very popular textbooks and were translated into several other languages. In reality, however, they were revisions of his father's *Institutiones anatomicae* (1611). Although the illustrations differed from edition to edition, few of them were original. Most were after Vesalius, Casserio, Vesling, Bauhin, Ruysch, and others. This edition contains eight folding plates and sixty-six copperplates of uneven workmanship. This second edition also contains the sixth edition of two letters of Johannes Walaeus, *De motu chyli et sanguinis*, which support Harvey's work. Bartholin has also added a final chapter, "De lacteis thoracicis et vasis lymphaticis," on the thoracic system and lymphatic vessels.

Choulant-Frank, pp. 245–247; Cushing B104 (1651 ed.); Wellcome II, p. 107.

*326. ——— and ERASMUS BARTHOLIN (1625–1698). *De nivis usu medico observationes variae. Accessit D. Erasmi Bartholini De figura nivis dissertatio*. 3 pts. in 1 vol. Copenhagen: Typis Matthiae Godicchii, sumptibus Petri Haubold, 1661. [26] 232 [14] 42 [15] pp., engr. plate. 14.6 cm. Vellum.

Chapter XXII of this historically important book makes the first known mention of the use of mixtures of ice and snow for freezing to produce surgical anesthesia. The author states that the technique was taught to him by one Marco Aurelio Severino of Naples (see No. 247). In order not to kill the tissues and cause gangrene, the ice-snow mixture was to be applied on the parts in narrow parallel lines. After a quarter of an hour, feeling would be deadened and the part could be cut without pain. This may be the first mention of such a technique since the time of Avicenna. The treatise on snow crystals, by Bartholin's younger brother, Erasmus, is the earliest publication on crystallography, and preceded Boyle on gems (1672) by eleven years. This interesting book also contains a list of Thomas Bartholin's works.

Cushing B114; Osler 1933; Waller 726; Wellcome II, p. 107.

327. ROYAL COLLEGE OF PHYSICIANS OF LONDON. *Pharmacopoeia Collegii Regalis Medicorum Londinensis*. Dublin: Impensis P. Wilson et J. Esdall, 1746. 176 pp. 15.5 cm. Calf.

The College of Physicians was incorporated by charter during the reign of Henry VIII in 1518. The idea of preparing an official pharmacopoeia was first considered by the College in 1585, but it was not until 1618 that it finally appeared in print. Updated revisions of the *Pharmacopoeia* were issued in 1650, 1677, 1721, 1746, 1788, 1809, 1824, 1836, and 1851. The present revision of 1746 was begun in 1738, and most of the next eight years was spent in conducting the necessary chemical and pharmaceutical experiments. This *Pharmacopoeia* was a great improvement over the previous revision of 1721 with great reduction in the number of simples, preparations, and compounds. This revision contained only 272 simples as contrasted with the 1,028 in the 1618 work, and only 378 preparations and compounds as compared with the 932 in the 1618 work.

Cushing R277 (1618 ed.); Garrison-Morton 1821 (1618 ed.); Waller 7386; Wellcome 4983 (1618 ed.).

328. ———. *The new pharmacopoeia of the Royal College of Physicians of London*. 2nd ed. London: Printed by J. W. Galabin for T. Longman, 1788. xvi, 350 pp. 20.4 cm. Calf, rebacked.

English translations of the *Pharmacopoeia* had been made since the mid-1600's, but it was not until the 1788 edition that a translation was officially authorized by the College. Thomas Healde (d. 1789), Lumleian lecturer at the College and senior physician of the London Hospital, made the translation.

329. ———. *The dispensatory of the Royal College of Physicians in London. . . . by John Quincy*. London: Printed by W. Bowyer, 1721. [18] 362 [15], front. 19.1 cm. Calf.

Two years after the *Pharmacopoeia Londinensis* was published, John Quincy (see No. 462) issued the first of two editions of his translation of the *Pharmacopoeia*. His work was simply an annotated translation with notes from his *Dispensatory* after the English text of the official preparations. The present work is most likely a 1721 reprint of the 1720 edition. The second edition appeared in 1727, some years after Quincy's death.

Gift of R. A. Kuever.

330. ———. ———. 3rd ed. London: Printed by T. Longman and J. Nourse, 1751. x, 414 pp. 19.2 cm. Modern cloth.

This third edition of the *Dispensatory* was translated into English by Henry Pemberton (1694–1771), a professor of physic in Gresham College, Fellow of the Royal Society, and one of the best chemists of his time. This edition also contains a lengthy narrative of the deliberations of the committee appointed by the College to review the previous *Pharmacopoeia*.

Osler 6089 (1746 ed.).

331. ———. ———. 4th ed. London: Printed by J. Nourse and T. Longman, 1760. x, 414 pp. 19.5 cm. Calf, rebacked.

The fourth edition of the *Dispensatory* appeared in 1760 and was again translated by Henry Pemberton who had been amply rewarded by the College for his work on the 1746 *Pharmacopoeia*. This edition also contains the lengthy narrative of the review committee.

Gift of J. M. Lindley.

*332. GIOVANNI ONORATO CASTIGLIONE (d. 1679) and BRANDA FRANCESCO CASTIGLIONE (fl. 1660). *Prospectus pharmaceuticus*. 2 pts. in 1 vol. Milan: Apud Joannem Baptistam Ferrarium, 1668. Pt. I: [24] 438 pp.; Pt. II: [6] 94 (misnumbered 102) pp., fold. plate. 29.8 cm. Limp vellum.

The authors, father and son, each physician to the Duke of Milan, were commissioned by the Milanese Senate to produce this extensive pharmacological compendium. Of simple format, with many recipes and formulas, it is a working pharmacopoeia. Of particular interest are the engraved title page illustrating the interior of a seventeenth-century apothecary shop and, at the end, a folding copperplate showing numerous figures of apothecary's vessels and chemical apparatus.

Wellcome II, p. 311 (1729 ed.).

*333. WALTER CHARLETON (1619–1707). *Onomasticon zoicon.* London: Apud Jacobum Allestry, 1668. [20] 309 [34] pp., illus., plates (part fold.). 20 cm. Contemporary calf.

Charleton was an unusually gifted physician, zoologist, and archeologist who studied physics, theology, and natural history. He was one of the founders of the Royal Society and later served as its president. This is the first edition of his encyclopedic work on all the then-known animals, snakes, insects, birds, fish, and fossils. Charleton includes the English, Latin, and Greek name for each species as well as brief remarks on their anatomy and paleontology.

The book also contains Sir George Ent's (1604–1689) first zootomical treatise, *Mantissa anatomica.* Ent was a friend and supporter of William Harvey and was one of the original members of the Royal Society. In this work, he describes and illustrates the anatomy of *Lophius piscatorius* (the toad fish or fishing frog) and *Glaeus piscis.* The book contains eight folding plates and there are several fine engravings in the text.

Garrison-Morton 292; Wellcome II, p. 329.

*334. ———. *De scorbuto liber singularis.* Leiden: Apud Felicem Lopez, 1672. 288 pp. 13.3 cm. Contemporary vellum.

This is the second edition of *De scorbuto* and was published the same year as the first London edition. Although Charleton was a brilliant individual and an active investigator, he believed in many of the classical concepts of disease, and this treatise on the causes and treatment of scurvy is written in that vein. Lind did a much better job one hundred years later (see No. 587).

Cushing C186; Osler 2294; Waller 1918 (London, 1672 ed.); Wellcome II, p. 329.

BRANDA FRANCESCO CASTIGLIONE (fl. 1660). *Prospectus pharmaceuticus.*

See No. 332.

*335. THÉOPHILE BONET (1620–1689). *Sepulchretum; sive, Anatomia practica.* 2 vols. Geneva: Sumptibus Leonardi Chouët, 1679. Vol. I: [40] 720 pp.; Vol. II: [4] 721–1706 pp., port. 33.6 cm. Contemporary vellum.

Bonet was born in Geneva, the son and grandson of physicians. He traveled widely as a young man and received his medical degree at Bologna in 1643. Bonet practiced for a time at Neuchâtel, then moved to Geneva where he developed an extensive and successful practice. Upon becoming deaf in 1670, he abandoned his clinical practice and devoted the remainder of his life to study and writing. In all, Bonet wrote or edited sixteen books on medical subjects. This is his greatest work and is the foundation upon which Morgagni based his *De sedibus* (see No. 498). The first edition appeared after he had been in practice over thirty years; it contains references to more than 400 writers and is based on some 3,000 autopsies. He includes diseases from ancient to contemporary times with emphasis on the sixteenth and seventeenth centuries. Book I concerns the head, Book II deals with the chest, Book III with diseases of the abdominal cavity, and Book IV with fevers, tumors, fractures, ulcers, and assorted other diseases.

Cushing B485 (1700 ed.); Garrison-Morton 2274; Osler 2077; Waller 1278; Wellcome II, p. 198.

*336. HENRICUS EYSSONIUS (1620–1690). *Tractatus anatomicus & medicus de ossibus infantis. . . . Accessit Volcheri Coiteri eorundem ossium historia.* Groningen: Typis Johannis Cölleni, 1659. [24] 216 pp. 12.7 cm. Vellum. Bound with No. 21.

Eyssonius, a Dutch physician, distinguished himself in osteology. This first edition of his treatise on children's bones is followed by the important tract of Volcher Coiter (1534–1576), *Tractatus anatomicus, de ossibus foetus abortivi, et infantis, dimidium annum nati,* which had been printed only once before, in a very rare collection of tracts issued in 1573.

Coiter, also Dutch, was a specialist in osteology and comparative anatomy. His studies of the formation of the bones in the fetus probably earn for him the place of priority as the father of modern embryological studies.

*337. BERNARDINO GENGA (1620–1690). *Anatomia chirurgica . . . & un breve trattato della circolazione del sangue.* Bologna: Il Longhi, 1687. [32] 332 [16] pp. 14 cm. Contemporary vellum.

An authoritative anatomist and surgeon in Rome, Genga stressed the importance of solid anatomical knowledge for the surgeon. This work, originally published in 1672, has been called the "first book devoted entirely to surgical anatomy" (Garrison-Morton 384) and remained a widely used manual for at least fifty years. In the tract appended to this work, Genga showed himself to be one of the first Italians to accept Harvey's theory on the circulation of the blood. But Genga also maintained that the discovery was made by Colombo and Cesalpino before Harvey. The parts played by those two Italian investigators and anatomists in the unfolding of the facts of circulatory physiology have long been a point of study and argument among medical historians.

Cushing G189 (1686 ed.); Garrison-Morton 384 (1672 ed.); Wellcome III, p. 102.

*338. ———. *Anatomia per uso et intelligenza del disegno; ricercata non solo su gl'ossi, e muscoli del corpo humano; ma dimostrata ancora su le statue antiche piu insigni di Roma.* Rome: Domenico de Rossi, 1691. 56 *ll.*, 40 plates. 47 cm. Vellum, in box.

This large atlas contains forty magnificent full-page engraved plates depicting the human figure in various poses, with and without dissection. As promised in the subtitle to the work, in some of the full-figure plates one recognizes engraved renditions of some of the celebrated antique statues in Rome. The plates, probably engraved by François Andriot after designs by Charles Errard, were intended primarily for the use of painters and sculptors, and they are still considered to be one of the best collections for the use of student artists. The text is by Giovanni Maria Lancisi (see No. 445).

Choulant-Frank, pp. 254–255; Garrison-Morton 386; Wellcome III, p. 102.

*339. ———. *Anatomy improv'd and illustrated with regard to the uses thereof in designing.* London: Republish'd by John Senex [1723]. 59 *ll.*, 42 plates. 46 cm. Paneled calf, restored.

This atlas is made up of copies of the plates used in the 1691 edition (No. 338), "now re-engraven," according to the lengthy subtitle, "by the ablest hands in England," and includes the text of Giovanni Maria Lancisi, translated into English.

Wellcome III, p. 103.

340. JOHANN JAKOB WEPFER (1620–1695). *Observationes anatomicae, ex cadaveribus eorum, quos sustulit apoplexia.* Schaffhausen: Impensis Onophrii a Waldkirch, typis Alexandri Riedingii, 1675. [16] 464 pp. 16.2 cm.

Wepfer, one of the most prominent Swiss physicians of the seventeenth century, studied medicine and the humanities at Basel and Strasbourg and traveled in Italy for several years before graduating from Basel in 1647. He was appointed city physician at Schaffhausen and some years later became personal physician to the Duke of Würtemberg. He also served as physician to the Marquis de Dourlach, Charles the Elector Palatine, and the army of Emperor Leopold. Wepfer's scientific works were characterized by keen insight, wide knowledge, and careful observation.

The present work was first published in 1658 and was followed by this and three later reprints. In it, Wepfer showed that apoplexy was a result of cerebral hemorrhage and described four cases with clinical and postmortem findings. He also clearly described the circular anastomosis of arteries at the base of the brain, later named after Willis. Although well-known in Europe, Wepfer's work does not seem to have been recognized in England and was not mentioned in Willis's *Cerebri anatome* (see No. 344) in 1664.

Garrison-Morton 2703 (1658 ed.); Waller 10220 (1658 ed.).

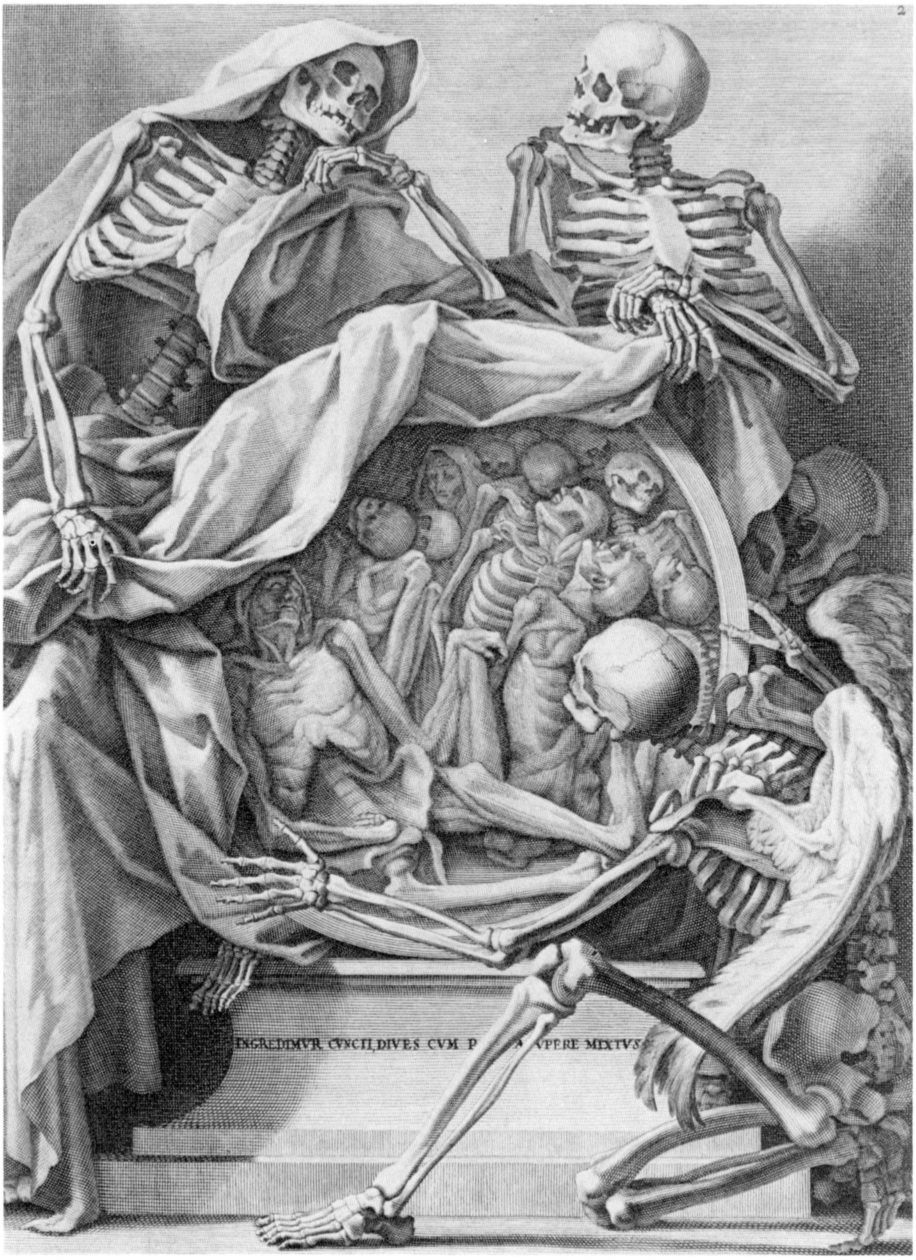

No. 338. Genga. *Anatomia.* The Angel of Death beholds the disinterred paupers.

341. ———. *Historia cicutae aquaticae.* Basel: Ex officina Episcopiana, 1716. [xvi] 336 [6] 24, 20 pp., illus., front., 2 plates. 20.2 cm. Calf.

In addition to his work on apoplexy, Wepfer published a number of important works in botany, zoology, and chemistry. This work on the effects of hemlock and other poisons contributed to the doctrine of vital force, for Wepfer showed that the heart and structure of the viscera were changed by the administration of poisons. He also demonstrated that a heart devoid of blood could be kept in motion for some moments after death by the action of substances such as *nux vomica tetanus* (strychnine), tobacco (nicotine), and hemlock (conium).

Garrison-Morton 974.1 (1679 ed.); Waller 10219 (1679 ed.).

*342. JOANNES VAN HORNE (1621–1670). *Μικρόκοσμος; seu, Brevis manuductio ad historiam corporis humani.* 2nd ed. Leiden: Apud Jacobum Chouët, 1662. [viii] 142 [16] pp. 13.2 cm. Contemporary calf. Bound with No. 393.

Van Horne, a Dutch physician and anatomist, was professor of anatomy at Leiden and numbered among his pupils Jan Swammerdam, Frederik Ruysch, and Nicolaus Steno. This small anatomy, first published in 1660, became very popular, despite its lack of illustrations, and was translated into Dutch, German, and French.

Cushing H456; Waller 4910; Wellcome III, p. 301 (1665 ed.).

*343. THOMAS WILLIS (1621–1675). *Diatribae duae medico-philosophicae.* Amsterdam: Apud Gerbrandus Schagen, 1663. [32] 376 pp., plate. 12.7 cm. Modern three-quarter morocco.

Willis, a graduate of Oxford, practiced medicine and taught there until 1666, when he went to London, where he attained a large practice and was known as an outstanding physician. In addition to his practice he carried on extensive research and published a number of important works on medicine, anatomy, and pharmacology. In this work Willis suggests that fermentation is an activity of the intestines, gives an early description of epidemic typhoid fever, and notes that urine has a sweet taste in diabetes mellitus. This work was first published in London in 1659, and this particular copy is one of the early editions published in Europe.

Cushing W212 (1662 ed.); Garrison-Morton 5020 (1st ed., 1659).

*344. ———. *Cerebri anatome: cui accessit Nervorum descriptio et usus.* London: Typis Ja. Flesher, Impensis Jo. Martyn & Ja. Allestry, 1664. [39] 456 pp., 15 plates (11 fold.). 19 cm. Contemporary boards, later calf back. Imprimatur leaf supplied from another copy. Four leaves of index in contemporary manuscript bound in at end. Marginal notes throughout in same hand.

Willis's *Cerebri anatome* was "the most complete and accurate account of the nervous system which had hitherto appeared. . . . Its illustrations are by Sir

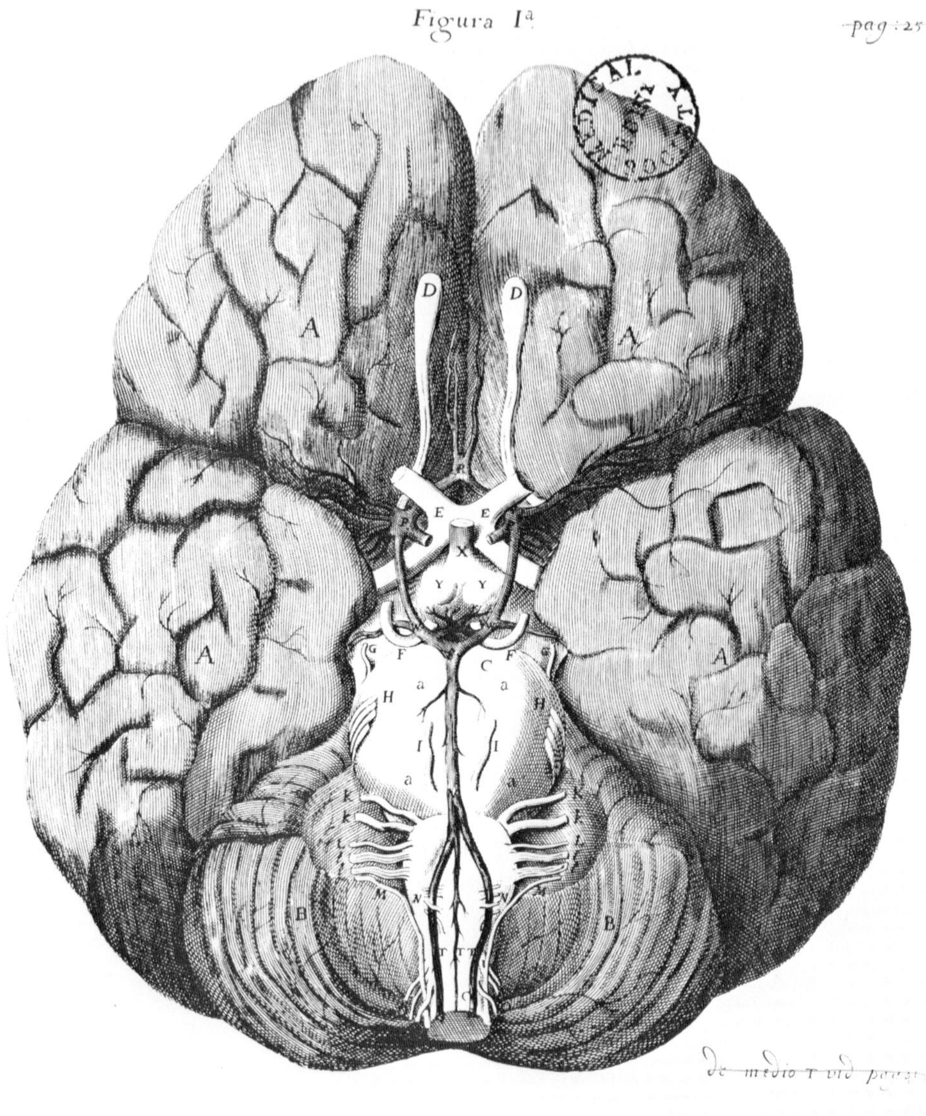

No. 344. Willis. *Cerebri Anatome*. The "circle of Willis."

Christopher Wren. Willis's classification of the cerebral nerves held the field until the time of Soemmering" (Garrison-Morton 1378). Included are his descriptions of the "circle of Willis" and the cranial nerve now called the "nerve of Willis."

Cushing W211; Garrison-Morton 1378; Osler 4249; Russell 866; Waller 10315.

*345. ———. *Pathologiae cerebri, et nervosi generis specimen.* Amsterdam: Apud Danielem Elzevirium, 1670. [12] 338 [19] pp., port. 13 cm. Vellum.

Willis followed up his anatomical account of the brain with this important work on its pathology and neurophysiology, first published in 1667. In it he develops a new theory of the cause of epilepsy and other convulsive diseases, and he makes a number of contributions to psychiatry. A second part of the volume is Willis's treatise on scurvy.

Cushing W215 (1st ed., 1667); Osler 4249A (1668 ed.); Waller 10333.

*346. ———. *De anima brutorum, quae hominis vitalis ac sensitiva est, exercitationes duae.* Lyons: Sumptibus Joannis Antonii Huguetan, 1676. [24] 298 [12] pp., 8 plates (part fold.). 22.9 cm. Newly rebound in antique paper over boards.

In this earliest English work on medical psychology, first published at Oxford in 1672, Willis describes the phenomenon now known as *paracusis Willisii*, based on his observation of a deaf woman who could hear only when a drum was beating. This is a typical example of Willis's ability to make application of isolated, but important, facts. The first clinical description of *myasthenia gravis* is also in this work.

Garrison-Morton 1544, 4793, 4966 (1st ed., 1672); Osler 4250 (1st ed.); Waller 10324.

*347. ———. *Pharmaceutice rationalis; sive, Diatriba de medicamentorum operationibus in humano corpore.* [Part I]. Lyons: Sumptibus Joannis Antonii Huguetan, 1676. [20] 180 [6] pp., 6 fold. plates. 22.5 cm.

One of the great books of seventeenth century English medicine, this is the first scientific work on pharmacology as well as a valuable epitome of the materia medica of the time. Willis describes the sweetish flavor of urine in diabetes mellitus, differentiating between it and diabetes insipidus. He gives a clear account of whooping cough and the first satisfactory figures on the structure of the lungs. The work was first published in Oxford in 1674.

Garrison-Morton 3926 and 5086 (1st ed., 1674); Osler 4251 (1677 ed.); Waller 10337.

*348. ———. *Opera medica & physica.* Lyons: Sumptibus Joannis Antonii Huguetan, 1676. [50] 694 [24] pp., plates (part fold.). 22.5 cm. Vellum.

This is the first collected edition of Willis's voluminous writings, containing a fine portrait of Willis, together with many folding plates, some of which are from his celebrated *Cerebri anatome.*

Also included in Willis's *Opera* is William Croone's (1633–1684) *De ratione motus musculorum* (1664), one of the earliest works on muscular action. Croone, a graduate of Cambridge and one of the original founders of the Royal Society, had a large and prosperous practice, and, in accordance with his wishes, his wife endowed after his death the Croonian Lectures at the Royal College of Physicians, London. In the treatise, he expresses his theory that the body of the muscle is responsible for its contractile power which is brought about by a nourishing fluid from the arterial system in combination with another fluid of nervous origin.

Cushing W214 (Geneva ed., 1676).

*349. JEAN PECQUET (1622–1674). *Experimenta nova anatomica, quibus incognitum hactenus chyli receptaculum, & ab eo per thoracem in ramos usque subclavios vasa lactea deteguntur.* Paris: Ex officina Cramosiana, 1654. [16] 252 [2] pp., illus. 20 cm. Contemporary limp vellum.

At the beginning of the seventeenth century, it was still widely believed that food was converted into blood as it passed through the digestive system. The blood was then carried to the liver where it was imbued with natural spirits and passed on to the heart for distribution throughout the body. Since only the blood vessels were known to the anatomists of that day, it was thought that chyle, the product of digestion, was transported to the liver by the venous system of the intestines. This notion was corrected by Gaspare Aselli (see No. 257) in 1622 when, quite by accident, he discovered the lacteal vessels in the mesentery of a dog. However, he incorrectly surmised that the lacteal vessels empty their contents into the liver.

It was not until 1651 that Pecquet reported his discovery of the receptaculum chyli and thoracic duct in *Experimenta nova anatomica*. Pecquet, a native of Dieppe, was a graduate of Montpellier and a Paris physician. In the book he accurately described the lacteal veins of Aselli and showed that they terminate in the receptaculum chyli and that the thoracic duct joins the venous system at the junction of the jugular and subclavian veins. Joannes van Horne (see No. 342) made the same discovery quite independently and corroborated Pecquet's findings in his *Novus ductus chyliferus* (1652). Only a short time later, Pecquet's work was confirmed and extended by Olaf Rudbeck (1630–1702) and Thomas Bartholin (see No. 324) to cover the entire lymphatic system.

Riolan (see No. 285) was as bitter a critic of Pecquet as he had been of Harvey, and in this second edition Pecquet answers Riolan's criticisms with further anatomical demonstrations and a sarcastic poem. Included with both the first and second editions are several letters of support from leading scientists of the day, some of which appear in this edition for the first time.

Cushing P192; Garrison-Morton 1095 (1651 ed.); Osler 3639 (1651 ed.); Waller 7280.

*350. RICHARD WISEMAN (1622?–1676). *Severall chirurgicall treatises.* London: Printed by E. Flesher and J. Macock, for R. Royston and B. Took, 1676. [15] 498, 79 [13] pp. 30.5 cm.

Wiseman was surgeon to both King James I and King Charles II and was the outstanding surgeon in seventeenth-century England. This large work discusses the cause, clinical appearance, and treatment of tumors, ulcers, diseases of the anus, the "King's Evil," wounds (including gunshot wounds), fractures, and venereal disease. Wiseman realized the difference between gonorrhea and syphilis and was the first to describe tuberculosis of the joints.

Cushing W250; Garrison-Morton 5573; Osler 4258; Waller 10368.

351. LAMBERT VAN VELTHUYSEN (1622–1685). *Tractatus duo medico-physici, uno de liene, alter de generatione.* Utrecht: Typis Theodori Ackersdijck & Gilberti à Zyll, 1657. [48] 162, 286 [1] pp. 12.8 cm. Contemporary vellum.

Velthuysen studied philosophy, theology, and medicine at Utrecht and later practiced there and taught at the University. This is apparently his only medical work and consists of two treatises—one on the spleen and the other on reproduction.

*352. THOMAS SYDENHAM (1624–1689). *Observationes medicae circa morborum acutorum historiam et curationem.* London: G. Kettilby, 1676. [56] 425 [54] pp., front. (port.). 16.1 cm. Polished calf.

In the later half of the seventeenth century, internal medicine took an entirely new turn in the work of one of its greatest figures, Sydenham, who revived the Hippocratic methods of observation and experience. He was one of the principal founders of epidemiology, and his clinical reputation rests upon his firsthand accounts of malarial fever, scarlatina, measles, dysentery, and numerous other diseases.

The present work is a third edition of Sydenham's book on fevers, first published in 1666 under the title *Methodus curandi febres.* It is the first definitive edition, being entirely rewritten and about four times larger than the earlier editions. It contains his important study on epidemiology and is one of the fundamental texts in this branch of medicine, with numerous observations on epidemics in London from 1661 to 1675.

Garrison-Morton 2198; Osler 994; Waller 9402.

353. ———. *The whole works of that excellent practical physician Dr. Thomas Sydenham.* 3rd ed. London: Printed for R. Wellington, 1701. [16] 453 pp. 18.9 cm.

Contrary to the title of this work, it does not contain all of Sydenham's writings. The book is actually an English translation of his *Methodus curandi febres* (see No. 352). It was first translated from the Latin by John Pechy (1655–1716) in 1697 and went through eleven editions.

Gift of R. A. Kuever.

354. ———. *Praxis medica. The practice of physick.* 3rd ed. By William Salmon, M.D. London: Printed for J. Knapton, 1716. [16] 580 (misnumbered 480) [4] pp. 19.4 cm. Paneled calf, rebacked.

Sydenham's posthumously published *Processus integri* [Advances in healing] (1695) constitutes his therapeutic system and was the customary handbook for English physicians for more than a century. It appeared in many editions and translations. This translation is by William Salmon (see No. 429), an "irregular" who wrote many astrological and semi-popular medical works as well as many translations into English of medical works originally in Latin.

Cushing S494.

Gift of Lucetta J. Tobie.

355. ———. *Opera medica*. 2 vols. in 1. Geneva: Apud Fratres de Tournes, 1716. Vol. I: [46] 815 [25] pp.; Vol. II: [8] 170 [14] 88 pp. 22.2 cm. Old calf. Bound with No. 449 and No. 450.

This is the first of nine Latin editions of selections from Sydenham's collected medical observations. It is interesting to note that Sydenham prepared his manuscripts in English and then had them translated into Latin for publication in accordance with the tradition of the time. After publication, someone invariably made an English translation of his Latin work.

*356. ———. ———. Venice: Ex typographia Balleoniana, 1735. [16] 574 [6] 82 pp. 39.5 cm.

This edition of Sydenham's collected works also contains treatises by Joannes Coccius (fl. 1670), Bartolomeo Boschetti (d. 1744), and Antonio Celestino Cocchi (1699–1747), as well as a number of dissertations on epidemics in various cities and regions of continental Europe during the late seventeenth and early eighteenth centuries. Among the authors represented are Bernardino Ramazzini, Walther Harris, Martin Lister, Charles Drelincourt, David Hamilton, and many others. William Musgrave's two treatises on arthritis (see Nos. 449 and 450) and a supplement containing additional works on plagues and epidemics by Karl Friedrich Loew (1699–1741), Andreas Loew (ca. 1660–ca. 1710), Giuseppe Lanzoni (1663–1730), and Carlo Ricca (1690–1746?) are also included.

Osler 1004.

357. ———. *The entire works of Dr. Thomas Sydenham, newly made from English originals*. 3rd ed. London: Printed for E. Cave, 1753. [2] x [xxvi] 672 [20] pp. 20.2 cm.

This work, translated in 1742 from the Latin by John Swan (fl. 1745), contains not only Sydenham's *Methodus curandi febres* but a number of his other works as well. His very popular *Processus integri morbis fere omnibus corandis, Schedula monitoria, Treatise of the gout and dropsy*, and epistles on venereal disease and smallpox are also included.

Waller 9417.

358. ———. *The works of Thomas Sydenham, M.D., on acute and chronic diseases.* By Benjamin Rush, M.D. Philadelphia: Published by Benjamin & Thomas Kite, 1809. xl, 473 [10] pp. 21.2 cm.

The professional stature of Sydenham was such that his writings remained popular for many years. In this early American edition, Benjamin Rush edited Sydenham's works on acute and chronic diseases, adding notes and comments to adapt Sydenham's material to the diseases and climate of this country.

Austin 1845; Waller 9420.

ERASMUS BARTHOLIN (1625–1698). *De figura nivis dissertatio.*

See No. 326.

*359. CARLO CESI (1626–1686). *Cognitione de muscoli del corpo humano per il disegno.* Rome: Franco Collignon, 1679. 18 *ll.*, (incl. 16 plates). 41.2 cm. Contemporary half calf.

Cesi was an Italian painter and etcher of copperplates who lived in Rome where he maintained his own painting academy. He was a pupil of Pietro da Cortona (see No. 297), and his work is of lesser quality than that of his teacher. Neither the artistic quality nor the anatomical accuracy of this book are of special note. The book contains two plates depicting skeletons and fourteen muscle plates of which five are of full male figures. The text is scanty and is chiefly used to describe the plates.

Choulant-Frank, pp. 256–257; Wellcome II, p. 321 (1730 ed.).

*360. DOMENICO DE MARCHETTI (1626–1688). *Anatomia.* Harderwyck: Ex officina Societatis Typographicae, 1656. [16] 291 (misnumbered 289) [2] pp. 12.7 cm. Old vellum.

Marchetti was Johann Vesling's (see No. 303) assistant until he succeeded Vesling in the chair of anatomy at Padua in 1649. Son of the well-known Paduan professor and surgeon Pietro de Marchetti (1589–1673), he published the first edition of his *Anatomia* at Padua in 1652. He was one of the first anatomists in Italy to use the wax injection techniques of Swammerdam and Ruysch. This small book contains his anatomical studies of the complete human body and is without illustrations.

Cushing M137; Osler (1688 ed.); Waller 6241.

*361. GERARDUS BLASIUS (1626?–1692?). *Anatome animalium.* Amsterdam: Sumptibus viduae Joannis à Someren, Henrici & viduae Theodori Boom, 1681. [8] 494 [2] pp., 60 plates. 26.3 cm. Contemporary calf.

Blasius (or Blaes) was a Dutch anatomist and physician whose primary interest was in comparative anatomy. This work is "the first comprehensive manual of comparative anatomy based on the original and literary researches of a working anatomist" (Francis J. Cole, *History of comparative anatomy*. London, 1944. pp. 150–151). The sixty engraved plates in this work treat seventy-eight species of animals. An engraved title page, preceding the regular title page, contains figures that are of unusual allegorical interest.

Cushing B434; Garrison-Morton 296; Wellcome II, p. 179.

362. FRANCESCO REDI (1626–1698). *Opere*. 7 vols. in 6. Venice: Per Gio. Gabbriello Ertz, 1712–1745. Illus. 20.4 cm. Contemporary vellum.

Redi has been called the father of helminthology and his studies on the poison of vipers (1664) and on the generation of lower animals place him at the forefront of the biological investigators of his time. His *Osservazioni intorno agli animali viventi che si trovano negli animali viventi* (1684) is one of the earliest and best works on parasitology. He described more than 100 species of parasites and was an avid student of the development of snakes, pigeons, insects, and fish. Redi was also one of the earliest to challenge the doctrine of spontaneous generation. His *Consultations*, which describes the case histories of about one hundred of his patients, shows him to be an honest thinker and capable physician who showed great concern for the welfare of his patients. His *Opere* is well-illustrated and contains many plates depicting the objects he studied.

Garrison-Morton 65 (1762 ed.); Osler 3772 (1748 ed.); Waller 20160 (1809 ed.).

*363. ———. *Lettera intorno all'invenzione degli occhiali*. Firenze: Francesco Onofri, 1678. 14 pp. 21.2 cm. Old limp decorated boards.

This letter of Redi's concerning the invention of eyeglasses is rare and is not usually found as a separate work. Redi claims that glasses were not known to the ancient Jews, Arabs, Greeks, or Romans and he attributes their invention to a Friar Alessandro Spina of Pisa (d. 1313).

Waller 14691 (1690 ed.).

*364. ROBERT BOYLE (1627–1691). *Certain physiological essays*. London: Printed for Henry Herringman, 1661. [4] 105 [9] 107–249 pp. 19.1 cm. Contemporary calf, rebacked.

Physicist, physiologist, chemist, and philosopher, Boyle was one of the great scientists and intellects of the seventeenth century. In Boyle's bibliography, John Fulton lists more than three hundred items, including contributions in chemistry, physics, medicine, philosophy, and theology. Although he was not formally trained as a physician, Boyle was deeply interested in the medical sciences and was made a "Doctor of Physick" at Oxford in 1665. Boyle was also a leader in the movement to separate chemistry from alchemy and was among the first to define a chemical element. His interests were wide-ranging and included studies on the properties of acids and bases, hydrostatics, respiration, combustion, magnetism, electricity, and the chemical nature of the blood. In this first edition of his *Essays*, Boyle presents a summary of his views on physical laws and their relation to human physiology. It is here that he gives the first statement of his "corpuscular hypothesis," or mechanical theory of matter.

Cushing B550; Osler 939 (1669 ed.); Waller 10754; Wellcome II, p. 221 (1669 ed.).

*365. ———. *Memoirs for the natural history of humane blood*. London: Printed for Samuel Smith, 1683/4. [16] 289 [7] pp. 16.1 cm. Old calf, rebacked retaining original spine.

The present work is Boyle's most important medical contribution and is one of the first to deal with the scientific analysis of the blood. Bloodletting was still quite common at the time, so Boyle had little difficulty obtaining blood for his experiments. In his analysis of the blood, Boyle includes its properties of taste, temperature, combustibility, and weight and also mentions its serous and red portions, volatile and fixed salts, oil, mucus content, etc. He discusses human and animal blood, and describes a series of experiments to test the anticoagulating properties of various substances. Boyle also provides a series of remedies prepared from blood for a wide variety of ailments from hysteria and epilepsy to coughs and other respiratory complaints.

Cushing B579; Garrison-Morton 861 (1683 ed.); Waller 1388; Wellcome II, p. 223 (1684 ed.).

366. ———. *Of the reconcileableness of specifick medicines to the corpuscular philosophy. To which is annexed a discourse about the advantages of the use of simple medicines*. London: Printed for Sam. Smith, 1685. [14] 225 pp. 16.9 cm. Calf.

Among Boyle's scientific works, these two treatises have been the least studied, probably because they were highly theoretical and offered little in the way of medical advice. Medical practice, at the time, was almost totally an art, and Boyle designed this book to put some science into that art. In the first treatise, he presents his arguments in a series of six propositions illustrated by means of numerous experiments, showing what Boyle believed would happen in the body when specifics were administered. The other section of the book was intended to discourage the use of complicated prescriptions, which in those days often contained twenty or more ingredients. Boyle presents a number of arguments and propositions to support his contention and concludes with an enthusiastic endorsement of the efficacy of gems and stones from the heads of snakes—a medieval belief which persisted for centuries.

Cushing B589; Osler 949; Waller 1391; Wellcome II, p. 224.

*367. ———. *A disquisition about the final causes of natural things*. London: Printed by H.C. for J. Taylor, 1688. [xvi] 274 [6] pp. 16.7 cm. Half calf.

This work contains Boyle's discussion of many physiological matters, especially those concerning the eye and defective vision. Boyle recognized that the site of the cataract is in the optic lens, and he included a number of case histories to substantiate his findings. This work contains the famous passage in which Boyle relates his conversation with William Harvey on how he discovered the circulation of the blood.

Cushing B556; Waller 10766; Wellcome II, p. 224.

*368. MARCELLO MALPIGHI (1628–1694) and CARLO FRACASSATI (1630–1672). *Epistolae anatomicae.* Amsterdam: Apud Casparum Commelinum, 1669. [4] 260 pp., 5 fold. plates. 13.3 cm. Vellum.

Professor of anatomy at Bologna, Pisa, and Messina, Malpighi was the founder of the science of histology and one of the greatest microscopic anatomists. He was a friend and colleague of Fracassati at the University of Bologna.

This work contains four letters of Malpighi and two of Fracassati on the brain, tongue, adipose tissues, and skin, as well as five folding plates illustrating their microscopic investigations.

Cushing M102a; Waller 6206; Wellcome III, p. 50.

*369. MARCELLO MALPIGHI. *Dissertatio epistolica de formatione pulli in ovo.* London: Apud Joannem Martyn, 1673. [3] 42 pp., 4 fold. plates. 23 cm. Bound with No. 370.

This important work on the developmental stages of the chicken firmly established Malpighi's reputation as an embryologist. The four plates accompanying the text far surpass previous work in this area and show the development of such fine structures as the neural groove, cerebral vesicles, aortic arches, and the optic vesicles. Also included with this treatise are seven letters between Malpighi and Henry Oldenburg, secretary of the Royal Society of London.

Cushing M102; Garrison-Morton 469; Waller 6200.

*370. ———. *Dissertationes epistolicae duae; una de formatione pulli in ovo. Altera de bombyce.* London: Impensis Joannis Martyn, 1673. [12] 100 pp., 12 fold. plates. 23 cm. Bound with No. 369.

Although the title page indicates that there are two dissertations in this work, only *De bombyce* is present in this issue. Malpighi was interested in silkworms and their cultivation and in this treatise he discusses their external form, musculature, tracheae, nerves, heart, intestines, genitourinary tract, and silk-spinning apparatus. Much of the silkworm's external and internal anatomy is illustrated in the twelve folding plates that follow the treatise.

Cushing M101 (1669 ed.); Osler 984.

*371. ———. *Anatome plantarum.* Vol. I only of 2 vols. London: Impensis Johannis Martyn, 1675. Vol. I: [4] 82 [2] 20 pp., 61 tables, 91 plates. 35.9 cm. Old vellum, rebacked.

Malpighi was an anatomist, biologist, embryologist, microscopist, and pathologist, and an excellent botanist. This rare volume, a landmark in the development of plant morphology, contains more than sixty fine copper engravings of seeds, plant cells, plants and their parts, and an appendix of embryological subjects. Volume II, published in 1679, is not present here.

Cushing M97; Garrison-Morton 536; Osler 985.

*372. ———. *Opera omnia*. 2nd ed. 2 vols. in 1. Leiden: Apud Petrum vander Aa, 1687. Vol. I: [16] 170 [22] pp.; Vol. II: 379 [37] pp., plates (part fold.). 23.5 cm. Vellum.

This collection of Malpighi's works contains his famed work on the anatomy of plants, the embryonic development of the chick, the anatomy of the silkworm (the first monograph on an invertebrate), and one of his greatest contributions: the discovery of the existence of capillaries, which completed the chain of the circulation of the blood postulated by Harvey.

Garrison-Morton 66 (1st ed., 1686); Osler 986 (1st ed.); Waller 6202.

*373. NATHANIEL HODGES (1629–1688). *Loimologia; or, An historical account of the plague in London in 1665; with precautionary directions against the like contagion.* London: Printed for E. Bell . . . and J. Osborn, 1720. vi, 288 pp. 18.9 cm.

During the great plague of London in 1665, Hodges remained to tend the victims while many other physicians and laymen fled the city in fear for their lives. His descriptions of the clinical symptoms, means of prevention, and methods of treatment contained in this work are among the best records of this plague. Prepared in Latin and first published in 1672, it was translated into English by John Quincy (see No. 462) in this 1720 edition. Quincy has also added an essay on the causes of contagious diseases and how they are best cured. In addition, he includes some remarks about an epidemic in France and how it might best be prevented from spreading to England. On the flyleaf of the book is a brief handwritten account of the plague in Algiers with the date May 6, 1787.

Cushing H372 (1721 ed.); Garrison-Morton 5121 (1st ed., 1672); Osler 2978; Wellcome III, p. 281.

*374. JOHN SMITH (1630–1670). Γηροκομία Βασιλική. *King Solomons portraiture of old age.* London: Printed by J. Hayes for S. Thomson, 1666. [14] 266 [5] pp. 16.6 cm. Calf, rebacked.

In this small volume with a strong religious emphasis, Smith expounds on the description of old age found in Ecclesiastes 12:1–6. The book's chief medical significance is in the author's attempt to show that King Solomon knew of the heart's action and how the blood circulated through the body. Smith does this by interpreting and explaining the meaning of two expressions from verse 6: the pitcher at the fountain and the wheel at the cistern.

Osler 4768 (1676 ed.); Waller 9029 (1676 ed.).

CARLO FRACASSATI (1630–1672). *Epistolae anatomicae.*

See No. 368.

*375. MARTIN LIPEN (1630–1692). *Bibliotheca realis medica*. Frankfurt: Cura & sumptibus Johannis Friderici, prelo Johannis Nicolai Hummii, 1679. [19] 492 [42] pp. 34.8 cm. Contemporary blind-stamped pigskin with two clasps.

This comprehensive and well-printed early bibliography of medicine is arranged by subject and contains numerous cross references as well as a long and detailed author index. Lipen, a native of Brandenberg, was not a physician but prepared this volume as part of a six-volume series on various aspects of learning dating from the beginning of printing. The earliest bibliography on circulation is found in this volume, which contains some twenty-seven entries including the works of Harvey, Highmore, Primerose, Riolan, and Walaeus.

Garrison-Morton 6744.1; Waller 18679; Wellcome III, p. 528.

*376. RICHARD LOWER (1631–1691). *Tractatus de corde*. Amsterdam: Apud Danielem Elzevirium, 1669. [16] 232 pp., 7 fold. plates. 15.2 cm. Vellum. Bound with No. 388.

Lower, a Cornishman, was one of the foremost English physiologists of the seventeenth century. He first described many finer structures of the heart, including the scroll-like nature of the musculature; he gave an accurate description of tricuspid valve endocarditis; and his chief contribution was his proof that venous blood, dark in color, becomes bright red on passing through the lungs by virtue of being brought into contact with air. He was one of the first to perform a blood transfusion.

Lower was an ardent supporter of Harvey, and this classic on cardiac physiology is the first important work on experimental studies of the heart after Harvey. This Amsterdam edition appeared the same year as the London edition, which is usually considered to be the first.

Cushing L372; Garrison-Morton 761 (London ed., 1669); Osler 3277; Russell 541; Waller 6047; Wellcome III, p. 552.

*377. ANTHONY VAN LEEUWENHOEK (1632–1723). *Anatomica seu interiora rerum*. Leiden: Apud Cornelium Boutesteyn, 1687. [6] 3–78, 260 (misnumbered 258) pp., illus., fold. plates. 19.1 cm.

*378. ———. *Arcana naturae*. 3rd ed. of No. 377. Leiden: Apud Cornelium Boutestein, 1708 (misdated 1808). [6] 64, 260 (misnumbered 258) pp., illus., fold. plates. 19.1 cm. Bound with No. 380.

*379. ———. *Continuatio epistolarum*. Leiden: Apud Cornelium Boutestein, 1689. [8] 124 pp., plates (part fold.). 19.1 cm. Bound with No. 382.

*380. ———. *Continuatio epistolarum*. 2nd ed. of No. 379. Leiden: Apud Johannem du Vivie, Theodorum Haak, & Joh. Arn. Langerack, 1715. [8] 124 pp., plates (part fold.). 19.1 cm. Bound with No. 378.

*381. ———. *Arcana naturae detecta.* Delft: Apud Henricum a Kroneveld, 1695. [4] 568 [14] pp., front. (port.), illus., fold. plates. 19.1 cm.

*382. ———. *Continuatio arcanorum naturae detectorum.* Delft: Apud Henricum a Kroonevelt, 1697. 192 [8] pp., fold. plates. 19.1 cm. Bound with No. 379.

"To Antonio van Leeuwenhoek, of Delft, belongs the high merit of having been the first to use the microscope systematically and of having brought the construction of the simple microscope in his own hands to a high degree of perfection. . . . Self-taught and never having attended a university, ignorant of Latin and Greek and of the classical texts, he became one of the greatest and most expert microscopists, thanks to the sagacity of his observations and the perfection of his technique" (Arturo Castiglioni, *A history of medicine.* New York, 1946. pp. 528–529). Leeuwenhoek was a master lens-grinder and, during his lifetime, constructed several hundred microscopes, grinding a new lens for each new investigation which he undertook.

These volumes contain some eighty letters from among the several hundred in which Leeuwenhoek communicated the results of his microscopical investigations to the Royal Society in London and which were published in its *Philosophical Transactions* over many years. Though not a trained scientist and unable to follow up his hundreds of investigations, he opened up avenues of anatomy hitherto unknown and unseen, leading to accurate physiology and, in turn, to accurate therapeutics. One example is use of his perfected microscope by Malpighi (see No. 372) to define the ultimate structure of the capillaries, which closed the final link in Harvey's description of the circulation of the blood. Leeuwenhoek first described the individual plant cell, the individual striped muscle cell, spermatozoa, red corpuscles, and the crystalline lens of the eye. These works are richly illustrated with Leeuwenhoek's drawings, which are of fundamental importance to histologic anatomy.

Cushing L128; Garrison-Morton 98; Osler 1020, 1021; Waller 10876, 10877, 10880, 10882, 10884; Wellcome III, p. 477.

*383. ———. *Ontdeckte onsigtbaarheden.* [Leiden: Cornelius Boutesteyn, Daniel van Gaesbeeck, 1684–1686]. Various pagings, illus., plates (part fold.). 19.1 cm.

The Dutch edition of a number of the letters to the Royal Society of London.

Waller 10887; Wellcome III, p. 476.

WILLIAM CROONE (1633–1684). *De ratione motus musculorum.*

See No. 348.

*384. BERNARDINO RAMAZZINI (1633–1714). *De morbis artificum diatriba.* Modena: Typis Antonii Capponi, 1700. viii, 360 pp. 19.4 cm. Contemporary boards, uncut.

Like many prominent physicians of his day, Ramazzini was a highly versatile individual—clinician, epidemiologist, sanitarian, poet, philosopher, and scholar. He was a prolific author and wrote on such subjects as the water supply of Modena, cattle plague, personal hygiene, and the abuse of cinchona. The present work, an early treatise on occupational diseases and the history of industrial medicine and hygiene, is regarded as his most important work. He discusses the diseases of over fifty occupations including miners, potters, masons, wrestlers, farmers, nurses, soldiers, and many others. In discussing the etiology, treatment, and prevention of these diseases he often goes back to Hippocrates, Celsus, and Galen, and, after summarizing their observations, relates his own experiences with the various diseases.

Cushing R12; Garrison-Morton 2121; Osler 3760; Waller 7727.

*385. ———. *De morbis artificum . . . diatriba Mutinae olim edita.* Padua: Per Jo. Baptistam Conzattum, 1713. [16] 453 [27] pp. 16.5 Original paper boards, uncut.

At the age of eighty, Ramazzini revised his important contribution to industrial medicine and saw it published only a year before his death. He rearranged the latter portion of the book, adding many new case histories, and included a supplement of twelve new chapters on occupations he had not previously described.

Cushing R12 (1st ed., 1700); Garrison-Morton 2121 (1st ed.); Osler 3760 (1st ed.); Waller 7727 (1st ed.).

*386. ———. *L'art de conserver la santé des princes, et des persones du premier rang. . . . L'art de conserver la santé des religieuses, et Les avantages de la vie sobre, du Seigneur Louis Cornaro.* Leiden: Chés Jean Arn. Langerak, 1724. [16] 374 [5] pp. 16.5 cm.

Ramazzini's interest in occupational disease is evidenced here in the French translations of his two treatises on the health of the nobility and of the religious. In the sixteenth century another Italian, Luigi Cornaro (1475–1566), had written a curious treatise on personal hygiene and the simple life, which is here translated into French with Ramazzini's notes.

*387. MATHIAS TILING (1634–1685). *De febribus petechialibus tractatus curiosus.* Frankfurt: Impensis Jacobi Gothofredi Seyleri, 1676. [40] 362 [5] pp. 16.7 cm. Vellum.

Tiling received his medical degree at Wittenberg in 1663, practiced at Emden and Bremen, and became professor of medicine at Rinteln in 1669. Although he wrote several works on clinical medicine and therapeutics, the present treatise is little known. It is one of the earliest works on cerebrospinal meningitis and presents the symptoms of the disease and suggested methods of treatment. It was not until 1805 that Gaspard Vieusseux (1746–1814) gave the first definitive description of the disease, and it was not until 1887 that Anton Weichselbaum (1845–1920) discovered *Neisseria meningitidis,* the causative agent of cerebrospinal meningitis.

Waller 9591.

*388. JAN SWAMMERDAM (1637–1680). *Tractatus physico-anatomico-medicus de respiratione usuque pulmonum.* Leiden: Apud Danielem, Abraham. & Adrian. à Gaasbeeck, 1667. [14] 121 [22] pp., illus. 15.2 cm. Vellum. Bound with No. 376.

Despite his short life and a professional career of only about twelve years, Swammerdam of Amsterdam was one of the outstanding comparative anatomists of the seventeenth century. He was a pioneer in microscopic studies, investigating especially the anatomy of insects. At his death after seven years of illness and scientific inactivity, he left a mass of papers and reports of investigations, most of which remained unknown until they were published a century later.

The present work, a classic on respiration, was his inaugural dissertation at the University of Leipzig and one of only four works published during his lifetime. He first showed that the lungs of a newborn infant would float if the child had ever breathed, and this discovery was put to legal use in cases of infanticide. The engraved title page illustrates his ingenious, if complicated, device for the study of respiration.

Cushing S482; Garrison-Morton 1724; Osler 959 (1679 ed.); Waller 9385.

389. FRANÇOIS MAURICEAU (1637–1709). *Traité des maladies des femmes grosses, et de celles qui sont nouvellement accouchées.* 2nd ed. Paris: Chez l'auteur, 1675. [18] 501 [25] pp., illus. 23.5 cm.

Mauriceau, a Parisian, was an ordinary surgeon and not a doctor of medicine, but his close observation and detailed studies of the fetus, the pregnant uterus, the female pelvis, and the techniques of delivery made him a leading obstetrician of his time.

His famous work on pregnancy and delivery, here in second edition, was first published in 1668 and went through many editions and translations. "It established obstetrics as a science" (Garrison-Morton 6147).

Garrison-Morton 6147 (1st ed., 1668); Waller 6364 (1681 ed.).

Gift of Dr. Walter L. Bierring.

390. ———. *The diseases of women with child, and in child-bed.* 6th ed. London: Printed for T. Cox, J. Clarke; and T. Combes, 1727. xliv, 373 [7] pp. 2 copies. Copy 1: 19.7 cm. Copy 2: 19.7 cm.

Mauriceau's popular *Traité des maladies des femmes grosses, et de celles qui sont accouchées* (1668) (No. 389) went through many editions and was translated into English, German, Dutch, and Italian. It was first translated into English by Hugh Chamberlen (ca. 1630–ca. 1720) in 1673 and continued through nine editions until 1758. The Chamberlen family developed a practical obstetrical forceps in the late 1640's and kept its design secret for several generations while profiting greatly from its use in their practice.

Cushing M211 (1755 ed.); Waller 6361 (1736 ed.).

Copy 2: In memory of Robert D. Gauchat.

391. ———. *Observations sur la grossesse et l'accouchement des femmes et sur leurs maladies & celles des enfans nouveau-nez.* Paris: Par la Compagnie des libraires associez, 1715. [8] 572 [12] pp. 2 copies. Copy 1: 24.4 cm. Copy 2: 24.6 cm. Bound with No. 392.

The present work was originally issued as Volume II of the fourth edition of Mauriceau's *Traité des maladies des femmes grosses, et de celles qui sont accouchées* (1694). It is a compendium of seven hundred case histories dealing with pregnancy and childbirth as well as with the diseases and problems of the newborn. Mauriceau's case histories are models of clear and succinct description, revealing him to be a skilled and experienced practitioner.

Cushing M212 (1738 ed.).

Copy 1: Gift of Dr. Walter L. Bierring.

Copy 2: Gift of Dr. John Martin.

392. ———. *Dernières observations sur les maladies des femmes grosses et accouchées.* Paris: Par la Compagnie des libraires associez, 1715. [2] 77 pp. 2 copies. Copy 1: 24.4 cm. Copy 2: 24.6 cm. Bound with No. 391.

This smaller work of 150 case histories is included with Mauriceau's *Observations sur la grossesse et l'accouchement des femmes.* As the title indicates, these case histories are his final observations on the diseases of pregnancy and childbirth. It is likely that they were intended to complete and amplify his earlier work in obstetrics and gynecology.

Cushing M212 (1738 ed.).

Copy 1: Gift of Dr. Walter L. Bierring.

Copy 2: Gift of Dr. John Martin.

*393. NICOLAUS STENO (1638–1686). *Observationes anatomica.* Leiden: Apud Jacobum Chouët, 1662. [xii] 108 pp., 3 fold. plates. 13.2 cm. Contemporary calf. Bound with No. 342.

A Danish physician, geologist, and clergyman, Steno studied medicine at Copenhagen, Leiden, and Paris. He settled in Italy, first as professor of anatomy at Padua and then in Florence as house physician to Grand Duke Ferdinand II. He served for a brief time as professor and royal anatomist in Copenhagen. Dissatisfied, he returned to Florence where he abandoned his scientific career and entered the priesthood, eventually becoming bishop. As an anatomist, Steno devoted his studies primarily to the muscles and glands and made many important contributions. In his dissertation on the muscles and glands, *De musculis et glandulis observationum specimen* (1664), he clearly recognized that the heart was a muscle, which was a great advance in the knowledge of this organ.

In the present work he assembled a collection of the observations and studies he had made of the glands of the eye, vessels of the nose, salivary and lacrimal glands, and the duct of the parotid gland (Stensen's duct). The text is accompanied by three finely executed folding plates.

Garrison-Morton 973; Osler 4018; Waller 9226.

*394. MARTIN LISTER (1638?–1712). *Exercitatio anatomica.* London: Sumptibus Sam. Smith & Benj. Walford, 1694. xi, 208 pp., 8 fold. plates. 17.5 cm. Old calf, rebacked.

Lister, at one time ordinary physician to Queen Anne, published a few medical works and edited a 1703 edition of Hippocrates' *Aphorisms.* His chief interest, however, was in zoology and he published several works in this field. The present work contains his essays on the anatomy of snails and slugs with eight folding plates depicting his studies. This work was followed by a companion volume in 1695 which treated various animals, birds, fish, and selected marine life.

Osler 3252; Waller 11892; Wellcome III, p. 529.

*395. FREDERIK RUYSCH (1638–1731). *Observationum anatomico-chirurgicarum centuria.* Amsterdam: Apud Henricum & viduam Theodori Boom, 1691. [16] 138, 120 pp., plates (part fold.). 23 cm. Contemporary vellum.

Ruysch, a Dutch surgeon and anatomist and professor of anatomy at Leiden and Amsterdam, mastered (and probably invented) a method of minute injection of anatomical structures allowing detailed studies. The recipe for the injected substance has been lost, however. He made many anatomical investigations, including those of the valves in the lymphatics, the bronchial arteries, and the vascular plexuses of the heart, and was the first to point out the nourishment of the fetus through the umbilical cord.

In this text of practical observations in medicine and surgery, Ruysch presents the results of one hundred studies and illustrates many of them with excellent engravings, many of which are undoubtedly enhanced by his injection techniques. Also bound with this work is his *Museum anatomicum Ruyschianum,* a catalog of the specimens in his museum, which was purchased and moved to Russia by Peter the Great in 1717.

Waller 8337.

*396. ———. *Adversariorum anatomico-medico-chirurgicorum decas prima.* Vol. I only of 3 vols. Amsterdam: Apud Janssonio-Waesbergios, 1717. Vol. I: [3] 34 [2] pp., 2 plates. 20.4 cm. Contemporary wrappers.

This first printing is one of the earliest accounts of the cellular activity of the female reproductive system. Included are two engraved plates showing six illustrations of the anatomy of the ovaries and uterus (see also No. 397).

The following collection of twenty-four papers (Nos. 397 through 407) by or about Ruysch was apparently bound together by a contemporary. While they do not constitute his complete works, the ten parts of his *Thesaurus anatomicus* are especially noteworthy, and the engraved illustrations which accompany them deserve special mention for their whimsical, almost surrealistic, quality: quaintly posed skeletons surrounded by stuffed monsters, strange reptiles, dried plants, and sea creatures. Three supplementary parts and two indices to the *Thesaurus,* and several shorter papers involving controversies in which Ruysch was involved, complete the collection.

*397. ———. *Adversariorum anatomico-medico-chirurgicorum decas.* 3 parts. Amsterdam: Apud Janssonio-Waesbergios, 1729–1737. Part I: [2] 34, 18 pp.; Part II: [4] 46 pp.; Part III: [6] 36 pp., plates (1 fold.). 24.1 cm.

*398. ———. *Thesaurus animalium primus.* Amsterdam: Apud Janssonio-Waesbergios, 1725. 20 pp., 7 plates (2 fold.). 24.1 cm.

*399. ———. *Thesaurus anatomicus.* 10 parts. Amsterdam: Apud Janssonio-Waesbergios, 1726–1744. Plates (part fold.). 24.1 cm.

*400. ———. *Curae posteriores.* Amsterdam: Apud Janssonio-Waesbergios, 1738. [8] 31 pp., 3 plates. 24.1 cm.

*401. ———. *Curae renovatae.* Amsterdam: Apud Janssonio-Waesbergios, 1742. [10] 22 pp., 3 plates (1 fold.). 24.1 cm.

*402. ———. *Tractatio anatomica.* Amsterdam: Apud Janssonio-Waesbergios, 1742. [4] 20 pp., plate. 24.1 cm.

*403. JOHANN CHRISTOPH BOHL (1703–1785). *Dissertatio epistolica, ad . . . Ruyschium.* Amsterdam: Apud Janssonio-Waesbergios, 1744. 13 pp. 24.1 cm.

*404. FREDERIK RUYSCH. *Responsio, ad Dissertationem epistolicam . . . Jo. Christoph. Bohlii.* Amsterdam: Apud Janssonio-Waesbergios, 1727. 12 pp., illus. 24.1 cm.

*405. PHILIPPE HECQUET (1661–1737). *Epistola . . . de Ruyschiano uteri musculo.* Amsterdam: Apud Janssonio-Waesbergios, 1727. 8 pp. 24.1 cm.

*406. ABRAHAM VATER (1684–1751). *Epistola gratulatoria, ad . . . Fredericum Ruyschium* [followed by] RUYSCH. *Responsio.* Amsterdam: Apud Janssonio-Waesbergios, 1727. 16 pp., plate. 24.1 cm.

*407. HERMANN BOERHAAVE (1668–1738) and RUYSCH. *Opusculum anatomicum de fabrica glandularum in corpore humano.* Amsterdam: Apud Janssonio-Waesbergios, 1733. 81 pp., illus. 24.1 cm.

Lindeboom 343.

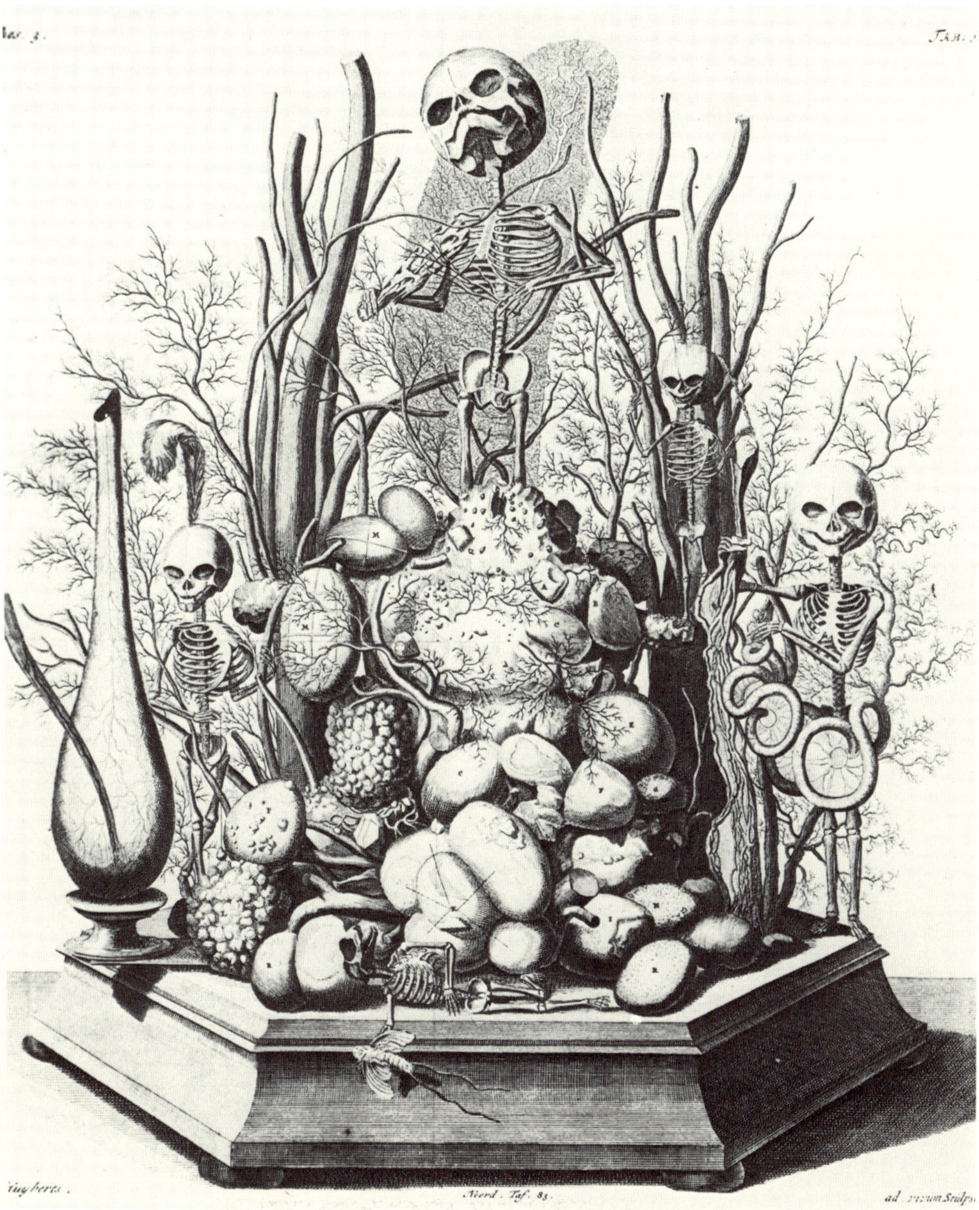

No. 397. Ruysch. *Adversariorum Anatomico-Medico-Chirurgicorum Decas.* Ruysch often portrayed anatomical subjects in an allegorical fashion.

*408. SEBASTIAN CHRISTIAN VON ZEIDLER (fl. 1680). *Somatotomia andropologica* [sic]. Prague: Typis Joannis Caroli Gerzabek, 1686. [8] 118 [2] pp., 28 plates, port. 29.3 cm. Limp vellum.

Little is known of Zeidler's life and work, although he was on the faculty at the University of Prague and was physician to the Emperor of Prussia. The text of this book fully explains the many anatomical figures depicted in the plates and refers chiefly to Greek authorities, although Vesalius, Fernel, and Bartholin, among others, are cited. The twenty-eight plates illustrate the human body, fetus, and many organs. They were widely borrowed from various sources including Vesalius, Spiegel, Casserio, and Rösslin.

*409. ———. *Somatotomia anthropologica.* Prague: Typis Joannis Caroli Gerzabek, 1686. [8] 118 [2] pp., 28 plates. 30.9 cm. Marbled boards, rebacked in calf.

In this printing of *Somatotomia anthropologica,* the title page has been reset to correct the spelling of the second word of the title from the original "andropologica." Moreover, this issue does not contain the portrait present in the first issue.

Waller 10462.

*410. JOHN MAYOW (1640–1679). *Tractatus duo, quorum prior agit de respiratione: alter de rachitide.* Leiden: Apud Cornelium Driehuysen [et] Felicem Lopez de Haro, 1671. 57 pp., 2 plates. 15.5 cm. Vellum.

Graduating from Oxford in 1670, Mayow was educated as a lawyer but made medicine his profession. Few details of his later life are known and no record of his medical studies has been found. He is said, however, to have practiced medicine during the summers at Bath, and he made a chemical analysis of its salt springs. The present work, his first publication, appeared in 1668 and includes an account of his experiments on respiration and his tract on rickets. Mayow visualized the heart as a muscular pump which circulates the blood and carries a substance he called *spiritus nitro-aereus* throughout the body. A century later Lavoisier identified *spiritus nitro-aereus* as oxygen. It was only after Lavoisier and Priestley made their discoveries that the significance of Mayow's work began to be recognized. His tract on rickets was only the second on the subject by an Englishman. In it he gives a clear description of the clinical symptoms of the disease and makes several useful suggestions concerning its management.

Osler 3358 (1668 ed.); Russell 565; Waller 6391.

*411. ———. *Tractatus quinque medico-physici.* 2 vols. in 1. Oxford: E theatro Sheldoniano, 1674. Vol. I: [42] 335 [1] pp.; Vol. II: 152 pp., port., 6 fold. plates. 18 cm. Contemporary calf, rebacked.

This historically important and rare book "is one of the best English medical classics" according to Garrison and Morton and is "one of the world's greatest masterpieces" according to John Ruhräh (*Pediatrics of the past.* New York, 1925. p. 344). In addition to the two treatises in *Tractatus duo* (No. 410), it includes his tracts on respiration in which he accurately describes the role of the intercostal muscles in breathing, a tract on respiration of the fetus *in utero,* and *De motu musculari* in which he gives what may be the first description of mitral stenosis. His work shows that he was much in advance of his time and that he was a conscientious researcher who based his results on close attention to detail in the manner of his contemporaries, Robert Boyle and Robert Hooke.

Cushing M236; Garrison-Morton 578; Osler 3359; Russell 566(b); Waller 6392.

*412. THEODOR KERCKRING (1640–1693). *Spicilegium anatomicum. . . . Osteogeniam foetuum.* Amsterdam: Sumptibus Andreae Frisii, 1670. [22] 280 pp., illus., 9 fold. plates. 22.2 cm. Vellum.

Kerckring, a physician at Amsterdam and a fellow-worker of Ruysch (see No. 395), added a number of original observations to anatomical knowledge. In this handsome volume, with its thirty-nine interesting and accurately drawn plates, he describes the *valvulae conniventes* (now sometimes called the "valves of Kerckring") of the small intestine. He also made noteworthy investigations of the fetal bones, described in the second section of this book.

Cushing K53; Garrison-Morton 383; Waller 5270; Wellcome III, p. 386.

*413. ———. *Anthropogeniae ichnographia.* Paris: Apud F. Leonard, 1672. [iv] 8 pp., illus. 23 cm. Quarter calf with marbled boards.

This work on fetal growth and bones, first published in 1671, is not as well known as his *Spicilegium anatomicum.*

Cushing K52 (1671 ed.); Waller 5268 (1671 ed.); Wellcome III, p. 387 (1671 ed.).

*414. GIDEON HARVEY (1640?–1700?). *The disease of London: or, A new discovery of the scorvey.* London: Printed by T. James, for W. Thackery, 1675. [14] 296 pp. 16.5 cm. Calf.

Though Harvey was a successful clinician, physician to Charles II and William III, as well as city physician of London, he was a medical outsider. He was a severe critic of and scourge to his contemporaries, whom he designated "dung-doctors," because of some of their clinical methods. Although he wrote almost endlessly on philosophy, diseases, cures, real or imagined quackery and charlatanry, with many of his books passing through two or three editions, the *Dictionary of national biography* (Vol. IX, p. 87) flatly states that "his works have no scientific value."

The present work on the scurvy deals with its causes, symptoms, and "several methods of curing the said disease by remedies, both Galenical, and chymical."

*415. GÉRARD AUDRAN (1640–1703). *Les proportions du corps humain.* Paris: Girard Audran, 1683. [7] pp., 28 plates. 41.7 cm.

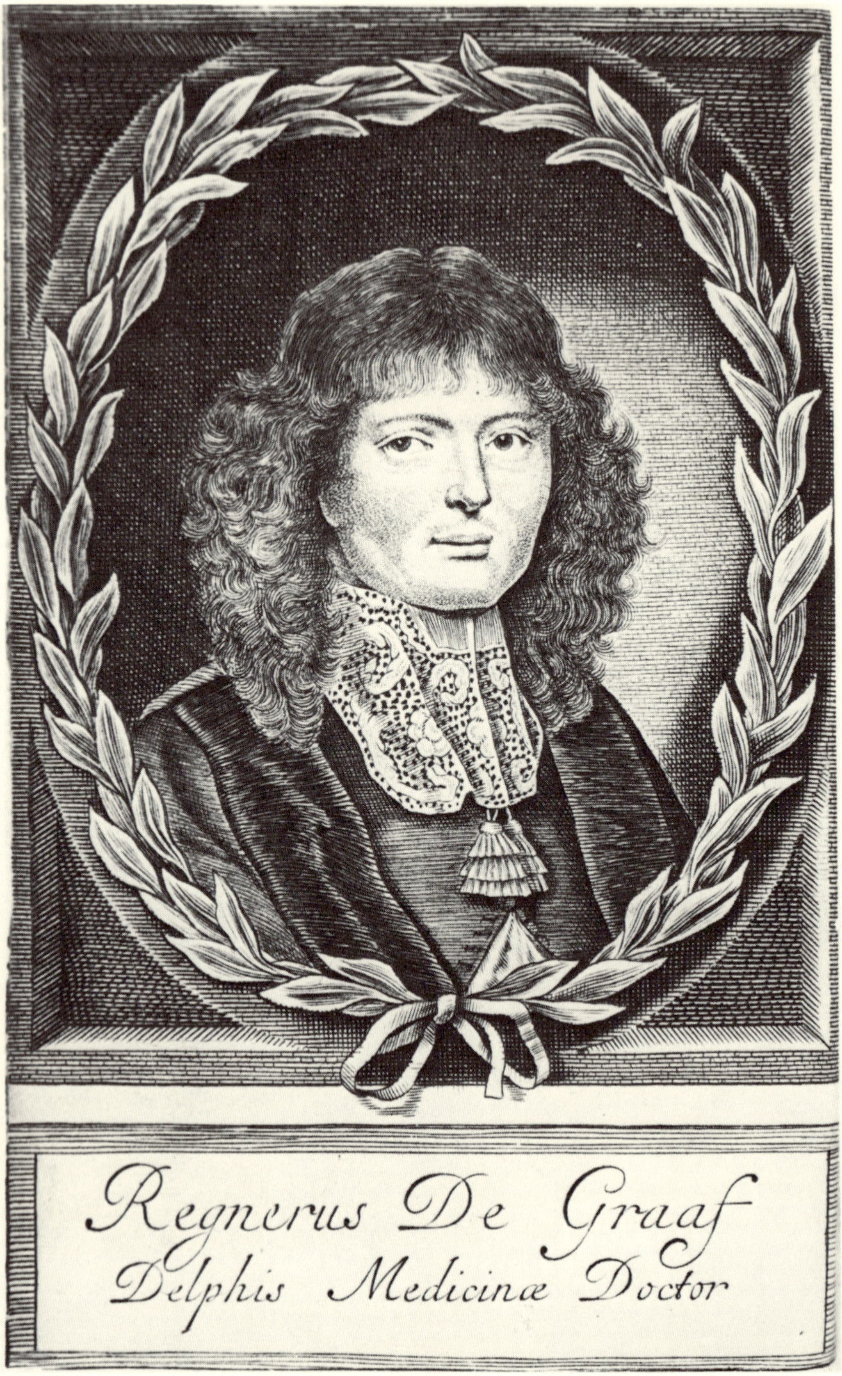

No. 418. De Graaf. *De Mulierum Organis Generationi Inservientibus.* The portrait frontispiece of the author at age 31.

From a noted family of French artists and engravers, Audran was one of its most distinguished members and was ultimately appointed engraver to King Louis XIV. This atlas of twenty-eight fine engravings was prepared by the author as an aid to artists and is based on classical statuary. The line drawings of such classical figures as Venus Aphrodite, Hercules, and Laocoön include detailed measurements to indicate precise proportions.

Choulant-Frank, p. 359; Wellcome II, p. 69.

416. REINIER DE GRAAF (1641–1673). *Tractatus anatomico-medicus de succi pancreatici natura & usu.* Leiden: Ex officina Hackiana, 1671. [22] 216 [14] pp., 3 fold. plates. 15.8 cm.

De Graaf, a Dutch anatomist and physiologist, was celebrated for his work on digestion as well as on the anatomy of the genital organs of both sexes. He was an early investigator of the pancreas and collected the pancreatic juice of dogs by means of artificially created pancreatic fistulae. In this work, he comments on the small quantity of juice secreted and its alkaline nature. The work also contains de Graaf's letter to Luca Schacht (1634–1689) on the reproductive system.

Cushing G348; Garrison-Morton 974 (1664 ed.); Waller 3678; Wellcome III, p. 142.

*417. ———. *De virorum organis generationi inservientibus. De clysteribus, et De usu siphonis in anatomia.* Leiden and Rotterdam: Ex officina Hackiana, 1668. [32] 234 [14] pp., front. (port.), 11 fold. plates. 16.2 cm. Contemporary paneled calf.

This small volume is the first edition of this classical and accurate account of the anatomy of the testicle. It contains also an account of the use of clysters and of experimental fistulae which far predates Claude Bernard and Beaumont. The eleven foldout plates of the anatomy of the male genitalia are interesting and original but of modest artistic attainment.

Cushing G345; Garrison-Morton 1210; Waller 3670; Wellcome III, p. 142.

*418. ———. *De mulierum organis generationi inservientibus tractatus novus.* Leiden: Ex officina Hackiana, 1672. [24] 334 [14] pp., front. (port.), 27 plates (9 fold.). 14.5 cm. Contemporary paneled calf.

De Graaf demonstrated ovulation anatomically, pathologically, and experimentally. He opposed the Aristotelian doctrine of the egg being formed in the uterus as a result of activation of the menstrual blood by the male semen, but held that generation takes place from the ovum pre-existent in the ovary. He herein gives the first description of ovarian ("Graafian") follicles and the corpus luteum. His was an advanced and accurate understanding of the anatomy of the female genitalia. The twenty-seven engraved plates illustrating de Graaf's anatomical research add interest to this small volume.

Cushing G344; Garrison-Morton 1209; Waller 3669; Wellcome III, p. 142.

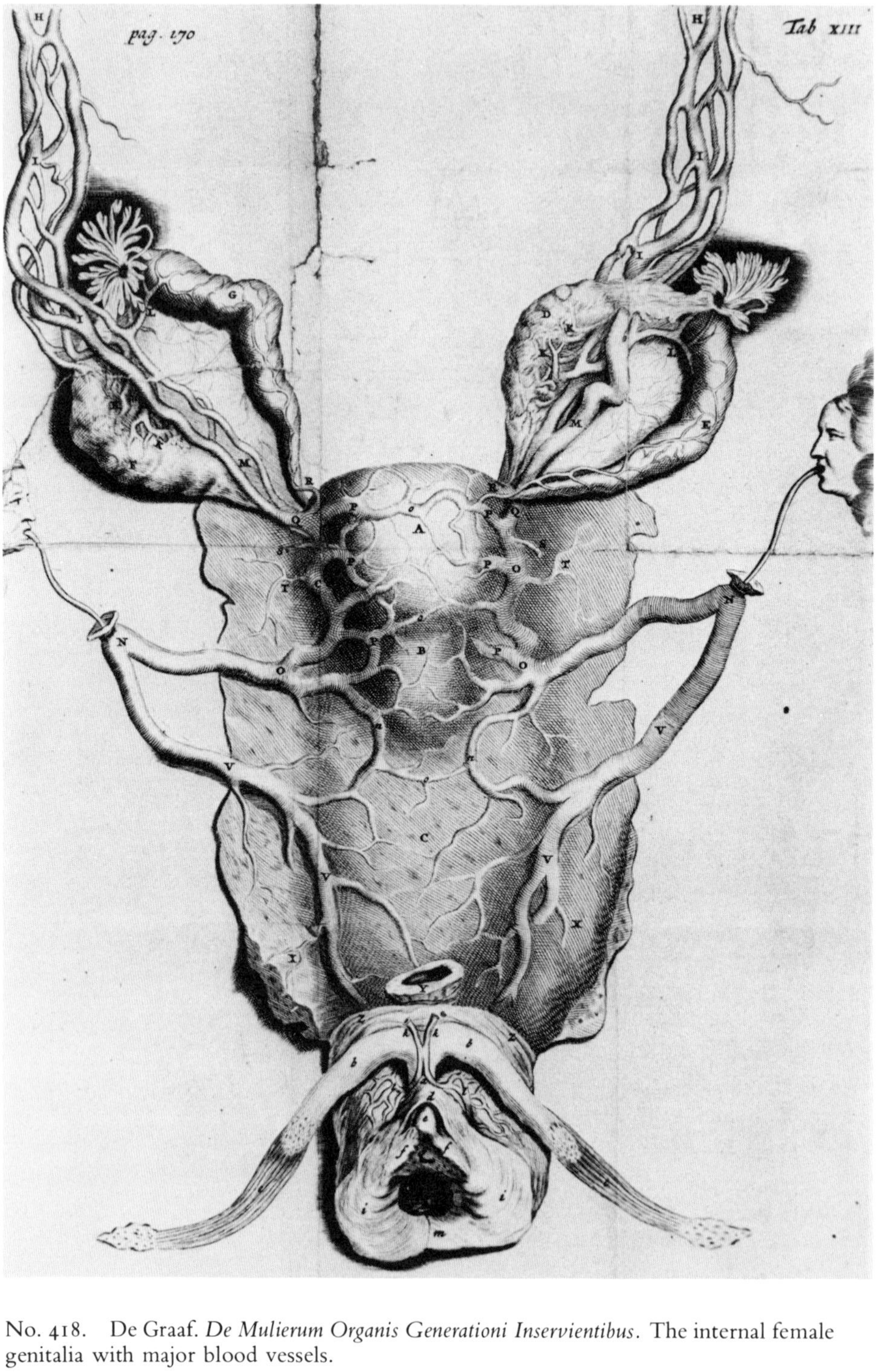

No. 418. De Graaf. *De Mulierum Organis Generationi Inservientibus.* The internal female genitalia with major blood vessels.

*419. ———. *Opera omnia.* 2nd ed. Leiden: Sumpt. Jo. Ant. Huguetan, 1678. xx, 390 pp., engr. port., fold. plates. 16.8 cm. Vellum.

This second edition of de Graaf's collected works contains all of his important works, including his books on the male and female genitalia and on the pancreas.

Waller 3675; Wellcome III, p. 142.

*420. NEHEMIAH GREW (1641–1712). *Musaeum Regalis Societatis; or, A catalogue & description of the natural and artificial rarities belonging to the Royal Society and preserved at Gresham Colledge. . . . Whereunto is subjoyned the comparative anatomy of stomachs and guts.* London: Printed by W. Rawlins, for the author, 1681. [12] 386 [4] 43 pp., front. (port.), 31 plates (1 fold.). 31.4 cm.

Grew, who was secretary of the Royal Society, compiled this catalogue of its museum. He was one of the early comparative anatomists to use the microscope and he introduced the term "comparative anatomy." His treatise on the comparative anatomy of stomachs and guts is an early classic in the field, and the thirty-one plates are particularly fine.

Cushing G402; Garrison-Morton 297; Wellcome III, p. 164.

*421. RAYMOND VIEUSSENS (1641–1715?). *Neurographia universalis.* Lyons: Apud Joannem Certe, 1685. [16] 252 [2] pp., illus., coat of arms, port., plates (part fold.). 34.3 cm. Contemporary blind-stamped vellum, rebacked.

The son of a French army officer, Vieussens did not receive adequate financial support for his education from his family, so provided his own support, studying philosophy at Rhodez and medicine at Montpellier. As physician to the hospital of Saint Eloy in Montpellier, he had occasion to perform over five hundred postmortem examinations during the course of which he made a number of anatomical discoveries. This well-illustrated compendium of the anatomy of the nervous system is based on these examinations and provides the most complete description of the brain and spinal cord to appear during the seventeenth century. Vieussens was one of the first anatomists to dissect out the internal capsule, corona radiata, cerebral peduncles, and pyramidal fasiculi of the pons. The twenty-two folding copperplates, printed on fine, thin paper, are in excellent condition in this copy.

Cushing V135; Garrison-Morton 1379; Osler 4171; Waller 9961.

*422. JOHN BROWNE (1642–ca. 1700). *A compleat treatise of the muscles, as they appear in humane body, and arise in dissection.* [London]: Printed by T. Newcombe for the author, 1681. [30] 237 (misnumbered 213) pp., front. (port.), 37 plates. 32.1 cm.

John Browne, physician to King Charles II, James II, and William III, was primarily a surgeon who practiced for a number of years at Norwich and later was surgeon to St. Thomas' Hospital, London. His most important contribution was one of the clearest early descriptions of cirrhosis of the liver.

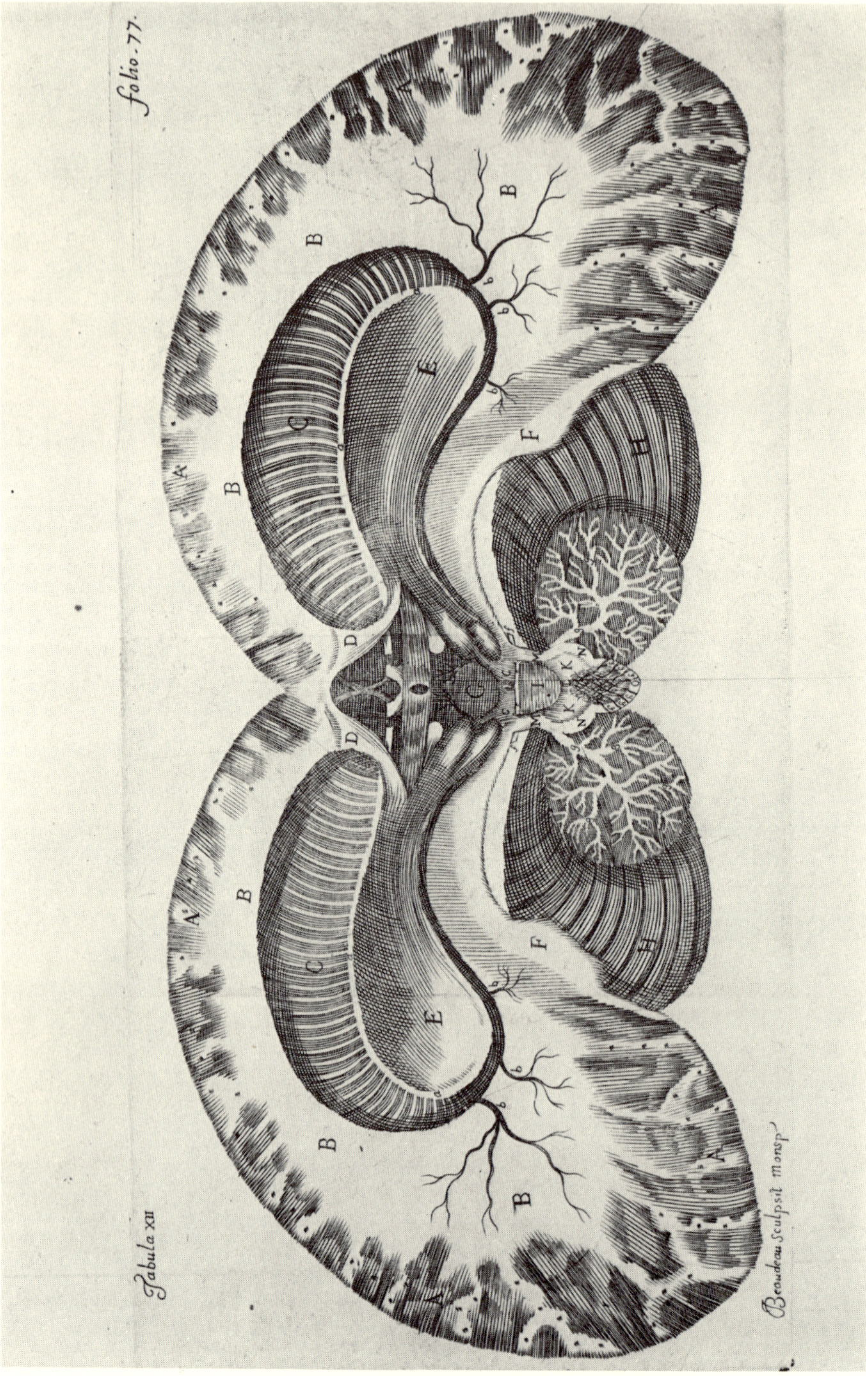

No. 421. Vieussens. *Neurographia Universalis.*

Browne was subjected to a scathing attack by James Young (1647–1721) in *Medicaster medicatus, or a remedy for the itch of scribling* (1685) in which the present work was shown to be plagiarized from works of Casserio (see No. 248) and William Molins (fl. 1640). The thirty-seven anatomical plates in which the poses and backgrounds of the figures had been altered were, with few exceptions, taken from Molins' *ΜΥΣΚΟΤΟΜΙΑ: or the anatomical administration of all the muscles of a humane body* (1648). Browne did not respond to Young's criticism, but did make extensive changes to his text and issued future editions of the book under the title *Myographia nova*. In spite of blatant plagiarism, his book was widely read and was translated into Latin and German, going through ten editions.

Cushing B762; Russell 101; Wellcome III, p. 251.

423. ———. *Adenographia; or, An exact anatomical treatise of the glandules*. London: Printed by Tho. Newcomb for Sam. Lowndes, 1684. [lxxvii] 207 pp. 16.2 cm.

Russell 111.

Bound with:

424. ———. *Chaeradelogia; or, An exact discourse of strumaes, or kings-evil-swellings*. London: Printed by T. N. for Sam. Lowndes, 1684. [xxii] 122 [8] pp. And bound with:

425. ———. *Charisma basilicon; or, The royal gift of healing strumaes, or kings-evil, swellings by contact, or imposition of the sacred hands of our kings of England and France, given them at their inaugurations*. London: Printed for Sam. Lowndes, 1684. [xl] 196 [12] pp.

Browne saw great importance in the glands, considering them even more significant then they really are. His descriptions of glandular tumors and "strumaes" are very vivid, and his case histories of patients cured by the king's touch are clear evidence of much of the foolishness which pervaded medicine of the seventeenth century.

Gift of D. H. Talbot.

*426. LORENZO BELLINI (1643–1704). *Gustus organum*. Bonn: Typis Pisarriani, 1665. [16] 247 pp. 12.8 cm. Contemporary vellum.

Bellini was a noted Italian anatomist and physiologist, a pupil of Borelli and Redi, and later became a strong supporter of the Iatro-mathematical School. At the age of only eighteen, Bellini published his best-known work, *Exercitatio anatomica de structura et usu renum* (1662), in which he showed that the kidney was not a solid organ but was composed of tubules, since known as Bellini's ducts. His *De urinis et pulsibus* (1683), in which he was among the first physicians to recognize the value of urine as an aid to diagnosis, was very successful and went through several editions. This small work on the sense of taste is one of Bellini's lesser writings, and in it he discusses the tongue and its role in the sensation of taste.

Wellcome II, p. 140.

*427. ———. *Opuscula aliquot.* Leiden: Apud Cornelium Boutesteyn, 1696. [20] 261 pp., 3 fold. plates. 20 cm. Late eighteenth century boards, rubbed.

Bellini dedicated this work to Alexander Pitcairn (1652–1713), the Scottish biologist and follower of Newton who tried to develop a mathematical theory of medicine. Because of Pitcairn's influence, Bellini's theories achieved an international reputation early in the eighteenth century.

In this work, Bellini expanded and more fully developed his mechanical theories of body functions. He applied his mechanistic theories to the action of the heart and respiration, the biliary system, the digestive process, and function of the glands. The three folding plates are filled with mathematical diagrams illustrating the application of his theories.

Osler 2003; Waller 870 (1714 ed.); Wellcome II, p. 140.

*428. PIERRE DIONIS (1643–1718). *Anatomia corporis humani, juxta circulationem sanguinis & recentiores observationes.* [1st Latin ed.]. Geneva: Sumptibus Cramer & Perachon, 1696. [22] 496 [23] pp., 19 plates. 17.8 cm.

Dionis, surgeon to the French royal house, was considered to be the most illustrious French surgeon of the seventeenth century. His *Anatomia* is considered a good text, but the illustrations, limited in number, are rather unimpressive copperplates.

Cushing D175; Osler 2469; Wellcome II, p. 471.

*429. WILLIAM SALMON (1644–1713). *Seplasium. The compleat English physician: or, The druggist's shop opened.* London: Printed for M. Gilliflower and G. Sawbridge, 1693. [70] 1207 pp. 17.3 cm. Contemporary calf, rebacked.

Salmon was one of the earliest and most successful writers on popular science and medicine. He had little or no scientific or medical background but nevertheless became very successful and had an impressive career as a self-styled physician. His personal library contained several thousand items, and he wrote widely on a variety of subjects. His remedies enjoyed great popularity and included Cordial Drops, Balsam, Elixir of Life, and Family Pills, all of which acquired a great reputation. The present work is one of several he wrote on popular medicine and is filled with advice for curing a wide variety of diseases with instructions for the preparation and use of all kinds of animal, mineral, and vegetable remedies.

Cushing S43; Waller 8426.

430. THOMAS GUY (1645?–1724). *Pharmacopoeia reformata in usum noscomii londinensis.* London: Brown [1782]. 60 pp. 13.2 cm.

The compilation of a pharmacopoeia by a hospital's physicians and pharmacists proved to be a great convenience to the many resident and consulting physicians who treated patients there. It was found that a great deal of time could be saved by simply requesting the desired medicine by name, and it was also possible for the pharmacy to prepare many medicines in advance and have them in stock for use when needed. Most of the formulae were for medicines that were regularly used to treat a particular set of symptoms. St. Bartholomew's Hospital, London, had its own printed pharmacopoeia as early as 1730, and other newly established hospitals were quick to develop their own pharmacopoeias. This pharmacopoeia was prepared by Guy and is one of the earliest produced for Guy's Hospital in London. Each printed leaf of the book is followed by two blank leaves for notes, and a prior owner of the book filled many of the leaves with handwritten prescriptions.

*431. THOMAS GIBSON (1647–1722). *The anatomy of humane bodies epitomized.* 2nd ed. London: Printed by J. Heptinstall, for Tho. Flesher, 1684. [14] 590 pp., 16 plates. 19.1 cm.

This popular handbook of anatomy was first published anonymously in 1682. Its author was Physician-General to the English army. Its popularity required this second, greatly revised and enlarged edition, the contents of which rely heavily upon Spiegel, Diemerbroeck, Thomas and Caspar Bartholin, Charleton, Glisson, Lower, Willis, Harvey, Malpighi, Wharton, Stenson, de Graaf, and other well-known anatomists.

Cushing G244; Russell 315; Waller 3532 (1703 ed.); Wellcome III, p. 113.

*432. LOUIS JOBLOT (1647–1723). *Observations d'histoire naturelle, faites avec le microscope, sur un grand nombre d'insectes, & sur les animalcules qui se trouvent dans les liqueurs préparées.* 2 vols. in 1. Paris: Chez Briasson, 1754–1755. Vol. I: Part I: xx, 38 pp., 14 plates; Part II: [2] 124 pp., 15 plates. Vol. II: Part I: vi, 78 pp.; Part II: 27 pp., 24 plates. 25.5 cm. Old boards, leather back.

This important work is of great interest in the history and development of the microscope as well as to the science of protozoology. In it, Joblot, a French contemporary of Leeuwenhoek, presented the first specialized treatise on the protozoa. The first edition was published in 1716, and this second edition contains many additional illustrations of minute animal organisms. The last twenty-four plates show the construction of the microscope which even then was a complex instrument.

Wellcome III, p. 356.

433. JOSEPH GUICHARD DUVERNEY (1648–1730). *A treatise of the organ of hearing, containing the structure, the uses, and the diseases of all parts of the ear.* London: Printed for S. Baker, 1737. xii, 145 [14] pp., 16 fold. plates. 16.5 cm.

Duverney was among the great anatomists of his time in Paris and is probably best known for his treatise on otology with its theories on sound and hearing, published in Paris in 1683.

The present work is the first English translation, and contains the sixteen plates of the original edition, though one is in electrostatic facsimile.

Waller 2667; Wellcome II, p. 506.

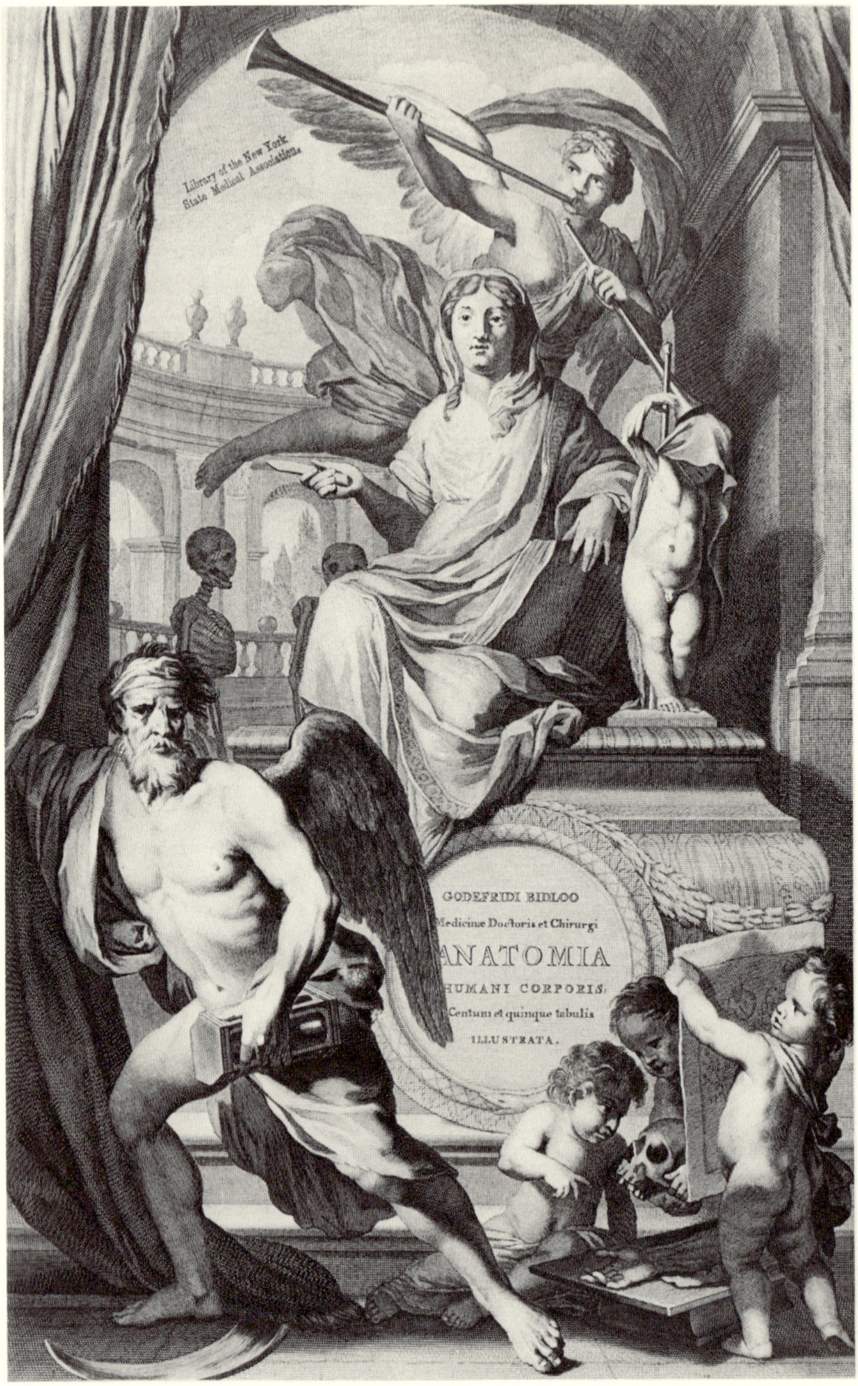

No. 435. Bidloo. *Anatomia Humani Corporis.* The title page, later plagiarized by Cowper (No. 468).

*434. ———. *Traité des maladies des os.* 2 vols. Paris: De Bure, l'Aîné, 1751. Vol. I: cciv, 454 pp.; Vol. II: [4] 541 [3] pp. 15.9 cm.

That Duverney was a good clinician, with a good anatomical base, is shown in this work of advanced understanding of the treatment of bone pathology, fractures, dislocations, etc.

Wellcome II, p. 506.

*435. GOVARD BIDLOO (1649–1713). *Anatomia humani corporis.* Amsterdam: Sumptibus viduae Joannis à Someren, haeredum Joannis à Dyk, Henrici & viduae Theodori Boom, 1685. [136] pp., front. (port.), 105 plates. 52.4 cm. Modern calf.

Bidloo, professor of anatomy at The Hague, was at one time physician to William of Orange. An English contemporary, William Cowper, furnished his *Anatomy of humane bodies* (see No. 468) almost completely with engravings plagiarized from this book by Bidloo, who promptly and publicly excoriated Cowper in a published communication to the Royal Society. Before the days of copyright, this is one of the most famous instances of plagiarism in the history of medicine.

This large folio contains not only 105 beautiful anatomical copperplates, but also a fine engraved portrait of the author. These plates are considered among the finest illustrations of the Baroque period, and the impressions in this copy are clean and bright, on heavy, well-preserved paper.

Cushing B376; Garrison-Morton 388; Wellcome II, p. 165.

436. Sir JOHN FLOYER (1649–1734). *A treatise of the asthma.* London: Printed for R. Wilkin, 1698. 247 pp. 16.3 cm.

Floyer was one of the most eccentric physicians of his time, and his works show great independence of thought as well as a true spirit of research. He was perhaps the first to measure the pulse with the aid of a specially adapted watch and to attempt to establish relationships between the pulse rate and conditions of health and disease. Floyer suffered from asthma for many years and often made himself a subject for investigation during his research into asthma. In this work, he discusses the influence of heredity in asthma and includes an early description of emphysema.

Cushing F213 (1717 ed.); Garrison-Morton 3166; Osler 2614; Wellcome III, p. 34.

*437. ———. *Medicina gerocomica; or, The Galenic art of preserving old men's healths.* London: J. Isted, 1724. xxii [2] 135 pp. 19.2 cm. Marbled boards, rebacked in leather.

One of the earliest works in English on geriatrics, it clearly demonstrates Floyer's independent approach to clinical investigation and establishes him as a pioneer in the field of geriatrics. He discusses diet therapy and its application to diseases of the aged, the use of hot and cold baths, and the importance of carefully recording

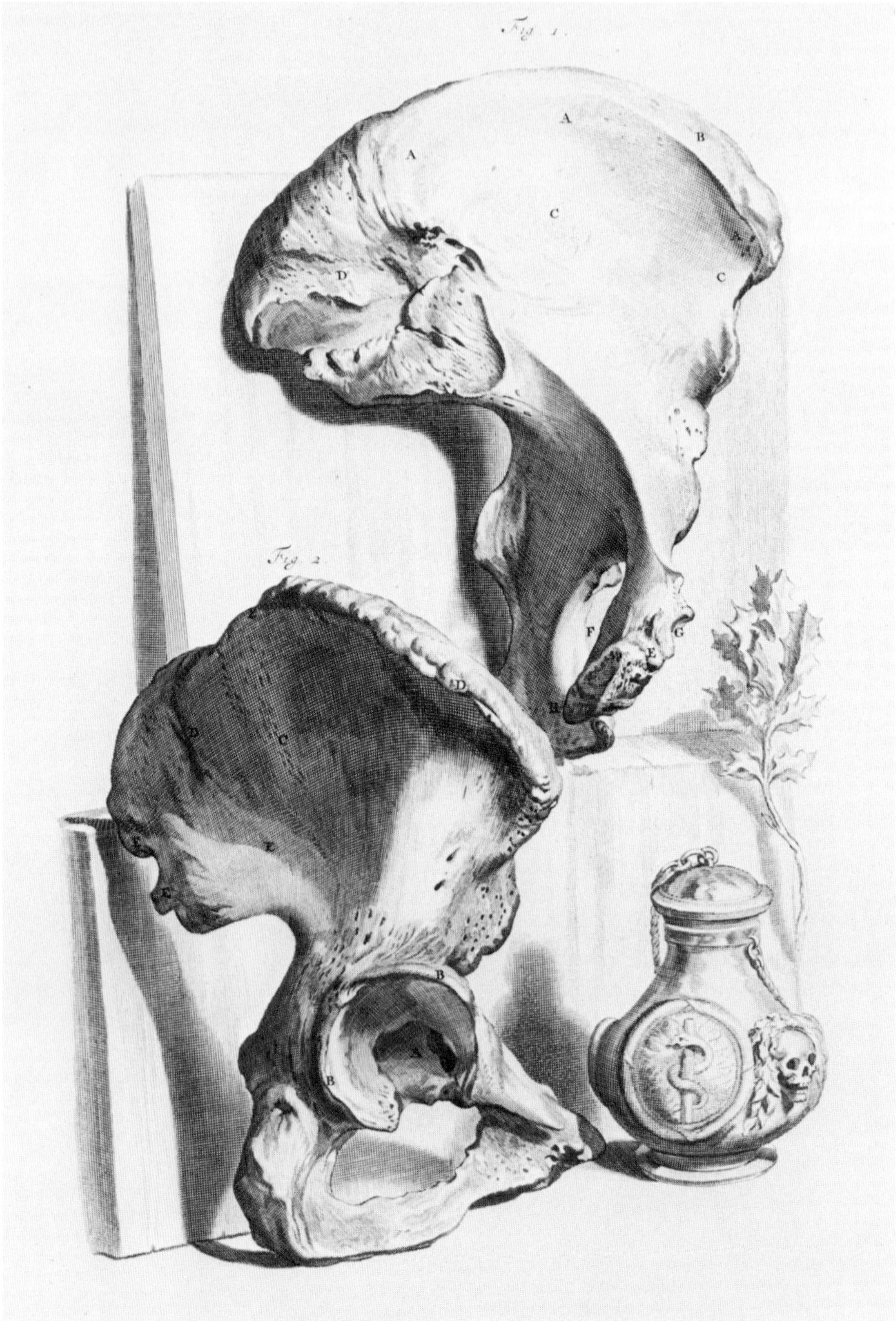

No. 435. Bidloo. *Anatomia Humani Corporis.*

the pulse. An appendix contains observations relating to the use of oils in preventing and curing many diseases.

Garrison-Morton 1595; Osler 2620 (1725 ed.); Waller 3091 (1725 ed.); Wellcome III, p. 35.

*438. ANTON NUCK (1650–1692). *Sialographia et ductuum aquosorum anatome nova.* Leiden: Apud Petrum vander Aa, 1690. [16] 158 [16] pp., 6 fold. plates. 15.9 cm. Vellum.

Nuck, first at The Hague and later professor at Leiden, was well known as an oculist, aurist, and dentist, and did his most important work in investigating the lymphatics and glands, in which he used the injection technique much as Ruysch had done with the blood vessels.

This book, first published in 1685 under the title *De ductu*, contains some of Nuck's best work on glands and ducts, especially the salivaries and tear ducts. The six large engraved folding plates were drawn by Nuck.

Osler 352 [i]; Waller 6919.

*439. ———. *Opera omnia anatomica, et chirurgica.* 3 works in one volume with general half-title page, each work having its own title page. Fold. plates. 15.6 cm.

Operationes et experimenta chirurgica. Leiden: Apud Samuelem Luchtmans, 1733. 170 [6] pp.

A late edition of an interesting book of surgical operations, containing several chapters on ophthalmology and otology, two on dentistry, three on hernia, on on blood transfusions, with illustrations.

Waller 6918.

Sialographia, et ductuum aquosorum anatome nova. [Leiden: Apud Samuelem Luchtmans, 1722]. [24] 158 [16] pp.

A late edition of No. 438.

Waller 6920.

Adenographia curiosa et uteri foeminei anatome nova. [3rd ed.]. [Leiden: Apud Samuelem Luchtmans, 1722]. [16] 152 [28] 64 pp.

This work on female anatomy contains the first description of the small structure now known as the "canal of Nuck."

Waller 6913.

*440. STEVEN BLANKAART (1650–1702). *Anatomia reformata, sive Concinna corporis humani dissectio, ad neotericorum mentem adornata.* Leiden: Apud Cornelium Boutestein [et] Jordanum Luchtmans, 1695. [12] 769 (misnumbered 759) [14] pp., illus., front. (port.), 84 plates. 19.4 cm.

The eighty-four anatomical plates in this work attest to the observational powers of the author, a Dutch anatomist who is possibly even better known for his medical dictionary published in Amsterdam in 1679. He used the injection technique to study the details of blood vessel distribution, this technique having first been suggested by Leonardo da Vinci and later used also by such prominent anatomists as de Graaf, Swammerdam, and Ruysch. There is a final chapter on the methods of embalming the human body. This edition is one of many published after the first edition of 1687.

Cushing B432; Wellcome II, p. 177.

441. HENDRIK VAN DEVENTER (1651–1724). *Observations importantes sur le manuel des accouchemens.* 2 pts. in 1 vol. Paris: Pierre François Giffart, 1734. Part I: xxxix [1] 368 pp.; Part II: [4] 371–431 [2] pp., plates (part fold.). 24.9 cm.

Deventer, born in The Hague, may be numbered among the founders of modern obstetrics. As a practitioner in his native city, he directed his greatest efforts to the practice of midwifery and to the study of its many unsolved problems. He was also interested in orthopedics and spent a great deal of time studying the bones of the pelvis. It was through his investigations of the normal and deformed pelvis and their effects on the course of labor that he was able to make significant contributions to the science of midwifery. The present work on obstetrics was first published in 1696 in the Dutch language at Leiden. A more elaborate Latin edition appeared in 1701, and this French translation was made from it. The book contains forty full-page illustrations of various aspects of delivery and other facets of midwifery.

Waller 2421; Wellcome II, p. 460.

*442. JEAN JACQUES MANGET (1652–1742). *Bibliotheca medico-practica.* 4 vols. Geneva: Sumptibus Joannis Anthonii Chouët, 1695–1698. Vol. I: [10] 1230 pp.; Vol. II: 1162 pp.; Vol. III: 872 pp.; Vol. IV: 1133 pp. 35.2 cm. Vellum.

Manget, a Swiss physician and savant, specialized in encyclopedic works and collections of the works of scientists and medical writers, but he also made some purely medical contributions, particularly on tuberculosis.

The present work is an encyclopedia of practical medicine and surgery, arranged alphabetically by disease. Almost nothing is omitted, ranging as it does from *abortus to vulnus,* and including even *stupidity*!

*443. ———. *Theatrum anatomicum. . . . Adjectae sunt . . . Barth. Eustachii Tabulae anatomicae, ab illustrissimô Joh. Maria Lancisio . . . explanatae.* 2 vols. Geneva: Sumptibus Cramer & Perachon, 1716–1717. Vol. I: [18] 434 pp.; Vol. II: [4] 452 [12] xvi, 34 [9] pp., front. (port., v. 1), illus., plates. 42.2 cm. Vellum.

In this compilation of contemporary anatomy, Manget systematically covers the anatomy of the human body, illustrated with 136 full-page engravings, some folded. The last portion of the second volume constitutes an authorized edition of Eustachi's *Tabulae anatomicae,* which had been first published only three years earlier in Rome. The plates, however, have been slightly reduced and some errors have crept in.

Although nearly all bibliographies and catalogues list this work as published in 1717, a close examination of the date on the title page of Volume I of this copy shows that the printed date is MDCCXVI and an additional I has been carefully inked in to make the date appear as 1717. The title page of Volume II carries the printed date MDCCXVII.

The Eustachian portion of Manget's work was also issued separately in the same year and appears in this catalogue as No. 202.

Choulant-Frank, p. 204.

444. [ROBERT PITT] (1653–1713). *The craft and frauds of physick expos'd.* London: Printed for Tim. Childe, 1702. [20] 192 pp. 17.4 cm.

During the seventeenth century, the Society of Apothecaries gained great wealth and esteem throughout England, and in many instances its members were also practicing medicine nearly full-time. This state of affairs ultimately led to open conflict with the physicians, and the situation was not resolved for more than a century. At the time this book was written, the quarrel centered on the opening of dispensaries by members of the College of Physicians and on the prosecution of apothecaries practicing medicine. Many pamphlets and books were written by both sides and this work by Pitt, an anatomist at Oxford and physician to St. Bartholomew's, London, is a direct attack on the apothecaries in which he defends the dispensaries and criticizes the practices of the apothecaries.

Cushing P295.

445. GIOVANNI MARIA LANCISI (1654–1720). *Translation of De subitaneis mortibus (On sudden deaths).* New York: St. John's University Press [1971]. xx, 212 pp. 25.3 cm. A facsimile.

Lancisi was one of the outstanding Italian clinicians of the early eighteenth century and was particularly skilled as a cardiologist. The present work on fatal illnesses was first published in 1707 and includes many postmortem findings, occasioned by the rash of sudden deaths that occurred in Rome during 1705 and 1706. Numerous diseases are mentioned in the autopsy reports, and Lancisi correlates many older classical ideas of disease with the newly-evolving clinical-pathological ideas which culminated in Morgagni's *De sedibus* in 1761 (see No. 501). This English translation was done by Alfred V. Boursy of Holy Cross College in Massachusetts at the request of Paul Dudley White, the well-known cardiologist, who assisted Boursy in preparing the book.

Cushing L34 (1709 ed.); Garrison-Morton 2731 (1707 ed.); Osler 3148 (1707 ed.); Waller 5542 (1708 ed.); Wellcome III, p. 441 (1707 ed.).

*446. ———. *Dissertatio de nativis, deque adventitiis Romani coeli qualitatibus. Cui accedit Historia epidemiae rheumaticae, quae per hyemem anni MDCCIX vagata est.* Rome: Apud Franciscum Gonzagam, 1711. [16] 258 [20] pp. 24.4 cm. Pasteboard, uncut.

Public health and epidemiology were also primary interests of Lancisi, and in this work he deals with the health conditions of Rome, its water supply, climate, etc. In the second part he describes the devastating epidemic of influenza which started in Italy in 1709 and swept over most of Europe.

Osler 3149; Waller 5543; Wellcome III, p. 441.

*447. ———. *De noxiis paludum effluviis, eorumque remediis. Libri duo.* Rome: Typis Jo. Mariae Slavioni, 1717. xxxii, 479 pp., fold. plate. 23.3 cm. Contemporary vellum over boards.

In this treatise, one of his most important contributions, Lancisi stressed the relationship of stagnant water to disease, opposed the destruction of forests because of the ecological value of trees and other vegetation, and maintained that quinine was to be employed in treating malaria. The book contains an engraved map which shows a drainage scheme for the marshy regions south of Rome.

Cushing L33; Garrison-Morton 5232; Osler 3151; Wellcome III, p. 441.

*448. ———. *De motu cordis et aneurysmatibus.* Leiden: Apud Philippum Bonk et Antonium Gerardum Steenman, 1740. xxxvi, 310 [22] pp., 8 fold. plates. 24.8 cm. Quarter calf, uncut.

This is a later edition (probably fourth) of an important work first published in 1728. Lancisi here classifies various cardiac diseases, gives a detailed description of valvular vegetations, describes cardiac syphilis, and establishes syphilis as a cause of cardiac aneurysm. The causes and characteristics of aneurysms were the chief interest of Lancisi's long professional life.

Cushing L32 (1st ed., 1728); Garrison-Morton 2973 (1st ed.); Osler 3152 (1st ed.); Waller 5541 (1738 ed.); Wellcome III, p. 441 (1st ed.).

449. WILLIAM MUSGRAVE (1655?–1721). *De arthritide symptomatica dissertatio.* Geneva: Apud Fratres de Tournes, 1715. [8] 170 pp. 22.2 cm. Old calf. Bound with No. 355 and No. 450.

Before studying medicine, Musgrave received a degree in law from Oxford in 1682. He then moved to London where he was elected a Fellow of the Royal Society for his knowledge and work in natural philosophy and medicine. He returned to Oxford in 1685 and received his medical degree in 1689, at which point he settled in Exeter where he practiced medicine with great success. Musgrave was highly acknowledged for his archeological investigations, and his *Antiquitates Britanno-Belgica* (1719–1720) received wide acclaim and special recognition from the King.

The present work, first published in 1703, was his major medical treatise and contains numerous case histories and many examples of symptomatic arthritis associated with venereal disease, asthma, fevers, scurvy, psoriasis, and podagra.

Waller 6782 (1723 ed.).

450. ———. *Arthritide anomala, sive interna, dissertatio.* Geneva: Apud Fratres de Tournes, 1715. [14] 88 pp. 22.2 cm. Old calf. Bound with No. 355 and No. 449.

In this treatise, first published in 1707, Musgrave deals primarily with arthritis as it is associated with other diseases.

Waller 6781 (1723 ed.).

*451. NICHOLAS ANDRY DE BOIS-REGARD (1658–1742). *De la génération des vers dans le corps de l'homme.* Paris: Chez Laurent d'Houry, 1700. [56] 468 [10] pp., 3 fold. plates. 16.2 cm. Old calf, badly wormed (perhaps appropriately, considering the subject matter of the work).

Andry, professor of medicine at Paris, was born at Lyons and studied and taught theology before becoming a physician in 1693. His first published works were in theology, and the present work on worms in the human body is his first medical book. Dealing with the effect and treatment of worms, the book became quite popular, went through several editions, and was translated into English and German.

Waller 417 (mistakenly indicates seven plates instead of the three present in this complete volume); Wellcome II, p. 45.

*452. ———. *L'orthopédie; ou, L'art de prevenir et de corriger dans les enfans, les difformités du corps.* 2 vols. Paris: Chez la veuve Alix, Lambert & Durand, 1741. Vol. I: [2] 47, xcviii (misnumbered cxviii), 345 [3] pp., front., 13 plates; Vol. II: [2] vi, 365 [5] pp., 1 plate.

Written late in Andry's life, this pioneering work is among the earliest to deal with the preventive and rehabilitative aspects of orthopedics. It was in this work that Andry coined the term orthopedics from the Greek words *orthos* (straight) and *paidios* (child) to express his adherence to the theory that many adolescent and adult deformities originate in childhood.

Following a long survey of human anatomy, there are instructions for the breast feeding of infants, directions for handling, dressing, feeding, and exercising children as well as specific treatment for diseases common to young children. Most of the work is concerned with preventing and correcting poor body posture and other defects caused by improper habits during the formative years. Andry also presents measures to be employed in correcting deformities such as curvature of the spine, club foot, stooped shoulders, etc. He places great emphasis on prevention and rehabilitation and offers sound advice for correcting not only bodily deformities but also deformities of the teeth and gums, speech defects, and mutism.

Garrison-Morton 4301; Waller 418; Wellcome II, p. 43.

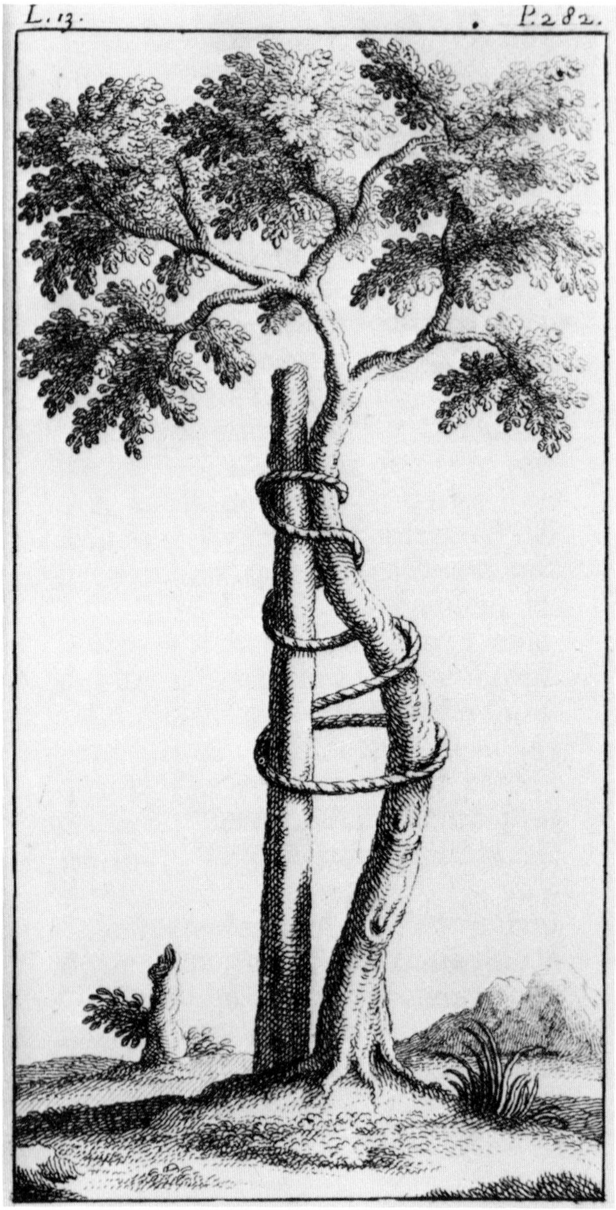

No. 452. Andry de Bois-Regard. *L'orthopédie.* A graphic representation of the orthopedic principle.

453. JAMES HARVEY (fl. 1700). *Praesagium medicum: or, The prognostick signs of acute diseases.* 2nd ed. London: Printed for G. Strahan, 1720. xvi, vii–xxix, 216 pp. 17.8 cm. Contemporary calf, rebacked.

Little is known of Harvey's life and work although it is clear that he was a practicing physician with great interest in symptomatology. Although the title page of this book states that it is a second edition, the work was first published in 1706 and another edition was published in 1713. Harvey carefully considers the symptoms caused by disorders in all parts of the body and cautions the physician to evaluate all physical signs before attempting to diagnose the patient's illness.

Waller 4087 (1st ed., 1706); Wellcome III, p. 219.

Gift of Dr. Robert E. Hardin.

*454. VINCENT DENIS DROUIN (1660–1722). *Description du cerveau.* Paris: Chez Guillaume de Lüyne, 1691. [16] 125 [3] pp., 9 fold. plates. 15.5 cm. Contemporary tree calf.

Drouin enjoyed an excellent reputation as a skilled surgeon in the French army and returned to private life to become chief surgeon at Des Petites Maisons in Paris. This work, important in the development of neuroanatomy during the late seventeenth century, is the result of keen observation and careful dissection. In it, Drouin discusses the skull, the brain and its circulation, and the structure of the nose, eye, tongue, and ear. The nine folding plates were engraved from Drouin's own drawings.

Wellcome II, p. 487.

*455. GEORG ERNST STAHL (1660–1734). *Sileni Alcibiadis, i.e. Ars sanandi, cum expectatione, opposita arti curandi nuda expectatione: satyra Harveana castigatae.* Paris: Veneunt apud Fr. Horth-hemels, 1730. 312 pp., front. 16.1 cm. Polished sprinkled calf.

Stahl, German chemist and physician, was the son of a Protestant minister and received his medical degree at Jena. He taught there until 1693 when he became professor of medicine at Halle. From 1716 until his death he was personal physician to Frederick I of Prussia who resided in Berlin. Stahl made his most important contributions in the field of chemistry and was among those who bridged the gap between alchemy and chemistry. He was also one of the propounders of the phlogiston theory and later became a major supporter of the animistic school of thought. The present work is Stahl's commentary on Gideon Harvey's (see No. 414) *The art of curing diseases by expectation* (1689) which was often issued with the Latin text of Harvey's work. Stahl's work is a biting and satirical commentary on Harvey, whose works had little scientific merit.

Cushing S383; Osler 2907; Waller 4082; Wellcome III, p. 219.

456. FRIEDRICH HOFFMANN (1660–1742). *Opera omnia physico-medica.* 6 vols. in 3. Geneva: Apud fratres De Tournes, 1740. Front. (port.). 35.4 cm.

———. ———. *Supplementum*. 2 vols. in 1. Geneva: Apud fratres De Tournes, 1749. Vol. I: [8] 313 [7] pp.; Vol. II: [4] 240, 32 [4] 80, 131 [1] pp. 35.4 cm.

———. ———. *Supplementum secundum*. 3 vols. in 2. Geneva: Apud fratres De Tournes, 1753. Vol, I: [12] 754 pp.; Vol. II: [4] 603 [1] pp.; Vol. III: [4] 194 pp. 35.4 cm.

Hoffmann, son of a prominent German physician, studied medicine at Jena, did postgraduate work in Holland, and then went to England where he worked with Robert Boyle. He practiced for a time at Halberstadt and in 1694 was appointed professor of medicine at the newly founded University of Halle. He spent several years as physician to Frederick I of Prussia but disliked court life and soon returned to his old activities at Halle.

Hoffmann was a prolific writer and in this work provides a comprehensive view of the medicine of his day. He was the chief designer of the mechanico-dynamic system, in which health is conceived of as normal movement and disease as disturbed movement. Hoffmann based his treatment on the use of sedatives, tonics, alteratives, and evacuants, according to the condition responsible for causing the disease. Apart from his system, Hoffmann was one of the premier practitioners of his day and one of the first to give good descriptions of appendicitis, chlorosis, rubella, and convulsive asthma with dropsy. He also wrote treatises on such subjects as pediatrics, physiology, pathology, medical ethics, and personal hygiene.

Garrison-Morton 72; Waller 4814–4816 (1761 ed.); Wellcome III, p. 285.

*457. ADRIAAN HELVETIUS (1661?–1727). *Traité des pertes de sang, de quelque espèce qu'elles soient, avec leur remède spécifique*. 2nd ed. Paris: Chez Laurent d'Houry, 1706. [16] 176 pp., fold. plate. 15.4 cm. Calf.

Helvetius, a Dutch physician, is credited with promoting the wide use of a new drug, the root of ipecacuanha, the therapeutic use of which had long been known by the natives of Brazil. With it, Helvetius cured Louis XIV from an attack of dysentery, and he acquired a large fortune when the French government subsequently purchased the cure from him. In this small volume, case histories are used to illustrate the benefits of, as well as the dangers from, the loss of blood, and how the dangers might be avoided.

Wellcome III, p. 243.

458. ANTONIO VALLISNIERI (1661–1730). *Opere fisico-mediche*. 3 vols. Venice: Appresso Sebastiano Coleti, 1733. Vol. I: [2] lxxxii, 469 pp.; Vol. II: [4] 551 pp.; Vol. III: [4] 676 pp., plates (part fold.). 35.7 cm. Contemporary vellum.

Vallisnieri was a pupil of Malpighi at Bologna and eventually became professor of practical medicine at Padua. Apart from his medical work, he was most active in entomology and continued the studies of the generation of insects begun by Redi. He also studied mammalian reproduction and correctly concluded that de Graaf's follicles were not true mammalian eggs, as de Graaf and others believed. This three-volume set of his collected works was edited by his son, Antonio, and contains his writings on medicine, entomology, zoology, and natural history.

Osler 4154.

*459. [DANIEL DEFOE] (1661?–1731). *A treatise concerning the use and abuse of the marriage bed.* London: Printed for T. Warner, 1727. vi, 406 pp. 19.5 cm. Modern calf.

Best known as a writer of novels, including *Robinson Crusoe*, and as a political pamphleteer, Defoe is credited with writing more than 500 works during his career as a merchant, political activist, and author. An accomplished writer with a plain and direct style, in this monograph he satirizes many aspects of marriage and sexual ethics. The book was published anonymously, and Defoe's name does not appear in it.

Wellcome II, p. 441.

*460. ———. *The history of the great plague in London, in the year 1665. . . . To which is added, A journal of the plague at Marseilles, in the year 1720.* London: F. and J. Noble, 1754. 376 pp. 18.9 cm. Modern half calf.

Defoe could scarcely have been "a Citizen, who lived the whole Time in London" as stated on the title page of the book since he was only four or five at the time of the plague of 1665. Nevertheless, this book gives a vivid description of the London plague as well as a later plague that struck Marseilles in 1720.

Cushing D100; Osler 4712 (1722 ed.); Wellcome II, p. 441.

PHILIPPE HECQUET (1661–1737). *Epistola . . . uteri musculo.*

See No. 405.

*461. JACOBUS HOVIUS (fl. 1702). *Tractatus de circulari humorum motu in oculis. . . . Epistola apologetica, in clarissimum virum D. D. Fredricum Ruyschium.* Leiden: Apud Joannem Arn. Langerak, 1716. [20] 203 [4] pp., 7 fold. plates. 19.2 cm. Contemporary boards.

This Hovius, a Dutch ophthalmologist and anatomist, is sometimes confused with another anatomist of the same name (1710–1786). The *Tractatus*, which was Hovius' graduation thesis at Utrecht, describes the *circulus venosus* (Hovius' canal). This structure, the *venae vorticosae*, consists of four veins which pierce the sclera and carry blood from the choroid coat of the eye to the superior ophthalmic vein. In the accompanying *Epistola*, Hovius defends his priority against Ruysch who described the same structure in 1706. The book contains seven folding copperplates illustrating the anatomy of the eye.

Osler 3015; Waller 4943; Wellcome III, p. 306.

462. JOHN QUINCY (d. 1722). *Pharmacopoeia officinalis & extemporanea; or, A compleat English dispensatory, in four parts.* London: A. Bell, 1718. xv, 618 pp. 19.1 cm. Blind-stamped sprinkled calf.

Quincy was an English apothecary and physician whose works had considerable influence on the practice of medicine and materia medica of his day. His medical writings included a translation and commentary of Santorio's *Medicina statica* (see No. 249), a popular medical dictionary, an account of the London plague of 1665 (see No. 373), and a series of medical essays. His *Dispensatory* had an exceptionally long and distinguished history and was the forerunner of Lewis's *Dispensatory* (see No. 579) and the *British pharmacopoeia*. The present work is the first edition of his *Dispensatory* which remained in print until 1782, reaching the fifteenth edition.

463. ———. ———. 11th ed. London: T. Longman, 1739. xvi, 700, lx pp. 19.5 cm. Calf.

The fourth edition of Quincy's *Dispensatory* was published in 1722, the year of his death. Later editions, such as this one, were published with few changes under anonymous editorship until the "twelfth edition" in 1749 (a twelfth edition had also been published in 1742). The "twelfth edition" underwent a major revision in order to modernize the theory section of the book which had become outmoded.

Waller 7714.

464. ———. ———. 15th ed. London: Printed for T. Longman, 1782. x [6] 656 [58] pp. 20.6 cm. Calf, rebacked.

The *Dispensatory* continued in its modernized form until 1782 when it ended with the present edition. However, the work had earlier been revised and improved by William Lewis in 1753 and issued as Lewis's *New dispensatory* (see No. 579), so Quincy's work was not concluded but continued under Lewis' guidance.

Cushing Q17.

465. [CHRISTOPH VON HELLWIG] (1663–1721). *Curieuser und vernünfftiger Urin-Artzt.* 2nd ed. Frankfurt and Leipzig: Verlegts Ernst Ludwig Niedt, 1725. [6] 198 [10] pp. 16.2 cm.

From time immemorial urine has been relied upon as a major diagnostic aid in one way or another. It was long recognized that a deviation from normal coloration pointed to a diseased condition somewhere in the body, and a collection of urine jars and color charts was once a standard item of equipment for anyone with any pretension to the art of healing by whatever means: divination, necromancy, astrology, magic, or medical science. Astrology, of course, has never died out completely, and the present work is an interesting example of the examination of urine and treatment of whatever disease or condition is indicated by means of astrological determinations. Hellwig wrote literally dozens of such popular pseudo-medical works, and this is one of his best-known and most widely-used.

Bound at the end of this volume is a work by Thomas Brian (fl. 1637), *Der englische Wahrsager*, a work similar to Hellwig's, which appeared originally in English as *The Pisse-Prophet*. These two works often appeared together.

Wellcome III, p. 240 (4th ed., 1748).

Gift of Dr. R. N. Larimer.

*466. ANTONI PACCHIONI (1665–1726). *De durae meningis fabrica & usu disquisitio anatomica*. Rome: Typis D. A. Herculis, 1701. [16] 139 pp., 5 plates (4 fold.). 16.2 cm. Soft boards, uncut.

"Antonio Pacchioni, . . . friend and pupil of Malpighi, with whom he collaborated in the publication of the anatomical plates of Eustachius, was particularly concerned with the anatomy and function of the dura mater. According to him, it was to be regarded as a muscular tissue whose contractions served to push the nervous fluid toward the periphery. He described in the dura mater the small bodies that bear his name and the incisura of the tentorium cerebelli" (Arturo Castiglioni, *A history of medicine*. New York, 1946. pp. 519–520).

Waller 7047.

467. WILLIAM COWPER (1666–1709). *Myotomia reformata; or, An anatomical treatise on the muscles of the human body*. London: Robert Knaplock, and William and John Innys, and Jacob Tonson, 1724. [14] lxxvii [5] 194 pp., front., illus., 67 plates. 44.7 cm. Modern quarter calf with marbled boards.

Cowper, British surgeon and anatomist, was admitted to the Company of Barber Surgeons in 1691 after serving his apprenticeship with two different London surgeons. According to Richard Mead, in the Advertisement to the present work, Cowper "was universally allowed to be as eminent an Anatomist as any of his Time."

Cowper first published this work in 1694, only three years after entering practice. A popular and well-received work, it is here edited by Richard Mead (see No. 485). Although it was meant to be a second edition of the 1694 issue, it is an entirely new publication. Greatly expanded and enlarged, it contains more than sixty well-executed copperplates and a lengthy introduction concerning the muscles and their action.

*468. ———. *Anatomia corporum humanorum*. [1st Latin ed.]. Leiden: Apud Joannem Arnoldum Langerak, 1739. [138] pp., 114 plates (part fold.). 52.1 cm. Paneled calf.

Cowper provided with this work, first published in English in 1698, one of the better-known stories of theft in medical history. Of the 114 plates in this collection, only nine were original with Cowper. All of the others were the work of Govard Bidloo and were published in his *Anatomia humani corporis* in 1685 (see No. 435). Cowper obtained three hundred sets of Bidloo's plates, pasted his own name over that of Bidloo on the title page, made a few corrections in ink, added nine

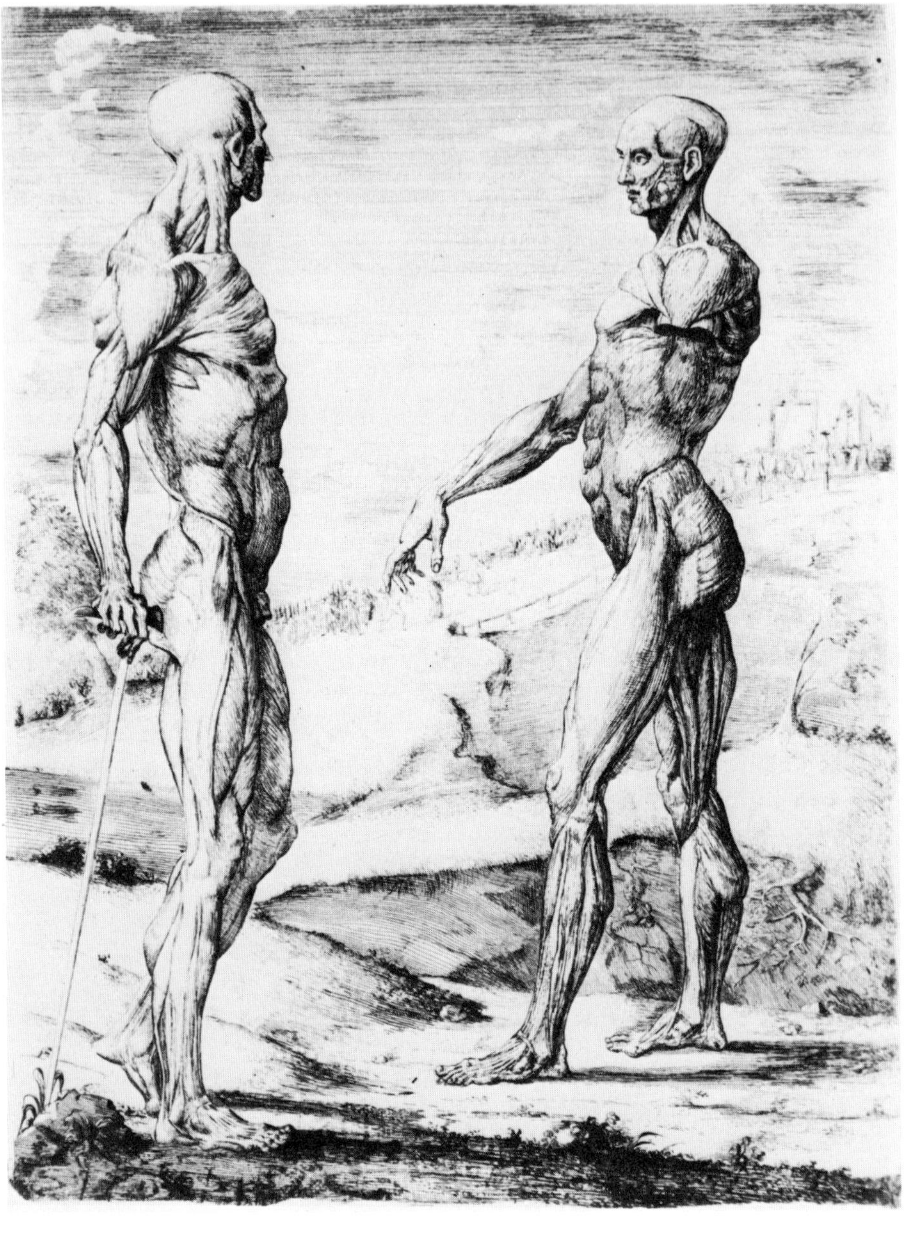

No. 467. Cowper. *Myotomia Reformata*. A partial dissection of the superficial musculature.

plates of his own, translated the text into English, and published the whole under his own name. Bidloo, naturally incensed over this plagiarism, arraigned Cowper before the Royal Society, and the two engaged in an exchange of polemical writings. Cowper's atlas was published again in the mid-eighteenth century in both an English edition (1737) and this Latin edition of 1739, with impressions taken from the old plates.

The atlas is, indeed, a handsome production, with its life-sized copperplates and striking engraved title page.

Choulant-Frank, pp. 252–253; Russell 213; Waller 2192 (1737 ed.); Wellcome II, p. 401.

469. JOHANN CONRAD BARCHUSEN (1666–1723). *De medicinae origine et progressu dissertationes.* Utrecht: Apud Gysbertum Paddenburg et Guilielmum Croon, 1723. [16] 679 pp. 20.5 cm. Old boards.

Barchusen, German chemist and physician, taught at Utrecht for many years. He received his medical degree while at Utrecht and discovered succinic acid during the course of his chemical studies and experiments. Although his major publications were in the field of chemistry and pharmacology, the present work resulted from his interest in history. It was first published in Amsterdam in 1710, and this is a revised and expanded edition. In a series of twenty-six essays he writes about the doctrines of Hippocrates, Paracelsus, Galen, and Celsus, ancient medicine, anatomy, magic and astrology, gymnastics, and important medical personages such as Fludd, Willis, Stahl, Le Boë, Severinus, and Helmont.

Waller 12600; Wellcome II, p. 99.

470. ANTONIO MARIA VALSALVA (1666–1723). *De aure humana tractatus.* Leiden: Apud Gisbertum Langerak & Johannem Hasebroek, 1735. [12] 143 [1] pp., 10 fold. plates. 21.2 cm. Paper.

Valsalva, student of Malpighi and teacher of Morgagni, is best remembered for his work upon the ear. This remarkable book, which became a standard on the subject for over a century, contains his anatomical, physiological, and pathological observations of the organ. In it he described and depicted even the smallest muscles and nerves of the ear, subdividing the ear into its internal, middle, and external parts, and he showed an original method of inflating the middle ear (Valsalva's maneuver) which is still practiced today.

Garrison-Morton 1546 (1704 ed.); Waller 9796.

471. ———. *Opera.* 3 vols. in 1. Venice: Apud Franciscum Pitteri, 1740. Vol. I: [38] 155 [1] pp.; Vol. II: [16] 531 [1] pp.; Vol. III: 504 [2] pp., fold. plates. 27 cm. Vellum.

Valsalva was deeply interested in pathology throughout his life, and Morgagni's great work, *De sedibus* (see No. 501), contains much material collected by Valsalva. In this work his beloved pupil, Morgagni, assembled and published posthumously his teacher's anatomical works.

Garrison-Morton 803; Osler 4159; Waller 9797 (1741 ed.).

*472. GIORGIO BAGLIVI (1668?–1707?). *De praxi medica ad priscam observandi rationem revocandi.* Rome: Typis D. A. Herculis, 1696. [20] 259, 119 pp., plates. 15.9 cm. Contemporary vellum.

Although Baglivi died at a comparatively young age, he was a master clinician with a wide circle of influence among colleagues in practice, students, and patients. And he was also a man of uncommon logic and common sense. "Let the young know," he wrote, "that they will never find a more interesting, more instructive book than the patient himself" (Preface). And, "To study medicine, it is necessary to compare disease with disease, moment with moment, and man with man, and to abandon forever those interminable discussions and logomachies, for which I find no other explanation than the anger of an outraged and avenging God who has inflicted them on man" (Preface). An iatrophysicist, Baglivi devoted much time to experimental physiology.

This small volume is the work for which Baglivi is usually remembered. Book Two contains the famous description of Marcello Malpighi's last illness and death, Malpighi having been Baglivi's teacher and colleague. Baglivi performed a postmortem examination of the body of Malpighi showing that death was caused by an acute spontaneous intracerebral hemorrhage.

Garrison-Morton 68 (1704 ed.); Wellcome II, p. 84 (later eds.).

*473. ———. *Opera omnia medico-practica, et anatomica.* 6th ed. Lyons: Sumptibus Anisson & Joannis Posuel, 1704. [56] 692 pp. 22.2 cm.

Garrison-Morton 68; Osler 1879 (1715 ed.); Waller 607–610 (later eds.); Wellcome II, p. 85 (later eds.).

474. HERMANN BOERHAAVE (1668–1738). *A method of studying physick.* [1st English ed.]. London: Printed by H. P. for C. Rivington, B. Creake and J. Sackfield, 1719. [48] 331 [28] pp., illus. 19.1 cm.

Boerhaave studied for the ministry, but, after promotion to doctor of philosophy, he took up the study of medicine, chemistry, and botany. He was appointed lecturer at the University of Leiden in 1701 and there began a career as one of the most admired teachers and best-known clinicians who ever lived. He wrote several important and lasting books, but he was first and last a clinician and a faithful Hippocratist who put the care of the patient above all considerations of theory. His influence on medical teaching and practice was enormous, as students flocked to his lectures from all over Europe and carried away his precepts and teachings to other medical schools and to their own practices.

The present work is the first English translation (except for a plagiarized work which did not bear his name) of his famed course of lectures, *Institutiones medicae*, first published in 1708. As was true of most of Boerhaave's works, it was published in scores of editions and translations, many of them without his authority, many of them lecture notes taken by students who sold them for publication under a bewildering array of titles.

Cushing B464; Lindeboom 87; Osler 1117; Waller 1190; Wellcome II, p. 188.

Gift of Dr. R. N. Larimer.

*475. ———. *Traité de la vertu des medicamens.* Paris: Chez les freres Osmont, 1729. [26] 471 [3] pp., illus. 16.8 cm. Calf.

A French translation of *Tractatus de viribus medicamentorum* (1719), which was a spurious edition, enlarged from lecture notes, of Boerhaave's *Libellus de materie medica* (1719). He had not originally intended to publish his collection of prescriptions, fearing that indiscriminate readers would bring harm to themselves and others by improper use of them. He finally felt obliged to issue his materia medica in order to correct the inaccurate works which were being published in his name from students' lecture notes.

Lindeboom 335; Wellcome II, p. 190.

476. ———. *Treatise of the materia medica.* London: Printed for G. Hawkins and E. Littleton, 1739. viii, 245, xxix pp. 16.2 cm.

This book is one of the earliest English translations of *Libellus de materie medica*—Boerhaave's popular collection of prescriptions. It was translated from a later Latin edition edited by Samuel Du Ry. Unlike many of the spurious editions then being published, this one was far more accurate because many of the earlier Latin editions had been edited by Boerhaave.

Lindeboom 309.

*477. ———. *Tractatus de viribus medicamentorum.* Paris: Apud Guillelmum Cavelier, 1740. lxx, 564 pp., illus. 15.9 cm.

One of the spurious Latin editions adapted from *Libellus de materie medica.*

Lindeboom 319; Waller 1228; Wellcome II, p. 189.

———. *Opusculum anatomicum de fabrica glandularum in corpore humano.*

See No. 407.

*478. ———. *Praelectiones academicae de morbis nervorum.* 2 vols. Leiden: Apud Petrum vander Eyk et Cornelium de Pecker, 1761. Vol. I: [32] 342 pp.; Vol. II: 343–850 [54] pp. 15.9 cm.

After Boerhaave's death several of his pupils published a number of his lectures, some of them taken down quite accurately in shorthand, particularly by Gerard van Swieten (see No. 540), one of the three contributors of Boerhaave's lectures to this work on nervous diseases.

Lindeboom 421; Wellcome II, p. 191.

*479. TOMMASO ALGHISI (1669–1713). *Litotomia; ovvero, Del cavar la pietra.* Venice: Appresso Alvise Pavino, 1708. 24, cx pp., 16 fold. plates. 22.2 cm. Vellum.

This tract on lithotomy, first published in 1707, is especially noteworthy for its sixteen folding plates illustrating diseased organs and surgical instruments.

Waller 351 (1707 ed.); Wellcome II, p. 30.

480. JACQUES BÉNIGNE WINSLOW (1669–1760). *Exposition anatomique de la structure du corps humain.* Paris: Chez Guillaume Desprez et Jean Desessarte, 1732. xxx, 740 [8] pp., 4 fold. plates. 2 copies. Copy 1: 25.3 cm. Calf. Copy 2: 25.3 cm. Calf.

A native of Denmark, Winslow studied in Holland and France and received his medical degree at Paris. He taught at the Jardin du Roi in Paris for a number of years and numbered Haller among his pupils. An expert anatomist, he was among the first to discard physiological details and hypothetical explanations from his writings in order to concentrate solely on descriptive anatomy. He was a leader in condensing and systematizing the anatomical knowledge of his time. This is reflected in the present work which is unusually well-organized with clear descriptions of individual anatomical structures. Popular among teachers and students, the book was widely used as a text for nearly a century after its publication. Winslow's foramen and Winslow's ligament commemorate his name.

Cushing W243; Garrison-Morton 394; Waller 10354.

Copy 2: Gift of Dr. John Martin.

481. GEORGE CHEYNE (1671–1743). *An essay of health and long life.* London: Printed for George Strahan and J. Leake, 1724. xx [24] 232 pp. 19.3 cm.

A Scottish physician and mathematician, Cheyne lived in Scotland for the first three decades of his life before moving to London in the early 1700's. His medical treatises on fevers and gout did not contribute appreciably to the advancement of science but were popular largely because Cheyne possessed a superior literary style. With the exception of his book on geometry, his works appear to have been prepared primarily for the lay reader. Much of the commonplace advice he gives in these works was based upon his own hypochondria, gouty arthritis, and continual struggle with obesity—at one time he weighed over 440 pounds. In this book, he sets forth his philosophy and rules for those who desire to live a long and healthy life.

Cushing C211; Osler 2303 (1725 ed.); Wellcome II, p. 338.

482. ———. *The English malady; or, A treatise of nervous diseases of all kinds.* London: Printed for G. Strahan and J. Leake, 1733. [6] xxxii, 370 pp. 19.4 cm. Paneled calf.

By "the English malady," Cheyne meant hypochondria or what was later known as neurasthenia. In this quite fascinating book, Cheyne describes his own case, supposed to be due to the vagaries of the English weather. He estimated that a third of all his patients were neurotic.

Cushing C210; Garrison-Morton 4840; Osler 2304; Waller 1950; Wellcome II, p. 339.

483. ———. *An essay on regimen.* London: Printed for C. Rivington and J. Leake, 1740. [4] xvi, iv [2] lxviii [2] 344 pp. 19.1 cm.

In the Preface to this work, prepared late in Cheyne's life, the author reveals his basic interpretation of and approach to philosophy. Viewing medicine as an integral part of philosophy, he felt it quite appropriate to address his remarks to the physician as well as to the lay public. In addition to the work on regimen, he has included five discourses on medicine, morals, and philosophy.

Cushing C214; Osler 2305; Wellcome II, p. 339.

*484. ———. *The natural method of cureing the diseases of the body, and the disorders of the mind depending on the body.* London: Printed for Geo. Strahan, and John and Paul Knapton, 1742. [20] 316 pp. 19.8 cm. Contemporary calf.

The present work is often considered to be the best of Cheyne's books because it summarizes his medical philosophy and doctrines. The book achieved immediate popularity and four editions were issued in English in the first year of publication; the book was soon translated into French, Italian, and Latin. Cheyne gave many useful and practical suggestions on healthful living during a time when such advice was urgently needed.

Cushing C216; Wellcome II, p. 339.

*485. RICHARD MEAD (1673–1754). *Medica sacra; sive, De morbis insignioribus, qui in Bibliis memorantur, commentarius.* London: Apud Joannem Brindley, 1749. xix, 108 pp. 20.6 cm. Contemporary calf.

Mead, an eminent London physician and early proponent of inoculation for smallpox, was also active in literary affairs. In eighteenth century England there was a profound change in the forms of medical practice and in the lot of the medical practitioner. Eminent physicians were no longer necessarily attached to royal courts or other noble households but were free to practice their profession independently, often with great honor and financial gain. (Mead is said to have made as much as £7,000 in a year.) The tendency toward literary and philosophical studies was accentuated and Mead was one of a number of physicians who also acquired a reputation in literature. Mead's purpose in this work was to account on natural grounds for the diseases mentioned in the Bible. He explains

Job's complaint as elephantiasis, Saul's as melancholia, Jehoram's as dysentery, Hezekiah's as an abscess, and so forth. He also discusses leprosy, palsy, and demoniacal possession.

Cushing M245; Osler 82; Waller 14234.

*486. ———. *Monita et praecepta medica.* London: Prostant apud Joannem Brindley, 1751. xii, 272 pp. 2 copies. Copy 1: 20.3 cm. Modern vellum, in box. Copy 2: 20 cm. Contemporary calf.

Mead's text of medicine covers a wide range of subjects: fevers, diseases of the skin, mental derangements, cardiovascular diseases, gastrointestinal complaints, apoplexy, afflictions of the eyes, and gynecological problems. The first edition is rare; the book is more common in Stack's English translation of 1751.

Osler 3367; Waller 6398.

487. ———. *Pharmacopoeia Meadiana.* London: Printed for John Hinton, 1756. vi, 108 pp. 20.4 cm.

An extremely active and able medical practitioner, Mead was often called upon by other physicians for advice and consultation, and undoubtedly prepared his *Pharmacopoeia* for their use as well as to assist in instructing students. Rather than the usual arrangement by remedy, the book is organized by disease entities, and within each disease category recipes are given as well as Mead's observations on the remedy's use and effect.

Gift of R. A. Kuever.

*488. ———. *Opera medica.* Naples: Ex typographia Benedicti Gessari, 1758. [viii] 202 [4] 56 pp., fold. plates. 22.7 cm. Contemporary vellum.

Mead's scientific curiosity, combined with his great learning and wide range of interests, resulted in a variety of works, as shown by this volume. Included here are his writings on the plague, principles of public health and control of contagious disease, medical numismatics, and comparative anatomy, as well as several other subjects. The book also contains Mead's Harveian Oration delivered before the College of Physicians on October 18, 1723. Mead based his lecture on the history of Greek and Roman medicine with passing reference to the medieval schools of medicine.

MATTEO BAZZANI (1674–1749). *Dissertationes quibus accedit alterius monstri historia.*

See No. 516.

489. JEAN LOUIS PETIT (1674–1750). *Traité des maladies des os, dans lequel on a représenté les appareils & les machines qui conviennent à leur guérison.* 2 vols. Paris: Méquignon l'aîné, 1784. Vol. I: [2] xxxvi, 430 pp.; Vol. II: [2] 574 pp., illus. 16.4 cm. Modern half cloth, marbled boards.

Petit was the leading French surgeon of the early eighteenth century and the first director of the Académie de Chirurgie in Paris. He invented the screw tourniquet, gave the first account of softening of the bones and of clot formation in arteries following ligation. He developed many new surgical procedures, including mastoidectomy, and he improved the techniques for performing amputations and herniotomy. This, his major work, was first published in 1705 as *L'art de guérir les maladies des os* and was translated into English in 1726.

Garrison-Morton 4300 (1705 ed.); Waller 7324 (1741 ed.).

*490. JOHN FREIND (1675–1728). *The history of physick; from the time of Galen, to the beginning of the sixteenth century. Chiefly with regard to practice.* 2 vols. Vol. I: 1st ed.; Vol. II: 2nd ed. London: Printed for J. Walthoe, 1725–1727. Vol. I: [4] 312 pp.; Vol. II: 415, 72 pp. 19.1 cm. Contemporary calf.

Freind was the first English historian of medicine, and this work, which went into numerous editions and translations, may still be read with benefit, particularly concerning English medicine during the Renaissance. Freind dabbled in politics, and it was during his imprisonment for alleged Jacobite activities that he wrote this history, intended, as he says in his introductory remarks, "to pass away a few leisure hours."

Garrison-Morton 6378; Wellcome III, p. 66.

*491. ———. ———. 2nd ed. 2 vols. London: Printed for J. Walthoe, 1725–1727. Vol. I: [4] 312 pp.; Vol. II: 415, 72 pp. 19.4 cm. Contemporary calf, rebacked.

The second edition of Freind's *History of physick* which has been corrected to include the errata printed in the first edition.

Wellcome III, p. 66.

*492. ———. ———. 4th ed. 2 vols. London: Printed for M. Cooper, 1750. Vol. I: 330 pp.; Vol. II: 415, 64 pp., front. (v. 1, port.). 20.4 cm. Contemporary calf.

The fourth edition of Freind's popular work, to which has been added his biography, an index of the authors cited in the text, and an index of medicines, diseases, and cures mentioned in the book.

Cushing F326; Osler 5894.

*493. ———. *Opera omnia medica.* London: Typis Johannis Wright; Impensis Gul. Innys, Ric. Manby & L. Gilliver, 1733. viii, 6, xxx [6] 591, 25, xi pp., front. (port.). 35.6 cm.

This collection of Freind's medical works was edited by John Wigan and contains a biography of Freind, also by Wigan. Freind's *History of physick* is included in a Latin translation, *Historia medicinae.*

Wellcome III, p. 66.

*494. STEPHEN HALES (1677–1761). *Statical essays.* 2 vols. Vol. I: 3rd ed. London: Printed for W. Innys and R. Manby; T. Woodward; and J. Peele, 1738. [6] x [4] 376 pp.; Vol. II: 1st ed. London: Printed for W. Innys and R. Manby; and T. Woodward, 1733. xxii [26] 361 [22] pp., plates. 19.7 cm. Contemporary calf.

Stephen Hales was an English clergyman with a curiously scientific turn of mind. His work not only threw original light on the hydrostatics of sap movement in plants, but, more importantly, it gave the first quantitative estimates of blood pressure. A glass tube inserted directly into the femoral artery of a horse permitted him to measure directly the height of the column of blood (arterial pressure). He was actually the inventor of the sphygmomanometer, and he studied as well the peripheral resistance, cardiac capacities, and blood velocity. This epochal work, so important to therapeutics ever since, was the most important step in the knowledge of the circulation between Malpighi and Poiseuille (1799–1869).

Cushing H36 (Vol. 2 only); Garrison-Morton 765; Osler 1081; Wellcome III, p. 194.

*495. GIOVANNI DOMENICO SANTORINI (1681–1736). *Observationes anatomicae.* Venice: Apud Jo. Baptistam Recurti, 1724. [12] 250 pp., 3 fold. plates. 27.4 cm. Contemporary vellum. Bound with No. 498.

At a time when the European universities were making great strides in anatomical discovery and publication, Santorini was considered by his contemporaries to be one of the greatest anatomists. This work records a number of new anatomical discoveries and corrects many errors of earlier anatomists. Santorini's skill and expertise were so outstanding that his name lives on in such anatomical structures as the accessory pancreatic ducts, risorius muscle, arytenoid cartilages, and duodenal papillae, several of which are described in this book. The text is accompanied by three folding copperplates which beautifully illustrate the musculature of the face, the pelvic musculature and genitalia of a sixteen-year-old girl with a tubal pregnancy, the external muscles of the ear, and detailed anatomy of the male genitalia and larynx.

Choulant-Frank, pp. 262–263; Garrison-Morton 392; Waller 8474.

*496. ———. ———. Leiden: Apud Gysbertum Langerak, 1739. [12] 254 (misnumbered 446) [4] pp., 3 fold. plates. 20.2 cm. Contemporary polished calf.

In this second edition of Santorini's *Observationes,* the text remains unchanged; the plates have been re-engraved although they are the same size as those in the first edition.

Choulant-Frank, pp. 262–263; Garrison-Morton 392 (1st ed., 1724); Waller 8475.

*497. ———. *Septemdecim tabulae, quas nunc primum edit atque explicat iisque alias addit de structura mammarum et de tunica testis vaginali Michael Girardi.* Parma: Ex regia typographia, 1775. [8] xxxv, 217 [2] pp., 42 plates. 31.9 cm. Half morocco.

Santorini worked as both a practicing physician and teacher-anatomist in Venice and was known to be one of the most careful and fastidious anatomists of his period. This work, edited by Michael Girardi (1731–1797) and issued thirty-nine years after Santorini's death, contains illustrations of many parts of the human body including the organs of smell and hearing, the pharynx, breasts, heart, stomach, liver, intestines, pancreas, and bladder. Of the twenty-one plates in the book, seventeen were by Santorini, and each plate is accompanied by a companion outline plate which is marked with reference letters. The book is one of the finest anatomies of the eighteenth century because of its excellent illustrations and comprehensive commentary.

Choulant-Frank, pp. 263–264; Cushing S66; Waller 8476.

*498. GIOVANNI BATTISTA MORGAGNI (1682–1771). *Adversaria anatomica prima [-tertia]*. 3 vols. in 1. Bologna: Typis Ferdinandi Pisarri, 1706–1717. Vol. I: [8] 48 pp., 4 plates; Vol. II: [6] 99 [1] pp.; Vol. III: [4] 111 [1] pp. 27.4 cm. Contemporary vellum. Bound with No. 495.

Morgagni's scholarly ability was apparent at an early age. At sixteen he was a pupil of Valsalva at Bologna, and there he received the stimulus to devote his life to pathology. By 1715 he took the chair of anatomy at Padua, a seat which he held with utmost distinction for many years. He was a brilliant and tireless investigator and, in addition to his work in medicine and anatomy, was a student of the classics and an archaeologist of repute.

The present work consists of the first three volumes of his research notes on microscopic anatomy. Volumes IV through VI were published in 1719 with complete sets being issued under the title: *Adversaria anatomica omnia.* Morgagni's studies furnished new and valuable information about the glands of the larynx, trachea and glottal regions, of the male urethra, and of the female genitalia. Also described here are those fine folds of the anal canal, still known as the "columns of Morgagni."

Osler 1182 (1719 ed.); Waller 6669 (1719 ed.).

*499. ———. *Adversaria anatomica omnia.* Venice: Ex typographia Remondiniana, 1762. xvi, 244 pp., 11 plates (1 fold.). 37.8 cm. Original vellum.

Morgagni's *Adversaria anatomica omnia,* of which this is a late but most complete edition, was first published as a unit in 1719. It was this series of publications that helped make him well known throughout Europe as an accurate anatomist, particularly as he corrected the errors of previous anatomists. Although the earliest of these writings was done in 1706, Morgagni was still vigorously active at the time of this edition, fifty-six years later, and his most famous work (see No. 501) had just appeared.

Osler 1182 (1719 ed.); Waller 6669 (1719 ed.).

*500. ———. *In Aur. Corn. Celsum et Q. Ser. Samonicum epistolae.* Hague-Comitum: Apud Rutgerum Alberts, 1724. 117 pp. 23.7 cm. Old mottled calf.

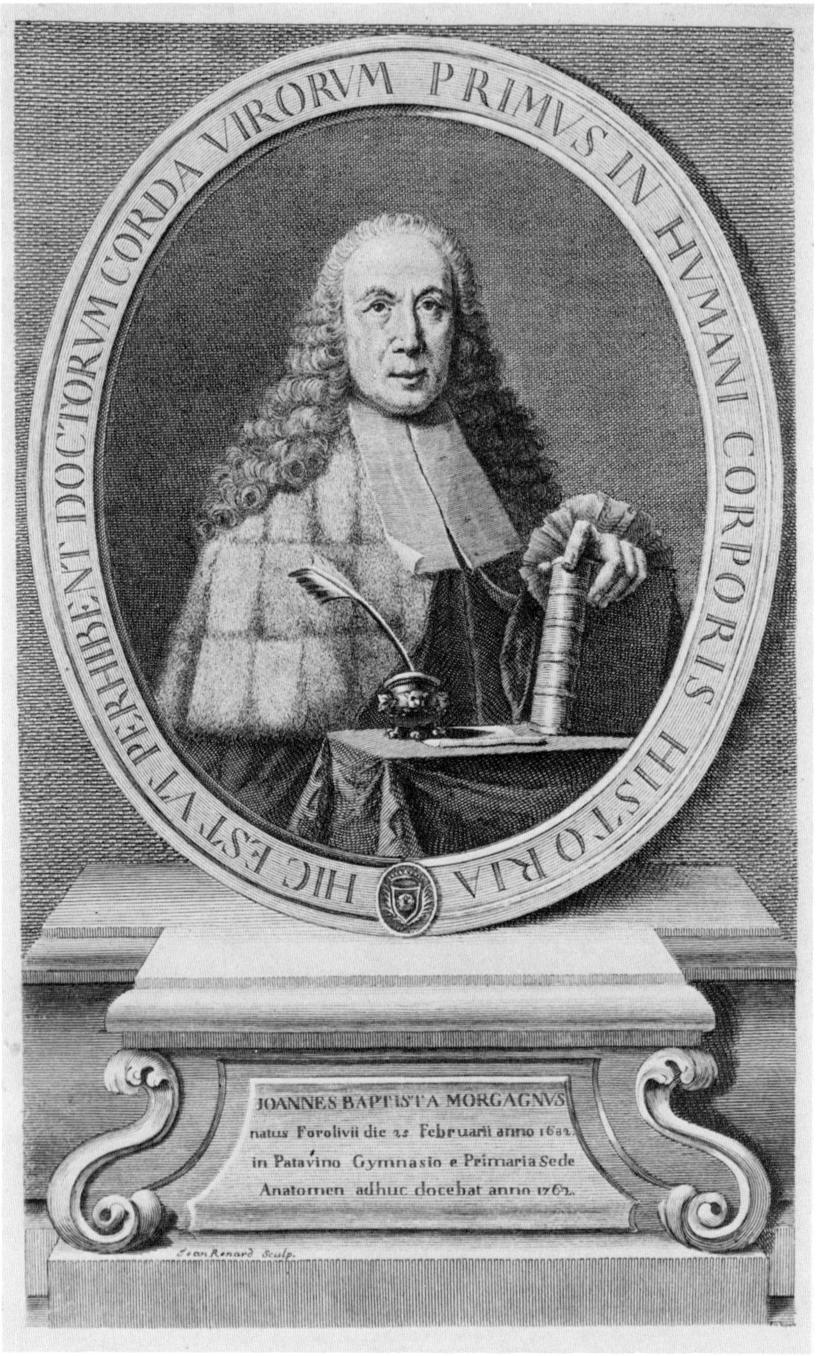
HIC EST VT PERHIBENT DOCTORVM CORDA VIRORVM PRIMVS IN HVMANI CORPORIS HISTORIA
JOANNES BAPTISTA MORGAGNVS
natus Forolivii die 25 Februarii anno 1682.
in Patavino Gymnasio e Primaria Sede
Anatomen adhuc docebat anno 1762.

No. 501. Morgagni. *De Sedibus et Causis Morborum*. The "cameo" portrait frontispiece.

This short work, dedicated to Lorenz Heister, contains four letters that Morgagni wrote to his friend and colleague, Giovanni Battista Volpi, during 1720 and 1721. Published for the first time in 1724, three of the letters are commentaries on the works of Celsus (see No. 9 ff) and one on the works of Quintus Serenus Samonicus (see No. 23).

Osler 1183 (1735 ed.).

*501. ———. *De sedibus, et causis morborum per anatomen indagatis libri quinque.* 2 vols. in 1. Venice: Ex typographia Remondiniana, 1761. Vol. I: xcvi, 298 pp.; Vol. II: 452 pp., front. (port.). 36.2 cm. Contemporary vellum.

Between his *Adversaria anatomica* of 1719 and *De sedibus, et causis morborum* of 1761, Morgagni had not published any major works. But the latter, published when he was seventy-nine years of age, had been years in preparation, and constitutes a foundation of modern pathological anatomy. Vast in scope, it is one of the most fundamentally important works in the history of medicine. In it he reports in precise and exhaustive detail his findings in nearly seven hundred autopsy dissections, introducing and insisting on the concept that diagnosis, prognosis, and treatment of disease must be based on an exact understanding of the pathologic changes in the anatomic structures. It put the final rout to the old humoral pathology. Morgagni's contribution to the understanding of disease may well rank with the contributions of Vesalius in anatomy and Harvey in physiology.

Garrison-Morton 2276; Osler 1178; Waller 6672.

*502. ———. ———. 2nd ed. 2 vols. Padua: Sumptibus Remondinianis, 1765. Vol. I: lxxxiv, 256 pp.; Vol. II: 338 pp., front. (port., v. 1). 38.1 cm. Vellum.

This second edition of Morgagni's landmark work contains additions and corrections to the first edition, but it is by no means a rewriting. Morgagni strove always to make simple what could have become complicated descriptions, and his Latin is utterly lucid.

Waller 6673.

*503. ———. *Epistolae anatomicae duae.* Venice: Ex typographia Remondiniana, 1762. viii, 96 pp. 39.9 cm. Modern quarter calf, uncut, in slipcase.

The two anatomical essays in this work constitute a detailed review of the anatomy and physiological functions of the liver. Although the historical aspects of the subject are emphasized, Morgagni includes many of his own observations.

Waller 6678.

*504. ———. *Opuscula miscellanea . . . tres in partes divisa.* 3 pts. in 1 vol. Venice: Ex typographia Remondiniana, 1763. Part I: vi, 120 pp.; Part II: 75 pp.; Part III: 84 pp. 39.4 cm. Original soft boards, uncut.

During his very long life, Morgagni was a prodigious worker and prolific writer, although most of his writings were very specialized, dealing with a single condition of pathological anatomy, a single portion of the anatomy, or classical and literary subjects. The present collection of some of his lesser writings includes tracts on gallstones, certain medico-legal matters, letters to Lancisi on the manner of Cleopatra's death, and Morgagni's biography of his teacher, Valsalva.

Cushing M508 and Waller 6680 (both in Naples ed. of same year).

*505. LORENZ HEISTER (1683–1758). *A general system of surgery in three parts.* 2 vols. in 1. 1st English ed. London: W. Innys, 1743. Vol. I: xvi, 476 pp.; Vol. II: 338 [10] pp., 38 fold. plates. 24.8 cm. Calf.

Heister, a German surgeon as well as an excellent anatomist, published his *Chirurgie* in 1718. It was the standard work on surgery in the eighteenth century, becoming one of the most translated, most used, and most respected texts ever written, and was still used as a standard text at Vienna as late as 1838. Heister had a sweeping knowledge of surgery, and the thirty-eight folding copperplate illustrations of braces and bandages were long followed and are prototypes of those still in use.

Waller 4234 (incomplete); Wellcome III, p. 237.

*506. ———. *Instituzioni chirurgiche.* 2 vols. Venice: Presso Francesco Pitteri, 1765. Vol. I: xx, 447 pp. 24.5 cm.; Vol. II: 400 pp., front. (port.), 38 fold. plates. 24.4 cm. Vellum.

An early Italian edition of Heister's well-known text on surgery. This one was translated from one of the many Latin editions of the work which first appeared in 1739.

ABRAHAM VATER (1684–1751). *Epistola gratulatoria.*

See No. 406.

507. JEAN ASTRUC (1684–1766). *De morbis venereis libri novem.* 2 vols. Paris: Apud Guillelmum Cavelier, 1740. Vol. I: [4] xl (misnumbered xxxvi) 536 [dxxxvii]–dcviii pp.; Vol. II: [4] 537–1196 pp. 25.4 cm.

Astruc, one of the most learned men of eighteenth-century France, was a scholar of the humanities as well as of almost every area of the medical sciences. He taught anatomy at Toulouse, was professor of medicine at Montpellier, and eventually occupied the chair of medicine at the Collège Royal de France in Paris. He is best known for this invaluable history of syphilis and venereal disease, which contains references to the writings of some six hundred authors and skillfully defends Astruc's contention that syphilis was introduced into Europe from America by the men returning with Columbus. The work was first published in 1736 and was translated into English the following year.

Cushing A294 (1741 ed.); Garrison-Morton 5195 (1736 ed.); Osler 1851; Wellcome II, p. 65.

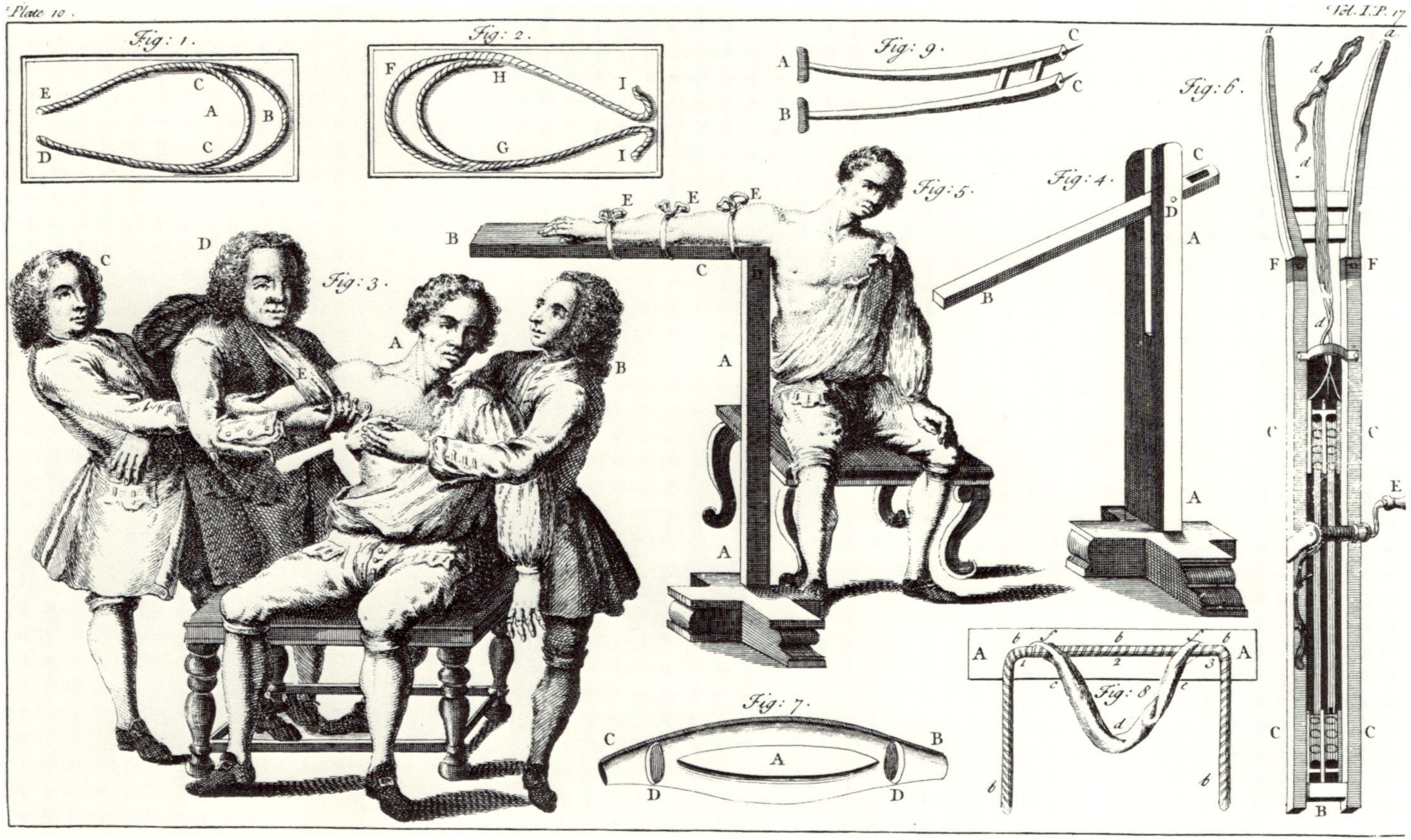

No. 505. Heister. *A General System of Surgery*. Apparatus used to reduce a dislocated shoulder.

*508. ———. *L'art d'accoucher réduit à ses principes, où l'on expose les pratiques les plus sûres & les plus usitées dans les difféntes especes d'accouchemens*. Paris: Chez P. Guillaume Cavelier, 1766. lxxxvii, 392 pp. 16.4 cm. Contemporary mottled calf.

Although this book was published as a separate work and is complete in itself, it is often considered the seventh and final volume of Astruc's extensive treatise on the diseases of women, *Traité des maladies des femmes* (1761–1765). The last two sections of the work bear intriguing titles: "Decision of the doctors of the Sorbonne on the validity of baptism by injection" (i.e., through the vagina on the undelivered fetus) and "Response to a letter from M.D.F.B. on the conduct of Adam and Eve regarding their first children."

Garrison-Morton 6019; Osler 1858; Waller 512; Wellcome II, p. 65.

509. GEORGE BERKELEY (1685–1753). *Philosophical reflexions and inquiries concerning the virtues of tar water, and divers other subjects connected together and arising one from another.* London: Printed for C. Hitch and C. Davis, 1744. 176 pp. 19 cm. Original paper.

Berkeley was an Anglican bishop who was active in several fields, but he is remembered chiefly as a philosopher and his major works were in the field of philosophy. He was born of English stock near Kilkenny, Ireland, and always regarded himself as a true Irishman in spite of his English parentage and religious affiliation. In his philosophy, Berkeley went beyond John Locke, who had argued that qualities such as color and taste arise in the mind while primary qualities of matter such as weight exist independently of the mind. Berkeley held that both types of qualities are known only in the mind and that matter does not exist independently of perception. He went on to demonstrate that qualities are perceived and that their perception is relative to the perceiver.

Several authorities believe that the present work is responsible for beginning the tar water fad that swept through England during the late 1740's. Berkeley discusses the preparation and use of tar water as well as the diseases and afflictions for which it is recommended.

Osler 1069; Wellcome II, p. 149 (2nd ed., 1744).

*510. [CÉSAR VERDIER] (1685–1759). *Abrégé de l'anatomie du corps humain.* 2 vols. in 1. Paris: De l'Imprimerie de P. G. Le Mercier fils, 1734. Vol. I: vi [4] 272 pp.; Vol. II: [6] 380 [4]. 16.2 cm. Original calf.

Verdier was a Parisian surgeon of great distinction, and this handbook of anatomy achieved great popularity and wide use. The book had reached six editions by 1768. It is primarily a reference work without illustrations and contains, as was common at the time, anatomical descriptions with some physiological background.

Waller 9870 (3rd ed., 1752).

*511. HENRI FRANÇOIS LE DRAN (1685–1770). *Parallèle des differentes manières de tirer la pierre hors de la vessie.* 2 vols. in 1. Paris: Chez Charles Osmont, 1730–

1756. Vol. I: [12] 195 [5] pp.; Vol. II: [4] 97 [3] pp., 8 fold. plates. 19.5 cm. Contemporary calf.

Le Dran, a French anatomist and surgeon, was a skilled lithotomist. In this work, he reviews the writings of his predecessors, discusses pelvic anatomy and pathology, describes his surgical techniques, and illustrates the instruments used to perform lithotomy.

Garrison-Morton 4283; Waller 5671; Wellcome III, p. 472.

512. WILLIAM CHESELDEN (1688–1752). *The anatomy of the humane body*. 2nd ed. London: Printed by S. Collins, 1722. xv, 326 pp., 31 plates (1 fold.). 19.4 cm.

This famous work, the first edition of which was published in 1713, was a standard text through a total of thirteen editions. This second edition contains thirty-one copperplates depicting both normal and pathologic anatomy. Cheselden won distinction as a physician and surgeon in London hospitals, but his chief claims to fame are his two important works on anatomy.

Choulant-Frank, p. 261; Cushing C205 (2nd U.S. ed., 1806); Garrison-Morton 390 (1st ed., 1713); Russell 149; Waller 1943 (7th ed., 1756); Wellcome II, p. 335.

*513. ———. *Osteographia; or, The anatomy of the bones*. London: [n. publ.] 1733. [53] pp., 56 plates, illus., coat of arms, front. 48.2 cm. Half calf.

This work, with its magnificent plates depicting the human skeleton, separate and articulated, still ranks among the best osteographic atlases. It shows normal adult, fetal, and some pathological bones with great accuracy and artistry. Cheselden lost a considerable amount of money on the production of his anatomical atlas because so few copies were sold. As a result, many of the sets were broken up so the plates could be sold separately in order to reduce the amount of his losses. Because of this, complete copies of the work are rare. All complete copies, as here, contain the text and a double set of plates. One of the sets is lettered and has descriptions on the verso of each plate; the other set is unlettered with no descriptive information.

Choulant-Frank, p. 261; Garrison-Morton 395; Russell 173; Waller 1941; Wellcome II, p. 335.

*514. ———. ———. Atlas only. London: [n. publ.] n.d. [1733?]. [1] *l*., 56 plates. 45.4 cm.

Only 300 copies of *Osteographia* were printed and 203 copies remained after the subscribers received their copies. Cheselden then broke up the sets and offered the plates of the human bones for 30 shillings a set and the plates of comparative osteology for 10 shillings a set. This undated issue with its specially printed title page and complete set of unlettered plates is undoubtedly part of one of the 203 copies that were broken up and sold.

Choulant-Frank, p. 261; Cushing C207; Garrison-Morton 395; Russell 175; Wellcome II, p. 335.

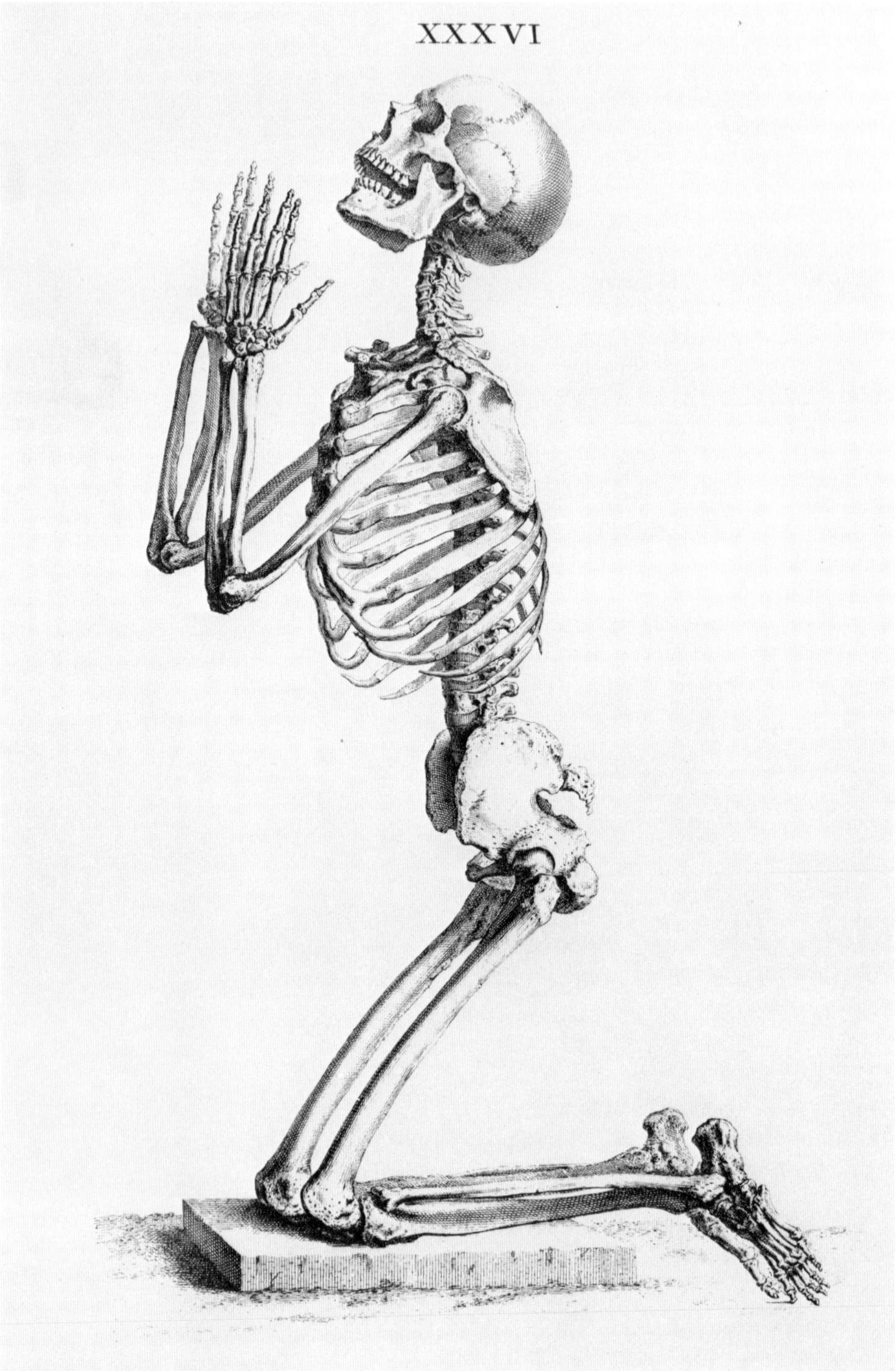

No. 513. Cheselden. *Osteographia*. The supplicating skeleton.

*515. EMANUEL SWEDENBORG (1688–1772). *The economy of the animal kingdom.* 2 vols. London: W. Newby, H. Baillière; Boston: Otis Clapp, 1845–1846. Vol. I: [8] 574 pp.; Vol. II: [8] 426 pp., illus. 21.2 cm. Calf.

Swedenborg, an eminent Swedish physicist and mining engineer, is better known as a theologian. His biological studies were largely confined to a few years of intensely concentrated effort in the European centers of anatomy (1736–1740) and immediately preceded the purely theological phase of his career. Being transitional in character, they must be classed apart from his earlier scientific accomplishments. The results of his studies reveal that his reasoning was based on the best scientific authorities of the day, and, although his efforts reached a highly speculative stage, it is evident that he possessed considerable intellectual prowess. He was among the first to recognize the cerebral cortex as the center of imagination, judgment, and will, and the source of motor volition.

The present work was first published in Latin in 1740 and is here translated by Augustus Clissold (1797?–1882) and edited by James J. G. Wilkinson (1812–1899). In it, Swedenborg presents his ideas about and investigations into the circulatory system, the functions of the brain, and the human soul.

Waller 9389 (1st Latin ed., 1740).

*516. GAETANO TACCONI (1689–1782). *De nonnulis cranii ossiumque fracturis eorumque conjunctione, itemque de osteocolla, de raris herniis quibusdam, de partu monstroso, naevis & maculis quae in foetibus imprimuntur dissertationes, quibus accedit alterius monstri historia a . . . Matthaeo Bazzani descripta.* Bologna: Typis Ferdinandi Pisarri, 1751. 70 pp., 5 plates (4 fold.). 24.7 cm.

Tacconi, surgeon at the hospital of Santa Maria della Morte, taught surgery at the University of Bologna and, after the death of Valsalva, took over the chair of anatomy there. This little-known treatise contains dissertations on cerebral lesions, fractures, hernias, and monsters. The added treatise on teratological lesions is by Matteo Bazzani (1674–1749), a physician and botanist of Bologna.

*517. GIAMBATTISTA MORANDI (fl. 1730). *Historia botanica practica, seu plantarum.* Milan: Ex typographia Petri Francisci Malatestae, 1744. [14] 32, 164 pp., 68 plates. 42.2 cm. Contemporary boards.

Morandi, who called himself "Botanicus, Galenicus, Pictor," was an Italian botanist and illustrator. The 544 illustrations of medicinal plants, drawn by Morandi, make this one of the most beautiful and important Italian herbals of the eighteenth century. Cardamom, anise, valeran, digitalis, and veronica, as well as many other plants, are described and pictured. Along with the detailed horticultural classification of each plant, Morandi includes information regarding its medicinal uses.

*518. JOHN HUXHAM (1692–1768). *Observationes de aëre et morbis epidemicis.* 2 vols. London: Impensis Joannis Hinton, 1752. Vol. I: 2nd ed. [4] xxx, 161 [1] 38 [6] pp.; Vol. II: [1st ed.]. [2] xix [1] 208 pp., 1 plate. 20 cm.

Huxham studied at Leiden under Boerhaave for three years and returned to England following his graduation, eventually settling in Plymouth where he developed an extensive practice and achieved considerable fame. His *Essay on fevers* (1739) and *A dissertation on the malignant ulcerous sore-throat* (1757) are his best-known works.

Volume I of the present work was first published in 1739 and contains Huxham's carefully recorded observations from 1728 to 1737 of the effects that weather has on various diseases. Volume I also contains his well-known *Opusculum de morbo colico Damnoniorum,* first published in 1739. An excellent work in clinical medicine, he erred only in that he ascribed the colic epidemic to the crude tartar contained in the apples and cider. In 1767, Sir George Baker (1722–1809) showed that it was actually lead poisoning caused by the lead used in the cider presses and vats. Volume II of the set contains additional observations Huxham made between 1738 and 1748. A third volume of fragmentary observations was published in 1770 from Huxham's notes.

Garrison-Morton 1675 (1752–1770 ed.); Waller 5040–5041; Wellcome III, p. 322.

*519. ———. *Medical and chemical observations upon antimony.* London: John Hinton, 1756. 78 pp. 20 cm.

The successful introduction of antimony as a therapeutic agent, chiefly as an emetic and purgative, is credited to Paracelsus. Its use was prohibited by royal decree in 1566 when a number of French physicians were convinced that it was a dangerous poison. Antimony came into use again in 1666 when Louis XIV rescinded the decree after being cured of an illness with emetic tartar which contained antimony.

In this treatise on antimony, for which he won the Copley medal in 1755 from the Royal Society, Huxham decrees that "it is without all Doubt a most excellent Mineral, when duly prepared, and judiciously administered" (p. 6). He gives directions for the preparation and use of antimony and briefly discusses its medical uses. The sweating, vomiting, and catharsis brought on by this powerful drug were believed to have beneficial effects on a variety of diseases, but Huxham cautioned that "whoever would give Antimonial Medicines with Safety and Success . . . should know what different combinations, Preparations, and Doses of them effect; otherwise it may prove a Poison, instead of a Remedy" (p. 6).

Wellcome III, p. 323.

*520. JEAN BAPTISTE SÉNAC (1693–1770). *Traité de la structure du coeur, de son action, et de ses maladies.* 2 vols. Paris: Chez Briasson, 1749. Vol. I: xliv [4] 504 [2] pp., 17 fold. plates; Vol. II: [4] 694 pp. 25.4 cm. Mottled calf.

A Jesuit priest, Sénac studied medicine at Rheims and was later appointed physician to Louis XV. He also served as councillor of state and eventually became a member of the Académie Royale des Sciences. Although he also wrote works on chemistry, anatomy, and the plague, they were overshadowed by this work on the heart. Here, in two volumes, is the first comprehensive and systematic treatise on the anatomy, physiology, and pathology of the heart and its diseases. Sénac described ossification of the coronary vessels, insufficiency of the cardiac valves, transfusion of blood, and the role of hydrothorax in circulatory failure. The first volume contains seventeen finely engraved plates of cardiac anatomy.

Garrison-Morton 2733; Osler 3960; Waller 8836 (1783 ed.).

*521. JOHANN ZACHARIAS PLATNER (1694–1747). *Institutiones chirurgiae rationalis tum medicae tum manualis in usus descentium.* Leipzig: In officina Fritschia, 1758. [xvi] 944 [16] pp., 6 fold. plates. 18.1 cm. Contemporary calf.

Platner, professor of anatomy and surgery at Leipzig from 1724 until his death, was able to affirm the tuberculous nature of hunchback which Hippocrates had suspected and Galen had confirmed. His surgical text, first published in 1745, passed through several editions and was translated into German and Dutch. The six folding plates depict several surgical appliances and instruments.

Waller 7502 (1747 ed.).

522. WILLIAM SMELLIE (1697–1763). *A sett of anatomical tables, with explanations, and an abridgement, of the practice of midwifery.* London: n. publ., 1754. [44] pp., 39 plates. 2 copies. Copy 1: 53.6 cm. Copy 2: 52.6 cm.

"The greatest figure in English obstetrics was William Smellie, who, after twenty years of village practice, came to London to devote himself to the teaching and practice of obstetrics. . . . To him are owed the first attempts to measure the fetal cranium *in utero,* and also important studies on the mechanism of delivery" (Arturo Castiglioni, *A history of medicine.* New York, 1946. pp. 629–630). It was Smellie who first laid down safe rules for the use of forceps, who separated obstetrics from surgery, and who imparted to obstetrics the stamp of science. His famed treatise on midwifery appeared in 1752, followed two years later by this set of plates, which is very rare and is said to have been issued in only 100 copies. The life-size plates are distinguished for their accuracy and are only to be compared with those of Smellie's pupil, William Hunter, whose *Anatomia uteri humani gravidi* (see No. 591) was one of the highest points in anatomical atlases.

Waller 9012.

Copy 1: Gift of Dr. E. D. Plass.

Copy 2: Gift of Dr. John Martin.

*523. ALEXANDER MONRO (1697–1767). *The anatomy of the humane bones. To which are added, An anatomical treatise of the nerves; An account of the reciprocal motions of the heart; and, A description of the humane lacteal sac and duct.* 2nd ed. Edinburgh: Printed for W. Monro, 1732. viii, 344, iv, 41 pp. 16.5 cm.

Monro *primus,* as he is usually called, was the first in the long line of the Monro family who held the chair of anatomy at Edinburgh uninterruptedly for more than 120 years. During the tenures of the Monros *primus* and *secundus,* the University of

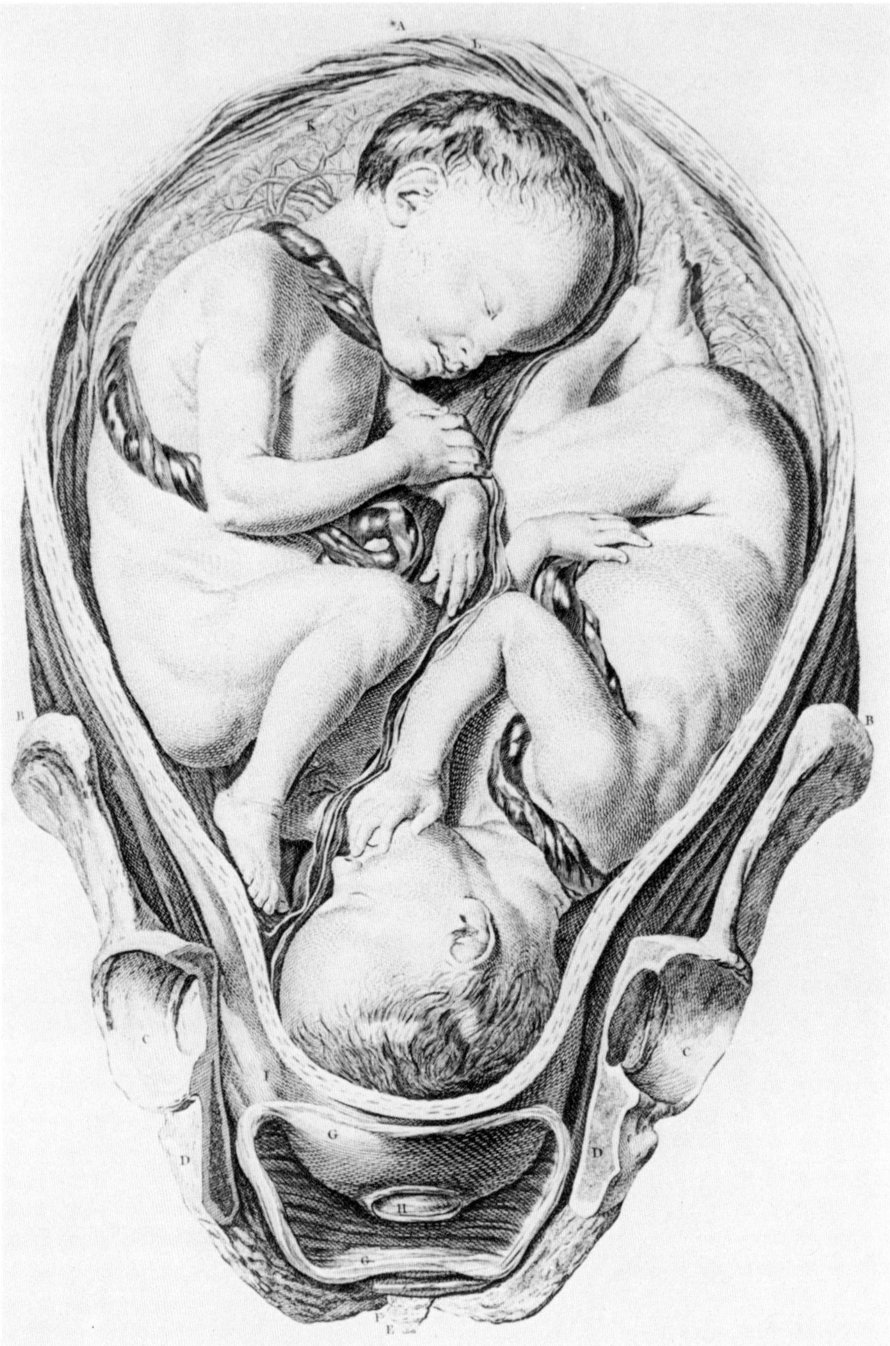

No. 522. Smellie. *A Sett of Anatomical Tables.* Twins in utero at the beginning of labor.

Edinburgh became a great center of medical teaching. Monro *primus* was a disciple of Boerhaave and William Cheselden, and his own teaching attracted hundreds of medical students.

The anatomy of the humane bones, first published in 1726, is his chief work and continued in use in successive editions for more than fifty years.

Russell 571.

524. ———. *Anatomy of the human bones, nerves, and lacteal sac and duct.* 7th ed. Edinburgh: Printed for G. Hamilton and J. Balfour, 1763. [vii] 410 pp. 16.8 cm.

Monro's *Anatomy* received wide acclaim and remained in print well into the early nineteenth century. Beginning with the second edition, all editions included Monro's separate treatises on the nerves and lacteal sac.

Russell 576.

Gift of Dr. Walter L. Bierring.

*525. BERNHARD SIEGFRIED ALBINUS (1697–1770). *Historia musculorum hominis.* Leiden: Apud Theodorum Haak & Henricum Mulhovium, 1734. 696 pp., 8 plates. 24.1 cm.

Albinus, a native of Frankfurt, was no doubt the finest descriptive anatomist of his day, and his works were especially endowed by the artistic copper engravings by the renowned Jan Wandelaer. He was a pupil of Bidloo, Rau, and Boerhaave and, with the latter, brought out a praiseworthy edition of Vesalius (see No. 176). In the present work on the muscles of the human body, the happy conjunction of Albinus and Wandelaer is seen in the lengthy and detailed text of the anatomist and the eight engravings of the artist.

Cushing A106; Wellcome II, p. 26.

———. *Dissertatio de arteriis et venis intestinorum hominis.*

See No. 530.

———. *Dissertatio secunda. . . .*

See No. 531.

*526. ———. *Icones ossium foetus humani.* Leiden: Apud Joh. et Herm. Verbeek, 1737. [4] 162 [2] pp., 32 plates. 26 cm. Quarter calf.

Albinus is particularly remembered for his descriptions of the bones, and this first edition of his treatise on fetal bones is one of his finest atlases. All of the fetal bones are illustrated with great detail and are finely lined in the sixteen plates and sixteen line drawings, but in no place is the total skeleton depicted. At the end of his preface, Albinus promises to see to it that only good prints are published and that the plates are not given away to anybody, to prevent the making of inferior prints for the sake of pecuniary gain.

Choulant-Frank, p. 280; Wellcome II, p. 26.

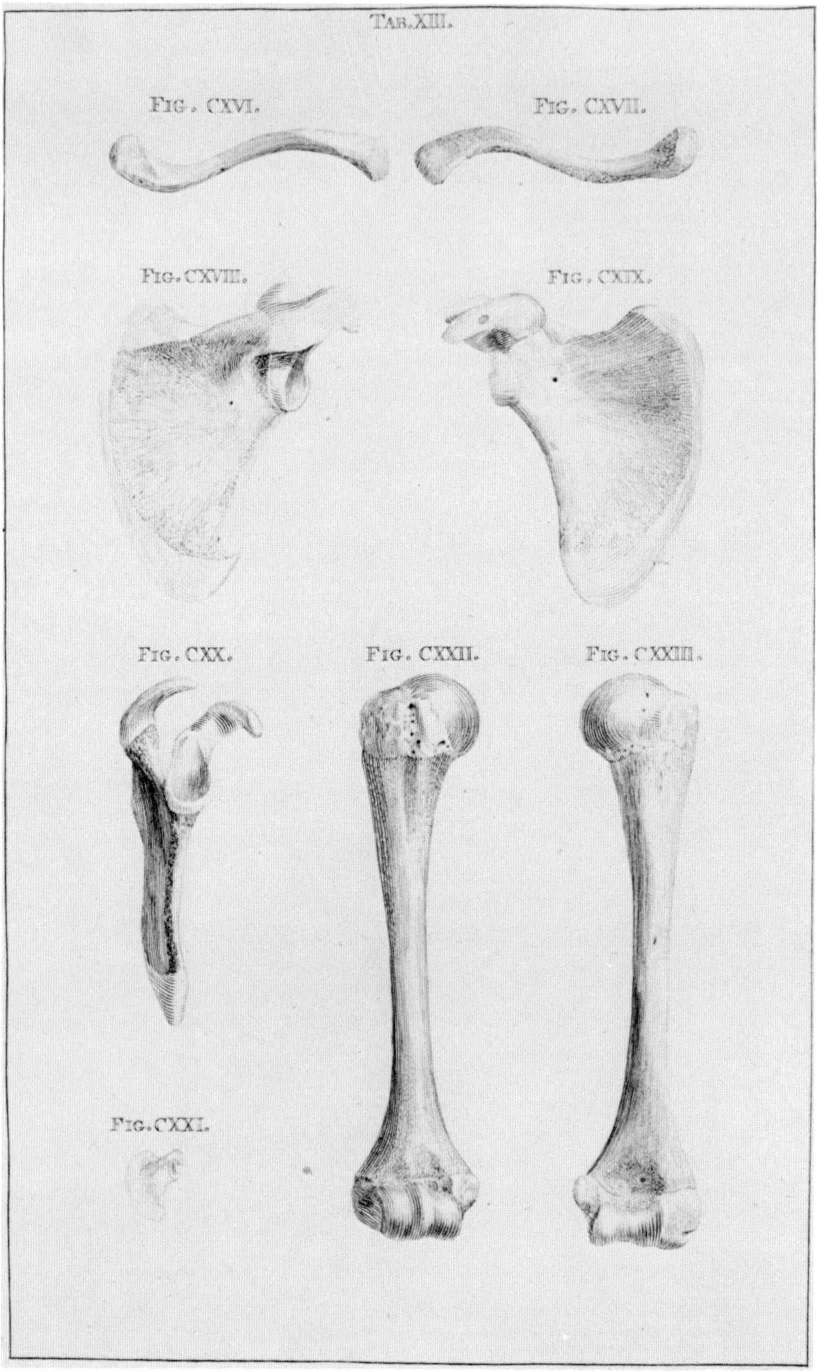

No. 526. Albinus. *Icones Ossium Foetus Humani*. The clavicle, scapula, and humerus.

*527. ———. *Tables of the skeleton and muscles of the human body*. Edinburgh: Printed by Balfour & Smellie, for Andrew Bell, engraver, 1777–1778. vi, 32 [2] 31 [sic]–86 pp., 41 plates. 44.1 cm. Half morocco.

Albinus' *Tabulae sceleti et musculorum corporis humani* (Leiden, 1748–1753) is perhaps the most monumental and finest anatomical atlas ever published. The plates, though probably derived from Vesalius, were drawn with painstaking accuracy, and Albinus described in his preface the methods used in the drawings of the skeletons and "muscle men." The Latin work was published in an English translation in 1749 with the plates reengraved. This Edinburgh edition of nearly thirty years later is a reprint of the London edition in smaller format. The twenty-eight plates and thirteen outline plates are taken from those done by Andrew Bell (1726–1809) for the London edition.

Russell 7; Waller 339; Wellcome II, p. 26.

*528. ———. *Academicarum annotationum liber primus [-septimus]*. 7 vols. (of 8) in 2. Leiden: Apud J. & H. Verbeek, 1754–1768. Plates. 25.2 cm.

This collection of miscellaneous treatises by Albinus, pertaining to anatomy, physiology, surgery, and the natural sciences, contains detailed anatomical descriptions, commentary on the works of other authors, and is beautifully illustrated by Jan Wandelaer. Volume Eight is not present in this set.

Choulant-Frank, p. 283; Cushing A102; Waller 336; Wellcome II, p. 26.

*529. ———. *Supellex anatomica*. [Leiden: Apud Petrum Delfos, 1775]. [8] 242 [30] pp. 20.3 cm. Bound with No. 586.

This posthumous publication was edited by Albinus' brother, Frederick Albinus with whose work, *De natura hominis libellus,* it is bound. It is a treatise on details of functional anatomy with frequent references to other publications of the author.

Wellcome II, p. 26.

JAN LADMIRAL (1698–1773).

Although the texts of two of the following six works are by Bernhard Siegfried Albinus (see No. 525), the collection belongs together because of the remarkable illustrations by Jan Ladmiral. Born in Normandy, Ladmiral and his younger brother were pupils of the German artist Le Blon while they were all working in London. Le Blon had invented a secret process for color mezzotinting which he taught to Ladmiral, but, because of carelessness in making the plates, little came of the process in Le Blon's hands and only one or two of his plates are known. Ladmiral, however, returned to the Continent and presented the invention as being new and his own, offering to make the colored anatomic plates for Albinus, who commissioned him to make the six plates that appear in this collection. They form the first series of full-color anatomical copperplates ever made and are extremely scarce. Harvey Cushing had three of the six in his collection, Erik Waller had only one, while Sir William Osler had none. The collection of six plates with accompanying text is as follows:

530. BERNHARD SIEGFRIED ALBINUS. *Dissertatio de arteriis et venis intestinorum hominis*. Leiden: Apud Theodorum Haak [et] Amsterdam: Apud Jacobum Graal & Henricum de Leth, 1736. 10 pp., mounted color plate. 28.6 cm.

Albinus praises the illustration which shows a portion of the intestine in which the arteries are shown as red and the veins blue. Ladmiral's signature appears on this plate and on the other five.

Cushing A104; Wellcome II, p. 26.

531. ———. *Dissertatio secunda. De sede et caussa coloris Aethiopum et caeterorum hominum*. Leiden: Apud Theodorum Haak [et] Amsterdam: Apud Jacobum Graal & Henricum de Leth, 1737. 16 [2] pp., mounted color plate. 28.6 cm.

The plate represents the skin and nails of a Negro woman, illustrating Albinus' text on skin coloring.

Cushing A105; Wellcome II, p. 26.

532. JAN LADMIRAL (1698–1773). *Icon durae matris in concava superficie visae*. Amsterdam: Apud Jacobum Graal & Henricum de Leth [et] Leiden: Apud Theodorum Haak, 1738. [4] pp., mounted color plate. 28.6 cm.

The texts of this and the balance of the collection consist only of explanations of the plates in Latin, French, and Dutch. The drawings for this and the following plate, both of the dura mater, are by Frederik Ruysch (see No. 395 ff.).

Cushing L4; Wellcome III, p. 428.

533. ———. *Icon durae matris in convexa superficie visae*. Amsterdam: Apud Jacobum Graal & Henricum de Leth [et] Leiden: Apud Theodorum Haak, 1738. [4] pp., mounted color plate. 28.6 cm.

Wellcome III, p. 428.

534. ———. *Icon membranae vasculosae*. Amsterdam: Apud Jacobum Graal & Henricum de Leth [et] Leiden: Apud Theodorum Haak, 1738. [4] pp., mounted color plate. 28.6 cm.

Wellcome III, p. 428.

535. ———. *Effigies penis humani*. Leiden: Apud Cornelium Haak [et] Amsterdam: Apud Jacobum Graal et Henricum de Leth, 1741. [6] pp., mounted color plate. 28.6 cm.

Waller 5483; Wellcome III, p. 428.

For a full description, see Choulant-Frank, pp. 267–269. And for another claimant to Le Blon's process see No. 589, Gautier d'Agoty, in this catalogue.

Gift of Dr. Henry J. Prentiss.

*536. [PIERRE LOUIS MOREAU DE MAUPERTUIS] (1698–1759). *Venus physique*. [N.p.: n. publ.] 1745. 194 pp. 15.1 cm. Marbled boards.

A rare first edition of Maupertuis' remarkable work on embryology and genetics. It is divided into two parts: "Dissertation sur l'origine des hommes et des animaux" and "Dissertation sur l'origine des noirs." The first part was originally published a year earlier under the title "Dissertation physique à l'occasion du Nègre blanc" and was written after an albino Negro appeared in Paris. A scientist, philosopher, and original thinker, Maupertuis was years ahead of his time in many aspects of biology, particularly embryology and genetics. His arguments against the then-prevailing theory of preformation and for epigenesis were so close to the idea of evolution that he is a true forerunner of Darwin and Mendel. His theories and observations are contained in this work, which he may have had published anonymously to avoid repercussions from Church authorities.

Osler 3350; Waller 6354 (1746 ed.).

*537. JOHANN FRIEDRICH CASSEBOHM (1699–1743). *Tractatus quatuor anatomici de aure humana*. Halle: Sumptibus Orphanatrophei, 1734. [12] 84 pp., 3 fold. plates. 21.2 cm. Vellum.

Cassebohm, a native of Halle, graduated from Frankfurt in 1730 where he prepared his doctoral dissertation on the human ear. He became professor of anatomy at Halle in 1738 and at Berlin in 1741, only two years before his death. Although this book has not received a great deal of attention, it is one of the earlier works containing highly accurate descriptions of the anatomy of the ear. The four tracts discuss the temporal bone, the external ear, the tympanic cavity, and the contents of the tympanic cavity.

Garrison-Morton 1547; Waller 1805; Wellcome II, p. 309.

538. JOHANN GOLDHAMMER (fl. 1740). *Compendieuser aber doch sehr offenhertzige Weiber- und Kinder-Artzt*. Leipzig and Nordhausen: Bey J. H. Gross, 1750. [12] 324 [28] pp., front. 16.3 cm.

In the first part of this early work on obstetrics and pediatrics, Goldhammer has presented his material in the form of 307 short questions with answers. A second part discusses the essential principles of obstetrical examination for midwives. And, in a third part, Goldhammer has assembled a collection of prayers with scriptural references for midwives and for expectant fathers and mothers.

Waller 3626 (1737 ed.).

Gift of Edna Dieman and Julia Bennett.

539. HENRY JACKSON (fl. 1740). *Reflexions concerning the virtues of tar water*. London: Printed for J. Robinson, 1744. 19 pp. 20 cm.

Jackson was a London chemist who had experimented with tar water and found it to be a remedy well worth using to cure a variety of complaints. This small pamphlet is largely a commentary on George Berkeley's treatise on tar water (see No. 509) in which Jackson provides, as the title pages states, "Hints for its improvement, so as to make it a most efficacious and pleasant Medicine."

Wellcome III, p. 336.

*540. GERARD VAN SWIETEN (1700–1772). *Commentaria in Hermanni Boerhaave Aphorismos, de cognoscendis et curandis morbis.* 5 vols. Paris: Apud viduam & filium Guillelmi Cavelier, 1755–1773. Front. (Vol. 1). 25.1 cm. Original mottled calf.

Swieten was one of Boerhaave's favorite and most famous pupils. He studied at Louvain and then at Leiden, where he received his medical degree in 1725. Swieten was Boerhaave's assistant in both the laboratory and the examining room, and his knowledge of shorthand made it possible for him to record Boerhaave's comments and remarks on his patients which he later published in this work. He became physician to Empress Maria Theresa in 1745 and after three years was made responsible for reorganizing and reforming medical education in Austria. As a result of his efforts, Vienna soon became one of the leading medical schools in the world. Swieten was not only a famous teacher and clinician, but he made many contributions to improve Austria's public health system and upgrade the practice of military medicine. His many activities left him little time to write, and this is his only medical work of note. Swieten labored over it for some thirty years, and it became one of the most widely read and frequently reprinted works of the eighteenth century. It is written in the Hippocratic manner, and the chapters on rheumatic fever, syphilis, and fevers are masterpieces of clinical description.

Cushing S487 (2nd English ed., 1771); Garrison-Morton 2200 (1742 ed.); Waller 9393 (1754 ed.).

541. [THOMAS REEVE] (1700?–1780). *A cure for the epidemical madness of drinking tar water, lately imported from Ireland by a certain R---t R----d doctor. In a letter to his L---p.* By T.R. M.D. London: Printed for J. and P. Knapton, 1744. 66 pp. 20 cm.

Reeve was physician to St. Thomas Hospital, London, for over twenty years and was also very active in the affairs of the Royal College of Physicians, serving as its president for nearly ten years. Although Reeve's name does not appear in the pamphlet, his initials do, and historians attribute it to him. His position of leadership in the College made him a likely individual to write this pamphlet in which he attacks George Berkeley's *Philosophical reflexions and inquiries concerning the virtues of tar water* (see No. 509).

*542. JOSIAS WEITBRECHT (1702–1747). *Syndesmologia; sive, Historia ligamentorum corporis humani.* St. Petersburg: Ex typographia Academiae Scientiarum, 1742. [xxviii] 276 pp., 26 fold. plates. 25.7 cm. Contemporary vellum.

Although he was born in Germany, Weitbrecht practiced and published his many anatomical works in St. Petersburg. At one time he catalogued the famous Ruysch museum of anatomical specimens, prefacing it with his own anatomical compendium. This, his chief work, has been translated into French and German. An exhaustive and fundamental treatise on the scientific study of the joints (syndesmology), it contains twenty-six large folding copperplates depicting the anatomy of the joints. The author is also remembered by Weitbrecht's ligament, a small ligament in the elbow.

Waller 10201.

*543. ANDRÉ LEVRET (1703–1780). *Observations sur la cure radicale de plusieurs polypes de la matrice, de la gorge et du nez.* Paris: Chez Delaguette, 1749. 500 (misnumbered 520) [3] pp., 6 fold. plates. 19.6 cm. Contemporary calf.

Along with Jean Louis Baudelocque (see No. 664), Levret was one of the two outstanding French obstetricians and gynecologists of the eighteenth century. He wrote on nearly every phase of obstetrics and gynecology, was active in championing the cause of male midwifery, and devised many obstetrical and gynecological instruments. He invented a special obstetrical forceps which he presented to the French Academy in 1747.

In the present work, Levret describes the surgical techniques used to remove uterine and vaginal polyps and records his experiences in more than thirty cases. Some of the instruments he devised for this type of surgery were prototypes for instruments later used to remove polyps from the nose and throat. The six fine copperplates depict a variety of the ingenious instruments he developed.

Wellcome III, p. 509.

*544. ———. *L'art des accouchemens, demontré par des principes de physique et de méchanique.* 2nd ed. Paris: Chez P. Alex. Le Prieur, 1761. [4] xvi, 466 [2] pp., port., 5 fold. plates. 19.3 cm. Contemporary mottled calf.

Levret first prepared this work as a text and guide for his students in 1753. A standard text for many years, it covers a wide range of subjects: female pelvic anatomy, conception, normal and pathological conditions, and the stages of gestation, parturition, and post partum period. There is also a section on the care of infants and small children. This edition includes Levret's views on the aphorisms of Mauriceau (see No. 389 ff.). The work is well-illustrated with five folding copperplates depicting the pelvis and uterus during various stages of fetal development.

Garrison-Morton 6153 (1st ed., 1753); Waller 5762; Wellcome III, p. 510.

*545. JOSEPH LIEUTAUD (1703–1780). *Essais anatomiques.* Paris: Chez Pierre-Michel Huart, 1742. xxi [3] 724 [16] pp., 6 fold. plates. 19.4 cm.

Pathological anatomy in France is said to begin with Lieutaud, physician to Kings Louis XV and XVI. This practical text of anatomy stresses the clinical implications of various structures and has been called the first surgical anatomy. Lieutaud is especially known for his descriptions of the heart and its cavities and the struc-

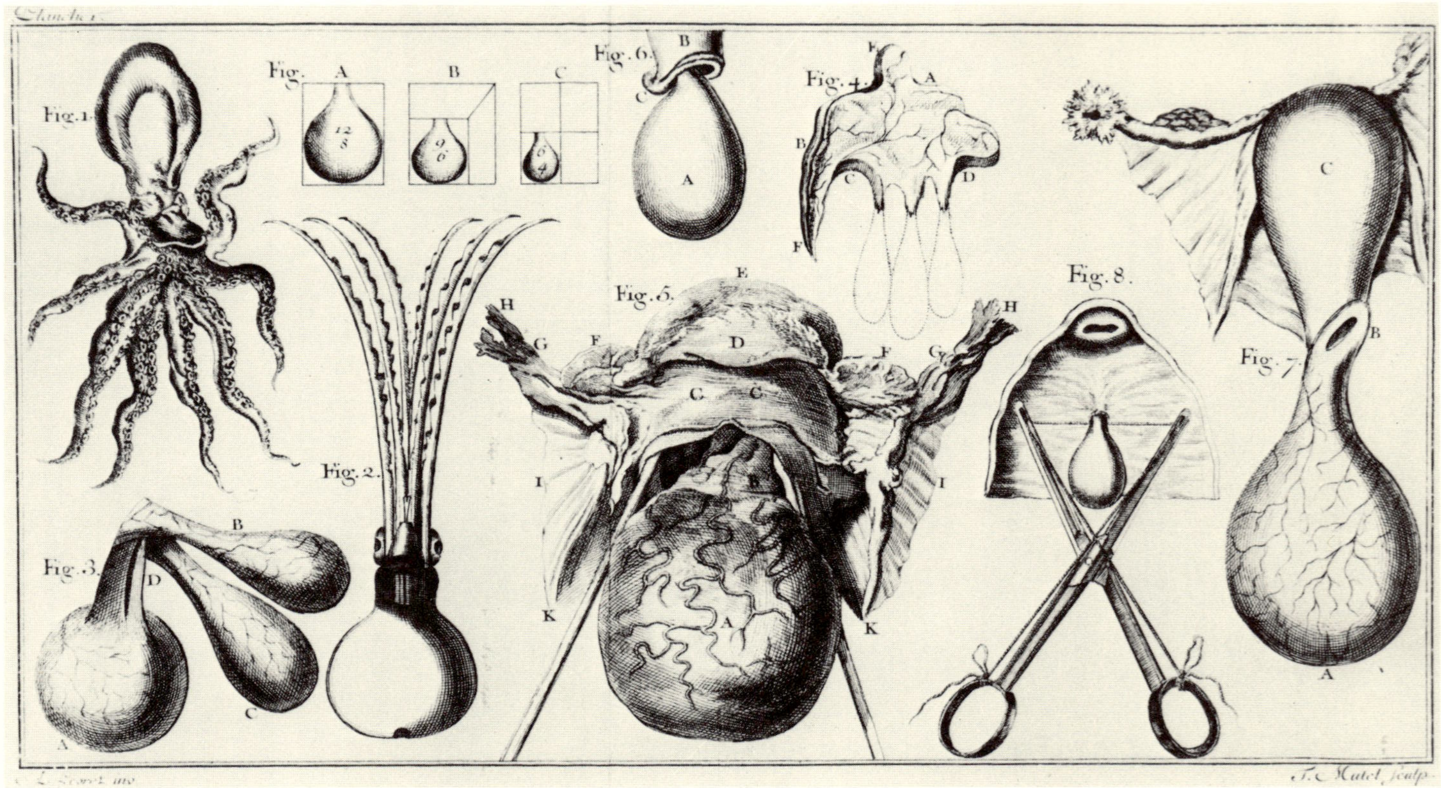

No. 543. Levret. *Observations sur . . . [les] Polypes.*

ture of the urinary bladder, as well as for numerous corrections of anatomical errors.

Garrison-Morton 396; Waller 5815; Wellcome III, p. 516.

*546. ———. *Précis de la matière médicale.* 3 vols. Paris: Chez P. Fr. Didot jeune, 1777. Vol. I: iv, xvi, 511 pp.; Vol. II: iv, 535 pp.; Vol. III: [4] 482 pp. 16.4 cm. Contemporary marbled calf.

This long, comprehensive work on pharmacology was widely used by Lieutaud's contemporaries and it went through at least four editions. In 1770, he published *Synopsis universae praxeos medicae* and the present work is his translation of the second part of that work. Part one was translated in 1765, and it, too, went through at least four editions. In the preface, Lieutaud indicates that he tried with each revision to bring his material up to date.

Wellcome III, p. 516 (1766 ed.).

JOHANN CHRISTOPH BOHL (1703–1785). *Dissertatio epistolica ad . . . Ruyschium.*

See No. 403.

547. JOHN WESLEY (1703–1791). *Primitive physic; or, An easy and natural method of curing most diseases.* 26th ed. Nottingham: Sutton, 1805. 118 pp. 17.6 cm.

Wesley, English evangelist, theologian, and founder of the Methodist Societies, was intensely interested in medicine and patterned many of his personal health care habits after the advice found in Cheyne's works, especially his *Health and long life* (see No. 481). As the Methodists' chief tutor, Wesley undertook to supply them with an abundance of inexpensive and worthwhile literature. He freely reprinted and abridged the writings of others or produced his own as circumstances warranted. In addition to his religious works, Wesley published this medical handbook, first in 1747, and followed by twenty-two other editions in his lifetime and nine after his death. An interesting combination of good sense and superstition, it is a collection of remedies for the treatment of diseases, symptoms, and accidental injuries. In this edition, Wesley's preferred remedies are marked with an asterisk.

Cushing W136 (1801 ed.); Osler 4214 (1st ed., 1747); Waller 10238 (1832 ed.).

548. JOHANN FRIEDRICH CARTHEUSER (1704–1777). *Fundamenta materiae medicae tam generalis quam specialis.* Venice: Apud Dominicum Deregni, 1755. 396 pp. 23.2 cm.

Professor of medicine, botany, and pharmacology at Frankfurt, Cartheuser wrote widely in the fields of chemistry, botany, pharmacology, pathology, and therapeutics. This work on the fundamentals of the materia medica was first published in 1749 at Frankfurt an der Oder. A popular work, it went through a number of Latin editions (this being the first one published in Venice) and was later translated into French.

Wellcome II, p. 306 (1749 ed.).

549. HIERONYMUS DAVID GAUBIUS (1705–1780). *Sermo academicus de regimine mentis quod medicorum est.* 2nd ed. Leiden: Apud Cornelium de Pecker, 1767. [2] 115 pp. 24.4 cm. Bound with No. 550.

Gaubius, a native of Heidelberg, succeeded his friend and teacher, Hermann Boerhaave, in the professorship of medicine at Leiden. He was an effective and successful teacher and his influence was widespread throughout Europe and America. Although he was deeply committed to chemistry, Gaubius did not allow that commitment to overshadow his interest in clinical medicine. In his most popular and well-known work, *Institutiones pathologiae medicinalis* (1758), he presented a modified humoral theory which ignored the body of pathological knowledge that had been accumulated during the previous century. This was unfortunate because his book went through many editions and translations and was used by countless students who had no knowledge of the work of Morgagni or Matthew Baillie. Gaubius did some of his best work in medicinal chemistry and many consider his treatise on prescriptions to be his finest work.

The present work is the first of two lectures given by Gaubius in 1747 and 1763, respectively, on the management and cure of mental diseases. During Gaubius' time a large proportion of the psychiatric cases showed no specific pathology. As a result, there was no reservoir of knowledge to draw upon and purely theoretical considerations were often introduced into the practice of psychiatry. In these lectures, Gaubius presents an approach to mental diseases in which he argues against the Leibnitzian theory of the supremacy of mind over matter and supports a more objective approach to the description of psychiatric conditions.

Waller 3432 (1747 ed.); Wellcome III, p. 95 (1747 ed.).

550. ———. *Sermo academicus alter de regimine mentis quod medicorum est.* 2nd ed. Leiden: Apud Samuelem et Joannem Luchtmans, 1769. [9] 94 pp. 24.4 cm. Bound with No. 549.

The second of Gaubius' two lectures on the management and cure of mental diseases.

Wellcome III, p. 95 (1763 ed.).

551. EBENEZER GILCHRIST (1707–1774). *The use of sea voyages in medicine.* 2nd ed. London: A. Millar, 1757. xi, 186 pp. 21.2 cm.

Gilchrist, a Scottish physician, spent his entire career in Scotland as a practicing physician, making several contributions to the literature on fevers as well as the present work on sea voyages. First published in 1756, it discusses the merits and benefits of the air at sea, histories of cures resulting from exposure to the sea air, and the proper use of sea voyages for health purposes. The author added an appendix concerning the use of the bath in fevers and a supplement containing additional observations on the use of sea trips for health purposes.

Osler 2731 (1771 ed.); Wellcome III, p. 115.

*552. CARL VON LINNÉ (1707–1778). *Clavis medicinae duplex, exterior & interior.* Stockholm: Impensis Laurentii Salvii, 1766. 29 [2] pp. 22 cm. In slipcase.

Linné (or Linnaeus) was both a physician and botanist and is perhaps better known for his work in the natural sciences than for his contributions in the practice and teaching of medicine. His *Systema naturae* (1735) remains as the basis of modern botanical classification and nomenclature. He excelled in his descriptions and was the first to introduce the binomial nomenclature and to classify man in the primate order as *homo sapiens*.

This small, concise treatise contains Linnaeus' medical system of classification. It is in outline form and classified quite rigidly. The book is rare and infrequently mentioned among his many publications.

553. Sir JOHN PRINGLE (1707–1782). *Observations on the diseases of the army.* 6th ed. London: Printed for A. Millar and T. Cadell, D. Wilson; T. Durham; and T. Payne, 1768. xxiv, 345, cxx [29] pp., illus. 19.3 cm. Modern half cloth with marbled boards.

Pringle, the founder of military medicine, served as Physician-General of the British Army from 1744 to 1752 and was also president of the Royal Society. In this book, first published in 1752, he outlined the basic principles of military sanitation and stressed the proper ventilation of military quarters regardless of their location. The preface of the book contains a brief account of the concept of neutrality for military hospitals on the field of battle. This idea was later embodied in the provisions of the Geneva Conventions. In an appendix to the book, Pringle includes a paper on septic and aseptic substances in which he recognizes the value of antisepsis and describes the effect of various chemicals in checking putrefaction. The last three pages of the index are missing from this copy.

Cushing P398; Garrison-Morton 2150 (1st ed., 1752).

*554. ALBRECHT VON HALLER (1708–1777). *Anatomen cadaveris virilis indicit ad diem XXIII Februar. MDCCXLI. et tabulam novam diaphragmatis addit.* [Göttingen: Typis Abram Vandenhoeck, 1741]. [8] pp., fold. plate. 36.8 cm. Original covers.

Albrecht von Haller was one of the intellectual giants of the eighteenth century and, indeed, one of the most accomplished men of all time. He was born in Bern, educated at Tübingen and Leiden; his accomplishments in medicine, surgery, anatomy, physiology, botany, literature, bibliography, and public service were simply enormous, and he achieved distinction in all of them. Any one of his major works, *Primae lineae physiologiae* (1747), *Elementa physiologiae corporis humani* (8 vols., 1757–1766), *Icones anatomicae* (8 vols., 1743–1756), or his exhaustive bibliographies in twenty volumes, would have been enough to occupy the lifetime of a lesser man, but Haller carried on a vast correspondence with hundreds of scientists, wrote thousands of reports, composed poetry which was a landmark in the development of German literature, wrote on the history of medicine, and was active in public affairs.

This brief and little-known anatomical work first appeared in the 1738 edition of Swammerdam's book on respiration (see No. 388) and was included in Haller's later anatomical treatises. The text has been prepared to correspond with the reference letters and numbers on the large foldout plate of the diaphragm drawn by Haller's fellow-physician, C. J. Rollinus.

Osler 1150; Waller 9386.

*555. ———. *Primae lineae physiologiae.* Göttingen: Ap. viduam Ab. Vandenhoeck, 1751. 567 (misnumbered 564) pp. 17.1 cm. Contemporary quarter calf.

Although Haller had many interests and talents, he was chiefly a physiologist, and one of his greatest contributions to physiology was his demonstration that irritability is a specific property of all muscle tissue and that sensibility is the exclusive property of nervous tissue. This work, first published in 1747, contains many of the ideas that Haller later developed more fully in *Elementa physiologiae corporis humani* (see No. 557), including his resonance theory, similar to that already advanced by Duverney (see No. 433) and to that of Helmholtz more than one hundred years later.

Garrison-Morton 585 (1747 ed.); Waller 4018 (1747 ed.); Wellcome III, p. 198.

*556. ———. *Deux mémoires sur le mouvement du sang, et sur les effets de la saignée.* Lausanne: Chez Marc-Mic. Bousquet et Paris: Chez David, 1756. viii, 343 pp., engr. front. 16.2 cm.

This work on the heart stamps Haller as a first-class investigator and experimental physiologist. His findings are based on animal experimentation and the experiments are carefully documented. The plate showing human blood transfusion is particularly interesting.

Cushing H65; Osler 747; Waller 3997.

*557. ———. *Elementa physiologiae corporis humani.* 8 vols. Vol. 1, Lausanne: Sumptibus M.-M. Bousquet; Vols. 2–5, Lausanne: Sumptibus F. Grasset; Vols. 6–8, Bern: Sumptibus Societatis Typographicae, 1757–1766. Front., 6 plates (part fold.). 24.3 cm. Mottled calf.

Historians agree that, of the vast amount of scientific literature produced by this gifted genius, this eight-volume work is his greatest and most important contribution. The work has had a lasting influence on the development of anatomy and physiology. In it Haller examined the entire body and in each section provided anatomical description along with data on the structure, physical properties, and chemical composition of the part under consideration. There are many physiological discoveries in this book that were forgotten, only to be rediscovered again years later. Two notable examples are the myogenic theory of the heart beat and the role of bile in the digestion of fat.

Garrison-Morton 588; Osler 1148; Waller 4007; Wellcome III, p. 199.

*558. ———. *Deux mémoires sur la formation des os, fondés sur des experiences.* Lausanne: Chez Marc.-Mich. Bousquet, 1758. [6] 267 pp., fold. table. 16.5 cm. Mottled calf.

Haller, in this work, first affirmed that bones form from cartilaginous anlage and not from the periosteum.

Wellcome III, p. 199.

*559. ———. *Sur la formation du coeur dans le poulet.* 2 vols. Lausanne: Chez Marc.-Mich. Bousquet, 1758. Vol. I: [6] 472 pp.; Vol. II: [8] 368 pp., plate. 16.3 cm. Contemporary calf-backed boards.

The first volume of this work is an excellent example of Haller's precise and detailed investigative methods, which are revealed here as he observed and recorded hourly the development of the vascular system in the hen's egg. The second volume deals with the muscular action and physiology of the respiratory system in humans and experimental animals.

Waller 11834.

*560. ———. *Opera minora emendata, aucta, et renovata.* 3 vols. Lausanne: Sumptibus Francisci Grasset, 1762–1768. Vol. I: xxii [2] 608 pp.; Vol. II: vi, 607 pp.; Vol. III: 388 pp., fold. plates. 26 cm. Original soft boards, uncut.

In these three volumes on anatomy, reproduction, and pathology, respectively, Haller collected various of his shorter writings which were scattered in other works and journals. They represent, with his *Icones anatomicae,* what he considered to be among his best works. The numerous plates contain his highly exact, clear, and striking representations of anatomic preparations.

Choulant-Frank, p. 289; Cushing H73; Osler 1156; Wellcome III, p. 199.

*561. ———. *Bibliotheca chirurgica.* 2 vols. Bern: Apud Em. Haller, & Basel: Apud Joh. Schweighauser, 1774–1775. Vol. I: iv, 593 pp.; Vol. II: viii, 695 pp. 23.9 cm. Contemporary calf.

In addition to his great achievements in anatomy, physiology, and botany, Haller found time during the last ten years of his life to prepare comprehensive retrospective bibliographies of the known literature on botany (1771), surgery (the present work), anatomy (see No. 562), and medicine (1776). They are still of considerable reference value in their respective fields and are landmarks in medical bibliography. These bibliographies contain an exhaustive summary of the important works in each field and are written in the clear, compact style so characteristic of Haller. Haller also includes a biographical sketch of each author and occasionally adds other bits of interesting information about the author or work.

Cushing H61; Garrison-Morton 5789; Osler 1162; Waller 18471; Wellcome III, p. 199.

*562. ———. *Bibliotheca anatomica*. 2 vols. Zurich: Apud Orell, Gessner, Fuessli, 1774–1777. Vol. I: vii, 816 pp.; Vol. II: iv, 870 pp. 25.1 cm. Original boards, uncut.

This bibliography of nearly all of the previously written work on anatomy is typical of Haller's erudition, thoroughness, and energy. He summarizes at least twenty percent of the works listed, some of the summaries running to a page or more, and comments on almost all of the important works.

Choulant-Frank, p. 290; Garrison-Morton 438; Waller 18469; Wellcome III, p. 199.

*563. FRANÇOIS MICHEL DISDIER (1708–1781). *Exposition exacte, ou tableaux anatomiques en tailles-douces, des différentes parties du corps humain*. Paris: Crepy, 1778. 60 *ll.*, 29 plates. 36.6 cm. Contemporary half calf.

According to Choulant, Disdier was a professor of surgery and also a drawing master at the Academy of Painting in Paris. The twenty-nine anatomical plates in this work are well-engraved but were most likely copied from the work of other anatomists. For example, the male and female figures depicted in the first plate bear a remarkable resemblance to a similar woodcut in Vesalius' *Epitome* of 1543. The entire book, including the text, was printed from engraved copperplates.

Cushing D186 (1758 ed.); Waller 2493; Wellcome II, p. 473 (1758 ed.).

*564. BALTHASAR LUDWIG TRALLES (1708–1797). *Usus opii salubris et noxius, in morborum medela, solidis et certis principiis superstructus*. 4 vols. in 1. Breslau: Sumptibus Caroli Godogredi Meyeri, 1757–1762. Vol. I: [12] 374 [2] pp.; Vol. II: [8] 356 pp.; Vol. III: [16] 272 pp.; Vol. IV: [20] 248 [24] pp., port. (v. 4) 21.8 cm. Contemporary calf.

Tralles, a German physician, studied at Leipzig and Halle and subsequently practiced and taught in Breslau. In addition to his medical works, he wrote several books on theology and philosophy. In this comprehensive treatise on the uses of opium, he reviews the history of its use as a therapeutic, gives a chemical analysis of its properties, and goes on to discuss its healthful and harmful applications in treating such problems as hemorrhages, fevers, pain, epilepsy, dysentery, and mental illness. He also describes the treatment of victims of accidental or intentional poisoning. Tralles' engraved portrait is the frontispiece of Volume Four.

*565. CHRISTIAN GOTTLIEB LUDWIG (1709–1773). *Institutiones pathologiae*. Leipzig: Ex officina Gleditschiana, 1754. [4] 172 [8] pp. 2 copies. Copy 1: 19.4 cm. Contemporary vellum. Copy 2: 19.4 cm. Quarter calf, sprinkled boards. Bound with No. 566.

After completing his medical education at Leipzig, Ludwig was appointed to the faculty as professor of medicine in 1740. He subsequently became professor of anatomy and surgery in 1747, of pathology in 1755, and of therapy in 1758. He also served as dean of the medical faculty for a number of years. The present work is a discussion of the physiological changes in the pathology of a wide range of diseases including apoplexy, asthma, cancer, gangrene, and tetanus. It is part of a series of six works on physiology, clinical medicine, surgery, pathology, therapeutics, and forensic medicine, each of which was published separately over a number of years.

Waller 6071; Wellcome III, p. 558 (1785 ed.).

*566. ———. *Institutiones therapiae generalis.* Leipzig: Ex officina Gleditschiana, 1754. [8] 162 [6] pp. 19.4 cm. Quarter calf, sprinkled boards. Bound with No. 565, copy 2.

This work on general therapy followed Ludwig's treatise on pathology in his series of six works on the fundamentals of medicine and is here bound with it. In this book, he discusses the rationale of treatment for a variety of diseases.

Waller 6072; Wellcome III, p. 558 (1785 ed.).

567. WILLIAM CULLEN (1710–1790). *Synopsis nosologiae methodicae.* 4th ed. 2 vols. Edinburgh: Apud Guilielmum Creech, 1785. Vol. I: iv, 368 pp.; Vol. II: [4] 417 pp. 20.4 cm.

Cullen, a Scottish physician, was instrumental in founding the school of medicine at Glasgow and later became one of the leading figures at the Edinburgh Medical School. Active as a practitioner, Cullen was also an outstanding teacher and attracted students from home and abroad. Benjamin Rush, William Shippen, Jr., Philippe Pinel, and Joseph Black were among his many pupils who later achieved fame and success. Cullen was one of the first teachers to deliver his lectures in English instead of the traditional Latin.

Although Cullen's classification of disease was incomplete and unnatural, it was a definite improvement over the efforts of his predecessors who included Boerhaave, Sauvages, Linné, and Vogel. He classified diseases by their symptoms, distinguishing four classes: pyrexias, neuroses, cachexias, and local diseases. He divided the classes into orders and further subdivided the orders into genera. For example, in the class of pyrexias he included the orders of fevers, inflammations, and hemorrhages. First published in 1769, his classification became extremely popular and remained in print until well into the nineteenth century.

Cushing C524 (1792 ed.); Garrison-Morton 2204 (1st ed., 1769).

568. ———. *Lectures on the materia medica.* Philadelphia: Printed for the subscribers, by Robert Bell, 1775. viii, 512 pp. 24.3 cm.

The present work, a collection of lectures on the materia medica delivered by

Cullen at Edinburgh, furnished the material upon which he based his *Treatise of the materia medica* in 1789 (see No. 571).

Austin 577; Cushing C522; Wellcome II, p. 412 (London ed., 1773).

*569. ———. *First lines of the practice of physic.* 4 vols. Dublin: Vol. I printed for Thomas Armitage, Vol. II printed by J. Williams, Vol. III printed for James Williams, Vol. IV printed for Luke White, 1777–1784. Vol. I: viii, 417 pp.; Vol. II: viii, 408 pp.; Vol. III: ix [1] 389 pp.; Vol. IV: vi, xlviii, 362 pp. (misnumbered 286). 21.1 cm. Contemporary calf.

"My duties, however, as a Professor, have necessarily produced the following sheets, intended chiefly as a text-book for the use of my students" (Preface). First published in Edinburgh in 1776, this work became very popular and was the authoritative work on medicine in the late eighteenth and early nineteenth centuries.

Wellcome II, p. 413.

570. ———. ———. 2 vols. in 1. New York: Printed by L. Nichols & Co. for Evert Duyckinck, 1801. Vol. I: 326 pp.; Vol. II: [2] 294 [10] pp. 21.3 cm.

Cullen's work exerted considerable influence on medical practice in Europe and the United States. His book was widely reprinted in this country and was translated into French and German.

Austin 570.

571. ———. *A treatise of the materia medica.* 2 vols. Edinburgh: Printed for Charles Elliot, 1789. Vol. I: xxiii, 432 pp.; Vol. II: [4] 610 pp. 2 copies. Copy 1: 26.8 cm. Cloth. Copy 2: 26.6 cm. Contemporary calf.

The present work resulted from a series of lectures (see No. 569) Cullen gave at Edinburgh. According to the author, "The Lectures on the Materia Medica formerly published in my name, though very incorrect, were so well received by the public, that notwithstanding my endeavours to prevent it, they have been several times reprinted, and even translated into foreign languages" (Preface). At first, Cullen considered revising his *Lectures* but concluded that it would be best to prepare an entirely new work and this treatise was the result. It, too, enjoyed great success and remained in print until the early nineteenth century.

Garrison-Morton 1838; Wellcome II, p. 413.

Copy 2: Gift of Dr. John Martin.

572. ———. ———. 3rd American ed. 2 vols. in 1. Philadelphia: Published by Mathew Carey, 1808. Vol. I: viii [9] 256 pp.; Vol. II: iv, 349 pp. 21.6 cm. Calf.

An immensely popular book, Cullen's treatise was first published in this country in 1789 and is here in the third edition.

Austin 589; Cushing C526 (1812 ed.); Garrison-Morton 1838 (Edinburgh ed., 1789).

Gift of H. C. Bulis and A. F. Barfoot.

*573. WILLIAM HEBERDEN (1710–1801). *Commentarii de morborum historia et curatione.* London: Veneunt apud T. Payne; Typis mandavit S. Hamilton, 1802. ix, 417 pp. 21.6 cm.

Called "the last of our learned physicians" by Samuel Johnson, Heberden was noted for his careful notes taken during a long practice. He spent the last twenty years of his life putting them in order and editing them for this work which was published by his son after the author's death. His most important contributions are his descriptions of angina pectoris, chicken pox, and the rheumatic nodules on the fingers now called Heberden's nodules. This work has been called the last important medical treatise written in Latin, and perhaps an indication of the disuse into which Latin had fallen may be seen in the fact that the work was immediately translated and published in English in the same year as this first edition.

Cushing H200; Garrison-Morton 2207; Waller 4173.

574. WILLIAM CADOGAN (1711–1797). *An essay upon nursing, and the management of children, from their birth to three years of age.* 2nd ed. London: Printed for J. Roberts, 1748. 34 pp. 20.1 cm.

Cadogan was born in London, studied at Oxford, and received his medical degree at Leiden during the declining years of Boerhaave's career. He maintained an active practice, for a time in Bristol and later in London. Because of the beneficial influence of this brief essay on the handling of infants, he was appointed physician to the Foundling Hospital in London. Published at a time when sensible practices of child care were largely neglected, the pamphlet became very popular and went through eight editions during the next eighteen years.

Cushing C9 (1752 ed.); Garrison-Morton 6322 (1st ed., 1748); Osler 2207 (1st ed.); Waller 1688 (1749 ed.); Wellcome II, p. 285 (1st ed.).

Gift of Robert D. Gauchat.

575. ———. *A dissertation on the gout.* 5th ed. London: Printed for J. Dodsley, 1771. 100 pp. 22.5 cm. Unbound, uncut.

Cadogan suffered from gout for many years, and this book is based upon his personal observations. It enjoyed great popularity although Cadogan was widely attacked and harshly criticized by those who disagreed with him. He believed that gout was not hereditary, seasonal, or curable, but was due to indolence, vexation, and intemperance. He recommended rational principles of diet and exercise, emphasizing a common sense approach to the management of gout.

Garrison-Morton 4489 (1st ed., 1771); Wellcome II, p. 285.

*576. THOMAS DIMSDALE (1712–1800). *The present method of inoculating for the small-pox.* London: Printed for W. Owen, 1767. 160 pp. 19.3 cm. Modern blue cloth.

Dimsdale, descending from a family that was prominent in English medical affairs, studied at St. Thomas' Hospital in London and received his medical degree from King's College in Aberdeen. In 1768 he was invited to Russia to inoculate Catherine the Great and the Grand Duke Paul against smallpox. In gratitude for this service, Catherine gave him an outright gift of £10,000 and a lifetime pension, as well as several other honors including elevation to baron of the Russian Empire. The present work, published a year before his visit to Russia, became highly successful and subsequently went through seven editions and was translated into several foreign languages. The treatise gives a full description of Dimsdale's methods and also includes twenty-nine case histories of individuals he inoculated.

Cushing D171 (1767 ed.); Garrison-Morton 5420; Waller 2470 (1772 ed.); Wellcome II, p. 470.

577. ROBERT WHYTT (1714–1766). *Observations on the nature, causes, and cure of those disorders which have been commonly called nervous, hypochondriac, or hysteric.* Edinburgh: Printed for T. Becket, 1765. viii [8] 520 pp. 20.2 cm.

Whytt, a pupil of Monro *primus* and predecessor of William Cullen in the chair of medicine at Edinburgh, was one of the foremost physicians of the eighteenth century because of his contributions to clinical medicine and particularly to the understanding of reflex action. His clear description of tuberculous meningitis, his explanation of the sentient (sensitivity) principle in involuntary action, and his discussion of the significance of emotions in the natural history of organic diseases easily offset his mistaken emphasis on the value of lime water in the treatment of calculi in the urinary tract. In this work, which Fielding H. Garrison calls "the first important English treatise on neurology after Willis" (*An introduction to the history of medicine.* 4th ed. Philadelphia, 1929. p. 326), Whytt discusses the significance of emotions in the pathogenesis of nervousness, hypochrondria, and hysteria.

Cushing W177 (1767 ed.); Garrison-Morton 4841; Waller 10277.

578. ———. *The works.* Edinburgh: Printed for . . . Balfour, 1786. [6] viii, 262 (misnumbered 762) [29] pp. 26.8 cm.

The present work was prepared by Whytt's son, Robert, and was published two years after his father's death. In addition to the previous treatise, the book contains some twelve additional monographs and papers as well as an appendix containing several letters relating to ulcers and an account of an epidemic of distemper in Edinburgh in 1758. Among the collection are his noteworthy *Essay on the vital and other involuntary motions of animals* (1751) in which he described reflex action in the pupil of the eye, as well as *Observations on the dropsy in the brain* (1768) which gives the first account of the clinical course of tuberculous meningitis in children.

Cushing W179; Russell 865.

579. WILLIAM LEWIS (1714–1781). *The new dispensatory*. London: Printed for J. Nourse, 1753. xii, 32, 664 pp. 20.6 cm.

Lewis, an English physician and chemist, received his medical degree from Oxford and is best remembered for his contributions to the literature of chemistry and pharmacy. Active both as a writer and a translator, he produced a number of successful works dealing with the practical aspects of chemistry and the pharmacopoeia, and translated the pharmaceutical and chemical works of several prominent German chemists.

This first edition of Lewis's dispensatory was intended to be a corrected and improved version of John Quincy's *Compleat English dispensatory* (see No. 462), which at that time had reached the twelfth edition. Lewis's work was of a wider scope in that he added to the translation useful notes on the materia medica and hospital prescriptions. The enlarged work quickly achieved prominence and new editions followed within a few years, reaching six editions by the late 1780's. The book was translated into German, and an edition was also printed in Dublin in 1768. The *Dispensatory* was continued by both Andrew Duncan, Sr. (1744–1828) and Andrew Duncan, Jr. (see No. 763), who further expanded and improved Lewis's work and continued to publish it through the twelfth edition in 1830.

Wellcome III, p. 511.

Gift of R. A. Kuever.

580. ———. *The Edinburgh new dispensatory*. 3rd American from the 4th Edinburgh ed. Walpole, New Hampshire: Printed by D. Carlisle, 1796. xxix, 622 pp., plates. 20 cm. Calf.

Lewis's *New dispensatory* has a long, complex, and interesting bibliographical history which can be traced from John Quincy's *Compleat English dispensatory* (see No. 462) to the first *British pharmacopoeia* in 1864. The present work is a vital link in that history, spanning the period from 1786 to 1801. The first few editions of the *Edinburgh new dispensatory* were edited by Andrew Duncan, Sr. and the remainder by John Rotheram (1751–1804), the editor of this edition. The work was very popular in Europe as well as in America and was reprinted in this country until 1818.

Austin 1145; Wellcome III, p. 511 (Edinburgh ed., 1791).

581. ———. *An experimental history of the materia medica, or of the natural and artificial substances made use of in medicine*. 2nd ed. London: Printed for R. Baldwin, 1768. xxiv, 622 [32] pp. 27.3 cm. Polished calf.

This work, first published in 1761, went through four editions and also was translated into German. In it Lewis discusses the natural history, pharmaceutical properties, and therapeutic value of a variety of medicines whose efficacy was known or could be deduced by logical reasoning.

Wellcome III, p. 512.

*582. PERCIVALL POTT (1714–1788). *Some few general remarks on fractures and dislocations.* London: Printed for L. Hawes, W. Clarke, and R. Collins, 1769. [iv] 126 pp., 2 plates. 20.5 cm. Modern half calf, marbled boards.

Pott was one of the busiest and most famous surgeons in England during the middle of the eighteenth century. His surgical writings were wide-ranging and included descriptions of congenital hernia, lacrimal fistula, hydrocele, fistula in ano, and cancer of the scrotum in chimney sweeps. This last work, a classic in industrial medicine, was one of the earliest examples of a specific type of neoplasm being related to a particular occupation. Pott's three best-known contributions were on tuberculosis of the spine (Pott's disease), puffy tumor (associated with osteomyelitis of the skull), and the present work on fractures. His discussion of fractures and dislocations included a common fracture of one or both bones just above the ankle, which some feel may have been the compound fracture of the leg that he suffered early in his career. His description of the physiology and pathological findings resulted in the eponym, Pott's fracture.

Garrison-Morton 4408; Waller 7602.

583. ———. *The chirurgical works of Percivall Pott.* 3 vols. London: Printed for T. Lowndes, J. Johnson . . . and S. Hayes, 1779. Vol. I: viii, 504 pp.; Vol. II: iv, 532 pp.; Vol. III: iv, 426 [16] pp., plates (part fold.). 21 cm. Contemporary calf, rebacked.

This three-volume set contains Pott's surgical writings and includes his treatises on fractures and dislocations, hydrocele, fistula in ano, congenital hernia, ruptures, and lacrimal fistula. Pott's writings were popular in America and an edition of the present work appeared in Philadelphia as late as 1819.

Cushing P354 (1783 ed.); Waller 7603 (1775 ed.).

*584. CAYETANO CABRERA Y QUINTERO (d. 1775). *Escudo de armas de Mexico.* Mexico: Impresso par la viuda de d. J. B. de Hogal, 1746. 17, 522 [24] pp., front., illus. 28.7 cm. Modern calf.

This beautifully printed work is among the relatively few eighteenth-century medical publications of Mexico. It describes the epidemic of "Matlazahuatl" (cholera) which swept that country in 1736–1737 killing forty thousand persons in Mexico City alone. In addition to the descriptions of symptoms and remedies, a recounting is given of the intervention of Our Lady of Guadalupe who, because of her act, was made Patron Saint of Mexico. The book also contains a wealth of material on local history including descriptions of the churches, local Indian tribes, religion, law, and the life of the capital.

*585. CARL FRIEDRICH HUNDERTMARK (1715–1762). *Liber singularis de incrementis artis medicae per expositionem aegrotorum apud veteres in vias publicas et templa.* 2nd ed. Leipzig: In officina Joannis Friderici Gleditsch, 1749. [8] 78 pp., 1 plate. 28 cm. Contemporary calf, gilt edges.

Hundertmark was professor of medicine and later professor of physiology, anatomy, and surgery at the University of Leipzig. He first published this work in 1739, and in it he discusses the ancient custom of exposing patients in the streets and temples in the hope of meeting people who had suffered and recovered from the same disease.

Osler 5981; Waller 4994; Wellcome III, p. 316.

*586. FREDERICK BERNARD ALBINUS (1715–1778). *De natura hominis libellus.* Leiden: Apud Petrum Delfos, 1775. x (misnumbered vi) 259 [39] pp., front. 20.3 cm. Bound with No. 529.

Frederick Bernard Albinus was the younger brother of the more famous Bernhard Siegfried Albinus, with whose *Supellex anatomica,* edited by the younger brother, this work is bound. It is a blending of anatomy and physiology.

Wellcome II, p. 26.

587. JAMES LIND (1716–1794). *A treatise on the scurvy.* 2nd ed. London: Printed for A. Millar, 1757. xvi, 476 pp. 2 copies. Copy 1: 20.3 cm. Calf. Copy 2: 19.6 cm. Quarter calf.

Scurvy had long been known as an often-fatal disease to which seamen on long voyages seemed to be particularly susceptible. As early as the sixteenth century, sailors themselves recognized the curative value of citrus fruit, and by the seventeenth century its use in the treatment of scurvy was medically recognized. But it was not until Lind's work in the eighteenth century that serious consideration was given to the regular supply of fresh fruit and citrus juices to seamen. Even so, the British Navy took no official recognition of it until after Lind's death.

Lind, a Scot, was a naval surgeon for most of his life. He was apprenticed to a surgeon when he was fifteen years old and, in 1739, entered the navy as a surgeon's mate. Lind left the navy in 1748 and completed his medical degree at the University of Edinburgh the same year. After ten years of private practice in Edinburgh, he became physician to the Haslar Naval Hospital near Portsmouth where he remained until he resigned in 1783. In addition to his important work on scurvy, he was also a pioneer in the field of tropical medicine.

Garrison-Morton 3713 (1st ed., 1753); Osler 3241; Waller 5828; Wellcome III, p. 520.

Copy 2: Gift of Dr. John Martin.

588. ———. *An essay on diseases incidental to Europeans, in hot climates, with the method of preventing their fatal consequences . . . To which is added, an appendix, concerning intermittent fevers; and a simple and easy way to render sea water fresh, and to prevent a scarcity of provisions in long voyages at sea.* 1st American from the 6th London ed. Philadelphia: William Duane, 1811. viii, 268 pp. 19.7 cm.

This work, Lind's third and last book, was published while he was serving as physician to the Naval Hospital in Haslar. In addition to discussing the diseases to which Europeans are susceptible in tropical climates and providing directions for their prevention and cure, Lind describes how fresh water may be collected by condensing the steam from boiling sea water. Lind also came close to recognizing the connection between mosquitoes and malaria in this important early work on tropical medicine.

Austin 1154; Garrison-Morton 2264 (1st ed., 1768); Waller 5829 (1st ed.); Wellcome III, p. 520 (1st ed.).

589. JACQUES FABIAN GAUTIER D'AGOTY (1717–1785). *Anatomie de la tête.* Paris: Chez le sieur Gautier, M. Duverney, Quillau, 1748. [22] *ll.*, 8 col. plates. 55.6 cm.

Gautier, a French printmaker, was, like Ladmiral (see No. 532 ff.), an assistant to Le Blon and, also like Ladmiral, claimed the color printing process as his own. He published some ten collections of colored plates of various portions of the anatomy, and he was the first person to print anatomical plates in color on a large scale. Although Choulant writes that "his anatomic illustrations . . . impress the critical observer with their arrogance and charlatanry and do not recommend themselves to the student of anatomy either for their faithfulness and reliability or for their technique" (Choulant-Frank, p. 270), they are of great interest from the point of view of book illustration and the history of anatomic illustration.

The dissections and preparations for the eight large figures in this atlas of the anatomy of the head were prepared by Joseph Guichard Duverney (see No. 433), and some of the plates are among the most elaborate produced by Gautier, especially notable for the intricate network of blood vessels which are meticulously indicated by direct color printing. This work is extremely rare.

Choulant-Frank, p. 271; Cushing G167; Wellcome III, p. 97.

Gift of Henry J. Prentiss.

590. ———. *Anatomie des parties de la génération de l'homme, et de la femme.* Paris: Chez J. B. Brunet et Demonville, 1773. 26 [4] pp., 8 col. plates. 39.4 cm.

The eight colored mezzotints in this collection show the anatomy of normal pregnancy, pathological female genitalia, and normal and diseased male genitalia. While vivid and startling, their importance is less to medicine than to the history of printing and illustration.

Choulant-Frank, p. 272; Wellcome III, p. 97.

Gift of Henry J. Prentiss

*591. WILLIAM HUNTER (1718–1783). *Anatomia uteri humani gravidi tabulis illustrata . . . . The anatomy of the human gravid uterus exhibited in figures.* Birmingham: Printed by John Baskerville, 1774. 40 pp., 34 plates. 63.5 cm. Cloth with leather back.

William Hunter, born in Scotland, was a London physician and obstetrician whose principal interest was in anatomy. Hunter served a three-year apprenticeship under William Cullen and received in 1750 his medical degree from the University of Glasgow. He was also a pupil of and then assistant to William Smellie (see No. 522) and later an assistant and dissector for James Douglas (1675–1742), the anatomist and obstetrician who discovered Douglas' pouch—the vesicouterine pouch. Upon becoming professor of anatomy of the Society of Navy Surgeons in 1746, Hunter initiated a series of lectures on anatomy, surgery, and obstetrics which became quite popular and well-attended. In 1768, he constructed an anatomical theater and museum on Great Windmill Street where many of the foremost surgeons and anatomists of the day, including his brother John (see No. 609 ff.), were trained. Hunter remained a bachelor and lived at his School of Anatomy where he practiced, taught, and developed his extensive collection of anatomical specimens.

This work, said to be "one of the finest anatomical atlases ever to be produced" (Garrison-Morton 6157), contains life-sized figures which not only are anatomically accurate but are themselves works of art. Hunter spent more than twenty-five years preparing this atlas, employed artists to prepare the engravings at enormous expense to himself, and entrusted the printing of the work to John Baskerville, the greatest English printer of the eighteenth century. This monumental work is, indeed, one of the great publications of world medical literature as well as a classic of book production.

Choulant-Frank, pp. 296–297; Cushing H522; Garrison-Morton 6157; Osler 3026; Russell 452; Waller 5004; Wellcome III, p. 319.

*592. ———. ———. London: Edward Lumley, 1815. iii, 19 pp., 34 plates. 49.5 cm. Half morocco.

This large folio edition is less ornate than the first, but the plates were made from those used in the first edition. As in the first edition, the text is in both Latin and English.

*593. CHARLES BONNET (1720–1793). *Considerations sur les corps organisés.* 2 vols. in 1. Amsterdam: Chez Marc-Michel Rey, 1762. Vol. I: xlii [2] 274 pp.; Vol. II: xx, 328 pp. 20.3 cm. Half calf.

It was Bonnet, a Swiss naturalist and philosopher, who first clearly worked out the theory of preformation of the embryo, or "incapsulation" (emboîtement), and in this he was supported by both Haller and Spallanzani. Parthenogenesis was widely accepted by philosophers and naturalists until the beginning of the twentieth century.

Garrison-Morton 472; Wellcome II, p. 200.

594. *Medicina flagellata; or, The doctor scarify'd.* London: Printed for J. Bateman and J. Nicks, 1721. xiv, 224 (misnumbered 214) pp. 18.3 cm. Blind-stamped calf.

During the seventeenth and eighteenth centuries quacks of every description flourished in London. Medicine still was more the pursuit of systems than the application of known principles of clinical pathology, so it is understandable that

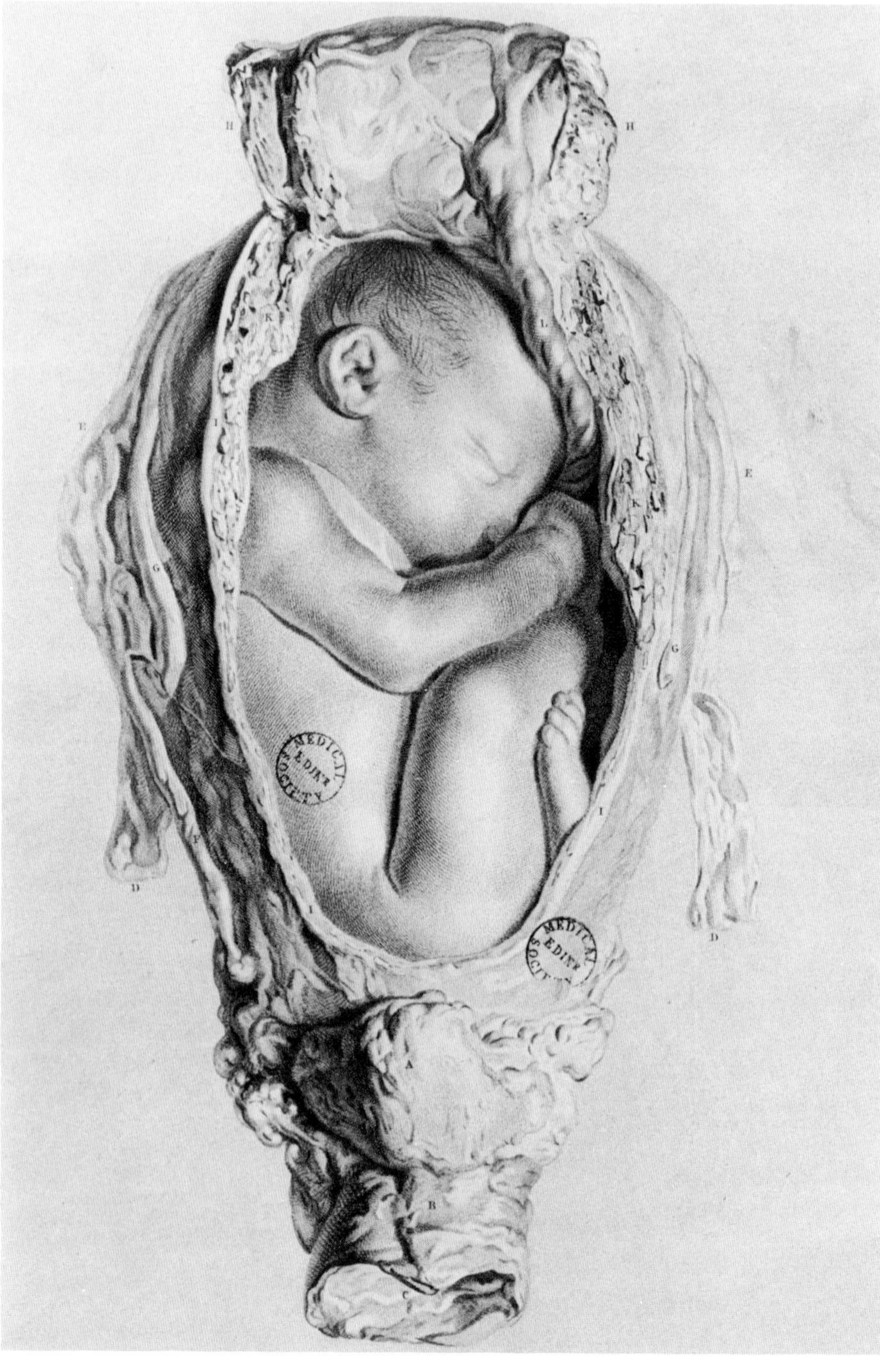

No. 591. William Hunter. *Anatomia Uteri Humani Gravidi.* Breech presentation of the term fetus.

quacks were ready to undertake what the legitimate practitioner could not cure. The contents of this work, by an unknown author, are best explained by its subtitle: *Laying open the vices of the faculty, the insignificancy of a great part of their materia medica; with certain rules to discern the true physician from the emperick, and the useful medicine from the noxious and trading physick. With an essay on health, of the power of a regimen. To which is added, a discovery of some remarkable errors in the late writings on the plague, by Dr. Mead, Quincey, Bradley, &c. With some useful and necessary rules to be observed in the time of that contagious distemper.*

Waller 6421.

Gift of Walter B. Mount.

595. [ANTOINE LE CAMUS] (1722–1772). *Abdeker; or, The art of preserving beauty.* London: Printed for A. Millar, 1754. vii, 220 pp. 10.3 cm. Contemporary calf.

Le Camus, a French physician, was professor of medicine and surgery at Paris and published several popular treatises on general medicine which were reprinted in multiple editions during his lifetime. The present work is an English translation of the French language work which went through three editions. According to the preface, this "is a translation of an Arabian manuscript, which Diamantes Utasto, physician to the Turkish Ambassador, brought to Paris in the year 1740." Abdeker, the Arabian author of this treatise on the cultivation and preservation of beauty, is known to have lived in the latter half of the twelfth century.

Wellcome III, p. 468 (French ed., 1754).

*596. THÉOPHILE DE BORDEU (1722–1776). *Recherches anatomiques sur la position des glandes et sur leur action.* Paris: Chez G. F. Quillau, 1751. xxiv, 520, 86 pp. 16.2 cm.

Bordeu, a graduate of Montpellier and the principal representative of clinical medicine in eighteenth-century France, was the chief representative if not the founder of the school of Vitalism. In the present work, the author sets forth his hypothesis of this vital power with regard to internal secretion: that every organ, tissue, and cell discharges, into the blood, products which influence the function of other parts of the body. In some ways a forerunner of the science of endocrinology, Bordeu's theory was based on speculation rather than rigid scientific investigation. But his theories were rather widely held and had their counterparts in similar "schools" and hypotheses in other European countries.

Waller 1306; Wellcome II, p. 203.

*597. PETRUS CAMPER (1722–1789). *Demonstrationum anatomico-pathologicarum.* 2 vols. Amsterdam: Apud Joann. Schreuder et Petrum Mortier Juniorem, 1760–1762. Vol. I: [6] 22 [2] pp.; Vol. II: [4] 24 [2] pp., 8 plates. 63.2 cm.

Camper, a Dutch physician, anatomist, and naturalist, was also an artist of great skill who illustrated all of his works. As an investigative anatomist, he made his mark as an anthropologist and craniologist. He made many original contributions to medicine, among them his discoveries of the *processus vaginalis* of the peritoneum and of the fibrous structures of the eye. Along with Albinus, Camper did much to influence trends in anatomic illustration toward making the figures lifelike and practical for the use of surgeons. The beautiful plates in this large volume are almost life-size.

Choulant-Frank, p. 285; Cushing C46; Waller 1723 (Vol. 2 only); Wellcome II, p. 293.

*598. ———. *Verhandeling over het natuurlijk verschil der wezenstrekken in menschen van onderscheiden landaart en ouderdom; over het schoon in antyke beelden en gesneedene steenen.* Utrecht: B. Wild en J. Altheer, 1791. viii, 108 pp., plates (part fold.). 27.9 cm. Original printed boards.

This work on cephalometry, in which Camper first described the facial angle (or Camper's line), probably has done more to perpetuate Camper's name than his work as an anatomist and artist. Loosely inserted in the book are five drawings of physiognomies referring to Camper's work presented in 1932 to a previous owner.

Choulant-Frank, p. 286; Waller 1740; Wellcome II, p. 293.

*599. LEOPOLD AUENBRUGGER (1722–1809). *Inventum novum ex percussione thoracis humani et signo abstrusos interni pectoris morbos detegendi.* Vienna: Typis Joannis Thomae Trattner, 1761. 95 [1] pp. 19 cm. Contemporary calf, in box.

This small book is one of the greatest of all medical classics and contains the results of Auenbrugger's experience with a new method of physical diagnosis—thoracic percussion. In the book, Auenbrugger describes the technique of percussion and the sounds made in various diseased conditions of the chest. Although his discovery was extremely important, it attracted little attention from the medical community. Maximilian Stoll (see No. 656), then director of the medical clinic at the Spanish Hospital, tried the new method and praised it in one of his books. After that, no more was heard of it until the late eighteenth century when Jean Nicolas Corvisart (see No. 701), while studying the works of Stoll, found a reference to Auenbrugger's discovery and began practicing percussion. Corvisart published a French translation of *Inventum novum* in 1808, a year before Auenbrugger died. Because of Corvisart's fame and the excellence of his translation, news of this classic discovery was quickly carried throughout the medical world. Although modern methods of clinical diagnosis have to a great extent replaced manual percussion, Auenbrugger's discovery is one of the milestones in the history of medicine.

This copy was once owned by Dr. Emil Wilhelm Mannkopf, a noted German physician who studied under Johannes Müller and Virchow.

Garrison-Morton 2672; Osler 1864; Waller 519; Wellcome II, p. 70.

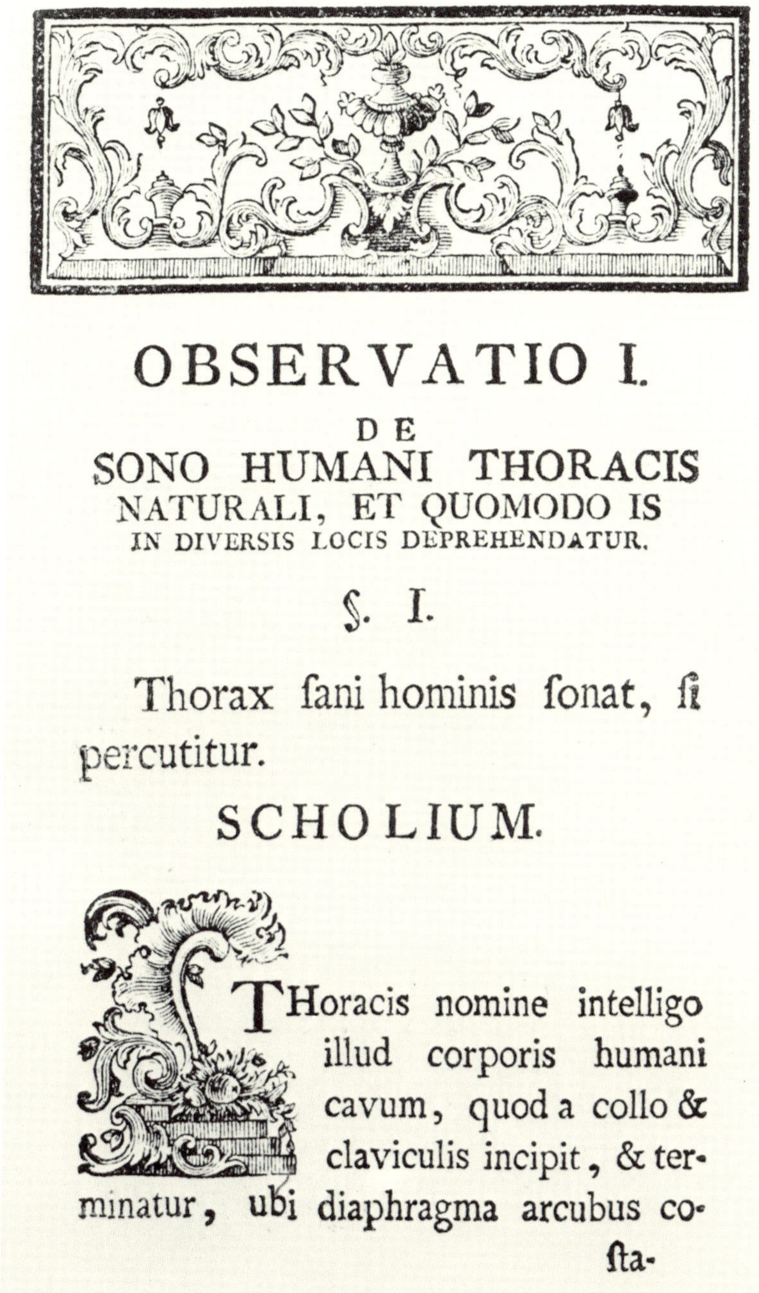

OBSERVATIO I.

DE
SONO HUMANI THORACIS
NATURALI, ET QUOMODO IS
IN DIVERSIS LOCIS DEPREHENDATUR.

§. I.

Thorax ſani hominis ſonat, ſi percutitur.

SCHOLIUM.

THoracis nomine intelligo illud corporis humani cavum, quod a collo & claviculis incipit, & terminatur, ubi diaphragma arcubus coſta-

No. 599. Auenbrugger. *Inventum Novum*. The first page of the text.

*600. GIOVANNI AMBROGIO MARIA BERTRANDI (1723–1765). *Trattato delle operazioni di chirurgia*. 2 vols. Venice: Presso Domenico Fracasso, 1786. Vol. I: 240 pp.; Vol. II: 264 pp., illus., 4 fold. plates. 18.4 cm.

One of the numerous treatises on surgery appearing in the eighteenth century when surgery had emerged from its somewhat inferior position with respect to medicine, this particular work by a little-known Italian surgeon seems to be unknown in most of the medical book collections.

Wellcome II, p. 156 (1763 ed.).

601. JOHANN FRIEDRICH MECKEL (1724–1774). *Tractatus anatomico physiologicus de quinto pare nervorum cerebri*. Göttingen: Apud Abram Vandenhoeck, 1748. [8] vi, 136 pp., 2 fold. plates. 21 cm. Modern half calf.

Often called "The Elder" to distinguish him from his grandson (see No. 815), Meckel was the first in a family of four noted German anatomists. He was followed by his son, Philipp Friedrich Theodor, and later by two grandsons. Meckel studied medicine at Göttingen where he was graduated in 1748. He returned to Berlin, became prosector in anatomy, and was the first to teach obstetrics at the Charité in Paris. He became professor of anatomy, botany, and obstetrics at Berlin in 1751. Meckel devoted much of his time to the study of anatomy and was the first to describe the submandibular ganglion. He also made important studies of the nerve supply of the face and the terminal visceral branches of the veins and lymphatics.

The present work was Meckel's doctoral dissertation and contains his description of the sphenomaxillary ganglion (Meckel's ganglion) and of the recess in the dura that lodges Gasser's ganglion (Meckel's cave).

Meckel was one of Haller's finest pupils and a commendatory letter from Haller is included at the end of the book.

Garrison-Morton 1249; Waller 6408.

Given in memory of Dr. John Roger Porter.

602. RUDOLPH AUGUSTIN VOGEL (1724–1774). *Historia materiae medicae ad novissima tempora producta in usum academicum*. Frankfurt and Leipzig: Apud Tobiam Goebhard, 1764. 404 pp. 16.6 cm.

Vogel, a German physician, taught and practiced in Erfurt for several years before joining the faculty at Göttingen. He wrote a number of works on chemistry, therapeutics, and pharmacy. In this work on the history of the materia medica, Vogel discusses the remedies then in use from an historical point of view by reviewing the literature of his time and presenting a synopsis of what the leading authorities thought about the uses of each remedy. In addition to medicines actively used in practice, Vogel includes remedies that were even then considered obsolete.

*603. IMMANUEL KANT (1724–1804). *Anthropologie in pragmatischer Hinsicht abgefasst.* 2nd ed. Königsberg: F. Nicolovius, 1800. xiv [2] 332 pp. 18.6 cm. Original boards.

Kant, the well-known German philosopher, was one of the most important thinkers of modern times. He was professor of logic and metaphysics at Königsberg for the greater part of his career and taught logic, metaphysics, moral philosophy, natural theology, and anthropology as well as mathematics, physics, and physical geography. He is, of course, best-known for his classic works in philosophy and the impact they had on modern philosophical systems. In this compact volume he attempted a classification of mental diseases. The book is divided into three parts: the first deals with sensation, memory, imagination, sagacity, wit, and originality; the second with pleasure and pain; and the third with the mental differences of the sexes and of the races of man.

Garrison-Morton 4969 (1st ed., 1798); Waller 19812 (1799 ed.); Wellcome III, p. 378 (1799 ed.).

*604. PIERRE TARIN (1725–1761). *Ostéo-graphie; ou, Description des os de l'adulte, du foetus, &c.* Paris: Chez Briasson, 1753. xxxiv, 24, 56, 126 pp., plates (part fold.). 25.1 cm. Contemporary marbled calf.

Tarin, a French anatomist, is better known for his *Dictionnaire anatomique* (1753) and his description of many anatomical structures in the brain. This atlas of the skeletal system of the fetus and adult contains many excellent detailed folding plates. Several of these plates were taken from the anatomical atlases of Albinus (see No. 525 ff.). Following a lengthy introduction to the study of human anatomy in French, the remainder of the text is presented in Latin and French on opposite pages.

*605. LEOPOLDO MARCO ANTONIO CALDANI (1725–1813) and FLORIANO CALDANI (1772–1836). *Icones anatomicae.* 3 vols. in 4. Venice: Ex calcographia Josephi Picotti, 1801–1813. Front., 264 plates and 229 outline plates. 68.7 cm. *Iconum anatomicarum explicatio.* 3 vols. in 5. Venice, 1802–1814. 33.7 cm.

Leopoldo Caldani succeeded Morgagni in the chair of anatomy at Padua, where he was already professor of theoretical medicine. In his later years he was assisted in the publication of his anatomical works by his nephew, Floriano Caldani, also a professor at Padua. They worked together on this massive and beautiful compilation of the best anatomic representations of past years. For example, the representations of bones and muscles follow Albinus, the teeth and sexual organs are after John Hunter, the lymphatics after Mascagni, etc. Some, however, were original preparations by the younger Caldani. A large and striking lithographic title page pictures a landscape with the flaying and opening of a cadaver. This volume is dated 1801 and, as lithography was invented in 1796 and came into use a few years later, this is one of the earliest lithographs used in book illustration.

Choulant-Frank, pp. 327–328; Wellcome II, p. 287.

*606. LEOPOLDO MARCO ANTONIO CALDANI. *Institutiones physiologicae*. Padua: Typis Cominianis, 1778. xvi, 471 pp. 18.5 cm. Original boards.

The Leyden jar became widely available in the mid-eighteenth century, and Caldani used it frequently for his studies of animal tissues. Although he was not successful in his attempts to stimulate the heart, he obtained a series of strong contractions in skeletal muscles with sparks from the jar. He first published this text on physiology in 1773 and prepared this revised edition five years later.

Waller 1693; Wellcome II, p. 287.

*607. JOHANN GOTTFRIED ZINN (1727–1759). *Descriptio anatomica oculi humani*. Göttingen: Apud viduam B. Abrami Vandenhoeck, 1755. [16] 272 pp., 7 fold. plates. 23.5 cm.

Zinn, one of Haller's best pupils at Göttingen, became professor of medicine there. Although he died very young, he produced this important book on the anatomy of the eye which is a fundamental work in the history of ophthalmology. His name is preserved in those of several of the finer structures of the eye: the central artery of Zinn, circulet of Zinn, zonule of Zinn, etc. Included in the volume are seven excellent folding plates.

Garrison-Morton 1484; Waller 10493.

608. WILLIAM HIRD (1728–1782). *Remarks upon pestilence and pestilential diseases*. London: Printed for W. Innys and J. Richardson, 1753. viii, 96 pp. 22.5 cm. Modern quarter cloth with marbled boards, uncut.

Hird was physician to Leeds Infirmary and is often remembered for his biographical tribute to the noted English physician, John Fothergill (1712–1780). The present essay was written as the result of a serious epidemic that killed many cattle in the Leeds region and in other parts of England. Hird discusses the disease at length and includes the results of his postmortem examination of a cow. He also considers other epidemic diseases, such as the plague, and gives suggestions for their prevention and cure.

Wellcome III, p. 276.

*609. JOHN HUNTER (1728–1793). *The natural history of the human teeth*. London: Printed for J. Johnson, 1771. [8] 128 pp., 16 plates each accompanied by a leaf of descriptive letterpress. 26 cm.

John Hunter, even more remarkable than his remarkable brother, William (see No. 591), was an anatomist and surgeon, practicing in London. He lacked the education and culture of his brother, yet his tireless energy helped him to overcome whatever obstacles his educational and cultural lacks may have provided. "Hunter remains one of the great all-round biologists like Haller and Johannes Müller, and with Paré and Lister, one of the three greatest surgeons of all time. . . . Hunter found surgery a mechanical art and left it an experimental

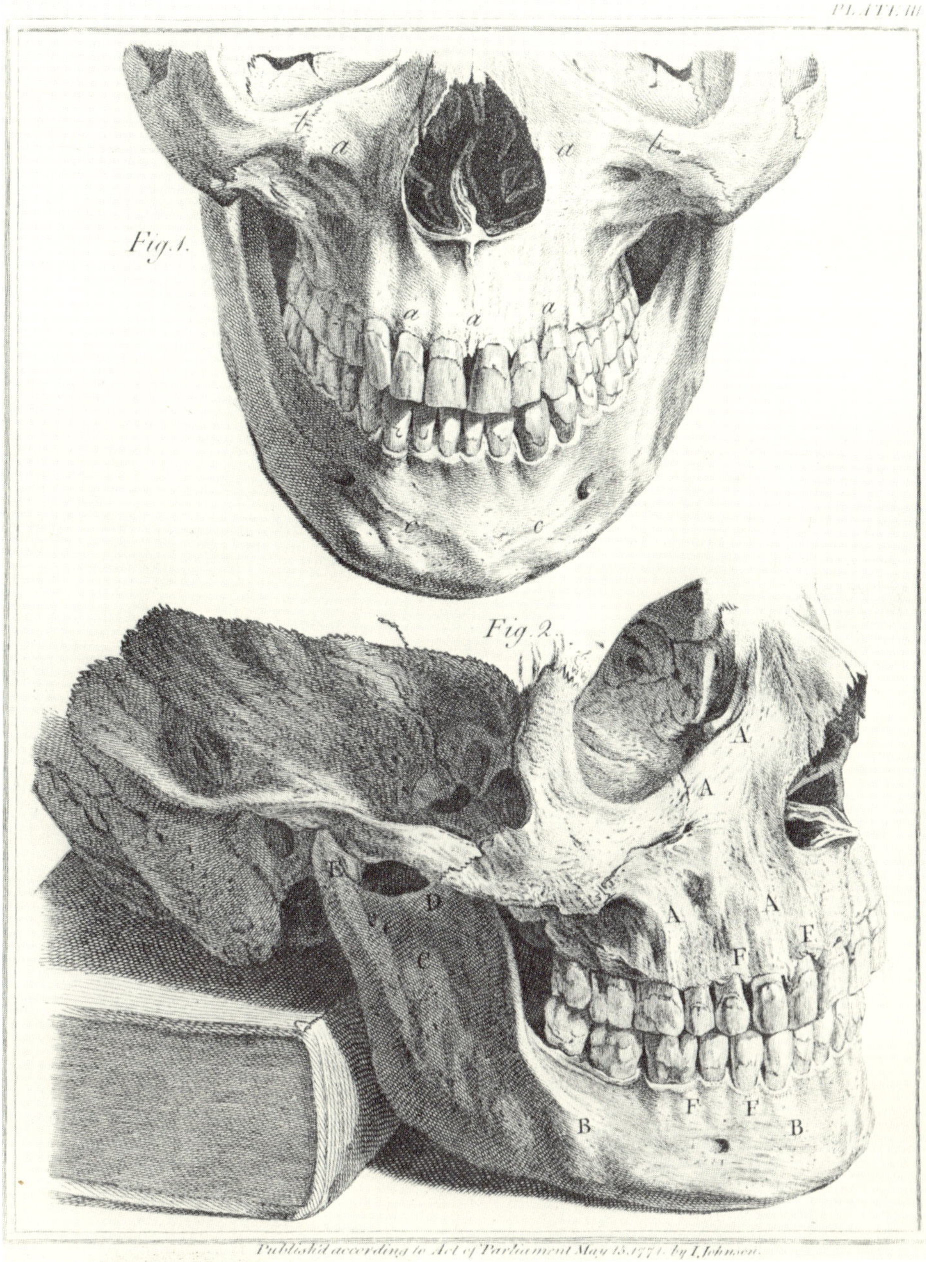

No. 609. John Hunter. *The Natural History of the Human Teeth.*

science" (Fielding H. Garrison, *An introduction to the history of medicine*. 4th ed. Philadelphia, 1929. p. 137).

One of Hunter's most important works was this treatise on the teeth. It was the first scientific study of the teeth and is basic to all modern dentistry.

Cushing H508; Garrison-Morton 3675; Waller 10650; Wellcome III, p. 317.

610. ———. *A treatise on the venereal disease*. London: [n. publ.] 1786. [12] 398 [26] pp., 7 plates. 26.1 cm. Calf.

During Hunter's time, venereal diseases were thought to be caused by a single pathogen. In order to test this theory, Hunter inoculated himself with matter taken from a patient who had gonorrhea; however, unknown to Hunter, the individual also had syphilis. As a result, Hunter contracted syphilis and concluded that the theory of a single pathogen was correct. Because of his reputation and authority, the experiment slowed for many years the development of knowledge about gonorrhea and syphilis.

Cushing H517; Garrison-Morton 2377; Osler 1227; Waller 4998; Wellcome III, p. 317.

611. ———. *Observations on certain parts of the animal oeconomy*. Philadelphia: Haswell, Barrington, and Haswell; New Orleans: J. J. Haswell & Co., 1840. 479 pp. 22.5 cm.

One of Hunter's major works, this book contains many of his studies and observations, including those on the descent of the testis into the scrotum, the structure of the placenta, the mechanism of digestion, the air sac in birds, the secondary sexual characteristics of the free-martin and pheasant, and his original description of the olfactory nerves.

Cushing H510 (1st ed., 1786); Garrison-Morton 309 (1st ed.); Osler 1222 (1st ed.); Russell 445 (1st ed.); Waller 11845 (1st ed.); Wellcome III, p. 317 (1st ed.).

*612. ———. *A treatise on the blood, inflammation, and gun-shot wounds*. London: Printed by J. Richardson, 1794. lxvii, 575 pp., 9 plates, port. 26 cm.

This remarkable, but typical, work of Hunter is based on his own observations during his military experience and is not in any way dependent on any other concepts. Its approach to physiology and pathology has a definitely modern ring. The book was finished but only about one-third through the press (in Hunter's own home) when Hunter died. It contains nine fine copperplates in the text as well as an engraved portrait and a biography of Hunter.

Cushing H515; Garrison-Morton 2283; Osler 1230; Waller 4997; Wellcome III, p. 317.

*613. ———. *The works of John Hunter*. 4 vols. London: Longman, Rees, Orme, Brown, Green, and Longman, 1835–1837. Front. (port.). 21.9 cm. Quarter calf, marbled boards.

Among his many accomplishments, Hunter was responsible for the establishment of some of the greatest medical museums in Europe, and the Hunterian museum of the Royal College of Surgeons of England was based on his own private collection. Unfortunately, much of the collection was destroyed during an air raid in 1941. Hunter's works were edited by Sir James Frederick Palmer (1804–1871), an English physician who later became mayor of Melbourne, Australia. Volume I includes a lengthy biography of Hunter by Drewry Ottley. An atlas containing sixty-one plates, normally included with the set, is not present.

Cushing H520; Garrison-Morton 78; Osler 1231; Wellcome III, p. 318.

614. ———. *Essays and observations on natural history, anatomy, physiology, psychology, and geology.* 2 vols. London: John Van Voorst, 1861. Vol. I: [2] xvii [1] 403 pp.; Vol. II: xii, 507 pp., port., facsim. 22 cm. Original blue cloth.

This collection of Hunter's papers and essays was prepared by Richard Owen (see No. 925 ff.). One of the founders of modern comparative anatomy, Owen was a surgeon, curator, and conservator, and he spent several years cataloguing and studying the Hunterian Collection. The material in this work came from Hunter's original manuscripts and was copied by William Clift (1775–1849), Conservator of the Museum of the Royal College of Surgeons, who had worked with Hunter for many years. Unfortunately, the bulk of the manuscripts were destroyed by Hunter's brother-in-law, Sir Everard Home (see No. 710).

Cushing H505; Osler 1233; Waller 10852.

*615. JOHANN GEORG RITTER VON ZIMMERMANN (1728–1795). *Von der Ruhr unter dem Volke im Jahr 1765.* Zurich: Füesslin, 1767. xii, 544 pp. 17.3 cm.

Zimmermann was born in Brugg, Switzerland, and studied medicine at Göttingen under the tutelage of Albrecht von Haller, in whose home he lived. Following graduation in 1751, he visited Amsterdam, Leiden, and Paris, after which he practiced in Bern for a year and was then appointed city physician in his native city. In 1768 he became court physician to the Duke of York in Hannover. He was one of the most popular and successful physicians of his time and was also a prolific writer. His books were reprinted many times and were translated into English and the major languages of western Europe. The present work contains the first description of bacillary dysentery, and it remained an authority on the disease for several decades after its publication.

Garrison-Morton 5090; Waller 10488.

616. SAMUEL AUGUSTE ANDRÉ DAVID TISSOT (1728–1797). *An essay on bilious fevers; or, The history of a bilious epidemic fever at Lausanne, in the Year MDCCLV.* London: Printed for D. Wilson and T. Durham, 1760. xii, 228 pp. 19.6 cm. Sprinkled calf.

Tissot, a Swiss physician, studied medicine in Geneva and Montpellier and settled in Lausanne, where his time was divided among practice, writing, and teaching. His medical works were numerous and include treatises on smallpox and inoculation, epilepsy, nervous diseases, migraine, popular medicine, onanism, and the present work on bilious fevers. Many of his works became very popular, were translated into English and the major European languages, and went through many editions. In this work on bilious fevers he recounts the history of an epidemic at Lausanne in 1755, including the etiology, symptoms, treatment, and prognosis of the fever.

617. ———. *De la santé des gens de lettres.* 6th ed. Lausanne: Chez François Grasset, 1795. xiv [2] 242 pp. 16.5 cm. Quarter calf.

In this work, Tissot writes of the diseases incidental to literary and sedentary individuals.

Cushing T122 (1768 ed.); Osler 4110 (1775 ed.); Waller 9610 (1768 ed.).

*618. ———. *Traité des nerfs et de leurs maladies.* 3 pts. in 6 vols. Paris and Lausanne: Chez P. F. Didot, 1778–1780. 15.9 cm. Calf.

Tissot collected material for many years for his important treatise on nervous diseases. His work is especially important because of his numerous condensations of previous literature and his precise references to many writers otherwise forgotten or overlooked. One of the most significant portions of this work is his monograph on epilepsy which had appeared separately several years earlier. Over all, Tissot's importance is due to his clear differentiation between diseases of the nervous system and the pathology of the other body systems, which laid the foundation of modern neurology.

*619. CHARLES WHITE (1728–1813). *A treatise on the management of pregnant and lying-in women.* London: Printed for E. and C. Dilly, 1773. xx, 353 pp., 2 plates. 20.5 cm. Contemporary calf, rebacked.

White, a contemporary of William Smellie and William Hunter, was the leading surgeon of his day in northern England. In 1752, at the age of twenty-four, he founded and became chief surgeon to the Manchester Infirmary and in 1790 he played a leading role in founding a lying-in charity hospital which later became St. Mary's Hospital, Manchester.

The present work is filled with practical suggestions, emanating as they do from an author of great experience, unusual powers of observation, and sound reasoning. White made substantial contributions to the etiology and prevention of puerperal fever in this treatise. He insisted on the necessity of maintaining absolute cleanliness in the lying-in chamber, adequate ventilation, and the isolation of infected patients. This book, translated into French and German and also printed in America, became a mighty force in the reform of medical practice at a time when it was sorely needed.

Cushing W164; Garrison-Morton 6270; Waller 10268.

*620. ———. *An inquiry into the nature and cause of that swelling, in one or both of the lower extremities, which sometimes happens to lying-in women.* Warrington: Printed by W. Eyres, for C. Dilly, 1784. 87 pp., 3 fold. plates. 20.6 cm. Boards.

A pioneer in aseptic midwifery, this work is White's other major contribution to obstetrics. In this short tract, he gave the first clinical description of *phlegmasia alba dolens* (thrombophlebitis of the lower extremities), as clinically accurate as any to be found in a modern text.

This particular copy has an interesting provenance in that it contains the bookplate of Dr. Irving S. Cutter, at one time Dean of Northwestern Medical School, and an inscription by Dr. William H. Welch, famous pathologist and bacteriologist at Johns Hopkins University, to whom the book was presented by Dr. Cutter in 1930.

Cushing W163 (1801 ed., Vol. 2 only); Garrison-Morton 6271; Waller 10269.

*621. LAZZARO SPALLANZANI (1729–1799). *De' fenomeni della circolazione osservata nel giro universale de' vasi.* Modena: Società tipografica, 1773. viii, 343 pp. 22.4 cm. Original limp boards.

A brilliant investigator in experimental physiology and the natural sciences, Spallanzani was not a physician; nevertheless, his contributions to the medical sciences exerted a lasting influence on the practice of medicine. He ranks equally with Haller in giving impetus to new avenues of physiological investigation and was one of the foremost scientists of the eighteenth century. Spallanzani was sent to the Jesuit college at Reggio at an early age and later studied law and the natural sciences at Bologna. After taking holy orders, Spallanzani was professor at Reggio, Modena, and subsequently at Pavia, where he enriched the museum by his collections from journeys along the shores of the Mediterranean. He studied the respiration, digestion, the senses of bats, the electricity of the marine Torpedo, the breeding of eels, the regeneration of different appendages of amphibia, and the biology of reproduction in animals.

In the present work, Spallanzani presented the results of his experiments on the circulation of the blood and the action of the heart. He showed that the impetus given the blood by the contraction of the heart was maintained throughout the entire arterial system down to the smallest capillary. As was true with most of his works, this one was later translated into a number of other languages.

Cushing S342.

*622. ———. *Opuscoli di fisica animale, e vegetabile.* 2 vols. in 1. Modena: Società tipografica, 1776. Vol. I: xvi, 304 [2] pp., 2 fold. plates; Vol. II: [4] 277 [3] pp., 4 fold. plates. 20.5 cm. Contemporary vellum.

A long controversy with John Turberville Needham (1713–1781) and Comte de Buffon (1707–1788) resulted in a series of essays, published in this two-volume work, in which Spallanzani rejected the then-popular theory of spontaneous generation. The work also contains two letters written to Spallanzani by Charles Bonnet (see No. 593), a well-known supporter of the theory of preformation.

Most of the experiments described in the *Opuscoli* consist of observations Spallanzani made on infusions of vegetable matter heated in closed vessels for various periods of time and set aside to await developments that would later be viewed with the eye or under the microscope. Although the matter of spontaneous generation was not resolved by this book, it clearly foreshadowed subsequent experiments by other investigators which culminated nearly a century later in Pasteur's epic work. The compilation contains six folding plates which depict over forty of Spallanzani's microscopic observations.

Garrison-Morton 102.

623. ———. *Dissertations relative to the natural history of animals and vegetables.* Vol. I only of 2 vols. London: Printed for J. Murray, 1789. Vol. I: [6] ii, 391 [14] pp. 21.1 cm. Calf.

Spallanzani's experiments on digestion were first published in 1780 in his native Italian and were translated into English for the first time in 1784. In this work he recorded the results of his experiments on the physiology of the digestive system. Spallanzani obtained specimens of gastric juice from many different animals and often experimented upon himself. He verified René Antoine Ferchauld de Reaumur's (1683–1757) conclusions concerning the digestive powers of gastric juice, proving in addition that it prevented putrefaction. Spallanzani observed that gastric digestion was neither putrefaction nor fermentation and erroneously concluded that it was not acid.

Cushing S343 (1784 ed.).

624. JOHN MOORE (1729–1802). *Medical sketches.* 1st American ed. Providence, Rhode Island: Printed by Carter and Wilkinson, 1794. vi [2] 271 pp. 20.6 cm. Calf.

Moore, a successful Glasgow physician and surgeon, is perhaps better known for his enormously successful book, *A view of society and manners in France, Switzerland, and Germany* (1779), which grew out of his experiences in western Europe as physician and traveling companion to Douglas, eighth Duke of Hamilton (1756–1799).

Moore originally prepared this work in manuscript to provide medical advice to a relative serving with the British forces in Virginia. He later improved the manuscript and first published it in England in 1786. In the first part of this two-part book, Moore discusses the basic physiological functions of the body and gives his views on the practice of medicine. The second part consists of a detailed discussion of the etiology, diagnosis, and therapy of various fevers common at that time.

Austin 1330.

Gift of Dr. R. N. Larimer.

625. WILLIAM BUCHAN (1729–1805). *Domestic medicine: or, A treatise on the prevention and cure of diseases by regimen and simple medicines.* 13th ed. London: Printed for A. Strahan; T. Cadell; and J. Balfour, and W. Creech, 1792. xxxvi, 712 [36] pp. 20.3 cm.

Buchan, a native of Scotland, practiced in Yorkshire for a time and later taught at Edinburgh where he had received his medical degree in 1761. He was unsuccessful in his bid for the chair of medicine at Edinburgh and, in 1778, moved to London where he soon gained a large practice. Buchan first published *Domestic medicine* at Edinburgh in 1769. It had an enormous circulation, no fewer than nineteen editions being published during the author's lifetime, and it continued in print until the mid-nineteenth century. Buchan gives simple and easily followed advice in this book and deals at considerable length with various matters that may affect the health, such as diet, ventilation, sleep, cleanliness, and infection. The greater part of the treatise is taken up with a description of the causes, management, and treatment of diseases, such as fevers, pneumonia, smallpox, whooping cough, and colic. His remarks are of lasting value and give valuable insight into the relationship between social conditions and disease in the eighteenth century.

Cushing B826 (Edinburgh ed., 1769); Wellcome II, p. 261.

626. ———. *Domestic medicine. . . . Revised and adapted to the diseases and climate of the United States of America.* Philadelphia: Printed by T. Dobson, 1795. xxxi, 757 pp. 20.8 cm. Calf.

Domestic medicine was translated into all the principal European languages and was even more popular on the Continent and in America than in Scotland. It was so highly esteemed in Russia that the Empress awarded the author a gold medal and a letter of commendation. It first appeared in America in 1771 and is here edited by the Philadelphia physician, Samuel Powel Griffitts (1759–1826).

Austin 317; Wellcome II, p. 261.

627. ———. *Advice to mothers.* Philadelphia: Printed . . . by John Bioren, 1804. [4] 344 pp. 20 cm.

After Buchan moved to London, he continued to write and published several other books dealing with various aspects of the preservation of health. This work was first published in London in 1803 and was reprinted the following year in Philadelphia. It went through several editions in the United States and England and was translated into several other European languages. In the book, Buchan provides practical advice on health matters to women before marriage, rules of conduct during pregnancy and childbirth, and recommendations for the nursing and rearing of children. An appendix is largely a reprint of William Cadogan's *An essay upon nursing, and the management of children* (see No. 574).

Austin 303; Wellcome II, p. 262 (London ed., 1803).

Gift in memory of Robert D. Gauchat.

*628. FELICE FONTANA (1730–1805). *Treatise on the venom of the viper; on the American poisons; and on the cherry laurel, and some other vegetable poisons. To which are annexed, observations on the primitive structure of the animal body; different experiments on the reproduction of the nerves; and a description of a new canal of the eye.* 2 vols.

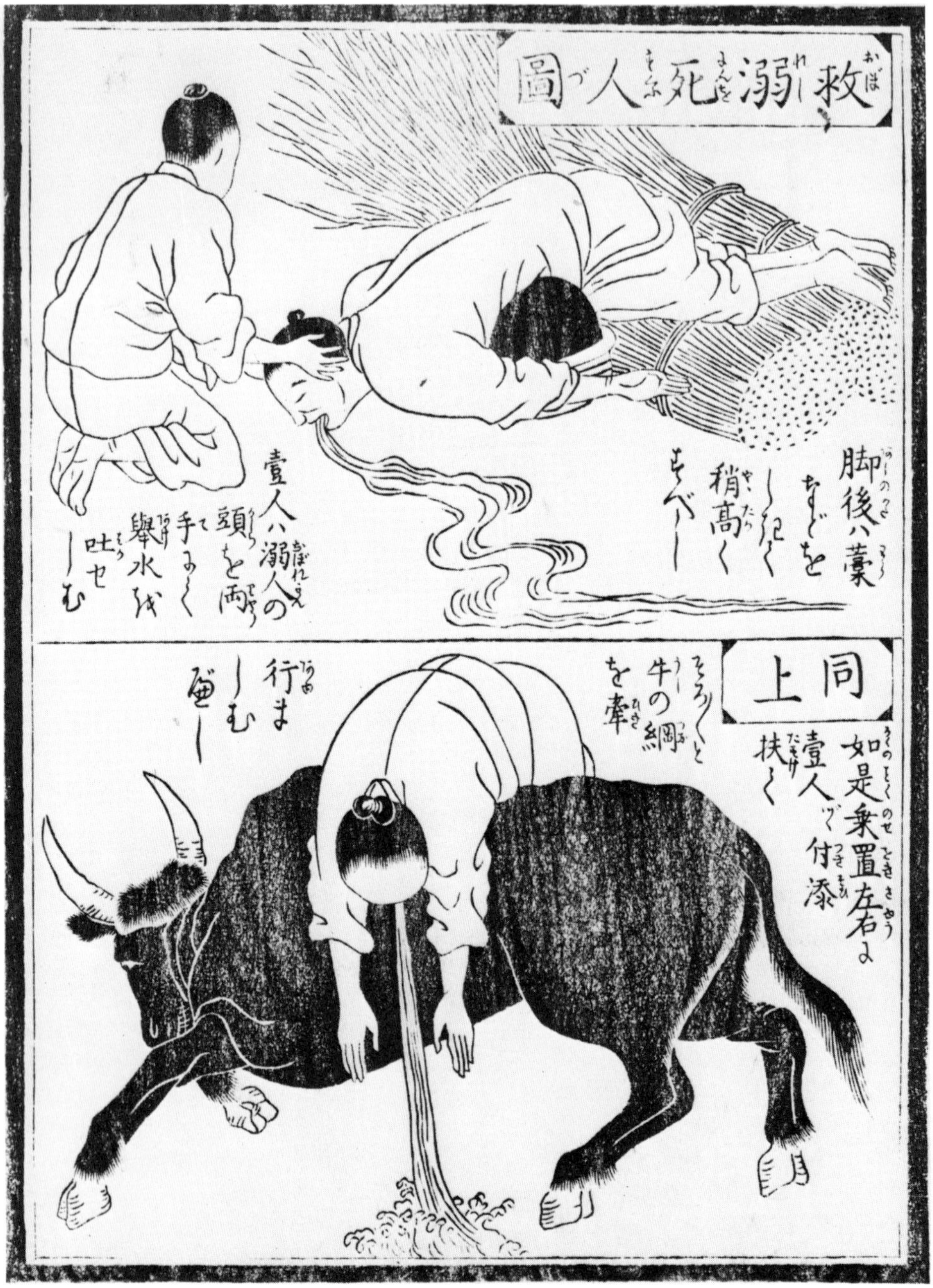

No. 630. Taki. *Kōkeisai Kyūhō*. Two methods of inducing vomiting.

London: Printed for J. Murray, 1787. Vol. I: xix, 409, xiv pp.; Vol. II: [4] 395, xxii pp., 10 fold. plates. 21 cm. Contemporary tree calf.

The Italian abbot, Fontana, was a distinguished naturalist and physiologist whose original and important researches on serpent venoms were published in Italian in 1767. In 1781 Fontana revised and enlarged his original treatise and added other essays, publishing the entire work in French. It is here in its first English translation and includes his letter in which he gives an account of his investigation of the space at the angle of the iris known as Fontana's space or canal.

629. ERASMUS DARWIN (1731–1802). *Zoonomia; or, the laws of organic life.* 2nd American from the 3rd London ed. 2 vols. Boston: Printed by D. Carlisle, for Thomas and Andrews, 1803. Vol. I: xxix [3] 466, 96 [1] pp.; Vol. II: xii, 524 pp., 6 plates (5 col.). 21 cm.

Darwin, physician, physiologist, philosopher, and poet, studied at Cambridge and Edinburgh and practiced medicine at Nottingham, Lichfield, and Derby. In the present work, first published in London in 1794–1796, Darwin stressed the concept of the gradual evolution of complex organisms and discussed the competition for existence, the idea of sexual selection, and the influence of environment. He thus anticipated by some sixty-five years the work of his renowned grandson, Charles (see No. 943 ff.).

Austin 619; Cushing D58 (1st ed., 1794–1796); Garrison-Morton 105 (1st ed.); Osler 2413 (1st ed.); Waller 10790 (1st ed.); Wellcome II, p. 433 (1st ed.).

*630. MOTONORI TAKI (1732–1801). *Kōkeisai kyūhō* [Emergency remedies for the benefit of the people]. 3 vols. Tokyo: [Published by Seijukan in the First Year of the Kansei-period] 1789. Vol. I: 101 *ll.*; Vol. II: 98 *ll.*; Vol. III: 104 *ll.* 26.7 cm. Original dark blue wrappers.

The author was a court physician famous in the annals of Japanese medicine. He was also known as Rankei Taki and Gentoku Tamba, combinations of his professional and personal names. Taki prepared this early Japanese home medical adviser at the request of the shogun Iyeharu in order to help disseminate medical knowledge among the common people. The three-volume set contains information on how to remedy maladies of various kinds and meet emergencies without the help of a physician. The work is illustrated with more than one hundred and thirty woodcuts of plants, animals, fish, and insects with medicinal uses, as well as illustrations of acupuncture sites, methods of reducing fractures, anatomical details, etc.

*631. RAPHAËL BIENVENU SABATIER (1732–1811). *Traité complet d'anatomie.* 3 vols. Paris: Chez Pierre-Franç. Didot le jeune, 1775. Vol. I: xxiv, 622 pp.; Vol. II: viii, 602 pp.; Vol. III: xii, 619 pp. 16.8 cm. Marbled calf.

Sabatier, a professor and member of the Académie des Sciences in Paris, devoted himself chiefly to anatomy and ophthalmology. Here in three volumes is his comprehensive treatise on human anatomy. A small work, it covers all the major systems of the body but is without illustrations.

*632. ———. *De la médecine opératoire.* 3 vols. Paris: De l'imprimerie de Didot le jeune, 1796. Vol. I: xviii, 365 pp.; Vol. II: xxxvii, 408 pp.; Vol. III: xxiv, 416 pp. 19.5 cm. Calf.

Sabatier's treatise on operative surgery was popular and well known during his day, for he was also a skilled and accomplished surgeon. It was widely adapted as a text and provides excellent coverage of the surgical art of the time.

Waller 8373 (incorrect pagination).

*633. JEAN JUVILLE (fl. 1773). *Traité des bandages herniaires.* Paris: Chez Belin, Hardouin & Gattey, et chez l'Auteur, 1786. [ii] [4] [iii]–xxxiv, 232 [8] pp., 14 fold. plates (13 col.). 19.5 cm.

The illustrations in this interesting book show a number of ingenious belts, straps, and other devices used in correcting various kinds of hernias and prolapses. While much of the apparatus would appear to be uncomfortable and cumbersome, some of it has a quite modern appearance.

Waller 5234; Wellcome III, p. 375.

*634. ALEXANDER MONRO (1733–1817). *Observations on the structure and functions of the nervous system.* Edinburgh: Printed for, and sold by, W. Creech, 1783. x, 176 pp., 41 (misnumbered 47) plates (part fold.). 49.9 cm.

Monro *secundus,* trained in anatomy by his father (see No. 523), was perhaps the greatest of the three Monros and, like his father, was a gifted and popular teacher as well as a distinguished physician. He received his medical degree at Edinburgh in 1755 and later studied with Hunter in London, Albinus in Leiden, and Meckel the Elder in Berlin. He is best known for his discovery of the foramen of Monro and for an incomplete description of the lymphatic system.

This massive text and atlas on human and comparative neurology is Monro's greatest work. The plates, though artistically sterile, are clear and accurate while the text contains a number of important descriptions, among them the interventricular foramen between the lateral and third ventricles (the foramen of Monro).

Garrison-Morton 1385; Russell 610; Waller 6645.

*635. ———. *A description of all the bursae mucosae of the human body.* Edinburgh: Printed for C. Elliot, T. Kay, and for Charles Elliot, 1788. 60 pp., 10 plates (part fold.). 47 cm. Half calf.

This classic work contains the first full anatomical description of the sacs between the tendons and bones which Albinus had named the *bursae mucosae.* They are illustrated on ten plates which for explicit clarity and accuracy have not been improved upon.

Russell 613.

*636. PAUL JOSEPH BARTHEZ (1734–1806). *Nouveaux éléments de la science de l'homme.* Montpellier: Chez J. Martel, 1778. xxvii, 348 [6] pp. 19.7 cm.

The author herein states those principles for which he is now best remembered, that is, that the "vital principle" (a term he introduced) is the basis of the phenomenon of life, and every abnormality of function of normal life—or of this "vital principle"—constitutes disease.

Wellcome II, p. 106.

*637. FRANZ ANTON MESMER (1734–1815). *Mémoire sur la découverte du magnétisme animal.* Geneva: P. F. Didot le jeune, 1779. vi, 85 pp. 17.2 cm. In box.

Mesmer, a German physician, maintained that an "animal magnetism" pervades the universe and exists in every living thing. He believed that its transmission from one person to another could cure various nervous disorders through its healing properties. Mesmer at first used magnets, electrodes, and other devices to effect his cures, but, after arousing suspicion among the Viennese physicians, he preferred to utilize his hands. Arriving in Paris in 1778, he set up a lucrative practice employing elaborate rituals to enhance his effect. His patrons included Louis XVI and members of the royal court. Eventually he was discredited by a committee of the French Academy of Sciences (including A. Lavoisier, J. Guillotin and B. Franklin) and in 1785 was forced to leave the city. Although many of his learned contemporaries regarded Mesmer's practice as quackery, his theory of animal magnetism laid the foundations of modern hypnosis and suggestion therapy.

This cheaply printed first edition is Mesmer's definitive work on animal magnetism.

Garrison-Morton 4992; Waller 6505.

638. ———. *Allgemeine Erläuterungen über den Magnetismus und den Somnambulismus.* Carlsruhe: [n. publ.] 1815. 78 pp. 20.1 cm.

This pamphlet on hypnosis, sleepwalking, and posthypnotic suggestion first appeared in 1812, three years before Mesmer's death and long after his medical practice had been put to an end.

Waller 6504 (1812 ed.).

*639. JOHANN GOTTLIEB WALTER (1734–1818). *Observationes anatomicae.* Berlin: Apud Gottlieb Augustum Lange, 1775. [viii] lxxxvii pp., 13 plates (part fold.), 2 accompanied by duplicate outline plates. 43.6 cm.

A skilled anatomist and dissectionist, Walter held the chair of anatomy at the

University of Frankfurt am Main and founded a huge anatomical museum later purchased by the University of Berlin.

The present work deals with developmental anomalies, such as conjoined twins, supernumerary limbs, and abnormalities in blood vessels and viscera. The nine large engravings are drawn from original dissections.

*640. ———. *Tabulae nervorum thoracis et abdominis.* Berlin: Litteris Georgii Jacobi Deckeri, 1783. [6] 17 pp., 4 plates, each accompanied by duplicate outline plate. 63.1 cm.

The four life-sized plates in this large atlas realistically depict the autonomic nerve supply to the abdominal viscera. Each plate is accompanied by an exquisitely detailed outline drawing keyed to the text.

Cushing W30 (1804 ed.).

*641. JOHN BROWN (1735–1788). *The elements of medicine.* 2 vols. in 1. Philadelphia: Printed by W. Spotswood for I. Thomas, 1791. xv, 295 pp. 21.3 cm.

Brown's unusual but immensely popular system of medicine (Brunonism) was based on the principle that life is maintained by a state of externally provoked excitability within living tissues. The disease state was seen as one in which this excitability fell above or below normal limits. After determining the degree and localization of the problem, appropriate stimulants or depressants were administered. In spite of its shortcomings, "the Brunonian theory . . . held the attention of Europe for a quarter-century and as late as 1802, a *rixa* or student's brawl between Brunonians and non-Brunonians at the University of Göttingen lasted two whole days and had finally to be put down by a troop of Hanoverian horse" (Fielding H. Garrison, *An introduction to the history of medicine.* 4th ed. Philadelphia, 1929. p. 314). Brown eventually died from his own cure, having administered to himself copious quantities of opium and alcohol to treat his gout. *The elements of medicine* is Brown's translation of his *Elementa medicinae* (1780) which expounds the basic Brunonian principles.

Austin 282; Cushing B705 (1803 ed.); Osler 2153 (1795 ed.); Wellcome II, p. 249 (1795 ed.).

*642. ANDREAS MAXIMINUS (fl. 1776–1783). *In Hippocratis Coi, medicorum omnium longe principis, librum De fracturis commentaria.* Rome: Apud B. Francesium, 1776. xxxvi, 304 pp., 5 plates. 27.5 cm.

Maximinus, also known for his edition of Eustachius' plates, is but one of many individuals who wrote commentaries on the works of Hippocrates. This commentary on fractures includes five full-page plates illustrating primitive methods used to reduce fractures. At the top of each page are several lines of Hippocrates' text in Latin followed by Maximinus' commentary.

Waller 4565; Wellcome III, p. 272.

643. HUGH SMITH (1736?–1789). *Letters to married women.* 3rd ed. London: Printed for the author, 1774. xvii, 256 pp. 16.5 cm.

First published in 1772, this popular work passed through six English editions and was translated into French and Dutch. In spite of its title, the work is on child rearing rather than marital hygiene. Smith was quite adamant in all his views, especially those concerning breast feeding. His florid prose, while in the style of the times, becomes at times quite melodramatic: "Believe it not when it is insinuated that your bosoms are less charming for having a dear little cherub at your breast." Smith was the first English writer to recommend breast milk as sole nourishment for the first six or seven months of life. He also helped draw attention to the high infant mortality rate by including the bill of mortality for London in the introduction to these *Letters.*

Waller 9028 (1792 ed.).

644. GEORGE FORDYCE (1736–1802). *A second dissertation on fever, containing the history and method of treatment of a regular tertian intermittent.* London: Printed for J. Johnson, 1795. 156 pp. 20.2 cm. In slipcase. Bound with No. 681.

After studying under Albinus and Cullen, Fordyce lectured on medicine and chemistry at St. Thomas' Hospital in London for almost thirty years. He confirmed Lavoisier's views against the phlogiston theory and, using himself as a subject, demonstrated that human beings maintain a constant body temperature at elevated external temperatures.

This is the second of his five works on fever published between 1794 and 1803.

Wellcome III, p. 41.

*645. MICHAEL UNDERWOOD (1736–1820). *A treatise on the diseases of children.* London: Printed for J. Mathews, 1784. xii, 288 pp. 16 cm.

This brief but well-written book is generally considered the best eighteenth-century English work on children's diseases. It contains the first description of *sclerema neonatorum* (Underwood's disease) and gives a superior account of both thrush and rickets. Underwood served at the British Lying-In Hospital and was one of the most respected obstetricians in London.

Garrison-Morton 4015; Osler 4144; Waller 9749 (1805 ed.).

*646. DOMENICO COTUGNO (1736–1822). *De aquaeductibus auris humanae internae anatomica dissertatio.* Naples and Bologna: Ex typographica Sancti Thomae Aquinatis, 1775. 116 pp., 2 fold. plates. 18.6 cm.

Born into a family of humble means, Cotugno underwent physical and economic hardships to secure his medical education. Before his thirty-first year he had written two books, made numerous important contributions to anatomy and pathology, and was made professor of surgery and anatomy at the University of Naples. An unselfish and generous man, Cotugno left a substantial endowment to the poor of the Neapolitan Hospital for Incurables where he was located during much of his early study.

Cotugno was the first to describe the fine anatomy of the inner ear. In this, his first major work, he identifies the aqueduct of the inner ear and the columns in the osseous spinal lamina of the cochlea, which are named after him. The work was originally published in 1761.

Garrison-Morton 1549 (1761 ed.); Waller 2165; Wellcome II, p. 398 (1761 ed.).

*647. ———. *De ischiade nervosa commentarius.* Naples: Apud fratres Simonios, 1764. [8] 88 pp., plate. 20.8 cm. Antique calf.

Cotugno was a keen observer and a fine clinician. In this, perhaps his most important work, he differentiates arthritis from nervous sciatica, gives the first detailed description of cerebrospinal fluid, and shows that the congealed protein in the urine of a nephrotic patient is a diagnostic sign.

Garrison-Morton 1382; Waller 2166; Wellcome II, p. 398.

*648. ———. *De sedibus variolarum σύνταγμα.* Naples and Bologna: Ex typographia Sancti Thomae Aquinatis, 1775. 171 pp., plate. 18.6 cm.

Extending his interests to preventive medicine and public health, Cotugno became a pioneer in epidemiology. In this work, first published in 1771, he gives a lucid description of the anatomy and pathology of smallpox pustules. It is regarded as one of the finest dermatological works of the eighteenth century.

Waller 2175; Wellcome II, p. 398 (1789 ed.).

649. JOSEPH JACOB VON PLENK (1738–1807). *De' morbi de' denti e delle gengie.* 2nd ed. Venice: Pezzana, 1786. 109 pp. 15.4 cm.

Possessed of an encyclopedic mind, von Plenk brought a multitude of knowledge and talents to every field he investigated. He is usually considered a member of the Viennese School together with de Haen, Stoll, Plenkiz, and Auenbrugger. So extensive were his talents that at one time or another he was professor of chemistry, botany, surgery, anatomy, and obstetrics at Vienna. Von Plenk is generally regarded as the founder of systematic dermatology and suggested the first practical system of dermatologic nomenclature in his *Doctrina de morbis cutaneis* (1776).

In the present work, von Plenk extends his dermatologic classification to the teeth and gums. It was originally published in Vienna in 1778 under the Latin title, *Doctrina de morbis dentium ac gingivarum.*

Waller 10689 (1790 ed.).

*650. WILLIAM HEWSON (1739–1774). *The works of William Hewson, F.R.S.* Edited with an introd. and notes, by George Gulliver. London: Printed for the Sydenham Society, 1846. lvi, 360 pp., port., 8 plates. 21.5 cm.

A pupil of William and John Hunter, Hewson made a number of important observations of fundamental significance in physiology and clinical medicine. He demonstrated the effectiveness of paracentesis of air for correction of pneumothorax, showed the existence of lacteal and lymphatic vessels in the lower vertebrates and, in his *An experimental inquiry into the properties of the blood* (1771), proved that fibrinogen is the clotting agent of the blood. After he died, his work was neglected for a time, but its essential importance later brought belated but well-deserved recognition.

This volume contains fine copies of Hewson's original figures and a portrait of the author.

Garrison-Morton 79; Osler 2955; Waller 4424; Wellcome III, p. 259.

*651. GENYŪ KAGAWA (1739–1779). *Sanron yoku* [Description of labor]. 2 vols. Kyoto, 1775. Vol. I: 41 *ll.;* Vol. II: 33 *ll.,* illus. 26.2 cm.

Kagawa is considered to be the father of modern Japanese obstetrics because of his many contributions and improvements to the art of childbirth. A skilled and accomplished obstetrician, he first published his work on obstetrics in 1765. In the work he discussed fetal development, the management of pregnancy and labor, the use of birth stools, the abdominal bandage, and version by external manipulation.

Although the present work, a commentary and explanation of the *Sanron,* has been attributed to Genyū Kagawa, some authorities believe that it was actually prepared by his adopted son, Genyū Okamoto.

652. ALEXANDER HAMILTON (1739–1802). *Outlines of the theory and practice of midwifery.* Worcester, Massachusetts: Isaiah Thomas, 1794. 302 pp. 19.3 cm.

Although the Edinburgh Royal Infirmary appointed its first professor of midwifery in 1726, it was not until 1783 that Alexander Hamilton actually established the Edinburgh School of Midwifery, complete with a separate maternity hospital. Hamilton was the first to distinguish and describe uterine and vaginal discharge and he promoted the concept of the perineum as supporting the pelvic structure.

Hamilton's *Outline* is actually a revision of his first major work on midwifery, *Elements of midwifery,* first published in 1775. The American edition of his later publication, *Treatise on the management of female complaints* (1793), is the first American publication devoted to the subject of gynecology.

Austin 862; Waller 4033 (1790 ed.); Wellcome III, p. 202 (1791 ed.).

In memory of Robert D. Gauchat.

653. THOMAS REID (1739–1802). *An essay on the nature and cure of the phthisis pulmonalis: or, Consumption of the lungs.* London and Philadelphia: Re-printed and sold by J. Crukshank, 1785. xi, 89 pp. 18.2 cm.

Of the many diseases which plagued Europe during the eighteenth and nineteenth centuries none was more dreaded than tuberculosis. It is estimated that one-fourth

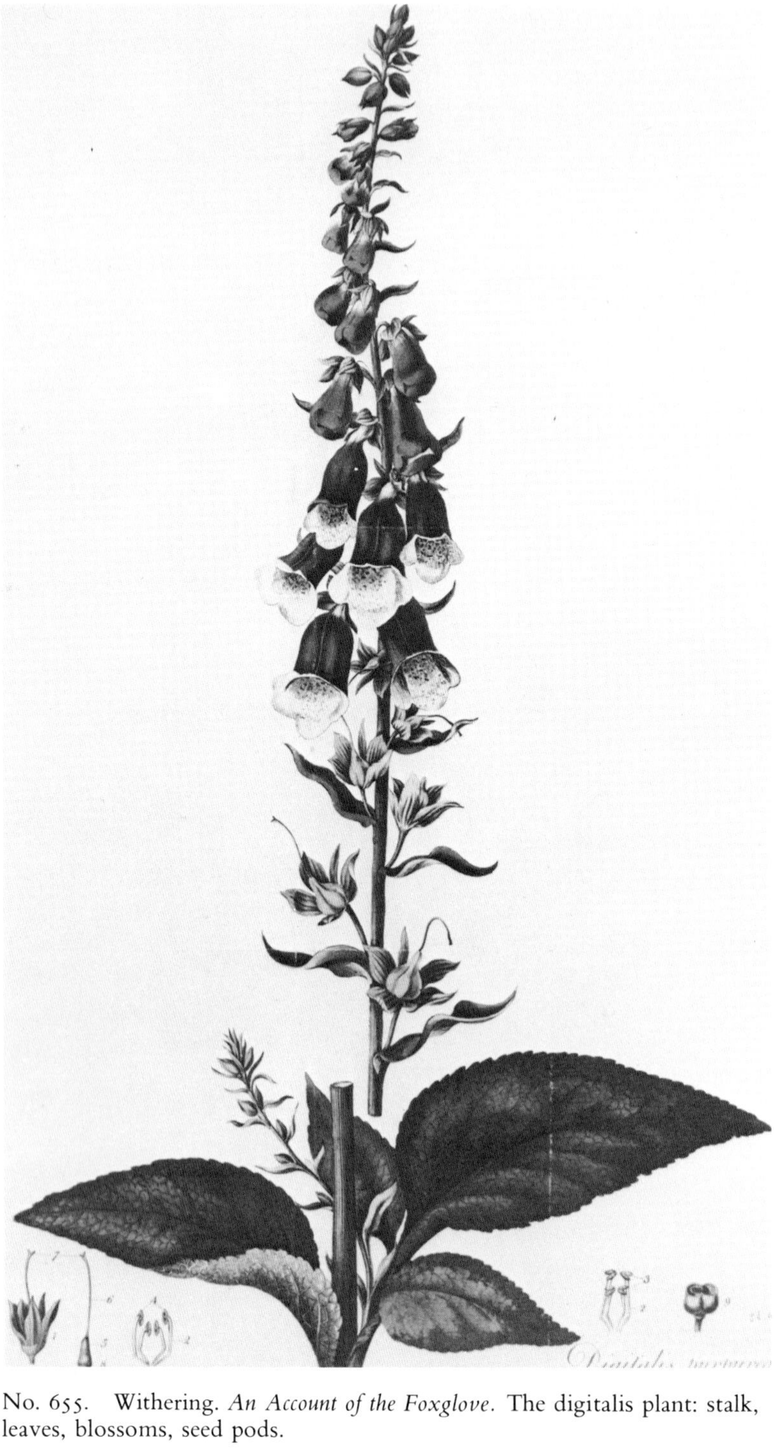

No. 655. Withering. *An Account of the Foxglove.* The digitalis plant: stalk, leaves, blossoms, seed pods.

of the population perished from it. Attempts to understand and cure the disease were largely unsuccessful. In his *Essay*, Reid reveals his belief that the origin of the disease is due to air obstructing the exhaling-vessels and recommends the evacuation of the lungs through vomiting as a treatment. His idea gained modest recognition and for a time daily vomits became the vogue.

Austin 1594; Waller 7862 (1782 ed.).

*654. HEINRICH AUGUST WRISBERG (1739–1808). *Descriptio anatomica embryonis*. Göttingen: Sumtibus viduae A. Vandenhoeck, 1764. [8] 80 pp., fold. plate. 22 cm. Modern boards, uncut and unopened.

Wrisberg, a well-known German anatomist, was a native of St. Andreasberg. He succeeded Johann Georg Roederer (1726–1763) as professor of obstetrics at Göttingen in 1764 and later became professor of anatomy at the University. A skilled and competent anatomist, Wrisberg did a great deal of research on the abdominal nerves. In addition, his name is eponymically associated with the cuneiform cartilages of the larynx, the ganglion of the superficial cardiac plexus, the posterior lateral meniscofemoral ligament, the set of filaments which connect the motor and sensory roots of the trigeminal nerve, the medial cutaneous nerve of the arm, and the nervus intermedius which arises from the geniculate ganglion and is the sensory component of the facial nerve.

Wrisberg was an active author and wrote many books during his career. The present work on the gross anatomy of the fetus is one of his earliest publications; therein he presents his observations on five cases in which he was able to perform postmortem examinations on fetuses (in various stages of development) that had either been aborted or died with their mother. The folding plate depicts each of the fetuses described in the text.

*655. WILLIAM WITHERING (1741–1799). *An account of the foxglove, and some of its medical uses: with practical remarks on dropsy, and other diseases*. Birmingham: Printed by M. Swinney for G.G.J. and J. Robinson, 1785. xx, 207 pp., fold. col. plate. 21.2 cm. Polished calf, gilt spine.

A man of wide-ranging talents and interests, Withering was one of the ablest clinicians of his day and one of the most famous men in Europe. He was graduated from Edinburgh in 1766 and soon enjoyed a successful practice in Birmingham. Despite his medical work, Withering found time to follow a number of other pursuits: he was a mineralogist, climatologist, inventor, cattle breeder, accomplished musician, and botanist. His first major scientific contribution, *A botanical arrangement of all the vegetables naturally growing in Great Britain* (1776), was a standard botanical work for many years. His fame, however, rests on his celebrated work with the foxglove plant (Digitalis). Beginning his research after hearing of an old country woman who used the herb to cure dropsy, Withering used foxglove to treat congestive heart failure with some success. Its introduction into the *Edinburgh Pharmacopoeia* in 1783 and its subsequent widespread acceptance eventually led to its overuse and Withering's classic *Account of the foxglove* was actually written as a protest against such abuse. The book includes 163 cases involving the use of digitalis and is regarded as one of the classics in pharmacology. In this copy, the famous colored illustration of the foxglove plant is in almost mint condition.

Cushing W254; Garrison-Morton 1836; Osler 426; Waller 10378.

*656. MAXIMILIAN STOLL (1742–1787). *Aphorismes sur la connaissance et la curation des fièvres.* Traduits en français par J. N. Corvisart. Avec le text latin. Paris: Régent et Bernard, 1797. xx, 581 pp. 20 cm.

Stoll was a member of the influential Viennese School which, during his lifetime, became one of the focal points of European medical inquiry. He is generally regarded as a systematist relying heavily on the work of Sydenham.

Stoll was one of the few physicians of the Viennese School who supported Auenbrugger's views on percussion. In this treatise on fevers he refers favorably to the practice and, in all probability, it was here that the translator, Corvisart, became acquainted with the subject. This prompted him to translate also Auenbrugger's classic work (see No. 599), which subsequently led to the general acceptance of percussion as a diagnostic practice.

Cushing S435; Osler 4040 (Latin ed., 1787); Waller 9286.

*657. ———. *Praelectiones in diversos morbos chronicos.* 2 vols. Vienna: Typis Christiani Friderici Wappler, 1788–1789. Vol. I: 425 pp.; Vol. II: 612 pp. 20.3 cm.

Stoll achieved considerable recognition as a pharmacologist, epidemiologist, and clinician. These lectures, published posthumously, attest to the depth of his knowledge of internal medicine.

Waller 9289.

*658. EDUARD SANDIFORT, editor (1742–1814). *Thesaurus dissertationum.* 3 vols. Leiden: Apud S. et J. Luchtmans [etc.], 1778. Vol. I: xv, 572 pp., fold. plates; Vol. II: xv, 575 pp., fold. plates; Vol. III: viii, 623 pp., fold. plates. 25.1 cm.

A pupil of Albinus, as well as his successor to the chair of anatomy and surgery at the University of Leiden, Sandifort directed his efforts to the development and perfection of the anatomy of disease and is sometimes called the father of pathological iconography. These volumes encompass a collection of theses and letters drawn from the works of Sandifort's contemporaries covering medicine, surgery, anatomy, pathology, and botany. The twenty-five folding copperplate engravings are of special interest.

Waller 8458.

*659. SAMUEL BARD (1742–1821). *A compendium of the theory and practice of midwifery.* New York: Printed and sold by Collins and Perkins, 1808. 239 pp., illus. 17.1 cm.

This was the first textbook of obstetrics written by an American and was a much respected work. The author, a graduate of King's College (Columbia) and of the medical school at Edinburgh, was a specialist in obstetrics. Long interested in medical education, he taught in the medical school in New York and, when it was united with Columbia College in 1792, became its dean.

Austin 117; Wellcome II, p. 99 (1812 ed.).

*660. ANTOINE LAURENT LAVOISIER (1743–1794). *Traité élémentaire de chimie, présenté dans un order nouveau et d'après les découvertes modernes.* 2 vols. Paris: Cuchet, 1789. Vol. I: xliv, 322 pp.; Vol. II: viii [323]–654 pp., 13 fold. plates. 20.2 cm. French calf.

A man of wide and varied interests, Lavoisier is generally regarded as the founder of modern chemistry. His discoveries and observations concerning the role of oxygen in combustion and respiration led to the downfall of the generally accepted phlogiston theory and the designation of a new chemical nomenclature. His later studies in respiration measurement laid the foundations for the study of human metabolism. In *Traité élémentaire de chimie,* Lavoisier gave a description of his new nomenclature and set out the lines along which he felt chemistry would have to develop in the future. The thirteen folding plates were drawn by his wife who assisted him in much of his work.

Despite Lavoisier's active attempts at prison reform and other humanitarian concerns, his position as tax collector led to his conviction and death by guillotine shortly after the French Revolution.

Cushing L91; Osler 1207 (1793 ed.); Waller 11177; Wellcome III, p. 460.

661. PIERRE JOSEPH DESAULT (1744–1795). *A treatise on fractures, luxations, and other affections of the bones.* Philadelphia: Printed by Fry and Kammerer, 1805. v, 413 pp., 3 plates. 20.5 cm.

Desault was chief surgeon at La Charité before moving to the Hôtel Dieu where he founded the school of surgery. He was the first to develop an effective method of ligating blood vessels for aneurysms and introduced a number of surgical instruments and techniques, most notably in the areas of fracture and dislocation. The present work is a translation of *Maladies des parties dures* originally published in Paris in 1798 as Part One of Desault's famed *Oeuvres chirurgicales.* The work was edited by Xavier Bichat (see No. 755), a pupil of Desault, and was translated by Charles Caldwell (1772–1853).

Austin 655.

*662. JOHN COAKLEY LETTSOM (1744–1815). *Observations on the cow-pock.* 2nd ed. London: Printed by Nichols and son for J. Mawman, 1801. vi, 88 pp., ports. 19.7 cm.

Although he made few original contributions to medical science, Lettsom is remembered as one of the founders of the Medical Society of London and for his

History of the origin of medicine (1778). Lettsom was a strong supporter of the new practice of vaccination and this book contains, in addition to Lettsom's general remarks on the subject, several interesting letters including those to Benjamin Waterhouse from John Adams and Thomas Jefferson.

Cushing L188; Wellcome III, p. 505.

*663. WILLIAM CRUIKSHANK (1745–1800). *The anatomy of the absorbing vessels of the human body*. London: G. Nicol, 1786. 192 pp., 3 plates (1 fold., 2 col.). 27.1 cm. Contemporary calf.

Educated at the Universities of Edinburgh and Glasgow, Cruikshank originally intended entering the clergy but his interest in anatomy and physics led him to medicine. Like William Hewson, Cruikshank became assistant to William Hunter (see No. 591) at his famous Windmill Street School, where his clinical prowess and teaching ability brought him the leadership of the school upon Hunter's death. Cruikshank was known as an outstanding practitioner who frequently opened his private office to the poor and indigent. His humanitarian nature moved Dr. Samuel Johnson, his most famous patient, to describe him as a "sweet blooded man."

Cruikshank's investigation of the lymphatic system in man was his chief contribution. The work was undertaken at Hunter's urging and with his assistance. Cruikshank also made notable observations on nerve regeneration and ovum migration.

This first edition of Cruikshank's treatise on the absorbing vessels established the modern understanding of lymphatics. Of special note is the large folding plate outlining the lymphatic system.

Cushing C504; Russell 231; Waller 2226; Wellcome II, p. 411.

664. JEAN LOUIS BAUDELOCQUE (1745?–1810). *An abridgment of Mr. Heath's translation of Baudelocque's Midwifery*. With notes by William P. Dewees. Philadelphia: Printed by Bartram and Reynolds, for Thomas Dobson, 1807. xiv, 658 pp., 7 plates. 21.3 cm.

One of the most influential obstetricians of the eighteenth century, Baudelocque refined and popularized many of the theories and practices of Smellie and Levret, and made a number of original contributions to the field. His fame rests primarily on the development of a technique for measuring the pelvis before delivery and the invention of a pelvimeter for this purpose.

His classic treatise on midwifery went through a number of editions and was widely translated. This abridgment retains several of the original plates including an engraving showing the proper use of the pelvimeter.

Austin 156.

665. BENJAMIN RUSH (1745–1813). *Medical inquiries and observations*. 3rd ed. 4 vols. Philadelphia: Published by M. Carey [etc.], 1809. Vol. I: [vi] 456 pp.; Vol. II: 453 pp.; Vol. III: 443 pp.; Vol. IV: vi, 427 [19] pp. 20.6 cm.

A Philadelphian, Rush was one of the signers of the Declaration of Independence, active in the Revolutionary War, and a leader in social betterment causes. He was on the medical faculty of the University of Pennsylvania after its creation in 1791 and also was treasurer of the U.S. Mint from 1797 until his death. While he was a diligent and devoted practitioner, his methods were sometimes called into question, particularly his excessive use of bleeding, or "depletion." Nevertheless, he was one of the most influential figures in the first hundred years of American medicine. His *Medical inquiries and observations,* first published from 1789 to 1793, was one of his major literary efforts.

Austin 1662; Garrison-Morton 80 (1st ed., 1789–1793); Osler 3859.

Gift of Dr. Julia Hill.

666. ———. *Sixteen introductory lectures . . . delivered in the University of Pennsylvania.* Philadelphia: Bradford and Innskeep, 1811. viii, 455 pp. 21 cm.

After Rush joined the medical faculty of the University of Pennsylvania in 1791, he regularly delivered these introductory lectures to beginning medical students.

Gift of the University of Iowa Foundation.

Austin 1683.

667. ———. *Medical inquiries and observations upon the diseases of the mind.* Philadelphia: Published by Kimber & Richardson, 1812. 367 pp. 22 cm. In slipcase.

Like Pinel, Rush strove to better the conditions of the insane and sought to establish American mental hospitals based on the best English institutions. His treatment, however, sometimes included profuse bleeding and total physical restraint, which frequently resulted in even greater misery for the patient. His work on diseases of the mind is the first, and for many years was the only, American work on mental illness.

Austin 1670; Cushing R327 (1830 ed.); Garrison-Morton 4924; Osler 3860.

*668. PHILIPPE PINEL (1745–1826). *Traité médico-philosophique sur l'aliénation mentale; ou la manie.* Paris: Richard, Caille et Ravier, 1801. lvi, 318 pp., 2 plates, fold. table. 19.7 cm. Original cloth.

Pinel, a Paris physician appointed as physician to a notorious mental hospital, found many of the patients in chains, some having been so for many years. Shocked by the conditions he uncovered, he insisted on humane treatment of the patients with specially selected physicians to treat them. He devoted the rest of his life to psychiatry and treatment of the insane. This classic book located the origin of mental disease in pathological changes in the brain and gave great impetus to the humanitarian treatment of the insane.

Cushing P286; Garrison-Morton 4922; Waller 7456.

669. ———. ———. 2nd ed. Paris: J. A. Brosson, 1809. xxxii, 496 pp., 2 plates, 2 fold. tables. 19.2 cm.

670. FRANÇOIS XAVIER SWEDIAUR (1748–1824). *Practical observations on venereal complaints.* 3rd ed. Edinburgh: Printed for Bell and Bradfute [1788]. 311 pp. 20.5 cm.

Swediaur practiced in Paris and London, producing works in both French and English. This edition of his first book on venereal diseases was published ten years before his definitive work on syphilis, *Traité complet sur les symptomes, la nature et le traitement des maladies syphilitiques* (1798). Also included in this volume is John Hunter's undated *A short review of a late treatise on the venereal disease.*

671. BENJAMIN BELL (1749–1806). *A treatise on the theory and management of ulcers.* Edinburgh: Printed for C. Elliot, 1789. 486 pp. 20.5 cm.

Bell was a prominent and successful surgeon in Edinburgh, where he studied under the famous Alexander Monro *secundus* (see No. 634). One of the first surgeons to emphasize the importance of preventing or diminishing pain during surgery, he introduced a number of improvements in amputation technique.

This treatise on the classification and treatment of ulcers was first published in 1778 and is considered one of the classics of eighteenth-century physiology.

Cushing B254 (Boston, 1791 ed.); Garrison-Morton 5578 (1st ed., 1778); Waller 846 (1st ed.); Wellcome II, p. 134 (1st ed.).

*672. ———. *A system of surgery.* 6 vols. Edinburgh: Printed for C. Elliot, 1783–1788. 99 plates. 21.3 cm.

A system of surgery was produced while Bell was on the staff of the Royal Infirmary and is his most famous work. The clarity and precision with which it was written provided a model for later nineteenth-century surgical works.

Garrison-Morton 5579; Waller 844; Wellcome II, p. 134.

673. ———. ———. 5th ed. 6 vols. Edinburgh: Printed for Bell & Bradfute, 1791. Plates. 21.1 cm.

Bell's *System of surgery* passed through seven editions, the last being published in 1801.

Wellcome II, p. 134.

674. ———. ———. Extracted from the works of Benjamin Bell, of Edinburgh, by Nicholas B. Waters. Philadelphia: Printed by T. Dobson, 1791. viii, 570, xxix pp., plates. 20.1 cm.

Waters' condensation was prompted by his concern that "we have had no work on this important branch of medicine, which gives a view of the present state of the art, in a moderate compass" (from the Preface). The work proved quite popular, the third and last edition appearing in 1814.

Austin 171; Cushing B252.

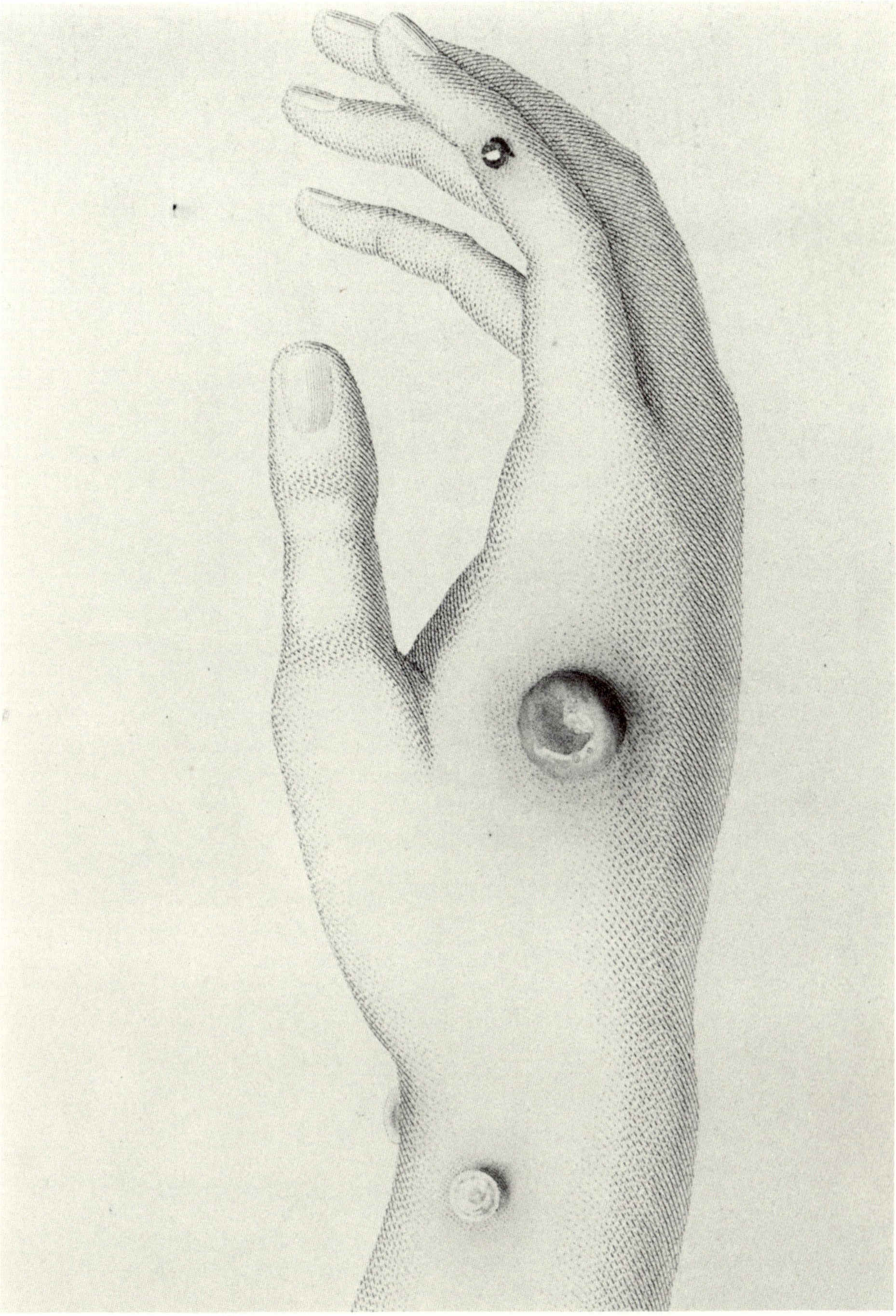

No. 677. Jenner. *An Inquiry into the Causes and Effects of the Variolae Vaccinae.* Cowpox lesion on a milkmaid's hand.

675. ———. *A treatise on gonorrhoea virulenta, and lues venerea*. 2 vols. in 1. Philadelphia: Printed for Robert Campbell, 1795. Vol. I: xii [17]–220 pp.; Vol. II: 250, xv pp. 21 cm.

Although chiefly regarded as a surgeon, Bell's interests extended to clinical medicine and pathology as well. In this treatise on gonorrhea which was first published in Edinburgh in 1793, he delineates the clinical distinction between gonorrhea and syphilis, although it remained for Ricord (see No. 906) to prove their separate identity. This is the first American edition.

Austin 177; Cushing B253; Garrison-Morton 5200 (1st ed., 1793); Waller 845 (1st ed.).

676. ———. *A treatise on the diseases of the bones*. Edinburgh: William Blackwood, and London: Smith Elder, 1828. xii, 294 pp. 19.7 cm.

This copy of Bell's important work on bone diseases has on the title page the signature of Valentine Mott (see No. 836), well-known nineteenth-century American surgeon.

*677. EDWARD JENNER (1749–1823). *An inquiry into the causes and effects of the variolae vaccinae, a disease . . . known by the name of the cow pox*. London: Printed for the author by S. Low, 1798. iv, 75 pp., 4 col. plates. 26.8 cm. Contemporary calf. Bound with No. 678.

On the basis of an old country tradition that milkmaids who had contracted cowpox were not susceptible to smallpox, Jenner, an English country physician, decided to experiment by injecting cowpox-infected lymph into a local boy. After inoculation the boy was found to be immune to smallpox and Jenner continued his experiments. In 1798 he published the present epochal work, the results of a long and successful series of case histories. By 1803 his work had been translated into numerous languages and his method of immunization was taken up with amazing speed, becoming almost universally adopted. Garrison has called Jenner's work "one of the greatest triumphs in the history of medicine" (Fielding H. Garrison, *An introduction to the history of medicine*. 4th ed. Philadelphia, 1929. p. 372). It is the foundation of all subsequent work in immunology and virology.

Cushing J42; Garrison-Morton 4523; Osler 1251; Waller 5136; Wellcome III, p. 351.

*678. ———. *Further observations on the variolae vaccinae, or cow pox*. London: Printed for the author by S. Low, 1799. 64 pp. 26.8 cm. Bound with No. 677.

This set of additional case studies was published with separate pagination and included as a supplement to the first edition. It appears again in the second edition (see next entry) with pagination continuous with the main text.

Wellcome III, p. 351.

*679. ———. *An inquiry into the causes and effects of the variolae vaccinae, a disease . . . known by the name of the cow pox.* 2nd ed. London: Printed for the author by S. Low, 1800. vii, 182 pp., 4 col. plates. 25.6 cm.

Jenner's early work met with strong opposition from among the medical profession, and in 1800 he published this second edition which contained, in addition to *Further observations on the variolae vaccinae,* "A continuation of facts and observations . . . " in order to strengthen his case.

Cushing J44; Osler 1252; Waller 5138; Wellcome III, p. 351.

680. JAMES HAMILTON (1749–1835). *Observations on the utility and administration of purgative medicines in several diseases.* 2nd ed. Edinburgh: J. Simpson, 1806. xv, 345 pp. 22.7 cm.

Hamilton was a student of William Cullen and Alexander Monro *secundus* at Edinburgh and for over thirty years a physician to the Royal Infirmary. After some early success with purgatives in treating typhus fever, he extended their use to a number of other diseases. His treatise on the subject went through eight British and three American editions.

Wellcome III, p. 203.

681. AUGUSTUS EVERARD BRANDE (fl. 1790). *Experiments and observations on the angustura bark.* 2nd ed. London: Printed by G. Stafford for T. Payne, 1793. [16] 133 pp. 20.2 cm. Bound with No. 644.

This series of case studies by Brande, who served as apothecary to the Queen, attests to the supposed remarkable qualities of the angustura bark in treating diarrhea, headache, fevers, and other assorted ailments.

Wellcome II, p. 230 (1st ed., 1791).

682. WILLIAM MOSS (fl. 1790). *An essay on the management and feeding of infants.* Philadelphia: Published by Benjamin Johnson, 1808. 104 pp. 19.6 cm.

Moss, surgeon to the Liverpool Lying-in Charity, had a great interest in the diseases of children and was an active participant in Liverpool's Inoculation Society which was founded in 1781 to inoculate the poor against smallpox. The first part of the present work is an abridgment of Moss's *Essay on the management and nursing of children,* first published in London in 1781. In the book he concentrates primarily on the feeding of infants and gives intelligent, well-reasoned arguments for the instructions and methods he espouses. The second and third parts of the book deal with vaccination and were separately published in Philadelphia in 1806 and 1807.

Austin 1346; Waller 6699.

In memory of Robert D. Gauchat.

*683. JOHN PUGH (fl. 1790). *A treatise on the science of muscular action.* London: Printed for C. Dilly, 1794. ix (misnumbered xi) vi–xvi, 106 pp. 15 plates, each accompanied by a duplicate outline plate. 31.6 cm.

John Pugh, a little known eighteenth-century anatomist and physiologist, was an advocate of a number of techniques and practices which might sound familiar to the modern physical therapist. He placed special emphasis on exercise in rehabilitating limbs affected by neuromuscular conditions and constructed an apparatus to aid in their restoration. Thomas Kirk, the artist responsible for the engravings, was well known for his portraits which were frequently exhibited at the Royal Academy. His rendering of the fifteen plates was produced by using stipple engraving, achieving a three-dimensional effect.

*684. PAOLO MASCAGNI (1752–1815). *Vasorum lymphaticorum corporis humani historia et ichnographia.* Siena: Ex typographia Pazzini Carli, 1787. [4] 138 pp., 27 plates, several accompanied by duplicate outline plates. 59.7 cm. Calf.

Mascagni, educated at Siena, was successively instructor in anatomy at Siena, Pisa, and Florence. This massive atlas contains twenty-seven plates and fourteen outline keys of the human lymphatic system which are masterful in their execution and leave little to be improved upon. They were drawn and engraved by the artist Ciro Santi (fl. 1787) of Bologna and form a landmark in anatomic illustration. Mascagni made several notable discoveries concerning the lymphatics, and this work contains his contribution with reference to the diapedesis of the corpuscles through the wall of the blood vessels in areas of inflammation.

Choulant-Frank, pp. 315–316; Garrison-Morton 1104; Waller 6295.

685. ANTONIO SCARPA (1752–1832). *Anatomicae disquisitiones de auditu et olfactu.* Ticino: In typographeo Petri Galeatii, 1789. [10] 101 pp., 8 plates, each accompanied by a duplicate outline plate. 42.4 cm.

Scarpa, a brilliant artist as well as a brilliant anatomist, was trained in anatomy by Morgagni at Padua and studied surgery at Bologna. At the age of twenty he became professor at Modena, and in 1783 he went to Pavia where he helped bring the University of Pavia to preeminence. His legacy includes works in otolaryngology, orthopedics, ophthalmology, neuroanatomy, and surgery.

In this work, Scarpa describes the auditory and olfactory mechanisms of fishes, birds, reptiles, and man. The eight plates were drawn by the author.

Choulant-Frank, p. 299; Garrison-Morton 1453; Waller 8532.

*686. ———. *Anatomicarum annotationum.* 2nd ed. 2 vols. Pavia and Milan: Apud Joseph Galeatium, 1792. Vol. I: 115 pp., 2 plates (1 fold.); Vol. II: 82 pp., 2 plates, each accompanied by a duplicate outline plate. 28.3 cm. Original wrappers, uncut, in slipcase.

Scarpa's *Anatomicarum annotationum,* first published in 1779, studies the nerve fibers in the ganglia, the plexuses, and the olfactory system. The four copperplate

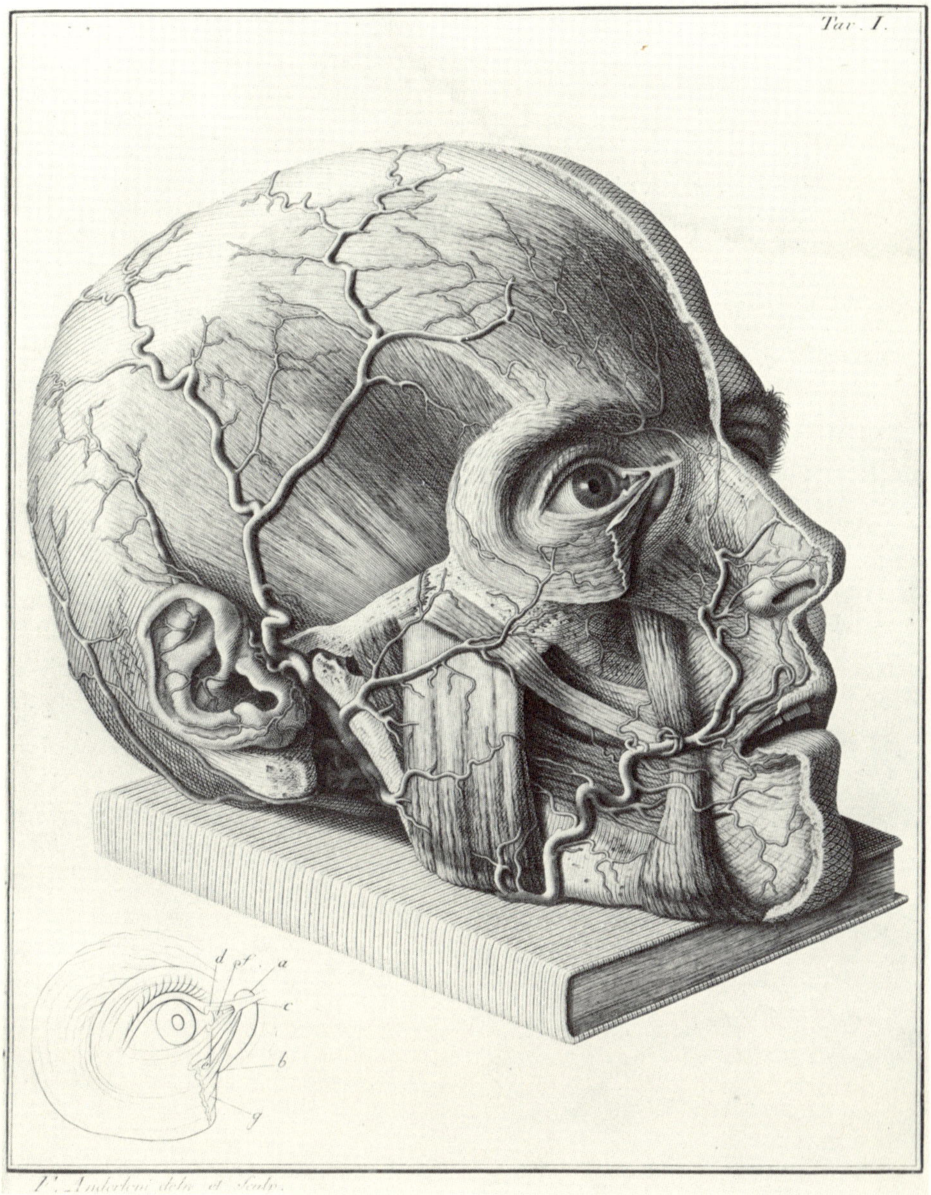

No. 688. Scarpa. *Saggio di Osservazioni . . . degli Occhi*. One of the most arresting of all anatomical illustrations.

illustrations are again examples of Scarpa's brilliant drawings of the finer anatomical structures.

Choulant-Frank, pp. 298–299; Waller 8533 (1st ed., 1779).

687. ———. *Tabulae neurologicae ad illustrandam historiam anatomicam, cardiacorum nervorum, noni nervorum cerebri, glossopharyngaei, et pharyngaei ex octavo cerebri.* 2 vols. Ticino: Apud Balthassarem Comini, 1794. Text: [3] 44 pp.; Atlas: 7 plates, each accompanied by a duplicate outline plate. 61.6 cm. Bound with No. 689.

This study of the nerves of the heart is Scarpa's most famous work and is illustrated with his outstanding life-size drawings. The plates were cut by Faustino Anderloni (fl. 1750) whom Scarpa had trained in order to realize his drawings as accurately and as meticulously as possible.

Choulant-Frank, p. 299; Cushing S111; Garrison-Morton 1253; Waller 8545.

———. *De penitiori ossium commentarius.*

See No. 874.

*688. ———. *Saggio di osservazioni e d'esperienze sulle principali malattie degli occhi.* Pavia: Presso Baldassare Comino, 1801. xi, 278 pp., front. (port.), 3 plates. 31.1 cm.

This classic work on ophthalmology remained the standard text for several decades, going through several editions and translations. It established Scarpa's reputation as a leading ophthalmologist and is especially notable for its copperplate engravings of the anatomy of the eye, drawn by the anatomist.

Garrison-Morton 5835; Waller 8543.

*689. ———. *Sull' aneurisma. Riflessioni ed osservazioni anatomico-chirurgiche.* 2 vols. Pavia: Tipografia Bolzani, 1804. Text: [4] vi, 114 pp.; Atlas: 10 plates, 5 accompanied by duplicate outline plates. 61.4 cm. Bound with No. 687.

In *Sull' aneurisma,* Scarpa makes the first distinction between true and false aneurysms. The ten accompanying plates drawn by Scarpa and engraved by Anderloni are exquisitely executed.

Garrison-Morton 2975.

690. ———. *Sull' ernie: memorie anatomico-chirurgiche.* Milan: Dalla Reale Stamperia, 1809. iv, 84 pp., 10 plates, each accompanied by a duplicate outline plate. 67.6 cm. Half vellum.

This authoritative work on hernia, from which are derived the eponyms "Scarpa's fascia" and "Scarpa's triangle" of the thigh, is enhanced by the ten life-size plates artistically drawn by Scarpa himself, depicting the operation and anatomical sections. Accompanying the principal plates are ten outline keys.

Garrison-Morton 3583; Waller 8544 (1819 ed.).

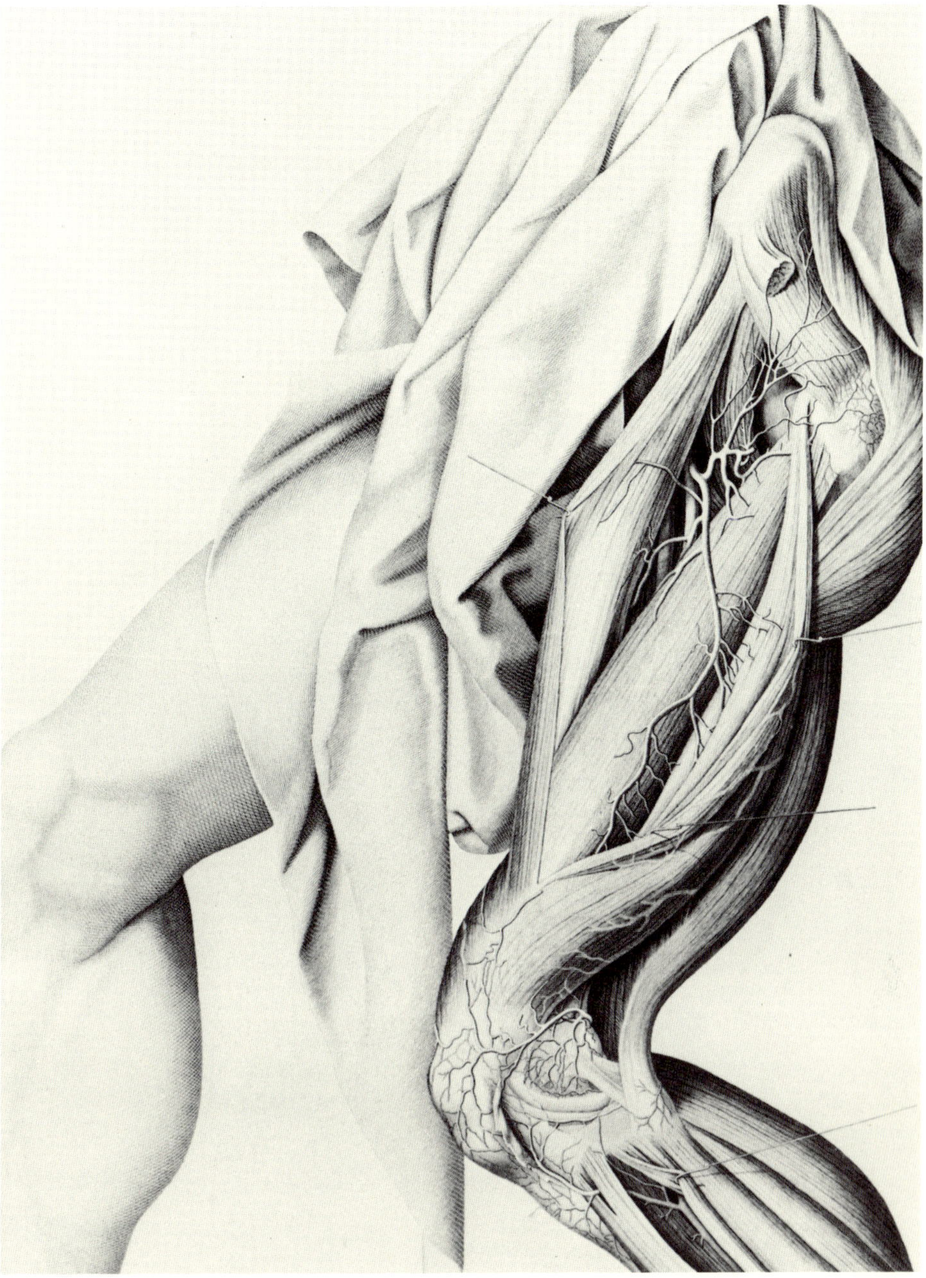

No. 689. Scarpa. *Sull' Aneurisma.*

691. ———. ———. 2nd ed. 2 vols. Pavia: Dalla stamperia Fusi, success. Galeazzi, 1819. Text: vi, 181 pp.; Atlas: 11 plates, each accompanied by a duplicate outline plate. 49.3 cm.

The plates from the first edition were also used in this second edition; however, each plate was printed on a single sheet and folded down the center before being bound into the atlas. An additional plate has been added to this edition.

Garrison-Morton 3583 (1809 ed.); Waller 8544.

Purchased from the James Emmett Conn Memorial Book Fund.

*692. JOHANN FRIEDRICH BLUMENBACH (1752–1840). *Institutiones physiologicae*. Göttingen: Apud Jo. Christ. Dieterich, 1786. xvi, 511 pp., 4 plates. 19.1 cm.

Physician, physiologist, historian, and bibliographer, Blumenbach is generally regarded as the founder of scientific anthropology. His classification of the subdivisions of the human race, which forms the latter part of this work, was the first to utilize facial configuration as well as skin color, and his system has survived to the present with but little modification.

Waller 1164; Wellcome II, p. 183.

*693. ———. *Geschichte und Beschreibung der Knochen des menschlichen Körpers*. Göttingen: H. Dieterich, 1807. xxi, 496 pp., 2 plates. 21.5 cm. Original wrappers, uncut.

Blumenbach's noteworthy book on human osteology contains his original description of the portion of the base of the skull immediately posterior to the sella turcica (clivus Blumenbachi). This interleaved copy contains scattered marginal notes believed to be in Blumenbach's hand.

Waller 1162 (1st ed., 1786); Wellcome II, p. 184.

694. ———. *Handbuch der vergleichenden Anatomie*. 2nd ed. Göttingen: Bey Heinrich Dieterich, 1815. xvi, 555 pp., 8 plates. 19 cm.

Blumenbach was the first German to lecture on comparative anatomy, and in this work he demonstrated the importance of comparative anatomy to the study of anthropology and human development.

Garrison-Morton 312 (1805 ed.); Waller 1163 (1805 ed.); Wellcome II, p. 183 (1805 ed.).

695. JAMES GREGORY (1753–1821). *A dissertation on the influence of a change of climate in curing diseases*. Translated from the original Latin, and enlarged with occasional notes, by William P. C. Barton. Philadelphia: T. Dobson, 1815. 212 pp. 23.3 cm.

Controversial, irritable, and sometimes vindictive, Gregory was nevertheless a brilliant lecturer and scholar, well-versed in language and art as well as medicine.

He did little original investigation but his *Conspectus* (1788), his best work, was widely read for its clarity and style. In 1800 Gregory touched off a famous scandal by accusing John Bell of incompetence and excluding him from the Royal Infirmary. Bell, in his rebuttal to the scathing attack (see No. 730), assesses the Gregory character: "I have one great consolation. . . . I am not wounding the reputation of a good nor the peace of an innocent man" (John Bell, *Letters on professional character . . . addressed to James Gregory, M.D.* Edinburgh, 1810. p. v).

Gregory's work on the influence of climate on disease received considerable attention during the first part of the nineteenth century and went through several editions.

Austin 841.

*696. JUSTUS CHRISTIAN VON LODER (1753–1832). *Tabulae anatomicae quas ad illustrandam humani corporis fabricam collegit et curavit-Justus Christianus Loder.* 2 vols. Weimar: Sumtibus Novi Bibliopolii vulgo Landes-Industrie-Comptoir dicti, 1803. Vol. I: 182 plates (part col., part fold.); Vol. II: various paginations. 41.7 cm.

A physician of wide experience and good reputation, Loder held professorships at Jena, Halle, and the University of Moscow. Like Caldani's *Icones anatomicae* (see No. 605), Loder's *Tabulae anatomicae* is a compilation of the best illustrations and representations of anatomy available at the time. Of the 1,434 figures included, 1,122 are copies drawn from the works of Albinus, John Hunter, Cheselden, Monro, Scarpa, Sandifort, and others, while 309 are original drawings. In many plates the vascular system is represented in color. This massive gathering is one of the most beautiful anatomical works of the nineteenth century.

Choulant-Frank, pp. 325–326; Waller III, p. 535.

697. JOSEPH PHILIPPE FRANÇOIS DELEUZE (1753–1835). *Histoire critique du magnétisme animal.* 2nd ed. 2 vols. Paris: Belin-Leprieur, 1819. Vol. I: xiv, 316 pp.; Vol. II: xiv, 362 pp. 19.5 cm.

Deleuze was assistant naturalist at the Paris Museum of Natural History and an early supporter of Mesmer's theory of animal magnetism, a subject on which he wrote numerous treatises including this historical survey.

Waller 2327 (1st ed., 1813); Wellcome II, p. 445 (1st ed.).

698. WILLIAM CURRIE (1754–1828). *A view of the diseases most prevalent in the United States of America, at different seasons of the year.* Philadelphia: J. & A. Y. Humphreys, 1811. 240 pp. 22 cm.

One of the founders of the Philadelphia College of Physicians and a surgeon in the Revolutionary War, Currie's place in American medical history stems largely from his heated disagreements with Benjamin Rush (see No. 665) as to the best method of containing the yellow fever epidemics in Philadelphia in 1797 and 1798. Rush believed the disease to be of domestic origin and that the use of mercurials and bleeding was the most efficacious remedy, while Currie thought the disease to be imported and was averse to bleeding. The controversy resulted in a great reluctance on the part of the citizenry to seek medical aid and a subsequent high mortality rate. Besides the present work on general medicine, Currie wrote a number of books and pamphlets on yellow fever.

Austin 608; Cushing C658.

699. JAMES THACHER (1754–1844). *The American new dispensatory*. 2nd ed. Boston: Thomas B. Wait & Co. and C. Williams [1813]. xxvii, 732 pp. 21.2 cm.

America's first medical historian and a practitioner of the first rank, Thacher is best known for his two-volume *American medical biography* (1828) and for his medical journal covering the American Revolution in which he gives a graphic eyewitness account of the struggle.

The popular *American new dispensatory,* Thacher's first work, is adopted from the *Pharmacopoeia of the Massachusetts Medical Society* (see No. 937) which was published previously by the Massachusetts Medical Society.

Austin 1878; Cushing T38.

700. ———. *Observations on hydrophobia, produced by the bite of a mad dog, or other rabid animal*. Plymouth, Massachusetts: Joseph Avery, 1812. 301 [1] pp., col. plate. 21.2 cm.

Of special interest in this work on hydrophobia is a hand-colored drawing of the "skull-cap," a plant which was used (unsuccessfully) in treating the disease.

Austin 1880; Cushing T40; Waller 4089.

*701. JEAN NICOLAS CORVISART DES MARETS (1755–1821). *Essai sur les maladies et les lésions organiques du coeur et des gros vaisseaux*. Paris: Migneret, 1806. lvi, 484 pp. 19.7 cm.

In this great classic of cardiac literature, Corvisart for the first time so ordered the symptomatology of heart disease that differentiation between cardiac and pulmonary disease was made possible. He distinguished between cardiac hypertrophy and dilatation, he divided the clinical course of cardiac failure into three phases, and he showed the relationship between cause and effect in valvular disease and cardiac failure. Corvisart was personal physician to Napoleon and enjoyed a close and loyal relationship with him.

Garrison-Morton 2737; Waller 2149.

*702. [JEAN ANTHELME BRILLAT-SAVARIN] (1755–1826). *Physiologie du goût; ou, méditations de gastronomie transcendante*. 2 vols. Paris: A. Sautelet, 1826. Vol. I: 590 pp.; Vol. II: 442 pp. 20.2 cm.

This famous work on eating was published anonymously by the author in the year of his death. A lawyer, writer, and musician, Brillat-Savarin fled during the French Revolution to the United States where he supported himself by giving French lessons and playing in an orchestra. He wrote a number of works on political economy and law after his return to France in 1796 but saved his most engaging style for his treatise on gastronomy on which he worked intermittently. Much of the work is written with mock grandeur covering such areas as taste, smell, diet, pleasures of the table, the history of cooking, recipes, and anecdotes of remembered feasts. Although there is a definite scientific approach to the material, the charm of the book lies in the personality and wit of the author which are apparent throughout.

Cushing B767; Osler 4394 (English ed., 1884); Wellcome II, p. 239 (1841 ed.).

*703. JOHN FLAXMAN (1755–1826). *Anatomical studies of the bones and muscles, for the use of artists*. London: M. A. Nattali, 1833. 13 pp., front. (port.), 21 plates. 48.9 cm.

"The first two plates were drawn and lithographed by William Robertson and contain six whole figures, viz.: the skeleton and the muscleman, each from three different viewpoints. . . . The nineteen plates following these were drawn by Flaxman and engraved by Henry Landseer. The first three are finished in aquatint and pertain to osteology. . . . The sixteen plates following are done in the easy, unconventional style of chalk-drawings and pertain wholly to myology. . . . Flaxman's drawings are all unconventional, clever, and true to nature" (Choulant-Frank, p. 341).

Choulant-Frank, pp. 341–342; Garrison-Morton 411; Wellcome III, p. 31.

704. SAMUEL THOMAS VON SOEMMERRING (1755–1830). *Icones embryonum humanorum*. Frankfurt am Main: Prostant apud Varrentrapp et Wenner, 1799. 10 pp., 2 plates. 57.7 cm.

Soemmerring, a German physician and anatomist, taught and practiced medicine at various cities and universities in Germany, but his chief fame rests on his series of incomparable anatomical atlases. "He aimed, like Albinus, at the discovery of the true and the beautiful in the form of every part of the human body and combined a perfect sense of artistic representation with the most exact perception of details. He endeavored, like Albinus, to have every part reproduced just as it exists in the living body, and not as it appeared after death from the treatment of the anatomist" (Choulant-Frank, p. 301).

In addition to the present work, Soemmerring's atlases of the eye (No. 705), ear (No. 706), tongue and male larynx—*Abbildungen der menschlichen Organe des Geschmackes und der Stimme* (1806)—and that of the olfactory organ—*Abbildungen der menschlichen Organe des Geruches* (1809)—are among his principal works.

Soemmerring intended this work as an appendix to Hunter's atlas of the gravid uterus (see No. 591). It covers the early phases of pregnancy, which were not included in Hunter's work. As in nearly all of Soemmerring's atlases, the drawings were done by Christian Köck (fl. 1750), whom Soemmerring trained especially for his anatomical works.

Choulant-Frank, p. 307; Garrison-Morton 473; Waller 9045.

*705. ———. *Abbildungen des menschlichen Auges.* Frankfurt am Main: Varrentrapp und Wenner, 1801. x, 110 pp., 8 plates, each accompanied by a duplicate outline plate, 1 in full color. 40.2 cm.

Choulant calls this "Soemmerring's most perfect work." Front and profile views are shown of the living eye of a male, female, Negro, and an albino. Other plates are anatomic and partly microscopic. Of the sixteen plates, eight are outline keys.

Choulant-Frank, p. 308; Garrison-Morton 1489; Waller 9046 (Latin ed., 1804).

*706. ———. *Abbildungen des menschlichen Hörorganes.* Frankfurt am Main: Varrentrapp und Wenner, 1806. x, 36 pp., 5 plates, 4 accompanied by duplicate outline plates. 40.6 cm.

This atlas on the human ear shows the parts in natural size and some much enlarged. The drawings are by Christian Köck.

Choulant-Frank, p. 308; Garrison-Morton 1554; Waller 9047 (Latin ed.).

*707. SAMUEL HAHNEMANN (1755–1843). *Organon der rationellen Heilkunde.* Dresden: In der Arnoldischen Buchhandlung, 1810. xlviii, 222 pp. 20.8 cm. Original boards, in black cloth box.

At the turn of the nineteenth century, a number of curative systems held the attention of the medical world. One of the more unusual of these was homeopathy, developed by Hahnemann, a German physician. Based on limited experimental evidence, he advanced the theory that many diseases could be cured by the administration of minute quantities of drugs which produced symptoms similar to the disease itself. Moreover, the smaller the quantity, the more potent its effect. At a time when drugs were normally used in large doses and sometimes indiscriminately, the infinitesimal doses of the homeopath did less harm than many conventional prescriptions. The system became quite popular, particularly in America where homeopathic practitioners may still be found. *Organon der rationellen Heilkunde* was Hahnemann's first and most important work on the subject.

Garrison-Morton 1966; Osler 2874 (1924 ed.); Waller 3960; Wellcome III, p. 191.

*708. JEAN GALBERT SALVAGE (fl. 1796–1812). *Anatomie du gladiateur combattant, applicable aux beaux arts.* Paris: Chez l'auteur, 1812. iv, 64 pp., front., plates (part col.). 56.8 cm.

This rare and beautiful book, with twenty-two large copperplates drawn by the author, uses several well-known classical sculptures for the anatomical subjects. Salvage was a French military surgeon whose studies of classical sculpture led him to the conclusion that the perfection of its execution was such that accurate bone and muscular structure could be illustrated in representations of the sculptures. "The 'Planche d'Instruction' and the fifteen plates immediately following it are struck off from two plates so as to bring out the bones in black and the body contours and muscles in red" (Choulant-Frank, pp. 333–334). The effect is striking and the text, engraved along with the plates, was printed in the same manner.

Choulant-Frank, pp. 332–334; Waller 8435.

*709. JAMES CURRIE (1756–1805). *Medical reports, on the effects of water, cold and warm, as a remedy in fever, and febrile diseases.* Liverpool: Printed by J. M'Creery, for Cadell and Davis, 1797. x, vii, 252, 45 pp. 22.6 cm.

Currie left his native Scotland for Virginia in 1771 but later returned to Britain where he became a political activist and abolitionist while maintaining a sizable medical practice in Liverpool. An early advocate of hydrotherapy, Currie was the first to use cold seawater baths to lower elevated body temperatures in typhoid fever.

Garrison-Morton 1988; Osler 2408 (1798–1805 ed.); Wellcome II, p. 420.

710. Sir EVERARD HOME (1756–1832). *Lectures on comparative anatomy; in which are explained the preparations in the Hunterian collection.* 6 vols. London: G. & W. Nichol, 1814–1828. Front. (port.), 371 plates. 34.6 cm.

A pupil and brother-in-law of John Hunter (see No. 609 ff.), and later his associate for over twenty years, Home was professor in the Royal College of Surgeons and, for thirty-four years, surgeon at St. George's Hospital. Upon Hunter's death, Home became custodian of his manuscripts, which included Hunter's own description of his anatomical collection. Thirty years later, Home deliberately burned the manuscripts and thereby began a controversy which remains to this day. Home claimed that Hunter requested him to destroy the papers, but it is suggested by some historians that Home later published much of the material (including portions of the present work) under his own name to further his reputation. Another, more charitable, explanation is that Hunter's unpublished views on comparative anatomy bordered on religious heresy and that Home, in a well-meaning but tragic gesture, burned the manuscripts to save Hunter's name.

In any case the six-volume work is a fine piece of scholarship and printing. Three of the volumes are comprised entirely of illustrations in the form of 371 expertly rendered plates.

Cushing H438; Garrison-Morton 315; Wellcome III, p. 294.

711. FRANZ JOSEF GALL (1758–1828). *Philosophisch-medicinische Untersuchungen über Natur und Kunst im Kranken und gesunden Zustand des Menschen.* Vienna: R. Gräffer, 1791. vii, 720 [6] pp. 21.5 cm.

Despite his notable contributions to the field of neuroanatomy, Gall is chiefly remembered as the founder of phrenology, a "science" he developed with his student-collaborator, Spurzheim (see No. 792). Unfortunately, the rapid rise of phrenology, its subsequent distortion, and eventual fall from favor, tend to obscure Gall's more deserving work, among which is this early treatise on philosophical anthropology.

*712. ——— and JOHANN GASPAR SPURZHEIM (1776–1832). *Anatomie et physiologie du système nerveux en général.* 4 vols. and atlas. Paris: F. Schoell, 1810–1819. Vols. I-IV: 28.7 cm. Atlas: 100 plates. 51.3 cm. Tree calf.

This elaborately produced work attests to the fact that, despite his later fall into disrepute, Gall was an excellent anatomist. A number of original anatomical observations are introduced in this five-volume work, including the concept of localization of brain function. Because Spurzheim parted with Gall in 1814, only the first two volumes were produced collaboratively. The one hundred plates which comprise the atlas are exquisitely rendered.

Garrison-Morton 1389; Wellcome III, p. 84.

*713. JOSEPH JAKOB VON MOHRENHEIM (1759?–1799). *Abhandlung über die Entbindungskunst.* St. Petersburg: Gedruckt bey der K. Akademie der Wissenschaften, 1791. [14] 216 [50] pp., 46 plates. 52.1 cm.

An Austrian, Mohrenheim became body-surgeon and accoucheur to Empress Catherine II of Russia, by whose order this now rare work was published. The book opens with a brief literary history of obstetrics, followed by an extensive text. The remarkable life-size engravings, many of them after Smellie (see No. 522), represent female genitalia, embryos, deliveries, and instruments.

Cushing M437 (1803 ed.); Garrison-Morton 6161; Waller 6594 (1803 ed.).

714. JOHANN CHRISTIAN REIL (1759–1813). *Rhapsodieen über die Anwendung der psychischen Kurmethode auf Geisteszerrüttungen.* Halle: In der Curtschen Buchhandlung, 1818. 500 pp. 22.2 cm.

Professor of medicine at the University of Halle and later Berlin, Reil is noted for his investigations into the causes and cures of insanity and was one of the first to advocate humane treatment for the mentally afflicted. He founded the first journal devoted to psychiatry, *Magazin für psychische Heilkunde.* Reil also made important strides in ophthalmology and neuroanatomy, his works on the structure of the crystalline lens and his description of the "island of Reil" in the brain being especially significant. This work on the "physical method of cure" of the insane focuses on Reil's belief that the minds of insane patients could be jarred through outside assaults on the senses such as the incitement of fear or loud noises. The work is considered by some to represent the beginnings of psychotherapy.

Garrison-Morton 4923 (1803 ed.).

715. VINCENZO CHIARUGI (1759–1820). *Abhandlung über den Wahnsinn überhaupt und insbesondere, nebst einer Centurie von Beobachtungen.* 3 vols. in 1. Leipzig: Bei Georg David Meyer, 1795. Vol. I: xii, 211 [1] pp.; Vol. II: [2] iv [2] 217–444 pp., fold. plate.; Vol. III: viii, x [2] 447–708 pp., fold. plate. 20.4 cm.

Deriving his concepts from an array of ancient and contemporary philosophers and scientists, Chiarugi labored at a definitive classification of mental illness, never knowing that his major contribution to the field lay elsewhere. In 1788, he was placed in charge of the hospital of Bonifazio where he published a set of regulations for the hospital staff, emphasizing the moral obligation and medical duty to respect the insane individual as a person. True to his own dictum, he instituted a program of humanitarian care, recreation, and daily visitation, and he ordered that physical restraint be minimized. Because of his oblique style and lack of ardent followers, Chiarugi did not receive the recognition he deserved, and he has been overshadowed by Pinel whom he anticipated and whose ideas paralleled Chiarugi's in virtually every respect.

This German translation of Chiarugi's 1793 Italian work on insanity includes his classification scheme and system of diagnosis.

Garrison-Morton 4921 (Italian ed., 1793); Waller 1954.

*716. GIUSEPPE DEL MEDICO (fl. 1800). *Anatomia per uso dei pittori e scultori.* Rome: Presso V. Poggioli, 1811. 52 pp., 38 plates. 37.3 cm.

Del Medico, professor of surgery at Rome, prepared this atlas of human anatomy for artists and sculptors. The thirty-eight copperplates with engraved explanatory captions include illustrations of muscles, internal organs, complete skeletons similar to those of Albinus, and two views of the Borghese gladiator.

Choulant-Frank, p. 331; Garrison-Morton 406.

717. THOMAS BEDDOES (1760–1808). *Observations on the medical and domestic management of the consumptive; On the powers of digitalis purpurea; and, On the cure of schrophula.* London: Longman and Rees, 1801. 270 [1] 132 (misnumbered 172) pp., plate. 20.6 cm.

Beddoes was a graduate of Oxford, and, after his appointment there in 1788 as reader in chemistry, he attracted audiences larger than any since the thirteenth century. His fervent belief was that true medical science must have a chemical basis, and, with this in mind, he set up a Pneumatic Institution where diseases were treated by the administration of gases. He appointed Humphry Davy (1778–1829), then a lad of nineteen, as superintendent, and it was here that Davy, in the course of his experiments on the medical properties of gases, discovered the anesthetic effects of nitrous oxide, or "laughing gas." Davy stayed at the Pneumatic Institution only three years, after which it became primarily a clinic for preventive medicine. Beddoes' theories as to inhalation may have been overdone but they have found some vindication in open-air treatment of tuberculosis and other respiratory diseases, and his general plan of inhalation therapy has become standardized as pneumotherapy.

Cushing B239; Wellcome II, p. 129.

Gift of Dr. R. N. Larimer.

718. EDWARD MILLER (1760–1812). *The medical works of Edward Miller, M.D. . . . Collected, and accompanied with a biographical sketch of the author; by Samuel*

Miller. New York: Printed and sold by Collins and Co., 1814. iv [4] [xi]–cxi, 392 pp., 2 port. (incl. front.). 21.2 cm. Original calf.

One of the early physicians of New York City, Miller achieved a wide reputation for his clinical competence and powers of observation. He was one of the first physicians to assert that yellow fever was not contagious, and he made extensive investigations of fever and cholera. Together with Samuel L. Mitchell and Elihu H. Smith, Miller began the *Medical repository,* America's first medical journal. The present collection of his works was gathered by Miller's brother Samuel (1769–1850) at the urging of Benjamin Rush.

Austin 1301.

719. MATHEW CAREY (1760–1839). *A short account of the malignant fever, lately prevalent in Philadelphia: with a statement of the proceedings that took place on the subject, in different parts of the United States.* 4th ed. Philadelphia: Printed by the author, 1794. 164 pp. 20.8 cm.

Born in Dublin, Carey emigrated to Philadelphia in 1784 after serving a prison sentence for revolutionary activities in Ireland. He became active in the Philadelphia publishing community and, in 1820, founded the *Philadelphia journal of the medical and physical sciences* which, after a change of title in 1824 to *American journal of the medical sciences*, is still being published.

The present work first appeared in 1793 and went through four editions within several months. Carey gives a graphic account of the great yellow fever epidemic that struck Philadelphia in 1793, with mention of the many measures adopted to combat the disease.

Austin 413; Cushing C90 (2nd ed., 1793); Garrison-Morton 5451 (1st ed., 1793); Wellcome II, p. 301.

*720. JEAN JOSEPH SUE (d. 1831). *The anatomy of the bones of the human body . . . copied from the elegant tables of Sue and Albinus.* By Edward Mitchell, engraver. With explanatory references by the late John Barclay. Edinburgh: Printed for Maclachlan & Stewart, 1829. [64] pp., 32 plates. 27.2 cm.

The thirty-two plates in this beautifully executed atlas were copied from the works of Sue and Albinus by the engraver, Edward Mitchell. John Barclay (1758–1826), who supplied the commentary, "appears to have been the first anatomist to use the suffix '-ad' indicating direction, *e.g.*, rotulad, tibiad, sternad" (Osler 1910).

Osler 1910.

*721. CASPAR WISTAR (1761–1818). *A system of anatomy for the use of students of medicine.* 2 vols. Philadelphia: T. Dobson, 1811–1814. Vol. I: xii, 422 pp.; Vol. II: viii, 453 pp., fold. tables. 21.6 cm. Rebound in modern buckram.

Wistar, a native Philadelphian, studied at the University of Pennsylvania and received his M.D. from the University of Edinburgh. He practiced medicine in

Philadelphia and, after 1792, taught anatomy at the University of Pennsylvania. His *System of anatomy* is the first American textbook on the subject and was in widespread use for many years, going through numerous editions. Although well-arranged for teaching, it is illustrated with only a few rather insignificant plates in Volume Two.

Austin 2082.

722. MATTHEW BAILLIE (1761–1823). *The morbid anatomy of some of the most important parts of the human body.* 1st American ed. Albany: Printed by Barber & Southwick for T. Spencer, 1795. viii, 248 [12] pp. 19.2 cm. In slipcase.

Baillie, a Scot, was the nephew and pupil of William Hunter (see No. 591). He performed postmortem examinations on several eminent men, including Dr. Samuel Johnson. Baillie was the last to own the famous gold-headed cane (see No. 825).

This work, first published in London in 1793, was the first systematic textbook of morbid anatomy and introduced the field as an independent science for the first time. This edition does not contain the fine illustrations found in the several English editions.

Austin 95; Cushing B41; Garrison-Morton 2281 (1st ed., 1793); Osler 1891 (1803 ed.); Wellcome II, p. 87 (1st ed.).

Gift of Dr. Everett D. Plass.

723. ———. *A series of engravings, accompanied with explanations, which are intended to illustrate the morbid anatomy of some of the most important parts of the human body.* 2nd ed. 2 vols. London: Printed by W. Bulmer, 1812. Text: 228 pp.; Atlas: 73 plates. 31.8 cm.

This atlas was intended to accompany Baillie's *Morbid anatomy*. The plates were drawn by William Clift, who became the first curator of the Hunterian Museum, founded by Baillie's uncle, John Hunter, at the Royal College of Surgeons (see Nos. 613 and 614).

Cushing B41; Garrison-Morton 2282 (1st ed., 1799–1802); Wellcome II, p. 87.

Gift of Dr. M. E. Barnes.

*724. NATHAN SMITH (1762–1829). *A practical essay on typhous fever.* New York: E. Bless & E. White, 1824. 88 pp. 21.2 cm.

When Dartmouth opened a medical department in 1768, Nathan Smith was appointed professor of anatomy, surgery, chemistry, and physics, and was, indeed, its entire faculty. A skilled surgeon, teacher, writer, and practitioner, Smith played a major role in the establishment of the medical schools at Yale and the University of Vermont, and the Jefferson Medical College at Philadelphia. His most important written contribution is this treatise on typhus fever, in which he gives the first clear description of the disease.

Cushing S291; Osler 3994.

*725. ———. *Medical and surgical memoirs.* Edited with addenda by Nathan R. Smith. Baltimore: Printed by W. A. Francis, 1831. vii [9]–374 pp., front. (port.), illus., plates. 21.1 cm.

Smith was the author of additional works on necrosis, fractures, lithotomy, and dislocations, and pioneered with a number of amputation techniques. His memoirs, edited by his son (see No. 898), contain nearly all of his notable works.

Cushing S290; Waller 9032.

726. JOHANN VALENTIN VON HILDENBRAND (1763–1818). *Über den ansteckenden Typhus.* Vienna: Gedruckt in der Degenschen Buchdruckerey, 1810. viii [2] 309 pp. 21.4 cm.

Hildenbrand studied medicine under Maximilian Stoll (see No. 656) at Vienna where he later was appointed professor of medicine. This classic treatise on typhus was widely translated in numerous editions. Hildenbrand's lucid description of the disease was so widely read that typhus is sometimes referred to in the French literature as "Hildenbrand's Disease."

Garrison-Morton 5375; Osler 2966 (English ed., 1829); Wellcome III, p. 263.

727. JOHN BELL (1763–1820) and Sir CHARLES BELL (1774–1842). *The anatomy of the human body.* 4 vols. in 2. New York: Printed and sold by Collins, 1812. Vol. I: ix [v]–xxviii, 284 pp., illus., plates; Vol. II: xxiv, 309 pp., illus., plates; Vol. III: x, 308 pp., illus., plates; Vol. IV: xii, 246 pp., illus., plates. 20.6 cm. Calf.

An eminent Scottish anatomist and surgeon, John Bell exerted great influence on the development of British surgery, particularly through his work on surgical pathology. He had a special interest in surgery of the blood vessels and was the first to ligate the gluteal artery. An excellent artist, like his even more famous younger brother, Sir Charles Bell (see No. 777 ff.), he illustrated his own books, and his engravings of the different parts and organs of the human body are landmarks in the history of anatomic illustration.

Bell's *Anatomy of the human body* was first published from 1793 to 1803 and was reissued in 1811 with an additional volume by Sir Charles Bell and illustrations by the authors themselves. This first American edition, from the fourth London edition, is a worthy example of their joint efforts in the long line of editions of this work.

Austin 191.

Gift of Dr. C. R. Baker.

728. JOHN BELL. *Discourses on the nature and cure of wounds.* 3 pts. in 1 vol. Edinburgh: Printed for Bell and Bradfute, 1795. Part I: vi, 241 pp.; Part II: [1] 169 pp.; Part III: [1] 67 pp., front., illus., plates. 23.5 cm.

This work and Bell's *Principles of surgery* (see No. 729) are his most enduring contributions to surgery. The second "Discourse" is a particularly valuable historical discussion of surgery of the arteries. The frontispiece, drawn by Bell, is a beautiful engraving of the arteries of the thigh and groin.

Waller 863.

Gift of R. W. Lemley.

729. ———. *The principles of surgery.* Abridged by J. Augustine Smith. New York: Collins, 1810. 562 pp., illus., plates. 21.3 cm.

Like most of his works, this abridgment of Bell's famous three-volume *Principles of surgery* contains a number of skillfully executed plates drawn by the author.

Austin 195; Waller 866; Wellcome II, p. 138.

*730. ———. *Letters on professional character and manners . . . addressed to James Gregory, M.D.* Edinburgh: Printed by John Moir, 1810. xxiii [1] 636 pp. 21.5 cm. Modern boards.

Although Bell studied at Edinburgh under such eminent teachers as William Cullen (see No. 567 ff.), Alexander Monro *secundus* (see No. 634), and Alexander Wood (1725–1807), he nevertheless felt that anatomy was poorly taught at the University. Therefore, after entering practice, Bell began to give private lectures in anatomy primarily for surgeons. His lectures became so popular and so many students were attracted that he built an anatomical school to accommodate his classes. After teaching successfully for thirteen years, he was suddenly subjected to a vicious and apparently unwarranted attack led by James Gregory (see No. 695), professor of the practice of medicine at the University. All Edinburgh was torn by this bitter and acrimonious feud, and, as a result, Bell discontinued his lectures and devoted himself to a large and successful surgical practice.

Some ten years later, Bell published the present work in rebuttal to Gregory's malicious attacks. The book demonstrates Bell's highly polished skill in nonmedical prose and is filled with invective and righteous indignation resulting from a decade of controversy and professional strife. Ever the gentleman, Bell deftly castigates Gregory while at the same time presenting the principles and ideals which he espoused in the practice of medicine.

Cushing B273; Garrison-Morton 1765; Osler 2001; Waller 864.

*731. JOHN ABERNETHY (1764–1831). *Surgical observations.* 2 vols. in 1. [London: Printed for Longman, Hurst, Rees, and Orme, 1809–1810]. Vol. I: x, 292 pp.; Vol. II: 234 pp. 20.8 cm. Contemporary half calf.

John Hunter's (see No. 609 ff.) successor at St. Bartholomew's Hospital was John Abernethy, his devoted pupil and disciple. Continuing Hunter's work on ligation, Abernethy became the first to tie successfully the external iliac artery for aneurysm, and in 1798 he ligated the common carotid. Although he was a generous man and quite popular as a teacher, he deliberately assumed a brusque manner with his patients, assuming it would inspire their confidence.

Surgical observations, his primary work, actually contains two publications: *Surgical observations on the constitutional origin and treatment of local diseases and on aneurysms* and *Surgical observations on diseases resembling syphilis.*

Garrison-Morton 5584; Wellcome II, p. 3.

*732. ———. *Surgical observations on injuries of the head; and on miscellaneous subjects.* Philadelphia: Printed for T. Dobson, 1811. 299 pp., plate. 21.6 cm. Original tree calf.

Like the preceding work, this volume covers a large number of topics including head injuries, venesection, joint surgery, lumbar abscesses, and Abernethy's classification of tumors. This first American edition was published one year after the original British work.

Austin 3; Cushing A13.

733. JOHN HASLAM (1764–1844). *Observations on madness and melancholy.* 2nd ed. London: J. Callow, 1809. vii [1] 345 pp. 21.4 cm.

Haslam's place in the history of psychiatry is secure although not entirely unimpeachable. He served as medical officer to Bethlem Hospital, the largest asylum in England, where, with his chief, Thomas Monro, he had the opportunity to study a large number of patients. Although a keen observer with wide experience (he is sometimes regarded as the first to describe general paralysis of the insane), he advocated and allowed practices which can only be described as inhumane. In 1816, he and Monro were dismissed by the Governors of Bethlem for gross malpractice.

Haslam regarded *Observations on madness and melancholy* as his major accomplishment, and for some years it was regarded as the outstanding work in the field.

Garrison-Morton 4794 (1798 ed.); Waller 4135; Wellcome III, p. 221.

734. JAMES WILSON (1765–1821). *Pharmacopoeia chirurgica.* 1st American from the 3rd London ed. Philadelphia: Thomas Dobson and son, 1818. xii, 252 pp. 17.5 cm.

Until the first U.S. pharmacopoeia appeared in 1820, American physicians were forced to rely on a variety of drug compendia, most of which were limited in scope or authority. This work on surgical therapeutics was written by James Wilson, Surgeon at Guy's Hospital, and was introduced into the United States after having gone through three British editions.

Austin 2073.

735. M. A. SALMADE (1766–1838). *Le livre des mères et des nourrices.* Paris: Merlin, 1801. xvi, 212 pp. 16.5 cm.

Most of this work on infant care is devoted to childhood diseases and their treatment. The work became considerably longer in later editions. Salmade was physician to Louis XVIII and Charles X.

Given in memory of Robert D. Gauchat.

*736. DOMINIQUE JEAN LARREY (1766–1842). *Mémoires de chirurgie militarie, et campagnes.* 4 vols. Paris: J. Smith, 1812–1817. Plates (part fold.). 20 cm. New quarter morocco and marbled paper over boards.

"Larrey was the greatest military surgeon in history" (Garrison-Morton 2160). Chief surgeon to Napoleon, whom he supported loyally, Larrey's experiences as a military surgeon, his innovations in military medical therapeutics, and his adventures in the great campaigns of Napoleon make fascinating reading. This work may be considered the best account of military medicine up to the time of its publication.

Garrison-Morton 2160; Osler 3162; Waller 5610; Wellcome III, p. 451.

*737. ———. *Surgical essays.* Translated from the French, by John Revere. Baltimore: N. G. Maxwell, 1823. 335 pp., plate. 22.2 cm.

This lesser-known work by Larrey was originally published in French in 1821. The essays cover both military and non-military medicine including a lengthy account of the uses of moxa, an ancient Oriental cautery.

*738. JOSEPH WENZEL (1768–1808) and CARL WENZEL (1769–1827). *Über die schwammingen Auswüchse auf der äussern Hirnhaut.* Mainz: F. Kupferberg, 1811. xx, 138 [2] pp., 6 plates. 33.4 cm.

Carl and Joseph Wenzel practiced medicine at Mainz and Frankfurt, respectively. They co-authored several books on the anatomy and physiology of the brain including the present work on meningeal tumors published three years after Joseph's death. The six large copperplates are drawn from the authors' own cases.

Waller 10218.

*739. ———. *De penitiori structura cerebri hominis et brutorum.* Tübingen: Apud Cottam, 1812. xiv, 354 pp., charts (part fold.), 15 plates, each accompanied by a duplicate outline plate. 40.7 cm.

The finely produced engravings which comprise the last section of this volume are among the first to illustrate accurately the deeper cerebral structures.

Waller 10217.

740. Sir ASTLEY PASTON COOPER (1768–1841) and BENJAMIN TRAVERS (1783–1858). *Surgical essays.* 1st American from the 3rd London ed. Philadelphia: James Webster, 1821. xiii, 409 pp., 21 plates (1 col.). 21.2 cm.

A pupil of John Hunter (see No. 609 ff.), Cooper made great strides in surgical technique, most notably in the area of vessel ligation. As a teacher, he stressed practical demonstrations over didacticism and gained the respect and admiration of his students, many of whom eventually became famous in their own right.

Cooper was not a prolific writer, but his publications were of the highest quality and were the result of personal knowledge and observation gained from long hours of practice, dissecting, and experimentation. Among his several publications were two papers entitled "Observations on the effects which take place from the destruction of the membrana tympani of the ear" which he read before the Royal Society in the early 1800's. In the first paper he showed that two patients with perforations of both eardrums could hear perfectly well although it had always been thought that this condition resulted in deafness. In the second paper he demonstrated that deafness caused by obstruction of the Eustachian tube could be relieved by myringotomy which equalized the air pressure on each side of the tympanic membrane and restored the patient's hearing. Cooper was awarded the Copley Medal of the Royal Society, the highest honor the Society could bestow, for noteworthy contributions to medical knowledge. The present volume was written while Cooper was a surgeon at Guy's and Travers a vascular and ophthalmic surgeon at St. Thomas'.

Garrison-Morton 5587 (1st London ed., 1818–1819); Waller 2116 (2nd London ed., 1818–1820).

741. Sir ASTLEY PASTON COOPER. *A treatise on dislocations and fractures of the joints.* 2nd American from the 6th London ed. Boston: Lilly & Wait and Carter & Hendee [etc.], 1832. 516 [38] pp., 34 plates (part fold.). 22.6 cm.

First published in 1822, this comprehensive treatise on dislocation and fractures enjoyed a popular reputation, passing through nine British and two American editions.

Cushing C396; Waller 2107; Wellcome II, p. 387 (2nd London ed., 1823).

*742. ———. *On the anatomy of the breast.* 2 vols. London: Longman, Orme, Green, Brown, and Longmans, 1840. Text: vii, 193 [64] pp. 32.3 cm. Atlas: 27 plates (part col.). 37.5 cm.

One of Cooper's last works, this somewhat rare text covers the physiology as well as the anatomy of the breast. Many of the accompanying plates are in color, and those in this copy are unusually well-preserved.

Wellcome II, p. 388.

743. WILLIAM POTTS DEWEES (1768–1841). *A compendious system of midwifery chiefly designed to facilitate the inquiries of those who may be pursuing this branch of study.* 2nd ed. Philadelphia: H. C. Carey and I. Lea, 1826. 612 pp., illus. 20.8 cm.

Dewees had already established himself as an outstanding obstetrician by the time he received his medical degree from the University of Pennsylvania, where he later became one of the first professors of midwifery. Dewees was much in demand for his services, and Kelly notes that he "was so famous that no parturient woman of the time considered herself safe in other hands" (Howard A. Kelly, *Dictionary of American medical biography*. New York, 1928. p. 322). His *System of midwifery*, unlike other early American works on the subject, contains a good deal of original material, including several well-executed plates. It ran through twelve editions.

Wellcome II, p. 461 (London ed., 1825).

744. ———. *A treatise on the physical and medical treatment of children*. 2nd ed. Philadelphia: H. C. Carey & I. Lea, 1826. xiv [9]–508 pp. 21.4 cm.

Although chiefly an obstetrician, Dewees also published works on gynecology, general medicine, and this popular treatise on pediatrics, the first American textbook on the subject.

Garrison-Morton 6331 (1st ed., 1825); Waller 2428 (1st ed.); Wellcome II, p. 461 (1832 ed.).

CARL WENZEL (1769–1827). *Über die schwammingen Auswüchse auf der äussern Hirnhaut*.

See No. 738.

———. *De penitiori structura cerebri hominis et brutorum*.

See No. 739.

*745. GEORGES CUVIER (1769–1832). *Leçons d'anatomie comparée de G. Cuvier*. Recueillies et publiées sous ses yeux par C. Duméril. 5 vols. Paris: Baudouin [1800]–1805. 52 plates, 7 fold. tables. 19.8 cm. Contemporary half calf.

A French naturalist and professor of natural history at the Collège de France, Cuvier is generally regarded as the founder of modern comparative anatomy and vertebrate paleontology. He based his work on the essential regularity and orderliness of nature, which led to his theory of the correlation of parts, stating that each part of an organism was necessarily related to the other parts. Although Cuvier recognized and identified distinct sequences of life forms, he was no evolutionist, believing rather that each species was fixed from the beginning and that extinct species and variations observed in fossil forms were caused by a series of supernatural interventions, the latest of which was Noah's flood. Although the influence of Cuvier's authority caused this theory to be widely accepted, delaying the acceptance of Darwin's theory of evolution, his view that an animal's structure was due to its function and habits is common today.

This massive work, a classic in organization and clarity, very largely defined the state of knowledge of comparative anatomy during the early nineteenth century.

Cushing C667; Garrison-Morton 311; Waller 2254; Wellcome II, p. 423.

*746. ———. *Le règne animal distribué d'après son organisation, pour servir de base à l'histoire naturelle des animaux et d'introduction à l'anatomie comparée.* 4 vols. Paris: Déterville, 1817. Plates. 19.4 cm. Quarter cloth and marbled paper.

Cuvier was the first to devise a systematic classification of the animal kingdom. He presented it first in a lecture in 1796 and published it two years later; he continued to expand his work, culminating in these four volumes on the animal kingdom published in 1817. In them, he classified animal life into four main types: Vertebrata, Mollusca, Articulata, and Radiata, thus laying the foundation for the great expansion of comparative anatomy later in the century.

Garrison-Morton 327 (1836–1849) ed.); Waller 14796; Wellcome II, p. 423.

*747. LUIGI SACCO (1769–1836). *Osservazioni pratiche sull' uso del vajuolo vaccino, come preservativo del vajuolo umano.* Milan: Nella Stamperia italiana e francese [1801]. [8] 216 pp., 2 fold. plates. 18.7 cm.

Sacco was Italy's first and most enthusiastic supporter of vaccination and, in this work, the first of three he wrote on the subject, he gives a history of vaccination and his plan for the inoculation of the population of Lombardy. By 1809, 1,400,000 persons had been vaccinated by Sacco or his associates.

Cushing S6; Waller 8374a.

*748. ———. *Trattato di vaccinazione, con osservazioni sul giavardo e vajuolo pecorino.* Milan: Tipografia Mussi, 1809. 223 pp., front. (port.), 4 fold. col. plates. 29.4 cm. Quarter calf.

This treatise on the smallpox vaccination had an enormous effect in swaying professional and public attitude in favor of the procedure. An exceptionally fine portrait of Edward Jenner and four hand-colored plates showing vaccinia pustules add to the beauty of this work.

Waller 8375.

749. SAMUEL THOMSON (1769–1843). *A narrative of the life and medical discoveries of Samuel Thomson.* Boston: Printed for the author by E. G. House, 1822. 182 pp., front. (port.). 17.3 cm.

Through early curiosity and experimentation, Thomson developed a unique curative system based upon the extensive use of vegetables, herbs, and steam. Possessing no formal medical training whatsoever, he became a traveling doctor riding on horseback throughout New England and eventually gained a modest reputation. This small book, combination autobiography and herbal, passed through numerous editions. Copies of the first edition are scarce.

Cushing T96 (1829 ed.); Osler 7773 (1827 ed.).

750. ———. *New guide to health; or, Botanic family physician.* 9th ed. Columbus, Ohio: J. Pike, 1833. 229 pp. 14 cm.

The Thomsonian System, as it was termed, flourished in New England and Canada for over twenty years and was partially embraced by a few prominent physicians, including Benjamin Waterhouse. This guide is the Thomsonian textbook giving detailed descriptions for the selection, preparation, and administration of the vegetables used in treating various maladies.

Osler 4104 (1832 ed.).

*751. ALEXANDER VON HUMBOLDT (1769–1859). *Versuche über die gereizte Muskel- und Nervenfaser.* 2 vols. Posen: Decker, 1797. Vol. I: 495 pp.; Vol. II: 468 pp., 8 plates. 19.2 cm. Marbled boards.

Perhaps the greatest scientist of his time, Humboldt was one of the most famous men in Europe. His immense literary output reflects the quantity and variety of his work, which covered virtually every area of the natural and physical sciences. The present work on electrical physiology, while overshadowed by his accomplishments in other fields, is nonetheless of fundamental significance. Taking as a starting point Galvani's discovery of muscular irritability, Humboldt describes and illustrates his own experiments in this field and translates his findings into the language of practical chemistry.

Cushing H495; Waller 10851; Wellcome III, p. 314.

*752. SAMUEL SCOFIELD (fl. 1810). *A practical treatise on vaccina or cow pock.* New York: Printed by Southwick and Pelsue, for Collins & Perkins, 1810. 139 pp., col. plate. 17.5 cm.

Jenner's work on smallpox inoculation received strong support from Scofield, a physician assigned to the New York City Dispensary and the person responsible for that city's inoculation program. In this work he describes the vaccination procedure and gives an interesting history of its use in various countries.

Austin 1712; Cushing S164.

*753. JULIEN JEAN CÉSAR LEGALLOIS (1770–1814). *Expériences sur le principe de la vie.* Paris: d'Hautel, 1812. xxiv, 364 pp., fold. plate. 19.2 cm.

A pupil of Magendie (see No. 818), Legallois was one of the earliest neurophysiologists. In this, his most celebrated work, he describes the role of the vagus nerve in cardiac and pulmonary functioning, gives the location of the medullary center for respiratory control, and revives the neurogenic theory of the heartbeat, last expounded by Borelli (see No. 315).

Cushing L131; Garrison-Morton 928; Waller 5679; Wellcome III, p. 479.

754. ALEXANDER PHILIP WILSON PHILIP (1770–1851). *A treatise on the nature and cure of those diseases, either acute or chronic, which precede change of structure; with a view to the preservation of health, and, particularly, the prevention of organic diseases.* Baltimore: E. J. Coale, 1831. 328 pp. 21.3 cm.

As one of the most popular physicians in Worcester, England, Philip enjoyed a successful and lucrative practice. He also managed to write a number of medical works on a variety of subjects, those on the therapeutic value of mercury being, perhaps, best known. This work on the diagnosis of various premorbid states was one of Philip's best.

Gift of Dr. Craig D. Ellyson.

*755. XAVIER BICHAT (1771–1802). *Traité des membranes en général et de diverses membranes en particulier.* Paris: Chez Richard, Caille et Ravier [1800]. [8] 326 pp. 19.9 cm.

Bichat deserves the term "one of the fathers of histology." Without benefit of the microscope, this French anatomist and physiologist established a system of normal and pathological structure based on the individual tissues rather than on organs as the important biological units.

This notable contribution to the understanding of tissues is considered by many to be Bichat's best work. His classification and description of the various kinds of membranes led to a better understanding of the nature of disease.

Garrison-Morton 537; Waller 1032 (1802 ed.); Wellcome II, p. 164.

756. ———. *Anatomie générale, appliquée à la physiologie et à la médecine.* 2 pts. in 4 vols. Paris: Chez Brosson, Gabon et Cie, 1801. Part I: cxii, 636 pp., fold. tables; Part II: xxxiii, 828 pp. 20 cm.

In the present work, Bichat presents a detailed description of the body's tissues in their healthy and diseased states. He discovered and named twenty-one kinds of tissues: nervous, vascular, mucous, serous, connective, etc., each considered elemental and having its own vital characteristic. Bichat's work had a significant impact on pathology as well as on clinical medicine. This is an important book, since it is a palpable step toward modern medicine.

Cushing B371; Garrison-Morton 403; Osler 1301; Waller 1027; Wellcome II, p. 164.

*757. ———. *Traité d'anatomie descriptive.* 5 vols. Paris: Gabon [et] Brosson, 1801–1803. 20.4 cm. Half calf, gilt spine.

Bichat died of tuberculosis at the age of thirty-one, having finished the first three volumes of this, his last great work. François Régis Buisson (1776–1805?) compiled the fourth volume and Philibert-Joseph Roux (1780–1854) the fifth.

Garrison-Morton 404; Osler 1302; Waller 1031; Wellcome II, p. 164.

*758. ———. *Pathological anatomy.* Translated from the French by Joseph Togno. Philadelphia: J. Grigg, 1827. 232 pp. 21.9. cm.

Although Bichat erroneously believed that each tissue had a specific and unique life-giving property, he held correctly that the disease of a tissue is essentially the

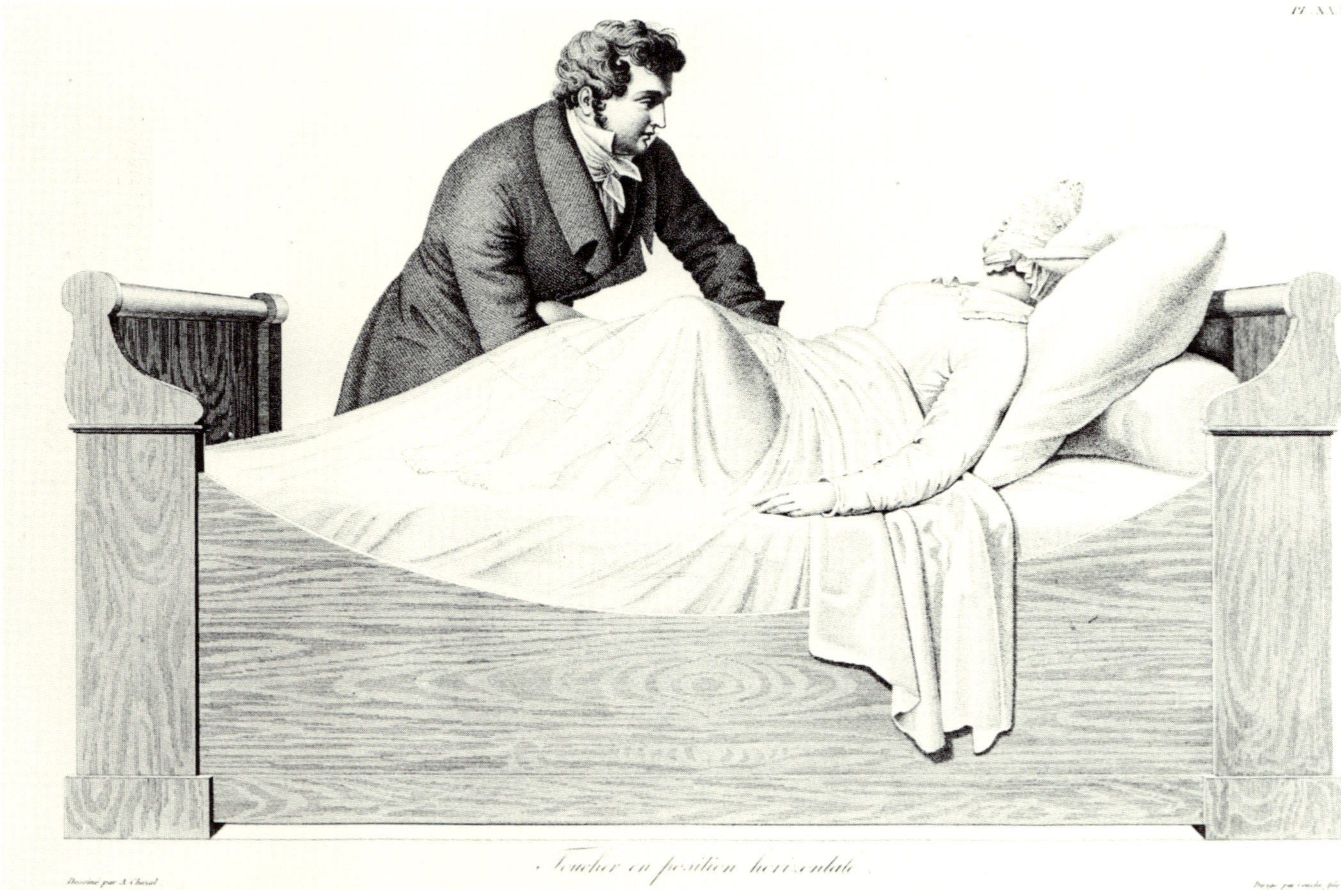

No. 759. Maygrier. *Nouvelles Démonstrations d'Accouchemens.* The man-midwife performs a prenatal examination.

same, in whatever organ it may be located. His observations are set forth in this, the last of his works, which may be regarded as a summary of his work in pathology.

Cushing B372.

*759. JACQUES PIERRE MAYGRIER (1771–1835). *Nouvelles démonstrations d'accouchemens, avec des planches en taille-douce.* Paris: Béchet, 1822. x, 80 pp., 79 (misnumbered 80) plates. 41 cm. Half polished calf.

Maygrier was one of a number of French obstetricians who followed the tradition of Jean Louis Baudelocque (see No. 664) in refining the science of midwifery. This textbook contains a series of eighty large engravings, most of which were drawn by Antoine Chazal (1793–1854). They cover virtually every phase of childbirth including pelvic deformities, pelvimetry, transverse presentations, cesarean section, the use of forceps, and even a section on infant feeding and lactation. Many of the illustrations were used again or adapted by later authors.

Cushing M230 (1840 ed.); Waller 6375.

760. ELISHA NORTH (1771–1843). *A treatise on a malignant epidemic, commonly called spotted fever.* New York: T. & J. Swords, 1811. xi, 249 pp. 20 cm.

North, a Connecticut native, received his medical education by studying with local physicians and with the noted Hartford physician, Lemuel Hopkins (1750–1801). He also studied for two years at the University of Pennsylvania but did not graduate. In 1817, he established the first eye infirmary in America at New London, where he enjoyed great success in treating diseases of the eye. Besides being one of the pioneers in the study of vaccination, North was one of the first to study cerebrospinal meningitis (at that time referred to as spotted fever) when it appeared in this country in 1807. The disease had only been recognized in Geneva in 1805, and this early American medical classic was the first book to be written on the subject. In it, North details his extensive experience with the disease and gives his views and methods of treatment as well as the views of other medical authorities around the country.

Austin 1425; Cushing N115; Garrison-Morton 4676; Osler 3507; Waller 6905.

Gift of Charles R. Baker.

761. JAMES MEASE (1771–1846). *An inaugural dissertation on the disease produced by the bite of a mad dog, or other rabid animal.* Philadelphia: Printed by T. Dobson, 1792. [6] 130 pp. 18.4 cm. Original calf.

Philanthropist, antiquarian, geologist, penologist, and physician, Mease was a notable figure in early nineteenth century America and was at the forefront of many of the intellectual and humanitarian causes of his time. He contracted yellow fever while combating epidemics, helped found the Philadelphia Athenaeum (an early public library), and led the fight for systematic instruction of pharmacists.

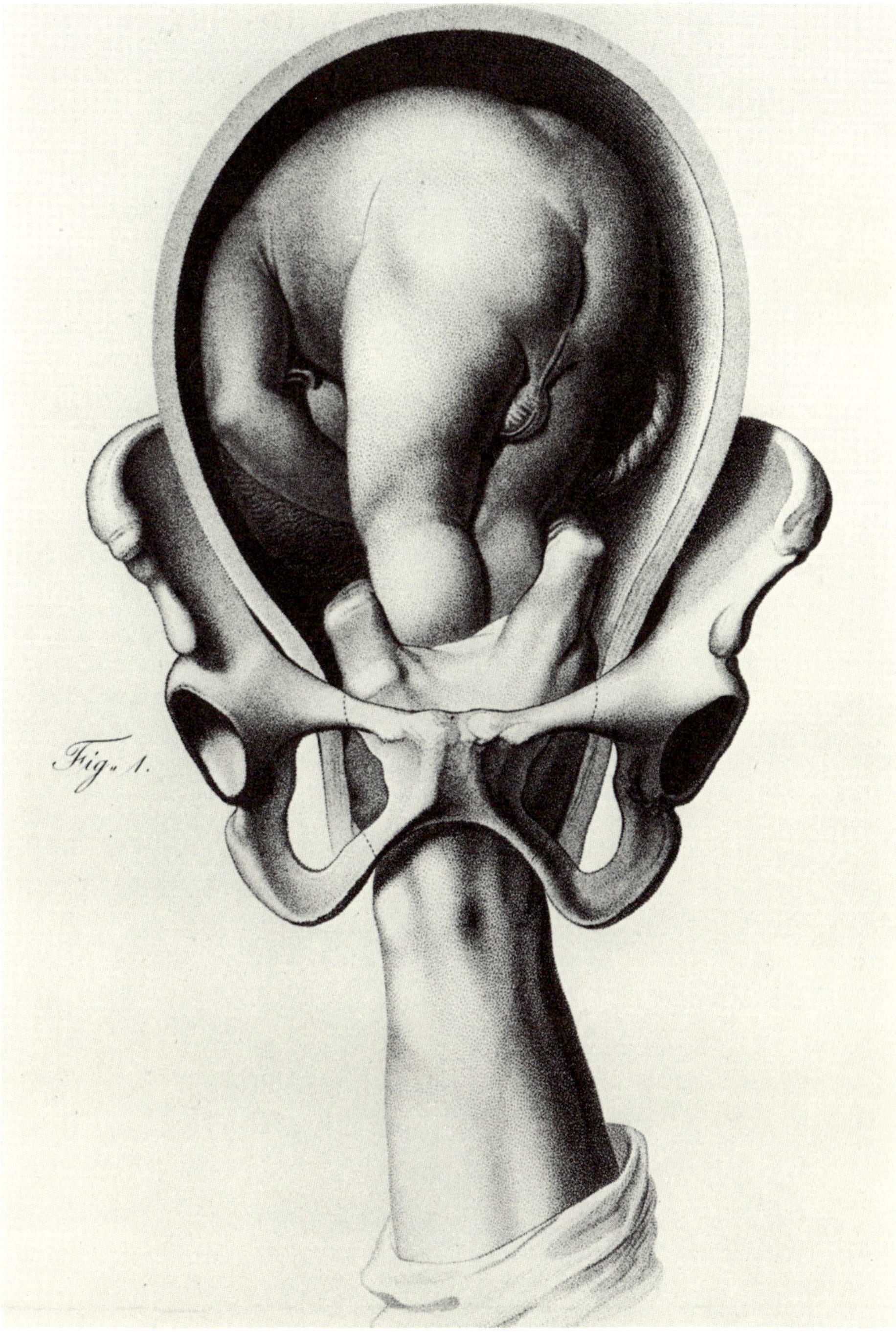

No. 759. Maygrier. *Nouvelles Démonstrations d'Accouchemens.* Podalic version and extraction.

This is Mease's first work on rabies, a subject on which he continued to write throughout his life. He was particularly active in exposing quackery in supposed cures of the dreaded disease.

Austin 1247; Cushing M252.

762. JOHN BLACKALL (1771–1860). *Observations on the nature and cure of dropsies.* 1st American from the 3rd London ed. Philadelphia: James Webster, 1820. xxii, 274 pp. 20.9 cm.

Blackall, physician to the Devon and Exeter Hospital, was one of the first to call attention to albuminuria in connection with dropsy. This work also includes several descriptions of angina pectoris.

Austin 208; Garrison-Morton 2209 (1st London ed., 1813); Waller 1097 (1825 ed.); Wellcome II, p. 173 (1st London ed.).

763. ANDREW DUNCAN (1772–1832). *The Edinburgh new dispensatory . . . including tr. of the Edinburgh pharmacopoeia, the Dublin pharmacopoeia and the London pharmacopoeia . . . from the eighth and last Edinburgh ed.* New York: James Eastburn, 1818. 793 pp. 20.4 cm. Modern cloth.

William Lewis (see No. 579 ff.) compiled the first edition of the *New dispensatory* in 1753. During the next century, the *New dispensatory* and its progeny, the *Edinburgh new dispensatory*, appeared in some thirty-five English, six American, and twelve foreign language editions or issues of one kind or another. Commonly referred to as the "Edinburgh Dispensatory," the various issues can be grouped into three main series. The present work falls into the third series which covers some twelve editions (1803–1830) and was edited by Duncan. Duncan was professor at Edinburgh and for many years editor of the *Edinburgh medical and surgical journal.* The dispensatory here was edited by Jacob Dyckman (1788–1822), a New York physician, who enlarged and adapted it to the American materia medica.

Austin 1148.

764. FRANÇOIS JOSEPH VICTOR BROUSSAIS (1772–1838). *A treatise on physiology applied to pathology.* Translated from the French, by John Bell and R. La Roche. Philadelphia: H. C. Carey and I. Lea, 1826. viii, 559 pp. 21.1 cm.

Surgeon of the armies of France and professor of general pathology at Paris, Broussais was the most celebrated French practitioner of his day, and, according to Castiglioni, the "most sanguinary physician in history" (Arturo Castiglioni, *A history of medicine.* New York, 1946. p. 699). Although he taught the importance of clinical observation, Broussais' rigid attitudes regarding his often erroneous theories hindered more often than helped the progress of French medicine. Broussais believed that the basis of all pathology was gastroenteritis and that debilitating treatment was called for in nearly every disease. His most common remedy was the application of leeches to the stomach or the head. The popularity of his methods is evidenced by the fact that during one year, over 35,000,000 leeches were imported into France.

This work on physiology, which incorporates many of Broussais' imaginative theories on the origin and nature of disease, was first published in France in 1822–1823.

Wellcome II, p. 248 (French ed., 1822–1823).

765. ———. *De l'irritation et de la folie.* Brussels: Librairie Polymathique, 1828. 56, xix, 431 pp., front. (port.). 20.2 cm.

". . . Although his follower, Bouillaud, was moved to let even greater torrents of blood, students had already begun to edge away from the elder vampire, whose extravagances were finally exploded by the good sense and temperate judgment of the clinician, Chomel, the statistical inductions of his pupil Louis and the sarcasms of Laennec, who slyly likened Broussais to Paracelsus" (Fielding H. Garrison, *An introduction to the history of medicine.* 4th ed. Philadelphia, 1929. p. 410).

Thus discredited, Broussais turned his attention to the field of mental illness. This treatise on irritation and insanity was written after he became president of the Society for Phrenology and is one of his last and lesser works.

Waller 1495; Wellcome II, p. 248.

FLORIANO CALDANI (1772–1836). *Icones anatomicae.*

See No. 605.

*766. JEAN ÉTIENNE DOMINIQUE ESQUIROL (1772–1840). *Des maladies mentales considérées sous les rapports médical, hygiénique et médico-légal.* 2 vols. Brussels: J. B. Tircher, 1838. Vol. I: vii, 393 pp; Vol. II: vi, 380 pp., 27 plates (1 fold.). 22.6 cm. Polished calf, gilt borders and spine.

As Pinel's most outstanding pupil, Esquirol so closely followed his teacher's works that the contributions of the two men are sometimes confused. Like Pinel, Esquirol did not attempt to analyze mental illness from a philosophical standpoint but sought to classify and describe the various kinds of insanity he encountered in his practice. Esquirol coined the term "monomania," a concept which anticipated the modern view of schizophrenia, and he was the first to distinguish hallucination from illusion. While at Salpêtrière, where he succeeded Pinel as chief physician, Esquirol introduced formal instruction in psychiatry and gained support for Pinel's humanitarian reform movements by lecturing throughout Europe.

Des maladies mentales, the work for which he is best known, served as a basic text in psychiatry for over fifty years.

Garrison-Morton 4798 (Paris ed., 1838); Waller 2817; Wellcome II, p. 531.

767. ROBERT HOOPER (1773–1835). *A compendious medical dictionary.* London: Printed for Murray and Highley, 1799. Unpaged. 17.9 cm.

Hooper was a successful London physician whose writings included works on

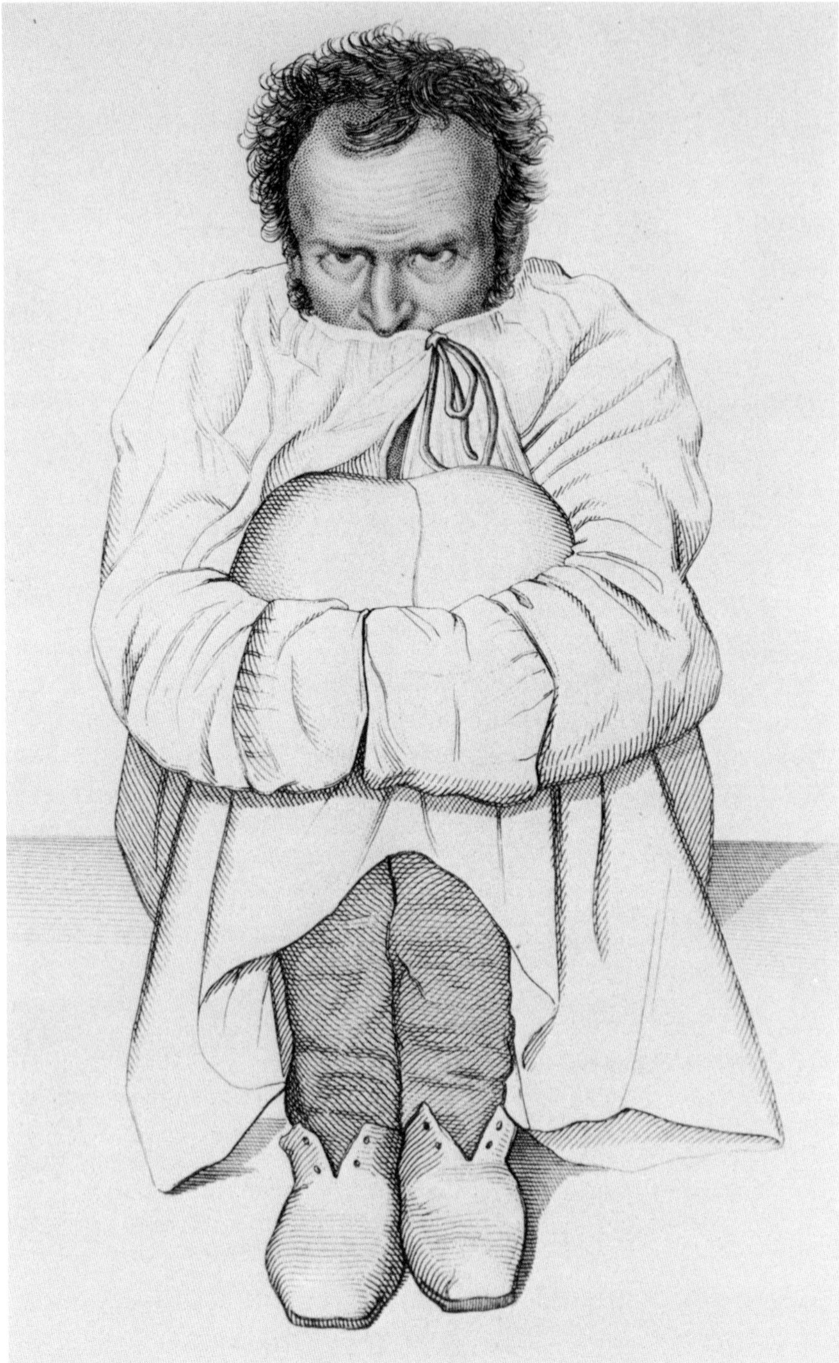

No. 766. Esquirol. *Des Maladies Mentales*.

botany, anatomy, and epidemiology. His medical dictionary was the most popular of the day, passing through numerous English and American editions.

Waller (1825 ed.); Wellcome III, p. 297 (1801 ed.).

*768. MARIE ANNE VICTOIRE BOIVIN (née GILLAIN) (1773–1841). *Mémorial de l'art des accouchemens.* 2nd ed. Paris: Chez Méquignon, 1817. xxxii, 398 pp., 4 fold. tables, 136 plates. 19.7 cm. Inscribed by the author.

Mme. Boivin, one of the most famous of the Paris midwives, made improvements on the vaginal speculum and wrote on hydatidiform mole. This and her other books were in sufficient esteem to go through several editions, and were used as texts at l'École d'Accouchemens.

Garrison-Morton 6165 (1st ed., 1812); Wellcome II, p. 195 (1st ed.).

769. JOHANN CHRISTIAN AUGUST HEINROTH (1773–1843). *System der psychisch-gerichtlichen Medizin.* Leipzig: C. H. F. Hartmann, 1825. xiv, 554 pp. 19.7 cm.

A pupil and disciple of Pinel, Heinroth was the first to bring mental institute reform to Germany. He divided his classification of the various types of mental illness into those affecting the feeling, the understanding, and the will. His acknowledged leadership of the spiritual school of psychiatry in Germany resulted in his being given a special chair of psychological medicine at Leipzig in 1811. This book on the medico-legal aspects of insanity is one of the first German works on the subject.

Garrison-Morton 1736.

*770. ALEXANDER MONRO (1773–1859). *Observations on the different kinds of small pox.* Edinburgh: Printed for A. Constable, 1818. vi, 281 [2] pp. 20.4 cm. Quarter-bound polished calf.

The last member of the famous Monro dynasty, Alexander Monro *tertius* did not rank with his father or grandfather as a teacher or scientist, choosing instead to make use of the notes handed down to him but adding little original work. His monograph on smallpox offers a history of the disease, a summary of the state of its treatment at the time, and a discussion on the effectiveness of vaccination.

771. ———. *The anatomy of the urinary bladder and perineum of the male.* Edinburgh: Maclachlan, Stewart & Co., 1842. ix, 90 pp., 5 plates. 21.9 cm.

This well-written anatomy of the male pelvic viscera was produced while Monro was professor of anatomy at the University of Edinburgh. The five engravings were taken from drawings made by E. Clarke, a pupil of Monro's.

*772. JOHN REDMAN COXE (1773–1864). *Practical observations on vaccination.* Philadelphia: Printed by James Humphreys, 1802. 152 pp., hand-col. front., 2 fold. tables. 23.1 cm. Original boards.

After studying medicine at Edinburgh and London, Coxe returned to his native Philadelphia, where he studied with Benjamin Rush (see No. 665) and eventually obtained his medical degree from the University of Pennsylvania. He was a personal favorite of Rush with whom he fought a yellow fever epidemic in 1793. Coxe did much to dispel ignorance and prejudice against vaccination in that area and was the first to use it in Philadelphia, inoculating both himself and his son, Edward Jenner Coxe.

The present work on vaccination was his first major medical treatise and appeared only four years after Jenner's celebrated work on the subject (see No. 677). He strongly supports the arguments for vaccination and presents many of his experiences and observations.

Austin 557; Cushing C457; Garrison-Morton 5425.

773. ———. *The American dispensatory*. Philadelphia: Printed by A. Bartram for Thomas Dobson, 1806. xvl, 787 pp., 6 plates. 21.7 cm.

Coxe was appointed professor of chemistry at the University of Pennsylvania in 1809 and was transferred in 1818 to the chair of materia medica and pharmacy. Active in the field even before joining the University, he is regarded by many as the father of pharmacy in Philadelphia. He introduced the jalap plant into this country and developed Coxe's hive syrup which he compounded largely with syrup of squill. The present work is one of the earliest American drug compendia.

Austin 552; Wellcome II, p. 402 (1818 ed.).

*774. ———. *An inquiry into the claims of Doctor William Harvey to the discovery of the circulation of the blood.* Philadelphia: C. Sherman, 1834. 258 pp. 22.4 cm.

Coxe objected to Harvey's receiving sole credit for discovering the circulation of the blood, and in this work he brings the reader's attention to the important contributions made by Galen, Servetus, Vesalius, and others in the understanding of the circulatory system.

Cushing C456; Osler 749.

*775. GASPARD LAURENT BAYLE (1774–1816). *Recherches sur la phthisie pulmonaire.* Paris: Gabon, 1810. xxiv, 439 pp. 19.9 cm.

Bayle studied both theology and law before turning his attention to medicine. During his lengthy tenure as Army physician and later as physician to the Charité, he made numerous investigations into the nature of tuberculosis. Bayle recognized and described six different kinds of consumption, was the first to use the term "miliary" in describing small tubercles, and successfully related tuberculosis of the lung to the same disease in other parts of the body. His efforts culminated in the present work which is generally accepted to have been the basis of Laennec's research.

Garrison-Morton 2322; Waller 798; Wellcome II, p. 121.

776. JEAN MARIE GASPARD ITARD (1774–1838). *Traité des maladies de l'oreille et de l'audition*. 2nd ed. 2 vols. Paris: Librairie médicale de Méquignon-Marvis fils, 1842. Vol. I: xxxii, 451 pp.; Vol. II: 538 pp., 3 fold. plates. 20.5 cm.

Itard was surgeon at Val de Grâce in Paris and later physician at the Institute for Deaf Mutes. Among his pioneering achievements were the invention of the eustachian catheter (Itard's catheter) and the publication of this, the first modern textbook devoted exclusively to diseases of the ear.

Garrison-Morton 3364 (1st ed., 1821); Waller 5080 (1st ed.); Wellcome III, p. 334.

*777. Sir CHARLES BELL (1774–1842). *Engravings of the arteries, illustrating the second volume of The anatomy of the human body, by J. Bell, Surgeon*. London: Printed by C. Whittingham, for T. N. Longman and O. Rees [etc.], 1801. 49 [2] pp., 10 col. plates. 25.4 cm. Calf, gilt rules and back.

Sir Charles Bell, a Scottish surgeon and anatomist, was one of the greatest scientists in medical history. Educated at the University of Edinburgh, he spent the major part of his professional career in London before returning to his alma mater as professor of surgery for the last few years of his life. Among his many contributions to medical science may be included his establishment of the existence of motor and sensory nerves and his showing the relationships of nerves to different parts of the brain and to different functions. All his discoveries were, in his own phrase, "deductions from anatomy." In addition to his preeminence as an anatomist, physiologist, neurologist, and surgeon, Bell was also an accomplished artist. All the drawings for the illustrations in his books were made by him, and they stand unrivaled for their facility, elegance, and accuracy.

This volume of engravings was intended, as the title states, to illustrate the work of Sir Charles' brother, John Bell (see No. 727 ff.), who had himself done the drawings to illustrate the first volume. The delicate shading and tinting of these engravings make it a work of beauty as well as of practical value for its painstaking detail and accuracy.

Wellcome II, p. 135.

*778. ———. [*Manuscript drawings of the arteries*]. New York: Editions Medicina Rara, 1971. [48] pp., 12 col. plates (part fold.). 26.7 cm. In slipcase. A facsimile.

Bell's original manuscript with colored drawings of the arteries is now in the National Library of Medicine in Bethesda, Maryland. The manuscript contains twelve vividly colored plates with holographic explanations for each. The drawings were probably made about 1798, and apparently were intended to illustrate Volume II of *The anatomy of the human body* (see No. 727), by Charles' older brother, John. Volume I of this work had appeared in 1797.

*779. ———. *The anatomy of the brain, explained in a series of engravings*. London: T. N. Longman and O. Rees [etc.], 1802. vii, 87 pp., 12 plates (11 col.). 28.6 cm. Rebound in modern buckram. Bound with No. 780.

In this work Bell displays both his descriptive and artistic capabilities. The twelve aquatint plates (eleven of them hand-colored) were engraved by Thomas Medland after Bell's own drawings and constitute what is probably Bell's most beautiful work on neuroanatomy and one of the most beautifully illustrated in the entire literature.

Cushing B264; Waller 860; Wellcome II, p. 135.

*780. ———. *A series of engravings, explaining the course of the nerves*. London: T. N. Longman and O. Rees [etc.], 1803. 49 pp., 9 plates (3 fold.). 28.6 cm. Rebound in modern buckram. Bound with No. 779.

This is a continuation of the work of Sir Charles' elder brother John's *Engravings of the bones, muscles and joints.* As with all of Bell's work, the nine plates in this volume are engraved after the author's own drawings and are notable for their detail and accuracy.

Cushing B264; Waller 849; Wellcome II, p. 135.

*781. ———. *Essays on the anatomy of expression in painting*. London: Printed for Longman, Hurst, Rees, and Orme, 1806. xii, 186 pp., illus., plates. 28.3 cm. Half calf and marbled paper.

In the opening Advertisement Bell states: "Anatomy stands related to the arts of design, as the grammar of that language in which they address us. The expressions, attitudes, and movements of the human figure, are the characters of this language; which is adapted to convey the effect of historical narration, as well as to show the working of human passion, and give the most striking and lively indications of intellectual power and energy." Both the text and the numerous illustrations in this unusual book make fascinating reading, and they drew the attention and praise of no less a person than Charles Darwin.

Choulant-Frank, p. 343; Cushing B257; Osler 1991 (1824 ed.); Wellcome II, p. 135.

*782. ———. *A system of operative surgery, founded on the basis of anatomy*. 2 vols. London: Printed for Longman, Hurst, Rees, and Orme, 1807–1809. Vol. I: xxxii, 448 pp., illus., 14 plates; Vol. II: xxiv, 385 pp., illus., 7 plates. 22.9 cm.

This work is a treatise on general surgery, largely from the anatomical point of view. The author was as much artist as anatomist and surgeon; typically, the book is illustrated by Bell himself, with twenty-one plates and ninety-three text figures.

Garrison-Morton 5583; Waller 851; Wellcome II, p. 136.

———. *Anatomy of the human body.*

See No. 727.

*783. ———. *Letters concerning the diseases of the urethra.* London: Printed for John Murray, 1810. xi, 149 pp., 6 plates. 20.9 cm. Contemporary calf, rebacked.

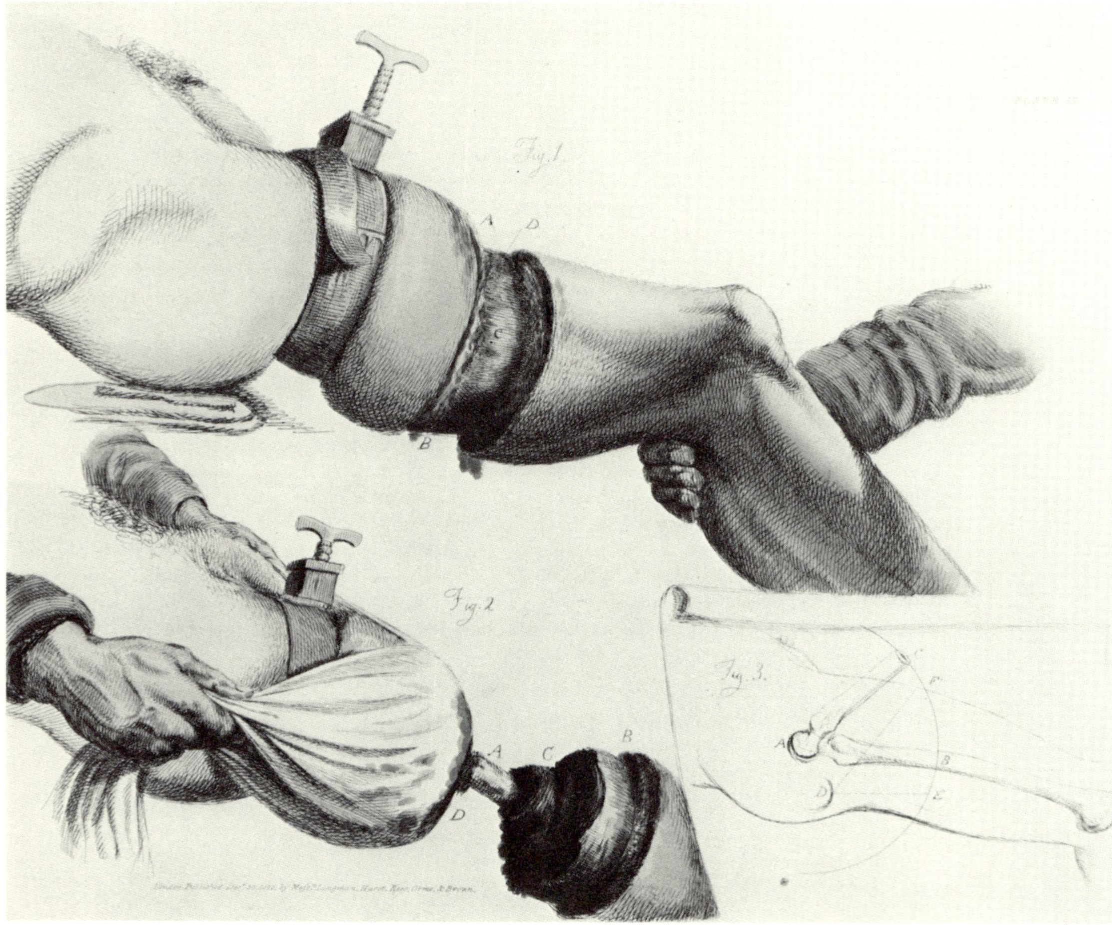

No. 785. Sir Charles Bell. *Illustrations of the Great Operations of Surgery*. Midthigh amputation with preservation of the skin flap.

Here, in a series of three letters, Bell presents his observations on various types of strictures in the urethra. He differentiates between simple, bridle, dilatable, spasmodic, callous, and ulcerated types of strictures and discusses their diagnosis, etiology, prognosis, and treatment. All six plates were drawn by Bell, and two were also etched by him.

Cushing B262 (Boston ed., 1811); Wellcome II, p. 136.

*784. ———. *An essay on the forces which circulate the blood; being an examination of the differences of the motions of the fluids in living and dead vessels.* London: Printed for Messrs. Longman and Co., 1819. viii, 83 pp. 17.5 cm.

A monograph of only eighty-three small pages, this book shows Bell to be not only a remarkable surgeon and artist, but a most literate and gracious writer as well. It is dedicated to Dr. John Abernethy (see No. 731).

Wellcome II, p. 136.

*785. ———. *Illustrations of the great operations of surgery: trepan, hernia, amputation, aneurism, and lithotomy.* London: Longman, Hurst, Rees, Orme, and Brown, 1821. viii, 134 pp., illus., 19 col. plates. 27 cm.

The surgical techniques herein described are surprisingly modern. The illustrations, drawn by the author, are mostly colored and are exceptionally graphic and instructive.

Cushing B260; Waller 857; Wellcome II, p. 136.

*786. ———. *Observations on injuries of the spine and of the thigh bone; in two lectures.* London: T. Tegg, 1824. xv, 101 pp., illus., 9 plates (2 fold.). 30.8 cm.

The text of these two lectures is, as usual, in Bell's typical lucid style, and the nine plates, drawn by the author, are remarkably effective. The first lecture is given over to a criticism of some views by another famous surgeon of Bell's time, Sir Astley Cooper (see No. 740). The second lecture is in support of his brother, John Bell, recently deceased, certain of whose findings had been claimed by Sir Astley Cooper as his own.

Wellcome II, p. 136.

787. ———. *The nervous system of the human body. Embracing the papers delivered to the Royal Society on the subject of the nerves.* London: Longman, Rees [etc.], 1830. xxiii, 238, clxxvi pp., 9 plates. 28.6 cm.

This work, containing nearly all of Bell's most important observations on the nervous system, includes his discovery of "Bell's palsy" and the first description of myotonia as well as two important essays, both taken from the *Philosophical transactions* of the Royal Society of London: "On the relations between the nerves of motion and of sensation, and the brain" and "On the functions of some parts of

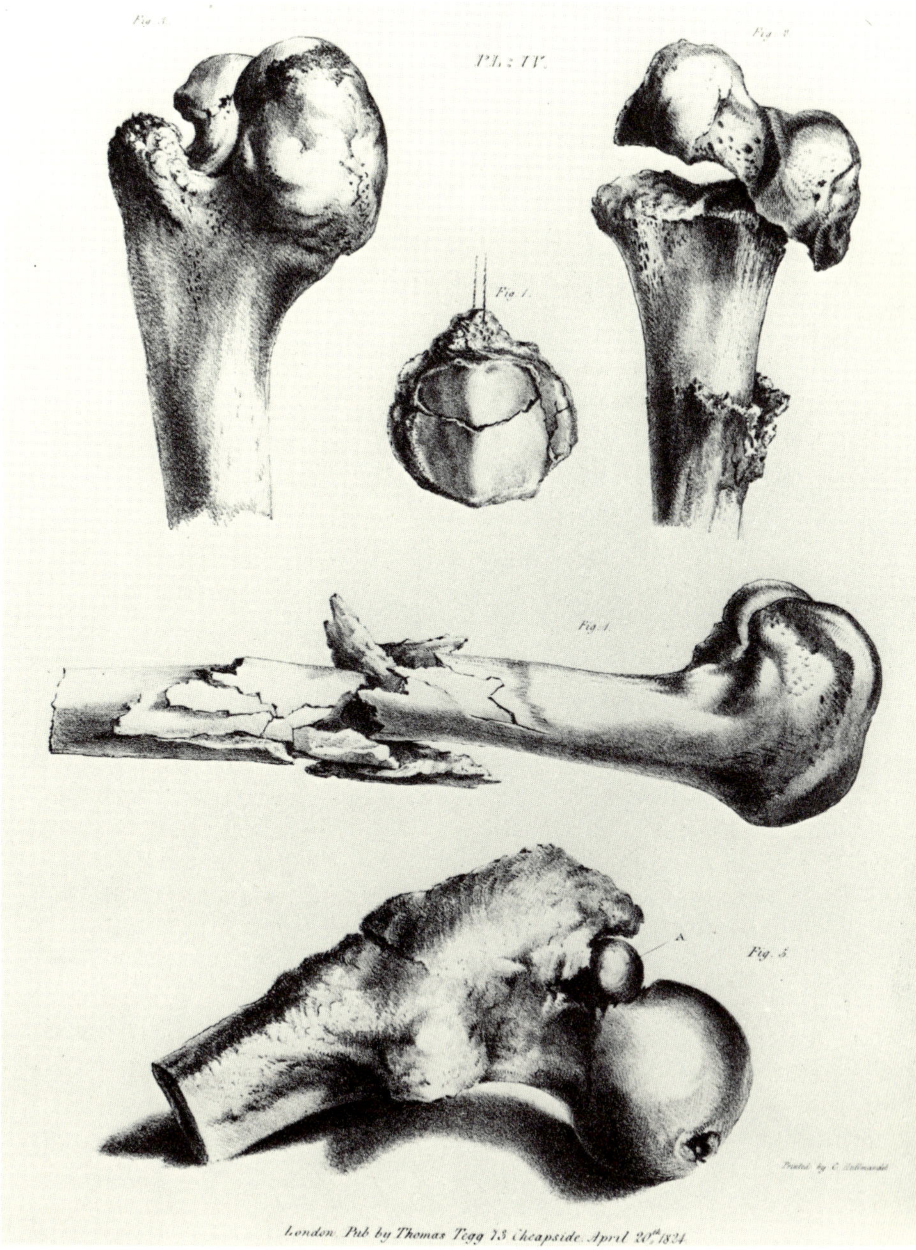

No. 786. Sir Charles Bell. *Observations on Injuries of the Spine and of the Thigh Bone.*

the brain, and on the relations between the brain and nerves of motion and sensation."

Cushing B263; Garrison-Morton 1258; Waller 862; Wellcome II, p. 136 (1844 ed.).

*788. ———. *The hand; its mechanism and vital endowments as evincing design*. London: W. Pickering, 1833. xvi, 314 pp., illus. 21.6 cm.

This monograph on the human hand, considered from the standpoint of comparative anatomy, is unusual and perhaps unique: illustrated by the author, written in clear language, and appealing to the non-scientific mind as well as to the anatomist. It was written as the fourth of eight treatises provided for under the terms of the will of the eighth Earl of Bridgewater, who left £8,000 for a series of scientific works called *The Bridgewater treatises on the power, wisdom and goodness of God, as manifested in the creation* (see No. 830). Bell's work was the best known of the Bridgewater Treatises and was frequently reprinted.

Cushing B258 (1834 ed.); Osler 1994 (1834 ed.); Waller 861 (1837 ed.); Wellcome II, p. 136.

*789. JOHN BURNS (1774–1850). *Obstetrical works*. New York: Collins and Perkins, 1809. viii, 256 pp., 2 plates (1 fold.). 21.1 cm.

Burns, educated at the universities of Glasgow and Edinburgh, was the first professor of surgery in Glasgow's school of medicine. At the time of his appointment in 1815, Burns had already had several years teaching experience at Anderson's College in Glasgow and had given clinical lectures in conjunction with his duties as surgeon to the Royal Infirmary. He was highly successful as a teacher and his classes drew large numbers of medical students. He wrote widely and at least two of his books on surgery and midwifery attained great popularity, going through numerous editions and being translated into several foreign languages.

The present volume contains his major obstetrical works: *The anatomy of the gravid uterus*, *Observations on abortion*, and *Practical observations on the uterine hemorrhage*.

Austin 360.

790. JULIEN JOSEPH VIREY (1775–1846). *Histoire naturelle du genre humain*. 3 vols. Paris: Crochard, 1824. Vol. I: [4] iii [1] xl, 514 pp.; Vol. II: [4] iii [1] 431 pp.; Vol. III: [4] iii [1] 534 [2] pp., plates (part col.). 20.4 cm.

Virey, French physician and biologist, was for many years chief pharmacist at Val de Grâce Hospital in Paris. An individual with wide interests, he taught, did research, and wrote a large number of books. Many of his writings were on philosophy and natural history although he also wrote several works on chemistry and pharmacy. This work, tracing the natural history of man, was first published in 1800.

*791. JOSEPH FOX (1776–1816). *The natural history and diseases of the human teeth.* 2nd ed. 2 vols. in 1. London: Printed for E. Cox, 1814. Vol. I: x, 100 pp., 13 plates; Vol. II: 179 pp., 10 plates. 28.5 cm.

As the first lecturer on dentistry at Guy's Hospital, Fox had an enormous impact on early nineteenth century dental practices. Though much of his theory of oral physiology and pathology was of dubious value, his operative procedures remained in vogue for more than fifty years. This treatise was, in its day, the most complete work of its kind and was the first to give specific operative procedures for correcting dental irregularities.

Garrison-Morton 3979 (1st ed., 1803); Waller 10626 (French ed., 1821); Wellcome II, p. 50.

*792. JOHANN GASPAR SPURZHEIM (1776–1832). *Phrenology: or, The doctrine of the mind, and of the relations between its manifestations and the body.* 3rd ed. London: C. Knight, 1825. viii, 303 pp. [15] leaves of plates. 21.5 cm.

Spurzheim's place in medical history, like that of his teacher-collaborator, Franz Josef Gall (see No. 711), is largely within the realm of pseudoscience. Together they invented and advanced the "science" of phrenology, a concept holding that the moral, sexual, and intellectual traits of an individual are linked to corresponding protuberances of the brain which in turn manifest themselves as lumps on the skull. After propagandizing with Gall throughout Europe, Spurzheim traveled to America where he found many adherents to the new theory, leading to the formation of secret phrenological societies throughout the country. Although phrenology was eventually discredited, the theory that the functions of the brain are localized within the cerebrum must justly be considered a major contribution to anatomy and physiology.

Spurzheim produced several English works on phrenology. In this book he presents the major tenets of the science, such as the belief that the brain is an "aggregation of organs," including such parts as the "organ of self-esteem," "organ of marvelousness," "organ of ideality," etc. Drawings of appropriately shaped craniums are included to demonstrate the dominance of the various traits and their corresponding protuberances.

Cushing S374.

———. *Anatomie et physiologie du système nerveux en général.*

See No. 712.

*793. GEORGE BELL (1777–1832). *A treatise on the cow-pox.* Edinburgh: Printed for W. Laing, 1802. 115 pp., 2 col. plates. 19.3 cm.

This scarce work, appearing four years after the epochal book on smallpox by Edward Jenner (see No. 677), includes the history of cowpox, its role in smallpox inoculation, and the methods of procuring and preparing the cowpox virus for inoculation. The two colored plates show the distinction between genuine and spurious cowpox. The author was the son of the noted surgeon, Benjamin Bell (see No. 671 ff.).

Cushing B270; Wellcome II, p. 137.

*794. DAVID DANIEL DAVIS (1777–1841). *Elements of operative midwifery.* London: Printed for Hurst, Robinson, 1825. [7] 345 pp., 20 double plates. 26.7 cm. Contemporary boards, rebacked.

Beginning as a general practitioner in Sheffield, Davis later went to London where he specialized in obstetrics and served as professor of midwifery at the University of London. He was physician-accoucheur at the birth of Queen Victoria in 1819 and was obstetric physician to University College Hospital from 1834 to 1841.

A practical and ingenious obstetrician, he introduced five new varieties of forceps which he describes and illustrates in the present work. The Davis forceps was the favorite instrument of Charles D. Meigs (see No. 865) who praised it highly in his *Obstetrics, the science and the art* (1849). The book contains twenty large lithographs depicting normal and abnormal fetal positions and deliveries, as well as a variety of obstetrical instruments including his new forceps.

Wellcome II, p. 435.

*795. WILLIAM FRÉDÉRIC EDWARDS (1777–1842). *De l'influence des agens physiques sur la vie.* Paris: Crochard, 1824. xvi, 654 pp., 1 fold. plate. 21.1 cm.

Edwards was born of English parents in Jamaica but eventually moved to France where he received his medical degree in 1815. He distinguished himself in a number of fields and founded the science of ethnology, but this classic treatise on environmental physiology constitutes his greatest achievement. Here Edwards describes and documents a mass of experimentation on the effects of air, water, heat, light, temperature, and electricity on the living organism. An English translation of the work was completed in 1832 by the pathologist, Thomas Hodgkin.

Garrison-Morton 1991; Wellcome II, p. 514.

796. JAMES JACKSON (1777–1867). *Letters to a young physician just entering upon practice.* 4th ed. Boston: Phillips, Sampson and Co., 1856. iv, 344 pp. 18.1 cm.

The first chairman of clinical medicine at Harvard and, while still a medical student, an ardent supporter of the newly-developed smallpox vaccination, James Jackson played an important role in the development of medical care and medical education in Massachusetts. Jackson studied under Sir Astley Paston Cooper (see No. 740 ff.) at Guy's Hospital in London where he formed a lasting friendship with another American student, John Collins Warren (see No. 802). Together they cooperated in a number of professional enterprises including the pharmacopoeia of the Massachusetts Medical Society and the founding of the Medical Improvement Society of Boston.

Letters to a young physician, dedicated to Warren, is both a philosophic and practical discourse on the practice of medicine.

Cushing J6 (1855 ed.); Osler 3062 (1855 ed.); Waller 5084 (1855 ed.).

797. ———. *Another letter to a young physician: to which are appended some other medical papers.* Boston: Ticknor and Fields, 1861. xii, 179 pp. 18.5 cm.

Another letter calls into question "whether there is any good to be derived from the practice of medicine" and cautions against the overuse of medicine in the alleviation of pain and disease. Among the appended papers is a fascinating "Memoir on the last sickness of General Washington and its treatment by the attendant physicians."

Cushing J5; Osler 3063.

798. JOHN MURRAY (1778–1820). *A system of materia medica and pharmacy.* 2 vols. Philadelphia: Dobson, 1815. Vol. I: vi [2] 399 pp.; Vol. II: iv, 384 pp. 21.6 cm. Calf.

Murray, a Scottish physician and chemist, taught chemistry, physics, pharmacy, and materia medica in London and Edinburgh. His major works were in these fields, and the present book is a more complete and comprehensive volume intended to replace an earlier work, *Elements of materia medica and pharmacy* (1804). The book was first published in London in 1810 and was designed as a textbook to accompany his lectures. In this first American edition, Nathaniel Chapman (1780–1835), noted professor of materia medica at the University of Pennsylvania, adapted it as a textbook for his lectures and added his notes throughout the text.

Austin 1353.

799. THOMAS BATEMAN (1778–1821). *A practical synopsis of cutaneous diseases, according to the arrangement of Dr. Willan.* 2nd American ed. Philadelphia: James Crissy, 1824. xxii, 320 pp., 1 col. plate. 21.3 cm.

Like Robert Willan (1757–1812), his celebrated teacher and collaborator, Bateman was born in Yorkshire and received his medical degree from Edinburgh. Willan is considered the founder of modern dermatology, and his classification scheme and nomenclature system for skin diseases are still in use today. However, his greatest work, *On cutaneous diseases* (1808), remained unfinished at his death. Bateman completed Willan's work with the present book in 1813. Based on Willan's classification of skin diseases, it became extremely popular, went through many editions, and was widely translated.

Garrison-Morton 4021 (2nd London ed., 1813); Waller 770 (2nd London ed.); Wellcome II, p. 113 (1st London ed., 1813).

*800. ———. *Delineations of cutaneous diseases.* London: Printed for Longman, Hurst, Rees, Orme, and Brown, 1817. vii, ii [72] *ll.,* 72 col. plates, each accompanied by a leaf of descriptive letterpress. 27.1 cm.

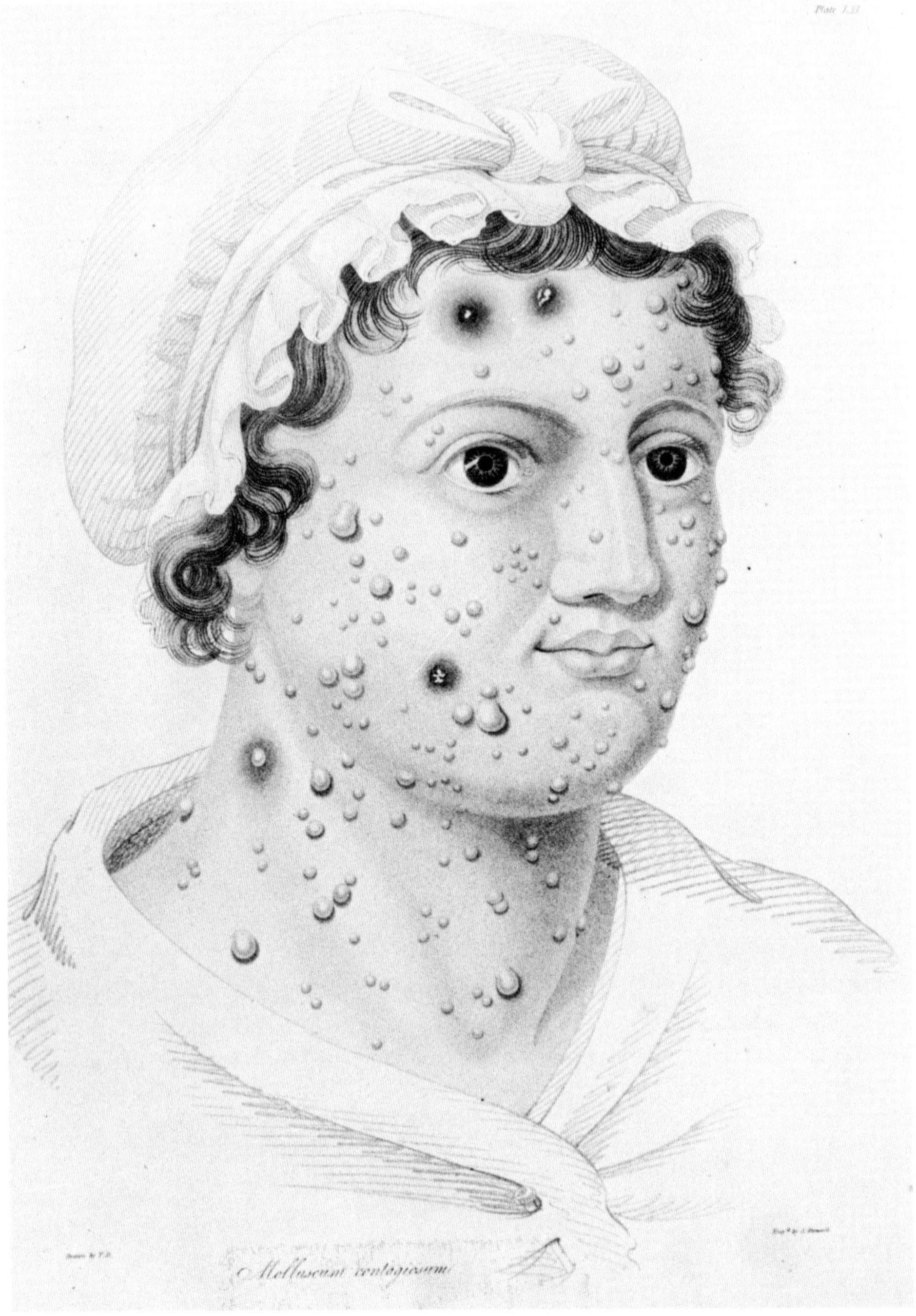

No. 800. Bateman. *Delineations of Cutaneous Diseases.* A young maiden suffering from *Molluscum contagiosum.*

Bateman and Willan worked so closely together that it is difficult, if not impossible, to identify correctly their individual scientific accomplishments. Bateman became, after Willan's death, the most noted dermatologist in London, and his practice and writings became largely dermatological. In addition to completing Willan's *On cutaneous diseases,* Bateman produced this magnificent atlas, which includes Willan's previously unpublished engravings. This compilation of seventy-two colored plates and accompanying description is the first dermatological atlas.

Garrison-Morton 3988; Osler 1963; Wellcome II, p. 114.

*801. FRANZ KARL NAEGELE (1778–1851). *The obliquely contracted pelvis, containing also an appendix of the most important defects of the female pelvis.* New York: [n. publ.] 1939. vi [5] 69 [1] pp., 16 plates (part col.). 28.6 cm.

Naegele was professor and director of the Obstetrical Hospital at Heidelberg, and it was there, in 1839, that he wrote this highly regarded and original work on the obliquely contracted pelvis. The work was of immediate value to practicing obstetricians; the ensuing years have added little information to his original observations. The beautifully rendered lithographs are reproduced faithfully in this, the first edition in English published 100 years later.

Garrison-Morton 6257 (1st German ed., 1839); Waller 6804.

*802. JOHN COLLINS WARREN (1778–1856). *A comparative view of the sensorial and nervous systems in men and animals.* Boston: J. W. Ingraham, 1822. 159 pp., 8 plates (4 fold.). 24.1 cm. Original covers.

John Collins Warren was the son of John Warren (1753–1815), a prominent Revolutionary War surgeon and one of the founders and early professors of the Harvard Medical School. The younger Warren received most of his medical education abroad, studying under the best teachers of his day. He was an excellent surgeon with a number of innovations and techniques to his credit. He was the first to operate for strangulated hernia, he introduced Hunter's operation for aneurysm, and he performed a number of successful operations for cataract. He is best remembered, however, for his tumor surgery for which he gained an international reputation. Warren's name is also linked with the founding of the American Medical Association and the establishment of the *New England journal of medicine and surgery* to which he was a frequent contributor.

This monograph on the comparative anatomy of the nervous system was read before the Massachusetts Medical Society in 1820 when Warren was professor of anatomy and surgery at Harvard. In his Foreword he states that "the want of books containing the previous labors of others is most deeply felt in the consideration of such a subject, on this side of the Atlantic." Several engravings supplement the text.

Cushing W51.

*803. ———. *Surgical observations on tumours, with cases and observations.* London: J. Churchill, 1839. xvi, 607 pp., 16 leaves of plates, col. illus. 23.5 cm. Original blind-stamped cloth.

Most of Warren's work in surgery was done before the era of anesthesia, a fact which makes his contributions in this field the more remarkable. *Surgical observations,* covering the signs, pathology, and excision of tumors, is his best work and attests to the high degree of scholarship and investigation with which he approached his art. The sixteen colored plates are of special interest.

Garrison-Morton 2611.1 (1837 ed.); Osler 4189; Waller 10122.

*804. ———. *Etherization; with surgical remarks.* Boston: W. D. Ticknor, 1848. v, 100 pp. 18.1 cm.

As director of the Massachusetts General Hospital, Warren allowed William Thomas Green Morton (see No. 1000) to perform his celebrated demonstration on the use of ether in surgery. Warren performed the operation (a surgical excision) while Morton served as anesthetist. Warren's support of the new development was in large part responsible for its subsequent worldwide acceptance. In this fascinating booklet, Warren gives a firsthand description of the early use of ether in surgery, including a detailed account of the famous operation mentioned above.

Cushing W53; Waller 10121.

*805. GERARD SANDIFORT (1779–1848). *Tabulae anatomicae.* Leiden: Apud S. et J. Luchtmanns, 1804. [4] 41 pp., 9 plates. 51.3 cm.

Like his celebrated father, Eduard Sandifort (see No. 658), Gerard was an anatomist and physician whose interests lay in the depiction and preservation of pathological specimens. He edited the thick volume of his father's famous *Museum anatomicum* (1793) and later produced the work for which he is best known, *Tabulae craniorum diversarum nationum* (1838–1843), a reproduction of skulls of various nationalities. *Tabulae anatomicae* is an atlas of pathological anatomy depicting the thoracic and abdominal viscera. The copperplates were drawn by the author and engraved by Robert Muys (b. 1742).

Choulant-Frank p. 313.

806. RICHARD CARMICHAEL (1779–1849). *An essay on venereal diseases, and the uses and abuses of mercury in their treatment.* Philadelphia: J. Dobson and A. Sherman, 1825. xiii, 360 pp. 21.5 cm.

Carmichael was one of the most active physicians in Ireland, holding a number of posts at various hospitals and medical schools, including the Richmond Hospital School of Medicine which he helped found. A strong advocate of professional education for physicians, Carmichael sought rigorous standards for physicians and the separation of pharmacy from medicine and surgery.

The present work is one of several which Carmichael wrote on venereal diseases. He made several improvements in treatment, most notably in the administration of mercury.

Austin 417 (1817 ed.); Wellcome II, p. 302 (London ed., 1825).

*807. A. P. BARRÉ (fl. 1820) and JEAN BAPTISTE LOUIS LETELLIER (fl. 1820). *Graphotomie humaine. Recueil lithographique représentant l'anatomie de l'homme; anatomie topographique.* Paris: Crévot, 1826. [4] pp., 40 col. plates. 33.3 cm.

Apparently but little known, this beautifully executed set of forty lithographic plates, partly colored, must have been privately issued in small quantity by the authors, who simply describe themselves as "docteurs en médecine." Index, preface, and explanations of the figures are entirely in lithography. There is no text.

*808. GIAMBATISTA MANFREDINI (fl. 1820). *Delle fasciature chirurgiche, e de' loro congrui apparecchi; trattato teorico-pratico.* 2 vols. Modena: Tipografia Camerale, 1828. Vol. I: [4] viii, 552 pp., Vol. II: [92] pp., 45 plates. 21.9 cm.

In this scarce and little-known work on surgical bandaging, Manfredini presents a comprehensive review of the theory, practice, and use of bandages, compresses, and other surgical apparatus. The second volume, an atlas, contains some 245 figures that illustrate a wide variety of bandages, splints, harnesses, trusses, and other devices for use in all types of medical situations where some type of binding or appliance was needed.

Waller 6212 (1823 ed.).

*809. GEORGE SIMPSON (fl. 1820). *The anatomy of the bones and muscles.* 2 pts. in 1 vol. Pt. I: London: Printed for the author by J. Johnson, 1825. v, iii, 65 pp., 14 plates; Pt. II: 2nd ed. London: Published for the author by J. Williams, 1834. [66]–140 pp., 16 plates. 29.5 cm.

This elegantly printed atlas includes thirty annotated plates (including seventeen life-size drawings) drawn and lithographed by various artists. Simpson, a member of the Royal College of Surgeons, was lecturer on anatomy to the Artist's Anatomical Society. He intended this work to exhibit "the parts as they appear on dissection, and more particularly in the living figure; as applicable to the fine arts. Designed for the use of artists and members of the Artist's Anatomical Society" (from the subtitle).

Choulant-Frank, p. 340.

*810. JOHN ABERCROMBIE (1780–1844). *Pathological and practical researches on diseases of the stomach, the intestinal canal, the liver, and other viscera of the abdomen.* Edinburgh: Printed for Waugh and Innes, 1828. xxiv, 396 pp. 21.3 cm.

Abercrombie, a member of the famous Edinburgh School of the eighteenth and early nineteenth centuries, was the first to treat neuropathology as a separate entity and is best known through his *Pathological and practical researches on diseases of the brain and the spinal cord* (1828). The present work, published in the same year, formed a companion volume in the presentation of his wide and important researches.

Wellcome II, p. 3.

*811. SÉBASTIEN GUILLIÉ (1780–1865). *Essai sur l'instruction des aveugles.* Paris: Imprimé par les aveugles, 1817. 224 pp., illus., front., 21 plates. 21.6 cm.

A native of Bordeaux, Guillié received his degree from the University of Paris in 1807. As a physician at Montolivet Hospital, he embarked on a study of the blind and thereafter devoted his life to this cause. He instituted the first French clinic for the blind in 1818 and helped form a large ophthalmological library in Paris. The present work outlines his methods for instruction of the blind. Various engravings are used to portray the crafts and occupations he thought suitable for his students. The book itself is the work of blind craftsmen.

Cushing G462; Waller 3858; Wellcome III, p. 180.

812. ALLAN BURNS (1781–1813). *Observations on the surgical anatomy of the head and neck.* 1st American ed. Baltimore: F. Lucas, jr., E. J. Coale, and Cushing & Jewett; Philadelphia: H. Carey & I. Lea, 1823. 512 pp., 10 plates. 21 cm.

Burns was one of the first to recognize mitral stenosis as a distinct disease entity, and he gave one of the earliest descriptions of the heart murmur mechanism. This highly regarded surgical treatise was written while Burns was on the anatomy and surgery faculty at Glasgow.

Garrison-Morton 405 (1st Edinburgh ed., 1811); Osler 2189; Waller 1663 (1st Edinburgh ed.); Wellcome II, p. 276 (1st Edinburgh ed.).

*813. RENÉ THÉOPHILE HYACINTHE LAENNEC (1781–1826). *De l'auscultation médiate, ou Traité du diagnostic des maladies des poumons et du coeur.* 2 vols. Paris: J. A. Brosson et J. S. Chaudé, 1819. Vol. I: xlviii, 456 [8] pp., 4 fold. plates; Vol. II: xvi, 472 pp. 20.3 cm.

Laennec was undoubtedly the most prominent French internist of his day. His ingenious use of a roll of paper as a first stethoscope opened an entirely new field of physical diagnosis, and by this means he virtually created the physical diagnosis of pulmonary diseases, giving clear, concise definitions of phthisis, pneumothorax, emphysema, etc. From his teaching came such terms as bronchial breathing; vesicular and cavernous respiration; mucus, bubbling, and sonorous rales; metallic tinkle; and egophony. Ironically, cirrhosis (his term) of the liver ("Laennec's cirrhosis") is perhaps more often associated with Laennec than the fact that his invention of the stethoscope was the most important advance in physical diagnosis between Auenbrugger's introduction of percussion in 1761 and Roentgen's discovery of X-rays in 1895.

Several folding plates in this landmark volume illustrate the construction of Laennec's primitive tubular wood stethoscope.

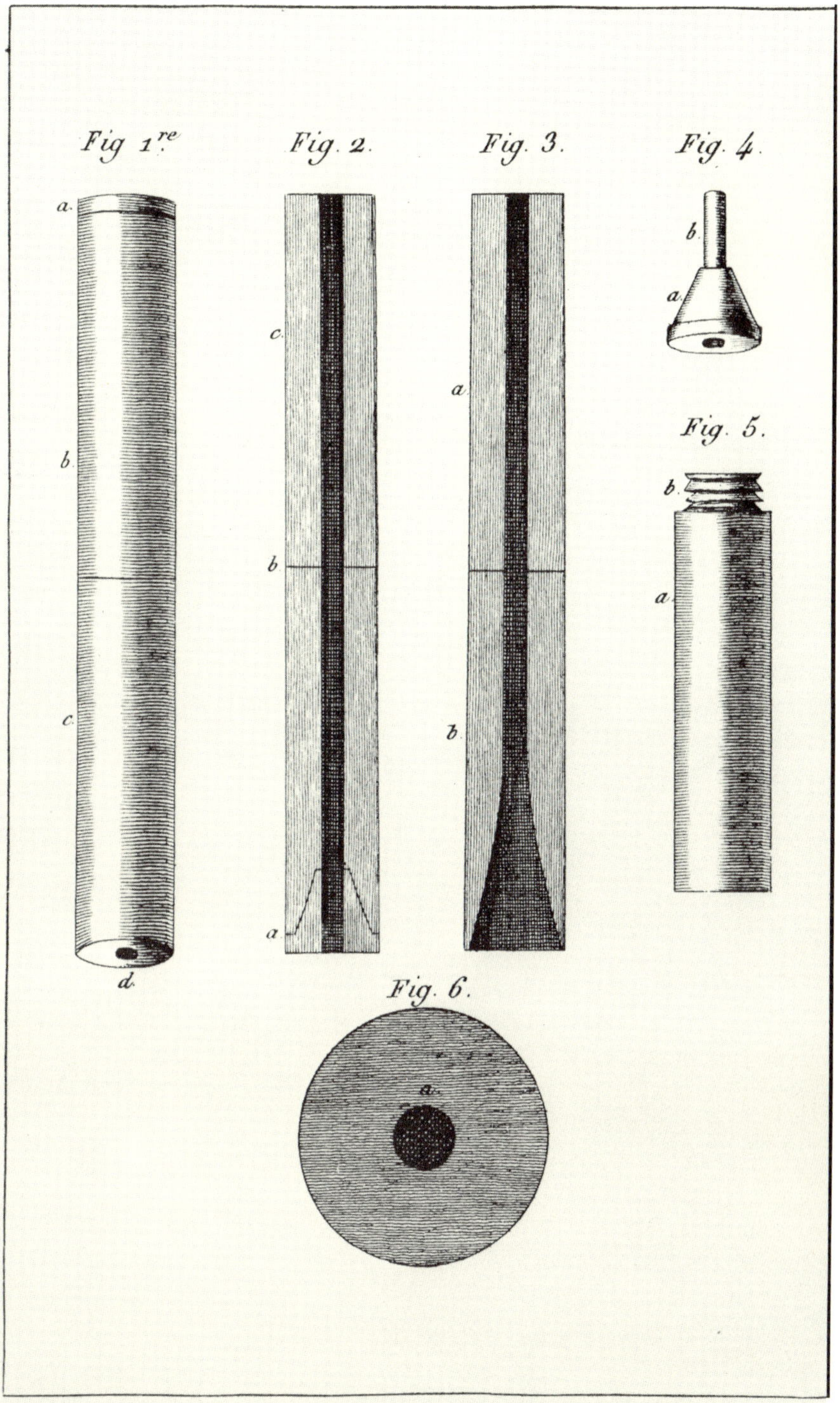

Planche Ire

No. 813. Laennec. *De l'Auscultation Médiate.* The primitive tubular wooden stethoscope.

Cushing L5; Garrison-Morton 2673; Osler 1318; Waller 5491; Wellcome III, p. 429.

814. ———. *A treatise on the diseases of the chest.* Translated by John Forbes. 1st American ed. Philadelphia: James Webster, 1823. viii, 319 pp., 8 plates. 21.8 cm.

This is the first of numerous American editions of Laennec's classic.

Cushing L10 (1830 ed.); Osler 1324 (1829 ed.); Waller 5489.

815. JOHANN FRIEDRICH MECKEL (1781–1833). *De duplicitate monstrosa commentarius.* Halle and Berlin: E librariis Orphanotrophei, 1815. vi, 98 pp., 8 plates (2 fold.). 32.7 cm.

Third in the line of the famous Meckels, Johann Friedrich was the leading comparative anatomist in Germany before Johannes Müller (see No. 909). He did much to clarify the misunderstandings concerning congenital malformations and other abnormalities, the subject of this work, and his work on comparative anatomy made Germany the center for this discipline in the first half of the nineteenth century.

*816. ———. *Handbuch der menschlichen Anatomie.* 4 vols. Halle: In den Buchhandlungen des Hallischen Waisenhauses, 1815–1820. 20.1 cm.

This four-volume unillustrated treatise on human anatomy is a fine example of the accuracy and scholarship which characterize all of Meckel's work.

Garrison-Morton 407.

817. JOHN SYNG DORSEY (1783–1818). *Elements of surgery; for the use of students.* 2 vols. Philadelphia: Edward Parker, 1813. Vol. I: vii, 407 pp.; Vol. II: vii, 388 pp., illus. 21.5 cm.

Dorsey was only nineteen when he received his medical degree from the University of Pennsylvania, and his early start allowed him to crowd a busy career into a brief but fruitful thirty-five years. He was the first American surgeon to perform a successful ligation of the external iliac artery. While professor of materia medica at his alma mater, Dorsey published this very successful textbook of surgery for which he prepared many of the illustrations.

Cushing D228; Waller 2533 (1818 ed.); Wellcome II, p. 481 (1823 ed.).

*818. FRANÇOIS MAGENDIE (1783–1855). *Précis élémentaire de physiologie.* 2 vols. Paris: Méquignon-Marvis, 1816–1817. Vol. I: vi, 326 pp.; Vol. II: 473 pp. 19.4 cm.

Magendie was the founder of the science of toxicology and a pioneer experimental physiologist in France and therefore the forerunner of such men as Claude Bernard and Louis Pasteur. He was the first to show conclusively that section of the anterior spinal nerve roots affected motility but not sensation, and vice versa as to the posterior roots. This same observation, partially described by Charles Bell, has long been known as the "fundamental law of Bell and Magendie." This *Précis* may be considered the prototype of later texts on physiology.

Waller 6135 (1825 ed.).

819. ———. *Formulary for the preparation and mode of employing several new remedies.* Philadelphia: J. Webster, 1824. 268 pp. 17.1 cm.

In this book, first published in French in 1822, Magendie introduced several newly-discovered alkaloids. Among the drugs he discusses are morphine, iodine, quinine, atropine, emetine, and strychnine. The present work was translated from the third French edition by Robley Dunglison (see No. 902).

Cushing M69 (1828 ed.); Garrison-Morton 1846 (French ed., 1822); Waller 6131 (French ed., 1836).

820. ———. *Lectures on the blood; and on the changes which it undergoes during disease.* Philadelphia: Haswell, Barrington, and Haswell, 1839. 276 pp. 21.5 cm.

The twenty-four lectures presented in this work were delivered by Magendie at the Collège de France in 1837 and 1838. In one of these lectures, he reports the first experiment in anaphylaxis in which he showed that rabbits who had tolerated a first injection of egg albumin died when given subsequent injections.

Garrison-Morton 2585.

BENJAMIN TRAVERS (1783–1858). *Surgical essays.*

See No. 740.

*821. Sir BENJAMIN COLLINS BRODIE (1783–1862). *Pathological and surgical observations on diseases of the joints.* London: Printed for Longman, Hurst, Rees, Orme, and Brown, 1818. vii, 329 pp., 6 plates (2 col.). 22.9 cm.

A pupil of Everard Home (see No. 710), Brodie lectured at the Great Windmill Street School for eight years before his appointment as surgeon at St. George's Hospital. His pioneering work in surgical techniques soon propelled him to the peak of his profession where, for over thirty years, he remained one of England's best-known physicians. He made contributions in a variety of areas including experimental physiology, subcutaneous surgery, digestion, and articular diseases. A tactful, self-effacing man, Brodie endeared himself to both colleagues and patients.

Brodie's treatise on diseases of the joints is his most important work and includes pathological observations and case studies on inflammation (including Brodie's abscess), ulceration, and tumors of the joints. The text is supplemented by six plates, two of which are in color.

Cushing B690 (1842 ed.); Garrison-Morton 4311; Wellcome II, p. 243.

*822. Sir WILLIAM LAWRENCE (1783–1867). *A treatise on ruptures.* 2nd ed. London: Printed for J. Callow, 1810. xiii, 484 pp., 2 plates (1 fold.). 21.5 cm.

Although Lawrence was best known as an eye surgeon whose practice was centered on St. Bartholomew's Hospital in London, he also contributed significantly to the understanding and management of ruptures. The present work, first published in 1807 as *A treatise on hernia,* remained for many years the standard work on the subject.

Garrison-Morton 3587 (1838 ed.); Wellcome II, p. 462 (French ed., 1818).

823. ———. *Lectures on physiology, zoology, and the natural history of man.* Salem: Foote, 1828. 495 pp., fold. plates. 23.7 cm.

With this lecture, originally delivered before the Royal College of Surgeons in 1819, Lawrence anticipated the doctrines of Darwinian evolution, arousing the anger of the conservative clergy who viewed his work as inconsistent with Scripture. The work was first published in London in 1819. This is the first American edition.

Cushing L93 (London ed., 1823); Wellcome III, p. 462 (London ed., 1822).

*824. ———. *A treatise on the diseases of the eye.* London: Printed for J. Churchill, 1833. xv, 730 pp. 21.6 cm.

"This comprehensive work marks an epoch in ophthalmic surgery. It is based on lectures delivered by Lawrence at the London Ophthalmic Infirmary" (Garrison-Morton 5849).

Garrison-Morton 5849; Wellcome III, p. 462.

*825. [WILLIAM MACMICHAEL] (1784–1839). *The gold-headed cane.* London: J. Murray, 1827. [7] 179 pp., illus., ports. 2 copies. Copy 1: 20 cm. Original boards, uncut. In slipcase. Copy 2: 20 cm.

A gold-headed cane was once a conspicuous part of the physician's adornment, and the particular gold-headed cane of this work was owned by Dr. John Radcliffe (1650–1714), an irascible London physician, who passed it on to a younger contemporary. The custom of passing on the cane continued through a series of five physicians, ending with Matthew Baillie (see No. 722), whose widow presented it to the Royal College of Physicians in 1823. The originally anonymous book is written as an "autobiography" of the cane and, in a series of charming essays, tells the story—actually biographies—of its several owners. Along the way there is much information concerning the state of medicine and its practice in England during the eighteenth century.

Cushing M48; Garrison-Morton 6709; Osler 6717; Waller 16091.

826. ———. ———. 2nd ed. London: John Murray, 1828. [7] 267 pp., illus., ports. 19.7 cm. Original cloth, uncut.

The second edition, following the first edition by only a year, was expanded in text and had added illustrations.

Cushing M49; Osler 6719.

Gift of Dr. R. N. Larimer.

827. GILBERT BRESCHET (1784–1845). *Mémoires chirurgicaux sur différentes espèces d'anévrismes, présentés a l'Académie Royale des Sciences le 8 octobre 1832.* Paris: J.-B. Baillière, 1834. 161 (misnumbered 169) pp., 6 plates (5 fold.). 26.3 cm. Half calf with marbled boards.

Breschet was professor of anatomy at the Faculté de médecine de Paris having succeeded Cruveilhier (see No. 863) to that position. Although he was primarily an anatomist, Breschet also performed research and wrote on pediatrics, otology, and the anatomy of the skin. This book on aneurysms was first presented as a lecture to the Académie Royale des Sciences and was also published in its *Mémoires.* Breschet discusses the different types of aneurysms that occur in various parts of the body and presents a number of case histories. The five folding plates accompanying the text are dissections that show aneurysms in the hand, foot, heart, and head.

Gift of the Sara (Conn) and Harold Lincoln Thompson Foundation.

*828. ———. *Études anatomiques physiologiques et pathologiques de l'oeuf dans l'espèce humaine et dans quelques-unes des principales familles des animaux vertébrés.* Paris: J.-B. Baillière, 1833. 144 pp., 6 leaves of plates: fold. illus. (1 col.). 27.2 cm. Plain wrappers, uncut.

This monograph is an extract from *Mémoires de l'Académie royale de médecine*, Tome II, 1833. In it, the author traces the development of the fetus from the time of conception until birth. He also includes descriptions of embryonic and fetal development which lead to parturition and birth defects. The six large leaves of lithographed plates depict the various stages of fetal development.

Waller 1446.

JOHN WATTS (1785–1831). *Medical and surgical register.*

See No. 991.

829. WILLIAM PROUT (1785–1850). *An inquiry into the nature and treatment of diabetes, calculus, and other affections of the urinary organs.* 2nd ed. London: Baldwin, Cradock and Joy, 1825. xii, 328 pp., fold. col. front. 22.5 cm.

Prout, an English physician and natural scientist, is associated with two important scientific achievements: the unitary hypothesis of atomic numbers (the idea that the atomic weight of an element is a multiple or fraction of the atomic weight of hydrogen) and the discovery of hydrochloric acid in the gastric juice of man and animals.

This book, Prout's first and only important monograph, was first published in 1821 and went through five English editions, two American editions, and two German translations. In it, Prout presents his observations on urinary diseases with other opinions and ideas then in vogue. The single folding plate contains colored illustrations of different types of urinary calculi.

Cushing P412 (Philadelphia ed., 1826).

830. ———. *Chemistry, meteorology, and the function of digestion.* London: William Pickering, 1834. xxiii [5] 564 [1] pp. 21.9 cm.

Natural theology was a subject of great popularity in the eighteenth and early nineteenth centuries until Darwin formulated his theory of evolution. It was while natural history or natural science was widely supported that the Bridgewater Treatises (see No. 788) were written. Authors of the treatises were to show that there is a unity of purpose in the physical world which is the result of the work of a beneficent and superior Creator.

The present work, the eighth and final Bridgewater Treatise, deals with three subjects which Prout was well-qualified to discuss by virtue of his extensive medical and scientific training. Although this is chiefly a book of apologetics which had little impact on the scientific community, in the work on chemistry Prout coined the word "convection" and clearly set forth what is today known as Avogadro's law. The section on meteorology is not particularly noteworthy, but the third section on the biochemistry of digestion was definitely in advance of its time. It was here that he discussed the three basic components of food—carbohydrates, fats, and proteins—and suggested that food was ultimately converted into blood.

*831. DANIEL DRAKE (1785–1852). *Natural and statistical view, or picture of Cincinnati and the Miami country, illustrated by maps.* Cincinnati: Printed by Looker and Wallace, 1815. 251 [4] pp., fold. plan, fold. map. 17.2 cm.

"The greatest physician of the west, and one of the most picturesque figures in American medicine, was Daniel Drake, who was the first after Hippocrates and Sydenham to do much for medical geography. . . . He was born in New Jersey in abject poverty and was reared in a log cabin among the Kentucky pioneers. . . . He was one of Osler's 'peripatetic physicians,' constantly moving from place to place in aid of the cause of medical education" (Fielding H. Garrison, *An introduction to the history of medicine.* 4th ed. Philadelphia, 1929. p. 441). Although ever on the move, Drake's center of activity was Cincinnati, where he founded a medical school as well as the important *Western journal of the medical and physical sciences.*

The present work on the city of Cincinnati and the Miami country provides ample evidence that Drake was more than a practicing physician. He describes the area from virtually every possible perspective, including its natural history, topography, political and demographic makeup, and weather. The appendix describing the 1811 earthquake is especially interesting.

Cushing D252; Osler 2500.

832. ———. *A practical treatise on the history, prevention, and treatment of epidemic cholera, designed both for the profession and the people.* Cincinnati: Corey and Fairbank, 1832. 180 pp. 19.4 cm.

This little book, "hastily compiled," as Drake says in the Preface, "in the midst of pressing engagements, and under continued ill health," remains one of the best accounts of the clinical picture of cholera which had visited Cincinnati in 1832.

Wellcome II, p. 485.

Gift of Dr. R. N. Larimer.

833. ———. *A systematic treatise, historical, etiological, and practical, on the principal diseases of the interior valley of North America.* First Series. Cincinnati: W. B. Smith & Co. [etc.], 1850. xvi, 878 pp., incl. tables, 19 plates (incl. fold. front., maps, diagrs.). 23.2 cm. Second Series. Philadelphia: Lippincott, Grambo & Co., 1854. xix [17]–985 pp., incl. tables. 23.2 cm.

Drake's "crowning achievement was the great work on the *Diseases of the interior valley of North America,* the result of thirty years' labor, based largely upon personal observation made during extensive travel. The first volume is a wonderful encyclopedia of the topography, hydrography, climate, and meteorology, plants and animals, population (including diet, habitat, and occupations) of the Mississippi Valley. The second volume, not published until after his death, treats of the autumnal malarial and other fevers, yellow fever, typhus fever, the exanthemata, and the unclassified 'phlogistic fevers,' in relation to topographic, meteorologic, and sociologic features. There was nothing like this book in literature, unless it might be Hippocrates on Airs, Waters, and Places" (Fielding H. Garrison, *An introduction to the history of medicine.* 4th ed. Philadelphia, 1929. p. 442).

Cushing D258, D259; Garrison-Morton 1777.

Gift of Dr. R. N. Larimer.

*834. WILLIAM BEAUMONT (1785–1853). *Experiments and observations on the gastric juice and the physiology of digestion.* Plattsburgh: Printed by F. P. Allen, 1833. 280 pp., illus. 22.2 cm. Original paper-covered boards. In slipcase.

Beaumont, an Army surgeon from Connecticut, was stationed at Michillimackinac, Michigan Territory, in 1822, when an accidental gunshot wounded a French-Canadian guide, Alexis St. Martin. Although the wound healed, it left a permanent fistula. Beaumont recognized the possibilities of studies of the gastric juice and the digestive process and, for the next ten years, made the most of them.

This unimpressive-looking little book, cheaply printed and bound, is a cornerstone of modern physiology and a great American medical classic.

Cushing B206; Osler 1972; Waller 805; Wellcome II, p. 123.

835. ———. *The physiology of digestion, with experiments on the gastric juice.* 2nd ed. Burlington [Vermont]: C. Goodrich, 1847. 303 pp., illus. 19.3 cm.

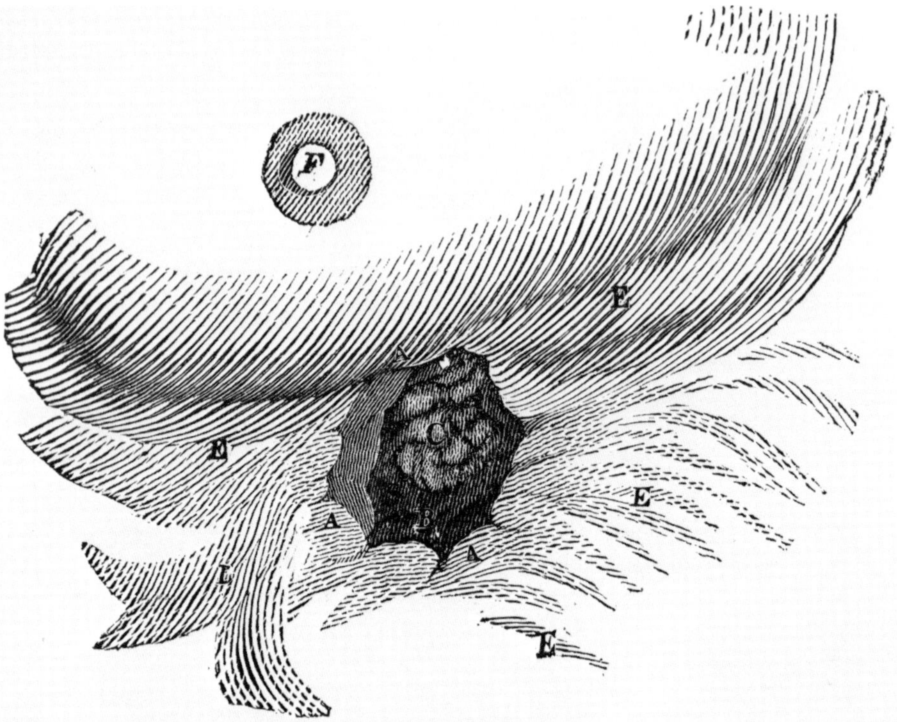

This engraving represents the appearance of the aperture with the valve depressed.

A A A Edges of the aperture through the integuments and intercostals, on the inside and around which is the union of the lacerated edges of the perforated coats of the stomach with the intercostals and skin.

B The cavity of the stomach, when the valve is depressed.

C Valve, depressed within the cavity of the stomach.

E E E E Cicatrice of the original wound.

F The nipple.

No. 834. Beaumont. *Experiments and Observations on the Gastric Juice.* The post-traumatic fistula of Alexis St. Martin.

This second edition of Beaumont's classic contains minor corrections by Samuel Beaumont, a cousin of the author.

Cushing B211; Waller 809; Wellcome II, p. 123.

*836. VALENTINE MOTT (1785–1865). *On hemorrhage from wounds, and the best means of arresting it.* New York: A. D. F. Randolph, 1863. 16 pp., illus. 22.7 cm.

Mott, the most renowned surgeon of New York in the nineteenth century, received his early medical education under local apprenticeship but later traveled to London where he studied under Sir Astley Paston Cooper (see No. 740). Mott returned to New York in 1809 and held various posts with Columbia College, Rutgers Medical College, and the College of Physicians and Surgeons. Mott's fame rests primarily on his achievements in vessel ligation, a subject which he investigated and about which he wrote extensively. In 1818 he became the first to ligate the innominate artery for aneurysm, and in 1821 he successfully ligated the common carotid.

This short pamphlet on hemorrhage, written for the Sanitary Commission of the U.S. Army during the Civil War, is one of Mott's last works and includes several diagrams illustrating the anatomy of the vessels and the use of the tourniquet.

———. *Medical and surgical register.*

See No. 991.

*837. JEAN GUILLAUME AUGUSTE LUGOL (1786–1851). *Mémoire sur l'emploi de l'iode dans les maladies scrofuleuses.* Paris: J.-B. Baillière, 1829. xviii, 78 pp. 20.1 cm. Bound with:

*838. ———. *Mémoire sur l'emploi des bains iodurés dans les maladies scrofuleuses.* Paris: J.-B. Baillière, 1830. viii, 52 pp., fold. table. 20.1 cm.

Waller 6079.

And bound with:

*839. ———. *Troisième mémoire sur l'emploi de l'iode dans les maladies scrofuleuses.* Paris: J.-B. Baillière, 1831. 219 pp. 20.1 cm.

Waller 6081; Wellcome III, p. 559.

Lugol made a number of important contributions in the classification, etiology, and treatment of tuberculosis including the employment of iodides, which he also used to treat goiter and other maladies. The iodide compound, "Lugol's solution," still bears his name. This work and the two which preceded it are papers originally delivered to the Académie Royale des Sciences in Paris. The last appeared in English translation the same year it was published in French.

840. WILLIAM PAUL CRILLON BARTON (1786–1856). *Vegetable materia medica of the United States.* 2 vols. Vol. I: 2nd ed. Philadelphia: H. C. Carey and I. Lea, 1825. xv, 273 pp., plates 1–24 (col.); Vol. II: 1st ed. Philadelphia: M. Carey and Son, 1818. xvi, 243 pp., plates 25–49 (col.). 26.9 cm.

Barton was a graduate of the University of Pennsylvania and a distinguished naval surgeon who, as Chief of the Bureau of Medicine and Surgery of the Navy Department in 1844, was instrumental in securing a number of reforms in naval medicine. Barton's fame as a botanist rests on this beautifully-produced atlas covering medicinal plants indigenous to the United States.

Austin 149 (1st ed., 1817–1818); Cushing B145; Garrison-Morton 1841 (1st ed.); Wellcome II, p. 110 (1st ed.).

841. MATTHIEU JOSEPH BONAVENTURE ORFILA (1787–1853). *Traité des poisons tirés des règnes minéral, végétal et animal; ou, Toxicologie générale.* 2nd ed. 2 vols. Paris: Chez Crochard, 1818. Vol. I: xvi, 658 [xvii]–xxxii pp.; Vol. II: xvi, 703 pp. 19.9 cm. Contemporary quarter sheep with marbled boards.

Orfila, a native of Minorca, studied at Valencia and Barcelona and was graduated at Paris in 1811. He was named professor of medicine at Paris in 1819 and became dean of the faculty in 1831. An eminent toxicologist, Orfila was also active as an epidemiologist and public hygienist. He was one of the founders of the Académie de Médecine in Paris and is considered by many authorities to be the founder of modern medico-legal toxicology.

His treatise on poisons was first published in 1814 and became a classic in the field. This second edition is a greatly enlarged version of the first edition.

Garrison-Morton 2072 (1st ed., 1814); Waller 7001 (1st ed.).

*842. JOHN LIZARS (1787?–1860). *A system of anatomical plates of the human body, accompanied with descriptions and physiological, pathological, and surgical observations.* Edinburgh: W. H. Lizars [1840?]. xxii [4] 241, xxxvi pp., 101 col. plates. 42.9 cm.

Although it contains no new discoveries, this superb atlas is certainly one of the most elegant works of the nineteenth century. The 101 colored lithographs were drawn by the author and his brother, William Home Lizars (1788–1859), from the author's dissections. Lizars was a pupil of John Bell and served as a naval surgeon before becoming professor of surgery at the Royal College of Surgeons in Edinburgh.

In this copy, the "Index to the letters of references," with their accompanying explanations, were cut out and mounted on the appropriate plates by a previous owner.

Cushing L313; Waller 5950; Wellcome III, p. 531.

*843. PIERRE CHARLES ALEXANDRE LOUIS (1787–1872). *Recherches anatomico-pathologiques sur la phthisie.* Paris: Gabon, 1825. xxiv, 16, 560 pp. 20.7 cm.

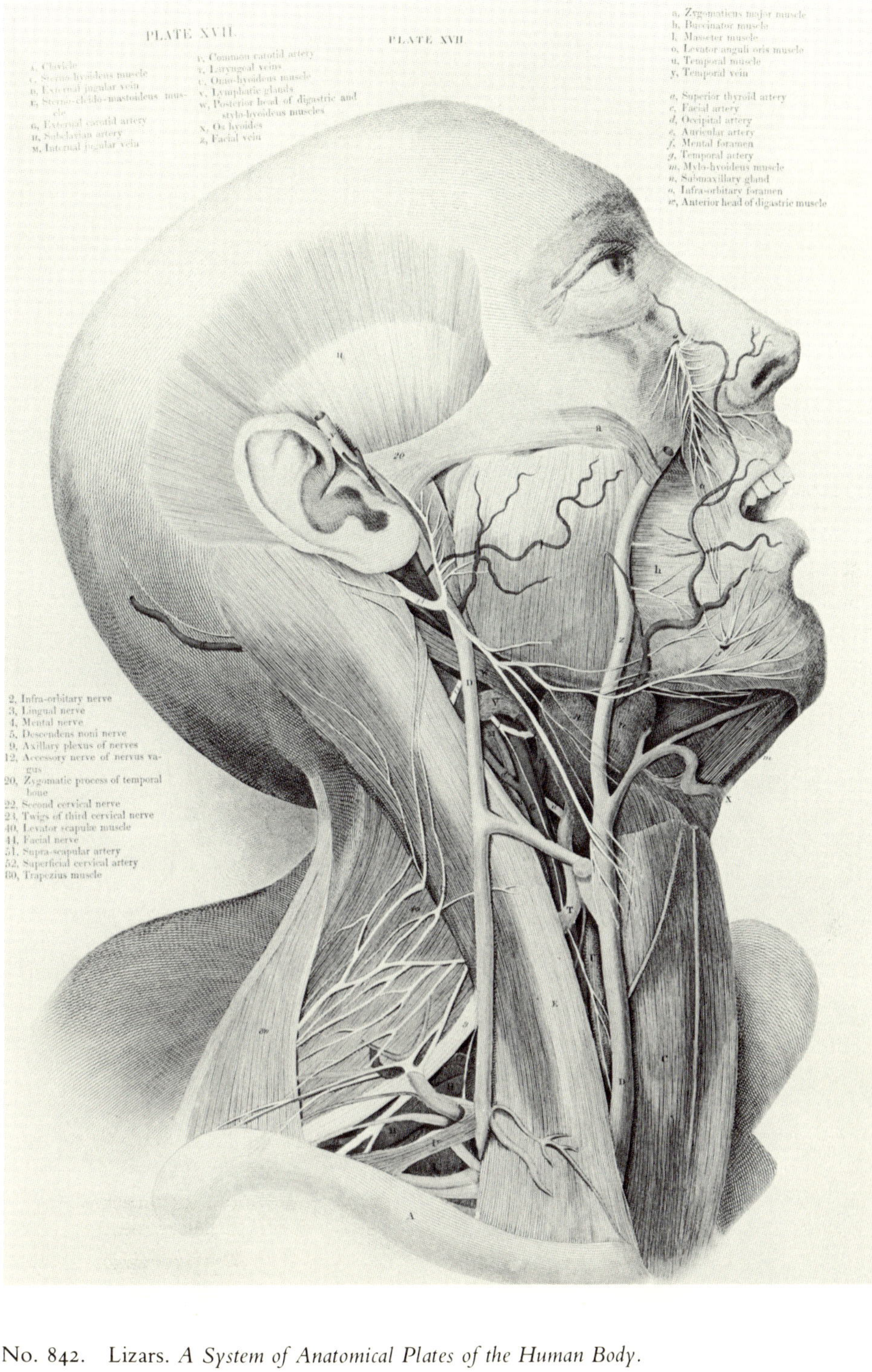

No. 842. Lizars. *A System of Anatomical Plates of the Human Body.*

One of the most influential figures in French medicine, Louis received his medical degree from the University of Paris in 1813. He practiced medicine for seventeen years in Russia but left to undertake further study after becoming distressed over the ineffectiveness of local measures taken to deal with a diphtheria epidemic. Returning to Paris, he embarked on the life-long study of the fatal diseases with particular emphasis on tuberculosis and typhoid fever. Working with a large number of patients, Louis collected detailed statistics on every case using the results as instruments of diagnosis and therapy. His reliance on the statistical analysis of disease, though sometimes faulty, helped put to rest the concept of *a priori* theories of medicine so pervasive at the time.

This work on tuberculosis, which established Louis' reputation as a clinician, gives a numerical study of extrapulmonary lesions based on 358 dissections and 1,960 clinical cases.

Garrison-Morton 3221; Wellcome III, p. 551.

*844. ———. *Recherches anatomiques, pathologiques et thérapeutiques sur la maladie connue sous les noms de gastro-entérite, fièvre putride, adynamique, ataxique, typhoïde etc., etc., comparée avec les maladies aigues les plus ordinaires.* 2 vols. Paris: J.-B. Baillière, 1829. Vol. I: xii, 458 pp.; Vol. II: 531 pp. 20.3 cm.

Although Louis did not clearly differentiate typhus from typhoid fever, he gave the first clinical-pathological description of the latter, and he was the first to use the term "typhoide" (meaning stupor) to indicate the mental condition of the patient. This two-volume treatise on the subject was based on a multitude of case studies.

Garrison-Morton 5023; Osler 3268; Wellcome III, p. 551.

*845. ———. *Recherches sur les effets de la saignée dans quelques maladies inflammatoires, et sur l'action de l'émétique et des vésicatoires dans la pneumonie.* Paris: J.-B. Baillière, 1835. 120 pp. 20.9 cm.

By publishing statistical evidence against the common practice of bloodletting in the treatment of pneumonia, Louis let loose a flood of controversy. Nevertheless, his attack marked the beginning of the decline of this time-honored, often lethal, procedure.

Garrison-Morton 1698; Wellcome III, p. 551.

846. JACOB BIGELOW (1787–1879). *American medical botany.* 3 vols. in 1. Boston: Published by Cummings and Hilliard, 1817–1820. Vol. I: xi, 197 pp., col. plates 1–20; Vol. II: xvi, 199 pp., col. plates 21–40; Vol. III: x, 197 pp., col. plates 41–60. 23.2 cm.

Considered one of the leading American scientists of his era, Bigelow achieved prominence as a physician, educational reformer, and botanist. A student of Rush, an associate of James Jackson, and professor of materia medica at Harvard, he managed an enormous consulting practice and played a prominent role in the great cholera epidemic of 1832, in which he convinced Boston authorities to adopt his stringent sanitary precautions. As a result, Boston's death toll was limited to 100 while 3,000 perished in New York. However, it was Bigelow's love of botany and the publication of this beautifully executed work that brought him most of his well-deserved acclaim. The sixty colored plates and the detailed but clearly written text mark it as one of the finest botanical treatises ever produced in America.

Austin 205; Cushing B384; Garrison-Morton 1842.

*847. ———. *A treatise on the materia medica, intended as a sequel to the Pharmacopoeia of the United States.* Boston: C. Ewer, 1822. 424 pp. 21.2 cm.

Trained as a physician, Bigelow was also a skilled botanist, and several of his works, notably *American medical botany* (see No. 846) and *Medical botany,* brought acclaim from both sides of the Atlantic.

This treatise on the properties of drugs is an attempt to describe and otherwise expand upon the items in the newly published *Pharmacopoeia of the United States.* Here Bigelow examines "the sources from which they are derived, the properties by which they are known, the objectives which they fulfill in practice, and the manner in which they are to be applied" (from the Preface).

Cushing B393; Wellcome I, p. 166.

*848. ———. *A discourse on self-limited diseases.* Boston: N. Hale, 1835. 48 pp. 22.3 cm.

This work was said by Oliver Wendell Holmes to have exerted more influence on medical practice in the United States than any other work that had been published in this country. Written as a reaction against the excessive use of pharmaceuticals by early nineteenth-century physicians, it had a profound and immediate effect on the profession.

Cushing B387; Garrison-Morton 2212; Osler 2034; Wellcome II, p. 166.

849. ———. *Nature in disease.* 2nd ed. Boston: Phillips, Sampson and Co., 1859. xii, 410 pp. 18 cm.

First published in 1854, Bigelow's *Nature in disease* is a collection of essays, many of which had appeared previously as journal articles or pamphlets "written or published at various times during a long and not inactive professional life" (from the Preface).

Cushing B392 (1st ed., 1854); Waller 1050 (1st ed.).

*850. FRÉDÉRIC JOSEPH BÉRARD (1789–1828). *Doctrine médicale de l'ècole de Montpellier.* Montpellier et à Paris: Librairie au Rabais, 1819. 516 pp. 19.4 cm.

Professor of hygiene at Montpellier, Bérard was one of the most respected physicians in France. Although a fine clinician, his most original work was done in the areas of medical philosophy and education. He was an avid supporter of public

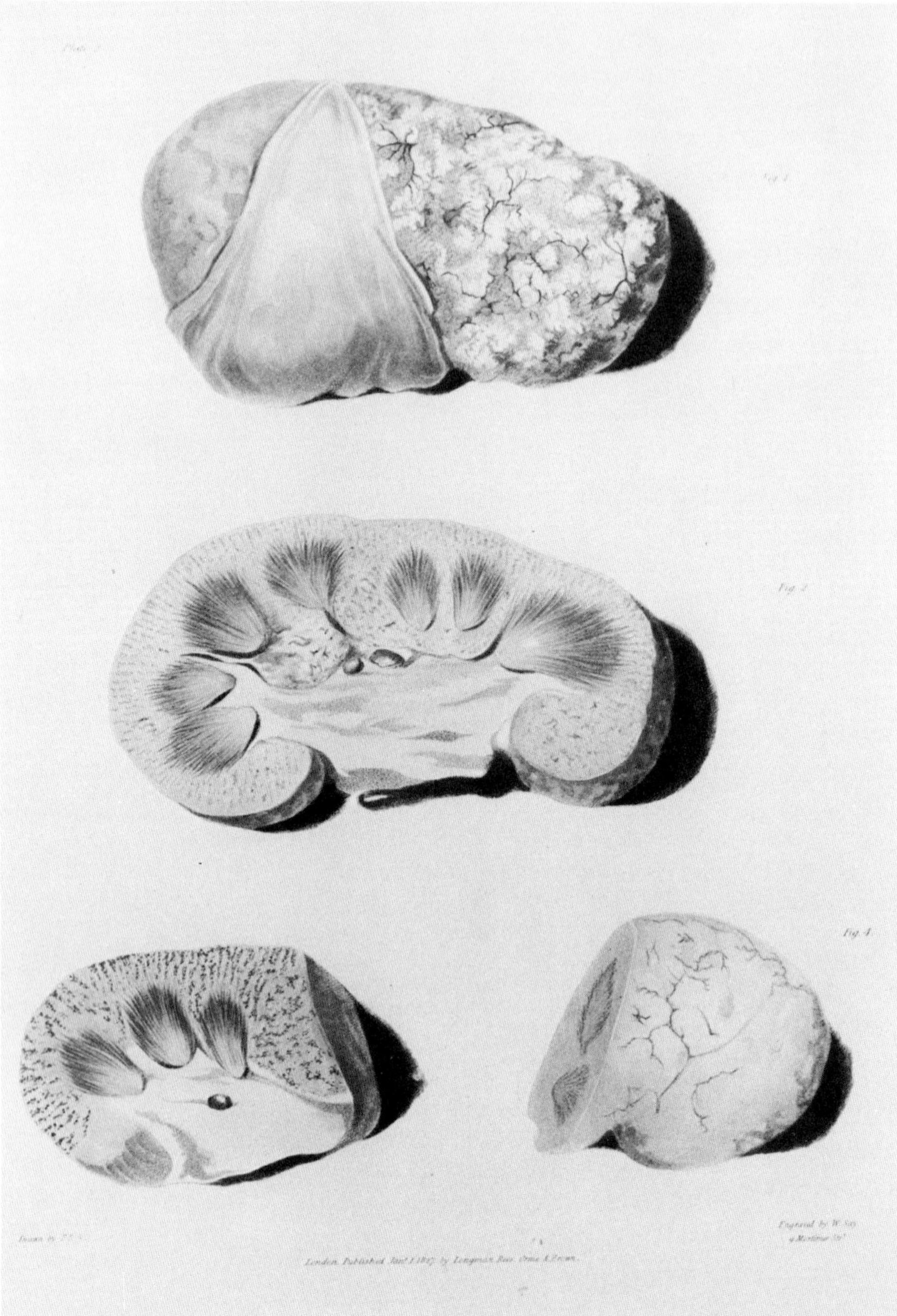

No. 851. Bright. *Reports of Medical Cases.* The kidney in dropsy.

health measures and was involved in a spirited debate with followers of Rousseau who believed civilization hindered the cause of health. Using statistics to support his view, Bérard produced a convincing argument.

The present work is Bérard's most lasting achievement—a comparison of teaching philosophies and methods in European medical schools.

Cushing B293; Osler 6220; Waller 12648; Wellcome II, p. 145.

*851. RICHARD BRIGHT (1789–1858). *Reports of medical cases.* Vol. I only of 2 vols. London: Longman, Rees, Orme, Brown, and Greene, 1827. xvi, 222 pp., 62 plates (part col., part fold.). 33.5 cm. Original boards, uncut.

In his day, Bright was the leading medical consultant in London and the most famous of the "great men of Guy's," a name given to the succession of eminent workers at Guy's Hospital. A student of Sir Astley Paston Cooper and James Currie, Bright's powers of observation marked him as a true follower of Sydenham. Although Bright advanced no new theories of disease and did little original classification in pathology, he collected and recorded an extraordinary amount of data from which he was able to draw his conclusions and to base his assumptions. The list of original descriptions attributed to Bright includes those for pancreatic diabetes, unilateral convulsions, laryngeal phthisis, condensation of the lung in whooping cough, and glomerulonephritis (Bright's disease). His *Report of medical cases,* covering a large number of diseases, is one of the most important books in nineteenth-century medical literature. The detailed case reports are models of clarity and conciseness and give ample evidence of Bright's skill as a clinician. The sixteen colored lithograph plates are among the finest medical illustrations and are beautifully preserved in this copy.

Garrison-Morton 2285; Osler 1340; Waller 1460; Wellcome II, p. 239.

852. ——— and THOMAS ADDISON (1793–1860). *Elements of the practice of medicine.* London: Longman, Orme, Brown, Green, and Longmans, 1839. [9] 613 pp. 21.5 cm.

This joint undertaking by two of the most famous physicians in nineteenth-century Europe is quite scarce. It was intended as a "work at once elementary and practical to which [teachers] might refer their pupils as a companion and assistant during the period of their studies" (from the Preface). More than sixty separate diseases and conditions are described, each accompanied by a lucid account of its history, causes, prognosis, diagnosis, and treatment. Though the style is obviously dated, the descriptions of many of the diseases excel in accuracy and conciseness. Originally issued in three parts from 1836 to 1839, the work is here complete in one volume. An intended second volume was never published.

Garrison-Morton 2215; Wellcome II, p. 239.

*853. FRANÇOIS JOSEPH MOREAU (1789–1862). *Traité pratique des accouchemens.* 2 vols. and atlas. Paris: G. Baillière, 1841 [atlas, 1837]. Vol. I: xiv, 564 pp.

20.5 cm.; Vol. II: 500 pp. 20.5 cm.; Atlas: 60 leaves of plates, each accompanied by a leaf of descriptive letterpress. 43 cm.

The art of obstetrics was advanced considerably in nineteenth-century France, and Moreau, a member of the Medical Faculty of Paris, was one of its most active clinicians and writers. This exhaustive text treats the problems of pregnancy, normal and abnormal delivery, and anatomical anomalies of the newborn. The sixty full-page lithographs which complement the text are exceptional and beautifully preserved in this copy.

ALEXANDER HODGDON STEVENS (1789–1869). *Medical and surgical register.*

See No. 991.

HIPPOLYTE BELLOC (fl. 1830). *A practical treatise on laryngeal phthisis, chronic laryngitis, and diseases of the voice.*

See No. 911.

*854. ALEXANDRE JEAN BAPTISTE PARENT-DUCHÂTELET (1790–1836). *De la prostitution dans la ville de Paris.* 3rd ed. 2 vols. Paris: J.-B. Baillière; New York: H. Baillière, 1857. Vol. I: xxiii, 731 pp., front. (port.), fold. chart, fold. diagr., fold. map; Vol. II: 892 pp. 20.8 cm. Half morocco, gilt spine.

With the rise of modern industry in early nineteenth-century Europe, public and occupational health became an issue of significance. In France, the physician Parent-Duchâtelet, as a member of the Council for Public Sanitation, undertook a number of studies which led toward the betterment of working conditions for large segments of society, most notably sewer workers and tobacco handlers. His detailed study of prostitution in Paris, however, is the work for which he is best known today. The treatise covers virtually every aspect of prostitution with emphasis on the life and health of the prostitute. The study was instrumental in organizing the government registration and supervision of brothels.

Garrison-Morton 1607 (1st ed., 1836); Osler 3615 (1st ed.); Waller 7195 (1837 ed.).

855. JACQUES LISFRANC (1790–1847). *Maladies de l'utérus, d'après les leçons cliniques.* Paris: G. Baillière, 1836. vi, 536 pp. 20.9 cm.

Lisfranc, French gynecologist and surgeon, devised many new operations including removal of the rectum, lithotomy in women, and amputation of the cervix uteri. This book on diseases of the uterus was prepared by one of his assistants, Jean Hippolyte Pauly (1806–1854). A comprehensive treatment of the subject, it includes many case histories from L'Hôpital de la Pitié in Paris where Lisfranc and Pauly practiced. The book was translated into German in 1838 and into English a year later.

Waller 7251; Wellcome III, p. 528.

856. MARSHALL HALL (1790–1857). *The principles of diagnosis.* 2nd ed. New York: D. Appleton, 1835. xxiv, 463 [5] pp. 21.7 cm.

Hall, a native of Nottingham, England, received his medical degree from Edinburgh. He studied abroad for a time, practiced in Nottingham for several years, and moved to London in the mid-1820's where he continued in private practice until his death. Although he had an extremely active and successful practice, he still found time to devote to serious physiological research. His most important discovery was the demonstration of reflex action and the fact that the spinal cord is composed of segments whose functional units are separate reflex arcs. Hall was a very active writer and wrote numerous papers on nervous diseases, artificial respiration, digestive diseases, and gynecology.

The present work resulted from an excellent course of lectures Hall conducted at the Royal Infirmary in Edinburgh just after his graduation. First published in 1817, the second edition appeared in England in 1834; both helped to establish his fine reputation.

857. ———. *Principles of the theory and practice of medicine.* 1st American ed. Boston: C. C. Little and J. Brown, 1839. iv, 724 pp., illus. 21.6 cm.

The third edition of Hall's *Diagnosis of disease* was published in London in 1837 under the present title. The present work is the first American edition, based on the third edition of Hall's textbook, edited by Jacob Bigelow (see No. 846 ff.) and Oliver Wendell Holmes (see No. 947 ff.) for use as a text in several American medical schools.

Cushing H56; Wellcome III, p. 197.

858. ———. *On the diseases and derangements of the nervous system.* London: H. Baillière, 1841. xxviii, 380 pp., 8 plates. 21.7 cm.

Hall's studies on reflex action were much more widely acclaimed in Europe than in Great Britain and were never given any recognition by the Royal Society. Hall did, however, develop and apply his ideas on the reflex to medicine and published several books concerning his research. He firmly established the concept of the reflex arc as a fundamental of neurophysiology and in this work applies it to the diseases of the nervous system.

Waller 3984; Wellcome III, p. 197.

*859. JULES GERMAIN CLOQUET (1790–1883). *De la squelétopée [et] Recherches sur les causes et l'anatomie des hernies abdominales.* [Paris: Méquignon-Marvis] 1819. 72, 176 pp., 10 plates. 25 cm.

As professor of clinical surgery and surgical pathology at the Medical Faculty of Paris, Cloquet produced a number of surgical and anatomical works, the most enduring of which is his *Anatomie de l'homme* (1821–1831), a five-volume atlas with more than 300 plates. He is also credited with the first description of the central canal of the vitreous (the hyaloid canal).

The present works were written in competition for the anatomy chair at Paris. The first gives directions for the preparation of a human skeleton from cadaver to mounted specimen, while the second covers the causes and anatomy of the abdominal hernia and contains a series of lithographs drawn by the author. The work is based on Cloquet's experience with over 500 hernia cases.

Garrison-Morton 3585.

*860. THEODORIC ROMEYN BECK (1791–1855). *Elements of medical jurisprudence.* 2 vols. Albany [New York]: Webster and Skinner, 1823. Vol. I: xxxiv, 418 pp.; Vol. II: viii, 471 pp. 21.3 cm.

The author of this first authoritative text on forensic medicine was a New York state physician and philanthropist.

Garrison-Morton 1735; Wellcome II, p. 126 (London ed., 1825).

*861. JOHANN LUDWIG CHOULANT (1791–1861). *Handbuch der Bücherkunde für die aeltere Medicin zur Kenntniss der griechische, lateinischen und arabischen Schriften im ärztlichen Fache.* Leipzig: L. Voss, 1828. xiv, 198 pp. 20.3 cm.

Choulant, a native of Dresden, was one of the greatest of medical bibliographers and historians. He was graduated from the University of Leipzig in 1818 and held a variety of posts there and at the Neustadt Medic-Chirurgial Academy where he eventually was made director. Choulant's rather uncouth and openly suspicious nature did not prevent him from establishing a sizable following among his students, and he was respected as a clinician of great ability with a large consulting practice. It is his numerous historical writings, however, that have endured, including a number of translations of early English works and extensive writings on Celsus (see No. 9 ff.), his favorite author.

Of Choulant's many historical bibliographies, the *Handbuch* is considered the greatest. It is a catalog of all the medical incunabula known to Choulant, and without it the study of Greek, Latin, and Arabic texts is nearly impossible.

Choulant-Frank, p. 7; Cushing C228; Garrison-Morton 6753; Osler 6973 (1841 ed.); Waller 18226; Wellcome II, p. 344 (1841 ed.).

*862. ———. *Geschichte und Bibliographie der anatomischen Abbildung.* Leipzig: R. Weigel, 1852. [17] xviii, 203 pp., illus., col. plates. 27.4 cm.

This combined history and bibliography covers anatomic illustration from the earliest time to Choulant's day. Special emphasis is placed on the pivotal works of the fifteenth and sixteenth centuries from which a number of illustrations have been included. Like all of Choulant's works, it is a model of accuracy and reliability.

Choulant-Frank, pp. 9–10; Cushing C226; Garrison-Morton 440; Osler 6975; Waller 12951.

*863. JEAN CRUVEILHIER (1791–1874). *Anatomie pathologique du corps humain.* 2 vols. and atlas. Paris: J.-B. Baillière, 1829–1842. Vols. I and II: various paginations; Atlas: plates (part col.). 44.1 cm.

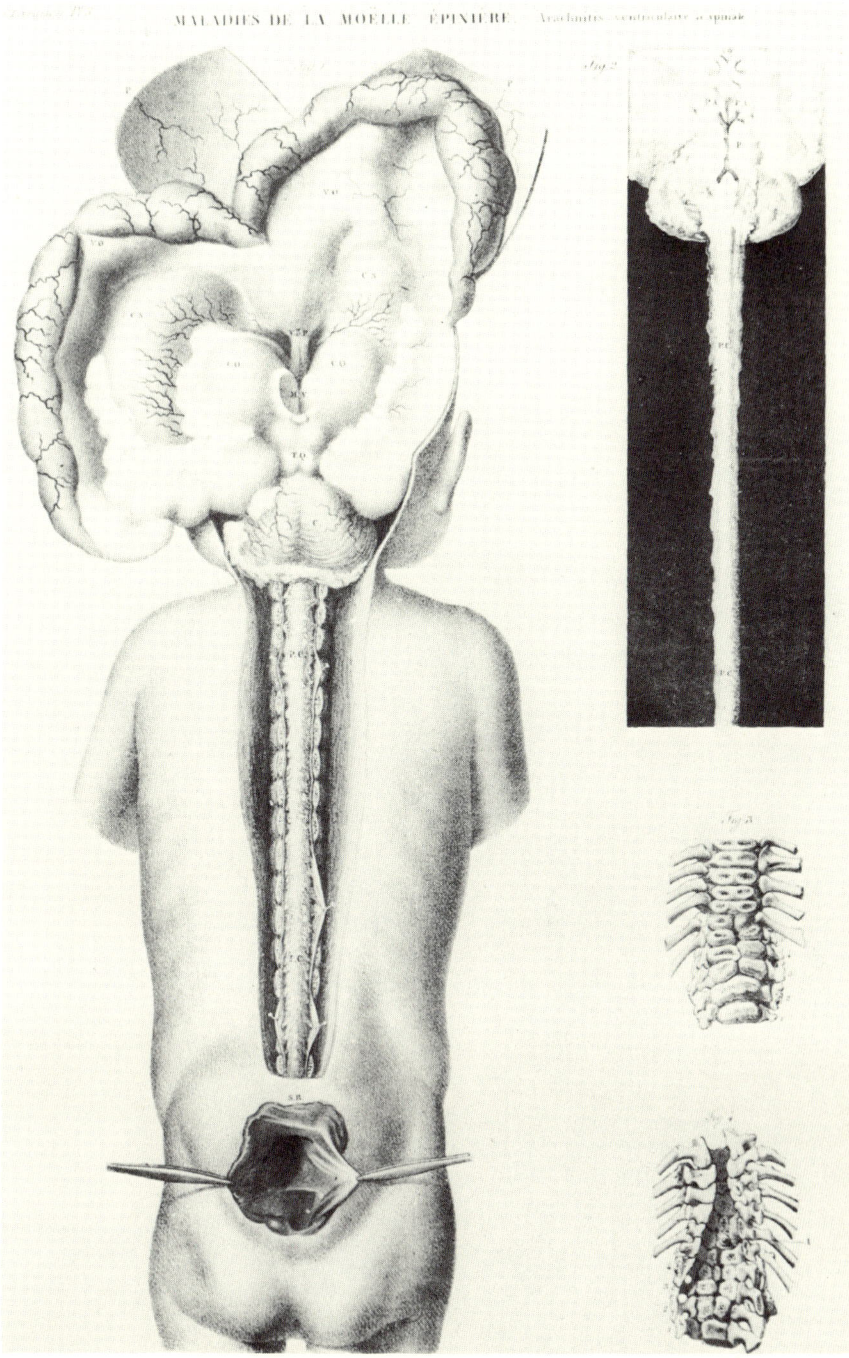

No. 863. Cruveilhier. *Anatomie Pathologique du Corps Humain*. Hydrocephalus, ventricular and spinal arachnoiditis, sacral meningocele.

In the nineteenth century pathology came into its own, being based for the first time on increasingly accurate knowledge of pathologic anatomy. Cruveilhier was the first occupant of the newly established chair of pathology at the University of Paris. In his day he was the leader, and he was the first to give an adequate description of disseminated sclerosis and of progressive muscular atrophy. He also described and named, for the first time, hypertrophic pyloric stenosis and ulceration of the stomach due to hyperacidity. His system of pathology, which erroneously taught that "phlebitis dominates all pathology," was permanently discredited by Virchow's later work. This atlas contains some of the finest illustrations of gross pathology ever made. They are colored lithographs, done by the anatomical illustrator, Antoine Chazal.

Cushing C511; Garrison-Morton 2286; Wellcome II, p. 412.

864. FRANKLIN BACHE (1792–1864). *A system of chemistry for the use of students of medicine.* Philadelphia: Printed and published for the author, 1819. xvi, 624 pp., illus. 21.5 cm.

Bache was for many years professor of chemistry at Jefferson College and played an important role in elevating the status of that school to its nineteenth-century prominence. He labored for thirty years on the *Dispensatory of the United States* and its various revisions; he contributed generously to the medical journals of his day, even editing for a time the *North American medical and surgical journal.* This chemistry text is his earliest work.

865. CHARLES DELUCENA MEIGS (1792–1869). *The history, pathology, and treatment of puerperal fever and crural phlebitis.* Philadelphia: Ed. Barrington & Geo. D. Haswell, 1842. 338 pp. 22.4 cm.

Meigs assembled the four reprints in this collection and also prepared the lengthy introductory essay. "A treatise on the epidemic puerperal fever of Aberdeen" by Alexander Gordon (1752–1799) is of special significance. The essay represents the earliest known suggestion that puerperal fever was carried by the attending physicians and midwives. Gordon wrote the work in 1795, more than fifty years before Holmes (see No. 948) and Semmelweiss (see No. 992) brought the problem to the attention of their contemporaries.

*866. ———. *A treatise on acute and chronic diseases of the neck of the uterus.* Philadelphia: Blanchard and Lea, 1854. iv, 17–116 pp., 22 plates (part col.). 23 cm.

Meigs was, in his time, one of America's most respected obstetricians and gynecologists and did much to establish norms of practice through his varied works. On the other hand, he was one of the most vocal opponents of Oliver Wendell Holmes's warnings on the contagiousness of puerperal fever (see No. 948).

This work is rather unusual in that it contains twenty-two colored lithographs, a number not often seen in American texts of this era. Meigs wrote the work while professor of midwifery at Jefferson Medical College.

*867. KARL ERNST VON BAER (1792–1876). *De ovi mammalium et hominis genesi.* Leipzig: Sumptibus L. Vossii, 1827. [4] 40 [1] pp., col. plate. 27.5 cm.

Baer was an early pioneer of modern embryology who, through painstaking and patient effort, investigated germ cell lineage of a variety of species, firmly establishing embryology as a comparative science. It was during his professorship at Königsberg that Baer wrote this most significant work, describing for the first time the mammalian ovum. In this epoch-making book Baer also made reference to the germ layer theory, suggested the similarity of the early stages of embryonic development in related species, and observed the first rudiment of the dorsal spine, later called the notochord. He broadened and confirmed his findings and observations in *Über Entwickelungsgeschichte der Thiere* (see No. 868). Baer is also considered to be one of the founders of modern morphology as a result of his work in comparative embryology.

Cushing B23; Garrison-Morton 477; Waller 594.

*868. ———. *Über Entwickelungsgeschichte der Thiere; Beobachtung und Reflexion.* 2 vols. in 1. Königsberg: 1828–1837. Vol. I: xxii, 271 pp.; Vol. II: 315 pp., 7 plates. 23.8 cm. Old half morocco.

Though Caspar Wolf (see No. 228) and others had previously observed the foldlike germinal development of various vertebrate embryos, it remained for Baer in this classic work on developmental anatomy to confirm the germ layer theory and to extend the concept to mammalian embryology. By studying the similarities and differences in the embryos of various species, Baer made a number of fundamental observations which provided the groundwork for modern comparative embryology. His discovery that embryonic homologues such as the fin of a fish and the hand of a man begin as nearly identical structures was cited later by Darwin to support his theory of evolution.

Cushing B27; Garrison-Morton 479; Waller 11772.

869. WILLIAM EDMONDS HORNER (1793–1853). *A treatise on special and general anatomy.* 2 vols. Philadelphia: H. C. Carey & I. Lea, 1826. Vol. I: xlvi, 491 pp.; Vol. II: [2] 524 pp. 21.1 cm.

A native of Warrenton, Virginia, Horner studied medicine at the University of Pennsylvania where he was graduated in 1814. He eventually settled in Philadelphia and became a member of the faculty at the University of Pennsylvania's medical school. In 1831 he succeeded Philip Syng Physick (1768–1837) as professor of anatomy and was elected head of the department. He was later appointed dean of the medical school, a post he held for more than thirty years. In addition to the present work, Horner was the author of two other monographs, one of which was the first treatise on pathological anatomy written in the United States. He made several advances in anatomy including the discovery of the *tensor tarsi* (muscle of Horner), a muscle in the lachrymal apparatus. The present treatise on anatomy, designed chiefly for the medical student, was later supplemented by Goddard's *Plates of the arteries* (see No. 955).

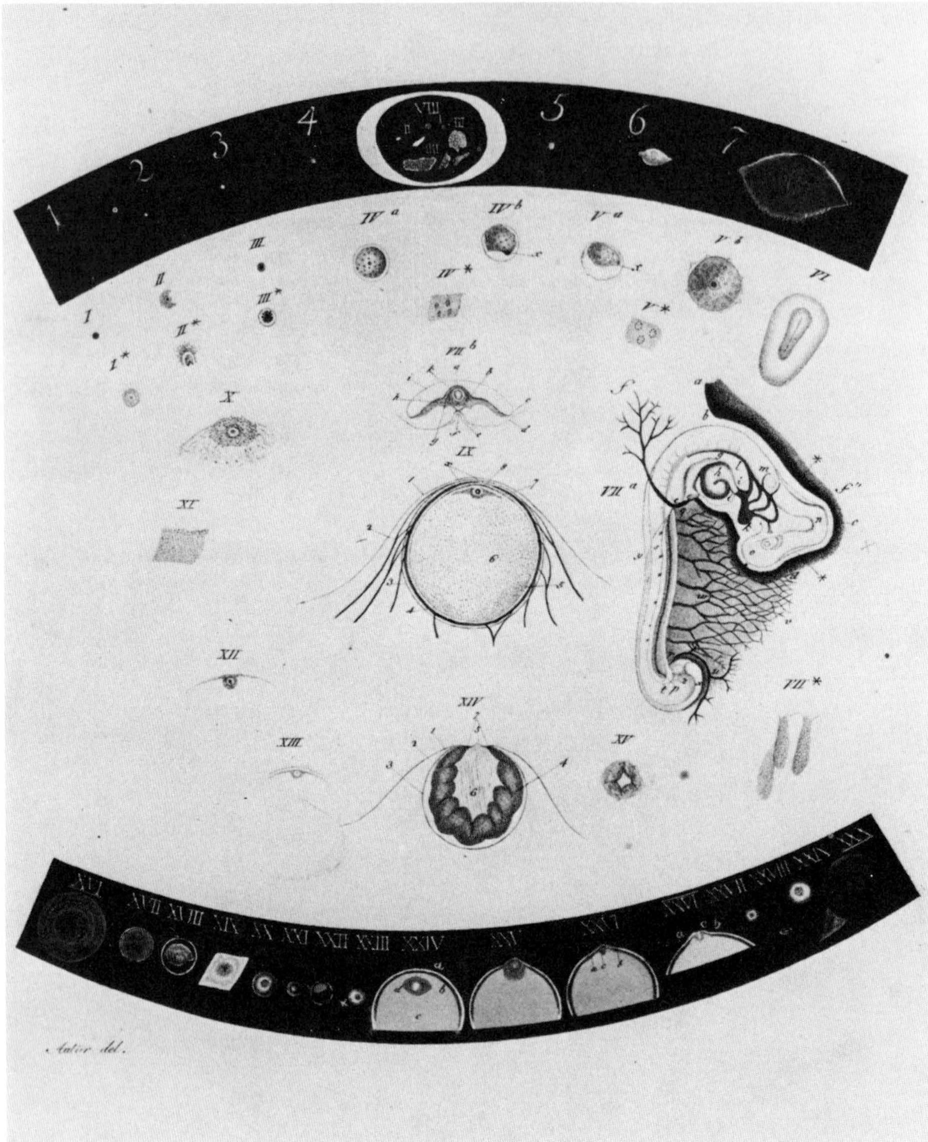

No. 867. Baer. *De Ovi Mammalium et Hominis Genesi*. The stages of development from fertilized egg to primitive embryo.

870. WILLIAM ZOLLICKOFFER (1793–1853). *A materia medica, of the United States, systematically arranged.* 2nd ed. Baltimore: J. Lovegrove, 1827. 245 pp. 23 cm.

Zollickoffer, a physician and botanist, was lecturer on medical botany, materia medica, and therapeutics at the University of Maryland. One of the first individuals in this country to write a materia medica, first published in 1819, his purpose was to acquaint American physicians with the medicinal plants of their own country. He follows the classification used by John Murray (see No. 798) and includes the opinions and observations of his colleagues and peers.

Austin 2106 (1st ed., 1819).

*871. Sir ROBERT CARSWELL (1793–1857). *Pathological anatomy. Illustrations of the elementary forms of disease.* London: Longman, Orme, Brown, Green and Longman, 1838. [218] pp., 48 col. plates. 36.3 cm. Contemporary half morocco.

This striking work is rightly regarded as one of the finest pathological atlases ever produced. It is rivaled for beauty and accuracy only by Cruveilhier's *Anatomie pathologique du corps humain* (see No. 863). The drawings are taken from a set of 2,000 watercolor paintings of diseased structures which remain at University College where Carswell was professor of anatomy. Osler said of the work: "These illustrations have, for artistic merit and for fidelity, never been surpassed, while the matter represents the highest point which the science of morbid anatomy had reached before the introduction of the microscope" (Osler 2250).

Garrison-Morton 2291; Osler 2250; Wellcome II, p. 306.

*872. THOMAS ADDISON (1793–1860). *On the constitutional and local effects of disease of the supra-renal capsules.* London: S. Highley, 1855. viii, 43 pp., 11 col. plates. 32.7 cm.

Possessed of rather rude demeanor, Addison nevertheless had a large practice. He was a brilliant lecturer and diagnostician and one of the most respected physicians at Guy's Hospital, devoting himself almost wholly to his students and patients. The present work is one of the truly remarkable medical books of the nineteenth century and has long been among the principal desiderata for medical book collectors. Addison describes here for the first time two chronic diseases of the adrenal gland: Addison's disease and pernicious anemia (Addison's anemia), the most important primary disease of the blood. The work is supplemented by several fine hand-colored lithographs. Addison's discoveries were never widely recognized by his contemporaries, yet today they are regarded as fundamentally significant in the study of the endocrine glands and the treatment of pleuriglandular diseases.

Garrison-Morton 3864; Osler 1744; Waller 225.

———. *Elements of the practice of medicine.*

See No. 852.

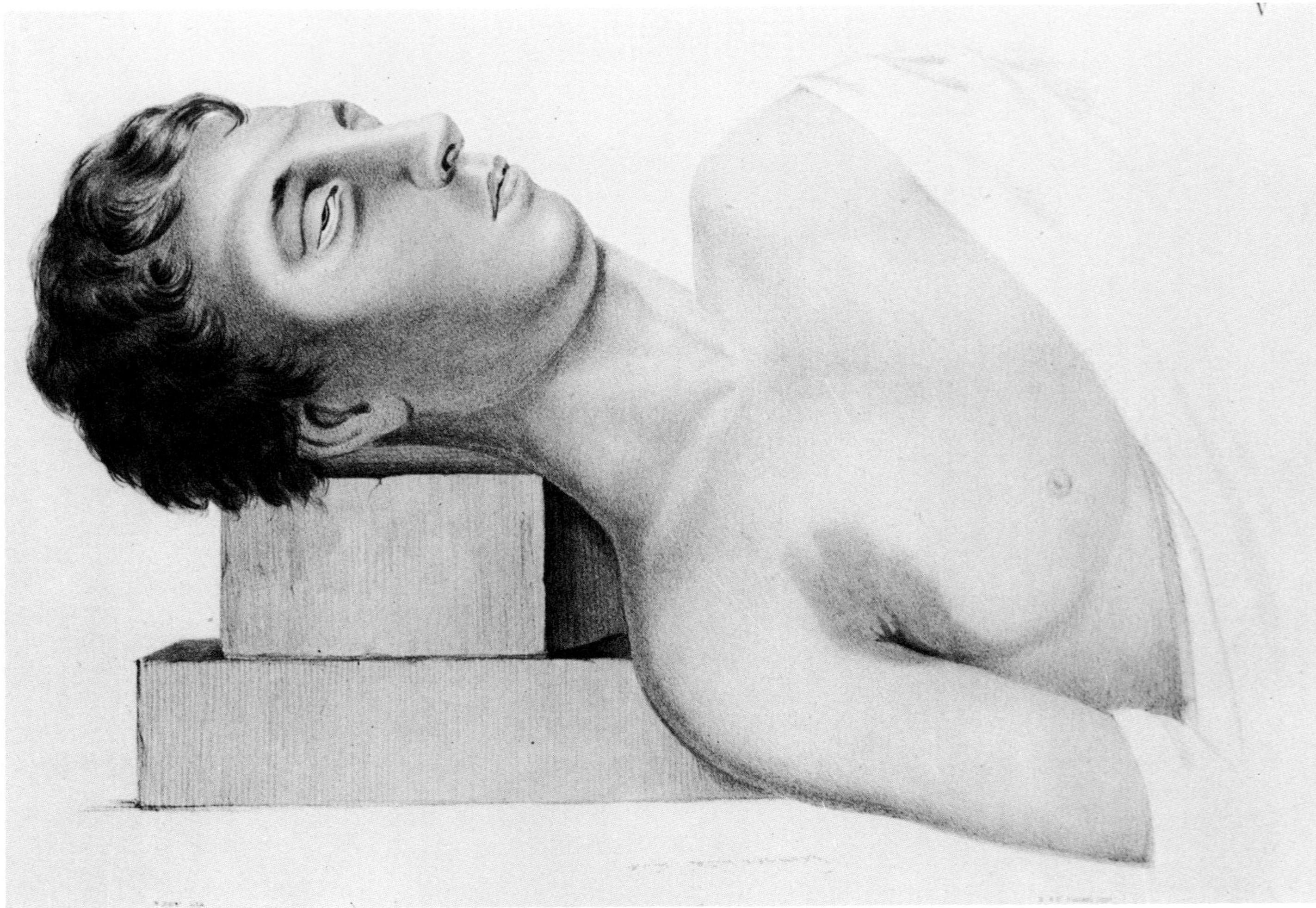

No. 872. Addison. *On the Constitutional and Local Effects of Disease of the Supra-renal Capsules*. The colors of the original plate show the typical bronze pigmentation in Addison's disease.

*873. HEINRICH RATHKE (1793–1860). *Entwickelungsgeschichte der Wirbelthiere.* Leipzig: W. Engelmann, 1861. viii, 201 pp., illus. 22.4 cm. Bound with No. 990.

Rathke is sometimes ranked with Baer (see No. 867) as a pioneer in vertebrate embryology. His discovery, in birds and mammals, of structures homologous to gill slits offered further evidence of ontogenic similarity among vertebrates. His name is perpetuated in the term "Rathke's pouch," a diverticulum which develops from the embryonic buccal cavity to become the anterior lobe of the pituitary gland. This highly praised work in comparative embryology was published posthumously by Kölliker (see No. 989) at the request of Rathke's son.

Waller 11933.

*874. JOHN DAVIDSON GODMAN (1794–1830). *Anatomical investigations, comprising descriptions of various fasciae of the human body.* Philadelphia: H. C. Carey and I. Lea, 1824. 134 pp., illus., plates. 21.8 cm.

Orphaned at six, cheated out of his rightful inheritance, and living the great majority of his days in poverty, Godman nevertheless accomplished a good deal within his short life. After brief employment as a printer's apprentice and sailor, Godman secured a medical education and subsequently held posts at the medical colleges of Ohio, Philadelphia, and Rutgers where he lectured with almost unparalleled popularity. His major work is the three-volume *American natural history*, published in 1826. Godman also founded the *Western quarterly reporter of medical surgical and natural sciences,* the first medical journal west of the Alleghenies.

The present work deals mainly with the anatomy and physiology of the various fasciae and is considered one of Godman's major achievements. A second part is Godman's translation of Antonio Scarpa's (see No. 685 ff.) *De penitiori ossium structura commentarius* [Treatise on the minute anatomy of the human bones].

875. ROBERT LISTON (1794–1847). *Elements of surgery.* Philadelphia: E. L. Carey and A. Hart, 1837. 540 pp. 21.7 cm.

Professor of clinical surgery at London's University College, Liston's brilliant knowledge of anatomy, coupled with the speed and dexterity of his scalpel, made him one of the finest surgeons of his day. He introduced a number of important surgical innovations, most notably in the area of dislocation reduction, amputation, and plastic surgery. Liston was the first European to use the newly discovered ether in surgery, employing it in an amputation of the thigh in 1846. *Elements of surgery,* first published in 1831, is one of Liston's most important works; it went through numerous editions.

Wellcome III, p. 530 (1st London ed., 1831).

876. JOHN CONOLLY (1794–1866). *An inquiry concerning the indications of insanity, with suggestions for the better protection and care of the insane.* London: Printed for J. Taylor, 1830. vi, 496 pp. 22.1 cm.

Conolly, a native of England, received his medical education at Edinburgh and was a private practitioner and professor of medicine at the University of London before he decided to devote himself to psychiatry. He began his work in psychiatry in 1839 when he became physician-superintendent of the Hanwell Asylum in Middlesex County. His name is inseparably linked to what is generally acknowledged as the major advance in the history of the medical care of the insane: the elimination of mechanical restraints. Conolly also made many first-rate contributions to the psychiatric literature, and in the present work, one of his most important, he discusses the condition of British asylums, insanity and its causes, and ways to improve the care of the insane.

Wellcome II, p. 382.

877. ———. *The treatment of the insane without mechanical restraints.* London: Smith, Elder, 1856. xii, 380 pp., port. 21.6 cm.

In this book Conolly summarizes the use of mechanical restraints in mental asylums and discusses the progress made in asylums where their use had been abandoned. Conolly's efforts on behalf of the non-restraint system marked the successful conclusion of a movement that began with Pinel. As a result, an entirely new approach to insanity was initiated throughout the civilized world.

Garrison-Morton 4933; Osler 2360.

878. PIERRE FLOURENS (1794–1867). *Recherches expérimentales sur les propriétés et les fonctions du système nerveux, dans les animaux vertébrés.* Paris: Chez Crevot, 1824. xxvi, 331 [2] pp. 19.4 cm.

Flourens was one of the French giants in the production of basic experimental neurologic researches for which the nineteenth century was so notable in France. He was firm in his conviction that the cerebrum controlled thought and motion, and that the cerebellum was the main organ of equilibration and coordination. This book, one of the nineteenth-century classics on experimental neurology, was published in a much enlarged edition in 1842.

Cushing F207; Wellcome III, p. 34.

879. JOHN WARE (1795–1864). *An introductory lecture delivered before the medical class in Harvard University, on the 16th of October, 1833.* Boston: Hilliard, Gray, 1833. 40 pp. 21.5 cm.

A Massachusetts physician, Ware was educated at Harvard Medical School where he became Hersey professor of the theory and practice of medicine. He published a noteworthy book on croup in which he was one of the first to recognize the characteristics of diphtheria. He also published essays on hemoptysis and delirium tremens in which he gave classic descriptions of their symptoms. With Walter Channing he edited the *New England journal of medicine and surgery* which eventually became the *New England journal of medicine.*

This introductory lecture to his course in the elements of medical science was published at the request of his class, and in it he expounds upon his views on the character, deportment, and conduct of the physician.

Gift of Dr. R. N. Larimer.

*880. ALFRED ARMAND LOUIS MARIE VELPEAU (1795–1867). *Traité d'anatomie chirurgicale, ou Anatomie des régions, considérée dans ses rapports avec la chirurgie.* 2 vols. Paris: Chez Crevot, 1825–1826. Vol. I: xxxi, 580 [12] pp., 6 plates; Vol. II: xvi, 664 [16] pp., 8 plates. 20.3 cm. Original wrappers, uncut.

Velpeau, a member of the faculty of the University of Paris, was considered the leading French surgeon of his time. He was one of the first to attack aneurysms of the great vessels.

This first edition of his work on surgical anatomy contains fourteen colored lithographic plates of much beauty and detail.

881. ———. *Nouveaux éléments de médecine opératoire.* 2nd ed. Atlas only. Paris: J.-B. Baillière, 1839. 32 pp., 22 plates. 31.3 cm.

First published in 1835, this atlas of surgery and its accompanying massive three-volume text (not present) was, in its time, the best French work on the subject. The first American edition appeared in 1847.

Garrison-Morton 5592 (1st ed., 1835); Waller 9850.

*882. ———. *Traité des maladies du sein et de la région mammaire.* Paris: V. Masson, 1854. xix, 727 pp., 8 col. plates. 21.9 cm. Original wrappers, uncut.

This long monograph on tumors of the breast was the most authoritative work of its time on the subject and includes an important account of hyperplastic cystic disease of the breast.

Garrison-Morton 5771.

*883. ERNST HEINRICH WEBER (1795–1878). *Anatomia comparata nervi sympathici.* Leipzig: Apud C. H. Reclam, 1817. 182 pp., 5 plates (part fold.), 2 of which are accompanied by duplicate outline plates. 20.9 cm.

Professor of anatomy and physiology at Leipzig for many years, Weber, together with his brother Eduard Friedrich, made what is regarded as one of the greatest physiological discoveries when they demonstrated the inhibitory powers of the vagus nerve on the heart. Weber did further work on the hydrodynamics of the circulatory system, including the first accurate measurement of the velocity of the pulse-wave. In 1846 he completed his classic work on touch and temperature sense (*Der Tastsinn und das Gemeingefühl*) in which he showed that sensation can be separated into visceral and muscular components.

The present work, an early exposition on the autonomic nervous system, provided the background for some of Weber's later discoveries.

Garrison-Morton 1316; Waller 10134.

884. ROBERT JAMES GRAVES (1796–1853). *Clinical lectures delivered during the sessions of 1834–5 and 1836–7*. Philadelphia: A. Waldie, 1838. xi, 405 [2] pp. 22.5 cm.

Graves was chief physician to the Meath Hospital in Dublin and a founder of the Park Street School of Medicine. He introduced the best types of the continental methods of clinical teaching and was also well known for his reforms in patient care. While at Meath Hospital he gave a series of clinical lectures which became well known and widely read. First published in journals in Great Britain, the series for two sessions were first collected and published together in this rare Philadelphia edition. His later clinical lectures, given at the Park Street School, introduced such innovations as the "pin-hole pupil," timing the pulse by the watch, and discarding the practice of "starving" fevers and replacing it with "feeding" fevers. In fact, he once requested that his epitaph be, "He fed fevers."

Osler 2818; Waller 3718.

Gift of Dr. R. N. Larimer.

*885. ———. *Clinical lectures on the practice of medicine*. 2nd ed. 2 vols. Dublin: Fannin, 1848. Vol. I: xx, 586 pp.; Vol. II: xii, 570 pp. 22.3 cm. Original cloth.

Graves first published his *System of clinical medicine* in 1843, and it became an immediate success because it reflected his superior abilities as a teacher, observer, and writer. At the request of his publisher, he agreed to undertake a second edition of the book, and, after considerable revision and enlargement, the present work was published.

Graves found himself so busy that he asked J. Moore Neligan (1815–1863), a faculty member at the Dublin School of Medicine, to edit the book. Neligan decided to rearrange the book and present its contents in the form of lectures which he felt more closely conformed to Graves' style of writing. Much new material was added to this edition, especially Graves' observations on the epidemiology of cholera. He was one of the first to clearly show that cholera was contagious and spread along the lines of human contact.

Garrison-Morton 2218 (1st ed., 1843); Waller 3717 (1st ed.); Wellcome II, p. 150.

*886. JEAN ZULÉMA AMUSSAT (1796–1856). *Mémoire sur la possibilité d'établir un anus artificiel dans la région lombaire sans pénétrer dans le péritoine*. Paris: Germer-Baillière, 1839. [6] 210 pp. 23.8 cm. Half calf with original printed wrappers pasted on sides.

Amussat was a prominent French general surgeon of the nineteenth century who taught and practiced in Paris. Although his surgical interests were varied, he concentrated on surgery of the bladder, prostate, and abdominal viscera. He won prizes for his contributions to lithotripsy, torsion of arteries, air embolus, and what was then called "artificial anus" (colostomy).

Extraperitoneal colostomy in the lumbar region for imperforate anus had been suggested some years earlier, and in this work Amussat reports on his success in adapting the method to the treatment of malignancies of the lower bowel and rectum where obstruction existed. His method of lumbar colostomy was popular until later in the century when anterior transperitoneal colostomy became the preferred method. Amussat devotes a considerable portion of the book to excerpts from earlier writers on the subject and includes his reflections on their writings.

Garrison-Morton 3442; Waller 393.

887. JONES QUAIN (1796–1865) and Sir ERASMUS WILSON (1809–1884). [*A series of anatomical drawings*]. 5 vols. in 2. London: Printed for Taylor and Walton, 1836–1842. Plates. 49.8 cm.

This elaborate series of anatomical plates and accompanying descriptions ranks with the best nineteenth-century representations. The five volumes cover, respectively, the muscles, blood vessels, nerves, viscera, and bones and ligaments. Quain was an anatomist and teacher of some note whose *Elements of descriptive and practical anatomy* (1828) went through eleven editions. Wilson, who co-edited the second through the fifth volumes, was a dermatologist and philanthropist whose fame rests largely on the role he played in the demise of flogging in the British army.

Choulant-Frank, p. 404.

*888. JOHN BELL (1796–1872). *Dietetical and medical hydrology. A treatise on baths.* Philadelphia: Barrington and Haswell, 1850. 658 pp., illus. 20 cm.

Hydrotherapy was a common form of treatment among the ancients, but it was not until the controlled experiments of James Currie (see No. 709) that such therapy was approached on a rational basis. Bell was a successful Philadelphia physician whose knowledge of bathing is readily apparent in this detailed work which covers not only the clinical application of bathing but also its historical and geographical aspects.

*889. GEORGE CATLIN (1796–1872). *The breath of life or mal-respiration. And its effects upon the enjoyment & life of man.* [3rd ed.]. New York: John Bradburn, 1865. 76 pp., illus. 21.6 cm.

Catlin was a famous explorer among the American Indians and, as he states in this curious, fact-filled little book, he visited and studied 150 tribes in North and South America. He was particularly impressed by the state of health of the mouths of these native peoples, which health he attributed largely to their good breathing habits, that is, with mouth shut.

Garrison-Morton 3267 (1st ed., 1861); Osler 2254 (1st ed.).

*890. VINCENT DUVAL (1796–1876). *Traité pratique du pied-bot.* Paris: J.-B. Baillière, 1839. xiv, 336 pp., illus., 10 plates. 20.9 cm.

Duval, a prominent Paris physician, published several works on orthopedics, this volume on clubfoot being the first. The many forms of the deformity are amply illustrated in the short atlas which concludes the work. This is a presentation copy containing Duval's signature.

Waller 2666.

*891. JEAN BAPTISTE BOUILLAUD (1796–1881). *Traité clinique et physiologique de l'encéphalite, ou inflammation du cerveau.* Paris: J.-B. Baillière, 1825. xxiv, 350 pp. 21.5 cm.

Although Bouillaud is rightly regarded as the last of the great bloodletters, he was a shrewd observer and responsible for a number of important discoveries, among them the localization of the speech center in the middle of the left cerebral hemisphere, an observation first reported in this early treatise on brain diseases. Bouillaud was dean of the Medical Faculty of Paris.

Wellcome II, p. 211.

*892. ———. *Traité clinique des maladies du coeur.* 2 vols. Paris: J.-B. Baillière, 1835. Vol. I: [xxxiii] 534 pp., 2 fold. plates; Vol. II: 632 pp., 6 fold. plates. 20.5 cm.

Other investigators had previously noted the relationship between rheumatism and heart disease, but Bouillaud was the first to demonstrate a "law of coincidence" which statistically confirmed the correlation. Also in this work is the first description of Bouillaud's disease (rheumatic endocarditis). The eight folding plates in this copy are in exquisite condition.

Garrison-Morton 2749; Waller 1350; Wellcome II, p. 211.

*893. FRANÇOIS LEURET (1797–1851). *Anatomie comparée du système nerveux.* 2 vols. and atlas. Paris: J.-B. Baillière; New York: H. Baillière, 1839–1857. Vol. I: xxxii, 592 pp.; Vol. II: [vi] 692 pp. 22.2 cm.; Atlas: 60 pp., 32 plates. 41.4 cm. Each volume and atlas individually boxed.

Leuret was a pupil of Esquirol and later the chief physician at Bicêtre. This extensive treatise on comparative neuroanatomy is a summary of what was then known on the subject. It is here that Leuret erroneously names the precentral and postcentral cerebral convolutions after Luigi Rolando (1773–1831), the well-known Italian neuroanatomist whom Leuret believed had first discovered them in 1829. Actually, they had been noted more than fifty years earlier by Felix Vicq d'Azyr (1748–1794).

*894. JACOB LODEWIJK KOENRAAD SCHROEDER VAN DER KOLK (1797–1862). *Anatomisch physiologisch onderzoek over het fijnere zamenstel en de werking van het ruggemerg.* Amsterdam: C. G. Van der Post, 1854. 90 pp., 3 plates. 27.3 cm.

Through careful microscopic studies of the brain, Schroeder confirmed the medulla as the seat of epilepsy. Impressed with its many reflex functions, he postulated "an exalted sensibility and excitability" of the ganglia of that region to be the cause of the disease. Schroeder was professor of anatomy at the University of Utrecht in the Netherlands. His work on the anatomy and physiology of the medulla provided the basis for Schroeder's later work on epilepsy.

This is a presentation copy bearing Schroeder's signature.

Garrison-Morton 4815 (German ed., 1859).

*895. CAMILLE MELCHIOR GIBERT (1797–1866). *Traité pratique des maladies spéciales de la peau*. 2nd ed. Paris: G. Baillière, 1840. viii, 483 pp. 20 cm.

Though primarily a dermatologist, Gibert also published several works on general medicine. In this book he describes in detail a condition then known as pityriasis, establishing as definite clinical entities the various forms of pityriasis rosea.

Garrison-Morton 4048 (1860 ed.).

*896. GABRIEL ANDRAL (1797–1876). *Clinique médicale*. 4th ed. 5 vols. Paris: Crochard, 1839–1840. 20.5 cm.

Andral was the founder of the science of hematology and is credited with the integration of that science into clinical and investigative medicine. A close friend and colleague of Pierre Louis (see No. 843 ff.), Andral supported his numerical method of case study and assisted in the campaign against bloodletting. Andral's powers of persuasion, his vigorous style of writing, and his skill at lecturing contributed significantly to his tremendous influence on European medicine.

The first volume of the first edition of *Clinique médicale* was begun while Andral was still a medical student and was first published in 1823. As a treatise on general medicine, it is representative of the best medical practices of the day.

Waller 405; Wellcome II, p. 43.

*897. ———. *Essai d'hématologie pathologique*. Paris: Fortin, Masson, 1843. 186 pp. 20.7 cm.

This short volume is one of the most important works in the history of hematology. Here Andral first uses the terms "anemia" and "hyperemia" and clearly describes a number of diseases of the blood including lead poisoning, septicemia, and polycythemia.

Garrison-Morton 3060; Waller 406; Wellcome II, p. 44 (1845 ed.).

*898. NATHAN RYNO SMITH (1797–1877). *Surgical anatomy of the arteries*. Baltimore: Toy, 1832. 104 pp., illus., col. plates. 27.3 cm.

Smith held the chair of surgery at the University of Maryland for fifty years and is best known for the development of an anterior splint for treating fractures of the femur, an apparatus on which he worked for over thirty years. He helped found or edit a number of early American medical periodicals including the *American journal of the medical sciences*.

Surgical anatomy of the arteries is Smith's greatest single work. The plates are copied from the *Anatomie de l'homme* of Jules Germain Cloquet (see No. 859).

899. BENJAMIN ELLIS (1798–1831). *The medical formulary.* 5th ed. Philadelphia: Carey, Lea & Blanchard, 1838. xvi, 231 pp. 22.6 cm.

Of the numerous formularies compiled during the nineteenth century in the United States, that of Benjamin Ellis must be included among the more popular, his version eventually passing through eleven editions. Ellis was professor of materia medica at Philadelphia College of Pharmacy.

Wellcome II, p. 519 (1831 ed.).

*900. PHILIPPE FRÉDÉRIC BLANDIN (1798–1849). *Traité d'anatomie topographique.* 2 vols. Paris: Chez Mme. A. Méquignon, 1826. Text: xliv, 690 pp. 21 cm.; Atlas: 28 pp., 12 leaves of plates. 33.3 cm.

Surgeon at Hôtel Dieu and professor of surgery of the Medical Faculty of Paris, Blandin was the first to describe the mixed glands of the tongue (Blandin's glands), and he developed a number of surgical techniques used in rhinoplasty. In *Traité d'anatomie topographique* he sought to integrate and show the relationship between anatomy and surgery. The twelve full-page lithographic illustrations in the atlas are by N. H. Jacob.

Cushing B431 (1834 ed.); Waller 1107 (1834 ed.); Wellcome II, p. 176.

901. ———. ———. 2nd ed. Atlas only. Brussels: Société Encyclographique des Sciences Médicales, 1838. 20 col. plates, each accompanied by a leaf of descriptive letterpress. 33.3 cm.

The number of plates in the second edition was increased to twenty, all in detailed color.

902. ROBLEY DUNGLISON (1798–1869). *Medical lexicon, a new dictionary of medical science.* 3rd ed. Philadelphia: Lea & Blanchard, 1842. [5] 749 pp. 23.5 cm.

A native of Keswick, England, Dunglison emigrated in 1824 to the United States when Thomas Jefferson offered him the chair of anatomy and physiology at the University of Virginia. Nine years later he moved to Jefferson Medical College where he remained for the duration of his career. Dunglison must rank among the most prolific of American medical writers and one of its finest lecturers. His works, while not offering much original material, were highly readable and accurate. Of his many books, his dictionary was probably the most popular, passing through twenty-three editions.

Waller 2642 (1874 ed.).

*903. SAMUEL GEORGE MORTON (1799–1851). *Illustrations of pulmonary consumption, its anatomical characters, causes, symptoms and treatment.* Philadelphia: Key & Biddle, 1834. xiii [4] 9-183 pp., 12 plates (part col.). 22.5 cm.

Morton, a native of Philadelphia and a graduate of the University of Edinburgh, did notable work in both natural history and clinical medicine. His investigations on the cranial anatomy of various races are considered milestones in anthropology.

This work on tuberculosis was the first of its kind to be published in the United States and is a summary of the contemporary knowledge regarding consumption. The descriptions of the disease are particularly vivid as are the twelve colored lithographic plates.

Garrison-Morton 3222.

904. JAMES SYME (1799–1870). *The principles of surgery.* Philadelphia: Carey & Lea, 1832. xxviii, 5–375 pp., plate. 21.1 cm.

Though he never earned a medical degree, Syme was a dominant figure in Scottish surgery throughout his career, most of which was spent in the Royal Infirmary. Syme's most important accomplishments lay in the areas of amputation and excision where his surgical skill was matched by his soundness of judgment and knowledge of pathology. In addition to introducing a number of surgical innovations, Syme was one of the first to recognize the value of ether in his operations. He was also an early supporter of the concept of antisepsis as taught by his pupil and son-in-law, Lord Lister (see No. 1035). *The principles of surgery* was published in the United States the same year it was released in Scotland and was one of a number of highly regarded surgical texts and atlases Syme produced during his career.

Cushing 5499 (Edinburgh ed., 1832); Waller 9436 (London ed., 1842).

JOSEPH E. PARKER (fl. 1840). *The anatomy, physiology and pathology of the human teeth.*

See No. 956.

*905. CHARLES MICHEL BILLARD (1800–1832). *Traité des maladies des enfans nouveaux-nés et à la mamelle.* Paris: Baillière, 1828. xv, 653 pp. 20.3 cm. Gilt, quarter morocco.

———. *Atlas d'anatomie pathologique, pour servir à l'histoire des maladies des enfans.* Paris: Baillière, 1828. 8 pp., 10 col. plates. 35.5 cm.

Billard was a prominent gynecologist at the time he wrote this pioneering work on pediatric pathology. Correlating his clinical observations with hundreds of autopsies on infants and children, he shed much needed light on an array of childhood illnesses, some of which had been thought to occur only in adults. Supplementing the text, which contains illustrative case histories, is a remarkable atlas containing ten colored plates showing various pathological conditions, including peptic ulcer, cerebral hernia, thrush, etc.

Garrison-Morton 6332; Waller 1060 (1835 ed.); Wellcome II, p. 167.

*906. PHILIPPE RICORD (1800–1889). *Traité pratique des maladies vénériennes.* Paris: J. Rouvier, 1838. 808 pp. Contemporary half calf. 21.5 cm.

Born in Baltimore of French parents, Ricord received his medical education in Paris. As surgeon to the Hôpital du Midi, which at that time was devoted solely to treating male venereal afflictions, Ricord gained international fame as a brilliant lecturer and scientist. In this, his major work, Ricord details the results of over 2,500 experiments proving the distinction between syphilis and gonorrhea, thus overthrowing the teaching of John Hunter (see No. 609 ff.) who considered the two to be identical. Ricord's descriptions of the three phases of syphilis and the accompanying case histories remain as accurate today as when he wrote them.

Garrison-Morton 2381; Waller 7974.

907. ———. *Traité complet des maladies vénériennes: clinique inconographique de l'Hôpital des vénériens*. Paris: J. Rouvier, 1862. 201 pp., 50 leaves of col. plates, col. illus., port. 34.9 cm.

Ricord's extensive work with venereal diseases at the Hôpital du Midi is chronicled here in sixty-six superb colored lithographs illustrating a multitude of conditions at various levels of infection in both sexes. The illustrations were drawn from nature by Bion and Beau and are accompanied by case histories and treatment modes.

Waller 7973 (1st ed., 1851).

908. JAMES HOPE (1801–1841). *A treatise on the diseases of the heart and great vessels*. 1st American ed. from the 3rd London ed. Philadelphia: Lea & Blanchard, 1842. xviii, 572 pp., plates (part fold.). 22.5 cm.

One of Europe's foremost authorities and teachers on morbid anatomy and heart pathology, Hope studied in London, Paris, Rome, and Florence before settling in London as a lecturer at St. George's Hospital. Hope was able to synthesize the work of his predecessors with his own observations, and his writings reflect a wealth of bedside experience. His *Treatise on the diseases of the heart and great vessels* was first published in 1831, but it was extensively revised before this first American edition appeared. Included in the work are some of the finest clinical descriptions of valvular defects ever written.

Garrison-Morton 2747 (1st ed., 1831); Wellcome III, p. 298 (1832 ed.).

*909. JOHANNES MÜLLER (1801–1858). *Ueber die phantastischen Gesichtserscheinungen*. Coblenz: J. Hölscher, 1826. x, 117 [1] pp. 20.7 cm.

Müller was one of the most brilliant leaders of the nineteenth-century school of physiology in Germany. Although he began his professional career as a practicing clinician, his interest and knowledge in the other sciences led to a career in investigative physiology during which he made important contributions in anatomy, neurology, embryology, chemistry, pathology, and botany. The strength of his influence can be measured by the number of important scientists who were fortunate enough to come under his tutelage. They include DuBois, Helmholtz, Henle, Schwann, and Virchow.

It is in the present work that Müller first enunciated his law of specific nerve energies (later propounded in detail in his *Handbuch*), stating that each sense organ, however stimulated, gives rise to its own characteristic sensation. This observation is probably his most important single contribution. The latter portion of the work deals with clairvoyance, hallucinations, and dreams—topics in which Müller remained interested throughout his life.

Cushing M570; Garrison-Morton 1456; Waller 6733.

*910. ———. *Handbuch der Physiologie des Menschen für Vorlesungen.* 2 vols. Coblenz: J. Hölscher, 1834–1840. Vol. I: viii, 852 pp.; Vol. II: vi, 780 pp., plate. 22.5 cm.

Müller's *Handbuch* is the great classic of the nineteenth century in the field of physiology. Here he summarizes the advances of the preceding decades and successfully integrates the contributions of other fields, notably comparative chemistry, physics, and psychology. It is largely through this work that physiology emerged as a medical discipline under Müller's leadership.

Garrison-Morton 601; Waller 6730.

———. *Observationes de canaliculis corpusculorum ossium atque de modo, quo terrea materia in ossibus continetur.*

See No. 961.

911. ARMAND TROUSSEAU (1801–1867) and HIPPOLYTE BELLOC (fl. 1830). *A practical treatise on laryngeal phthisis, chronic laryngitis, and diseases of the voice.* Translated by J. A. Warder. Philadelphia: A. Waldie, 1839. 186 pp. 22 cm.

Trousseau's immense skill as practitioner and clinician caused Garrison to compare him with men such as Bright and Addison. Although he discovered no new diseases, his descriptions of the common maladies of the day such as diphtheria, typhoid fever, and scarlet fever are unrivaled for their clarity and accuracy. As a leader of the French therapeutic renaissance, Trousseau was instrumental in creating new modes of treatment of croup, emphysema, pleurisy, goiter, and malaria. Trousseau received the prize of the French Academy of Medicine for this classic essay on laryngology which originally appeared in 1837.

Cushing T167; Garrison-Morton 3258 (1st French ed., 1837); Waller 9697 (1st French ed.).

*912. ———. *Clinique médicale de l'Hôtel-Dieu de Paris.* 2 vols. Paris: J.-B. Baillière et fils; New York: Baillière Bros., 1861–1862. Vol. I: lii, 772 pp.; Vol. II: 841 pp. 21.7 cm.

As professor of clinical medicine and physician to the Hôtel Dieu, Trousseau developed a well-deserved reputation as an exceptional lecturer and teacher and an advocate of bedside teaching through clinical demonstration. *Clinique médicale* contains the bulk of his most important writings and passed through three editions.

Garrison-Morton 2221; Waller 9696.

*913. EDWARD WILLIAM TUSON (1802–1865). *Myology.* 2nd ed. London: Callow and Wilson, 1828. [2] 8 *ll.*, 8 col. plates. 53.8 cm.

This unusual teaching atlas by the English anatomist, Tuson, depicts the somatic musculature in colored lithographs, printed on flaps and mounted in layers on figures of the skeleton. It is unusual to find the moving parts intact and preserved as in this copy.

Choulant-Frank, p. 234; Cushing T196.

*914. JULES SICHEL (1802–1868). *Traité de l'ophthalmie, la cataracte et l'amaurose.* Paris: G. Baillière, 1837. xi, 750 [2] pp., 4 col. plates. 20.9 cm. Gilt morocco.

Born in Frankfurt in 1830, Sichel came to Paris and established the first private eye clinic where he had a large and devoted clientele. He was justly recognized as one of the finest ophthalmologists of the nineteenth century. This early work on cataracts is an example of his exacting scholarship that helped establish Sichel's reputation. The several plates are similar in style to those in his atlas (see No. 915).

*915. ———. *Iconographie ophthalmologique.* 2 vols. Paris: J.-B. Baillière, 1852–1859. Text: xix, 823 pp.; Atlas: 80 pp., 80 plates (part col.). 30.7 cm. Half calf.

Probably the most massive and detailed nineteenth-century work on ophthalmology, this is Sichel's *magnum opus* and is said to have taken twenty-five years to complete. The eighty delicately executed colorplates illustrate virtually every eye malady known at the time and they remain accurate in nearly every detail. The accompanying text includes thorough discussions of the various diseases based on the case histories of Sichel's patients.

Garrison-Morton 5868; Waller 8910.

*916. PIERRE LOUIS ALPHÉE CAZENAVE (1802–1877) and HENRI ÉDOUARD SCHEDEL (d. 1856). *Abrégé pratique des maladies de la peau.* Paris: Chez Béchet jeune, 1828. xl, 526 pp. 20.6 cm. Calf back, gilt spine.

Both Cazenave and Schedel were pupils of the eminent Laurent Théodore Biett (1781–1840), and this authoritative text is based largely on his clinical lectures. By 1862, four French, three English, and two German editions had been published. Cazenave later founded the first journal devoted to dermatology, *Annales des maladies de la peau et de la syphilis.*

Garrison-Morton 3990; Waller 1835 (1847 ed.); Wellcome II, p. 317.

*917. GASPARD JOSEPH MARTIN-SAINT-ANGE (1803–1888). *Iconographie pathologique de l'oeuf humain fécondé en rapport avec l'étiologie de l'avortement.* Paris: J.-B. Baillière, 1884. viii, 188 pp., 19 plates., col. illus. 31.7 cm.

The nineteen colored plates in this atlas on fetal pathology were lithographed from drawings by the author, a French physiologist and pathologist.

918. ELISHA BARTLETT (1804–1855). *The history, diagnosis, and treatment of the fevers of the United States.* [2nd ed.]. Philadelphia: Lea and Blanchard, 1847. xxi, 547 pp. 23 cm.

Bartlett, a native of Rhode Island, was graduated from the medical department of Brown University in 1826 and spent the next few years in France where he was greatly influenced by Louis (see No. 843 ff.) and his practical approach to medicine. Bartlett returned to the United States and settled in Lowell, Massachusetts. Although he practiced there for many years, Bartlett held professional chairs at various times in nine different institutions, including Dartmouth College, Transylvania University, University of Maryland, Vermont Medical College, University of Louisville, and the College of Physicians and Surgeons of New York.

Bartlett was also an active writer, editor, and contributor to the medical periodicals of his day. The present work, discussing typhoid and typhus fever, was first published in 1842 and is his most notable contribution to the literature. In this second edition, he enlarged the sections on periodical and yellow fevers. According to Osler, "This work immediately placed Bartlett in the front rank of American physicians of the day. It had a powerful influence on the profession of the country" (Sir William Osler, *An Alabama student and other biographical essays.* New York, 1908. p. 132).

Cushing B130 (1856 ed.); Wellcome II, p. 109.

*919. JOHN HILTON (1804–1878). *On the influence of mechanical and physiological rest in the treatment of accidents and surgical diseases, and the diagnostic value of pain.* London: Bell and Daldy, 1863. xii, 499 pp., illus. 22.2 cm. Original cloth, recased.

Hilton received his professional education at Guy's Hospital and, when finished, became a member of the Royal College of Surgeons. He remained at Guy's and was, in turn, demonstrator of anatomy, assistant surgeon, and surgeon. Upon retirement, he was appointed consulting surgeon. He was active in the affairs of the Royal College of Surgeons and served on the council from 1854 until his death, serving as president in 1867.

In a series of lectures at the Royal College of Surgeons, Hilton introduced a new concept in the treatment of surgical disorders by urging removal only of those tissues which hindered nature's own healing process and by advocating rest as being of prime importance in this natural process. This classic work has been reprinted for more than a hundred years, and it still contains valuable and valid lessons.

Garrison-Morton 5609; Osler 2971.

*920. KARL VON ROKITANSKY (1804–1878). *Handbuch der pathologischen Anatomie.* 3 vols. Vienna: Braumüller & Seidel, 1842–1846. Vol. I: 572 pp.; Vol. II: xiii, 882 pp.; Vol. III: xiv, 632 pp. 21.1 cm.

Rokitansky rightly may be regarded as the finest anatomical pathologist of his age. It was largely through his influence that the Vienna School reblossomed into world prominence. Although he never practiced medicine, his studies and descriptions of structural changes in disease, based on over 30,000 autopsies performed while he was director of Vienna's Pathological Institute, had an enormous impact on clinical medicine.

The number of original observations in his *Handbuch* is staggering. Included here are the first differentiation between lobar and lobular pneumonia, the first pathological account of spondylolisthesis, the first accurate description of acute yellow atrophy of the liver, and the correct classification of patent ductus arteriosis as a congenital lesion. Not without its shortcomings, the work includes Rokitansky's anachronistic humoral disease theory which was criticized by Virchow (see No. 1011 ff.), then professor of anatomy in Berlin. Rokitansky admitted the error and rewrote the entire work. In spite of such theoretical miscalculations, Rokitansky revealed more clearly than any of his predecessors the natural history of disease and its structural manifestations.

Garrison-Morton 2293.

*921. ———. *Die Defecte der Scheidewände des Herzens.* Vienna: W. Braumüller, 1875. vi, 156 pp., illus. 32.1 cm.

An outstanding and popular teacher, Rokitansky was untiring in his efforts to provide clear and accurate descriptions of the various states of disease. He labored for more than a decade to produce this, his last work, an outstanding illustrated exposition of the defects of the septum of the heart.

Garrison-Morton 2778.

922. WILLIAM STOKES (1804–1878). *A treatise on the diagnosis and treatment of diseases of the chest. Part 1. Diseases of the lung and windpipe.* Dublin: Hodges and Smith, 1837. xx, 557 pp. 22.2 cm. Original cloth, uncut.

Stokes, a colleague and close friend of Robert Graves (see No. 884), was the son of Whitley Stokes, Regius professor of medicine at the University of Dublin and himself a distinguished and accomplished physician. Stokes succeeded his father as Regius professor in 1845. William studied chemistry at Glasgow and then went to Edinburgh where he received his medical degree in 1823. Before returning to Dublin in 1825, he published the first treatise on the stethoscope in the English language. After his return to Dublin, he was appointed physician to Meath Hospital, a position he held for nearly fifty years. In addition, he was one of the editors of the *Dublin journal of medical science*, taught at the University, and maintained an extensive private practice.

Stokes established his reputation in the history and development of internal medicine through the publication of this work. He describes the peculiar type of breathing known as Cheyne-Stokes respiration, a first stage of pneumonia not known before, and other findings of significance. The projected second part was never published.

Garrison-Morton 2213; Osler 4035; Waller 9280.

Gift of Drs. Robert and Janet Wilcox.

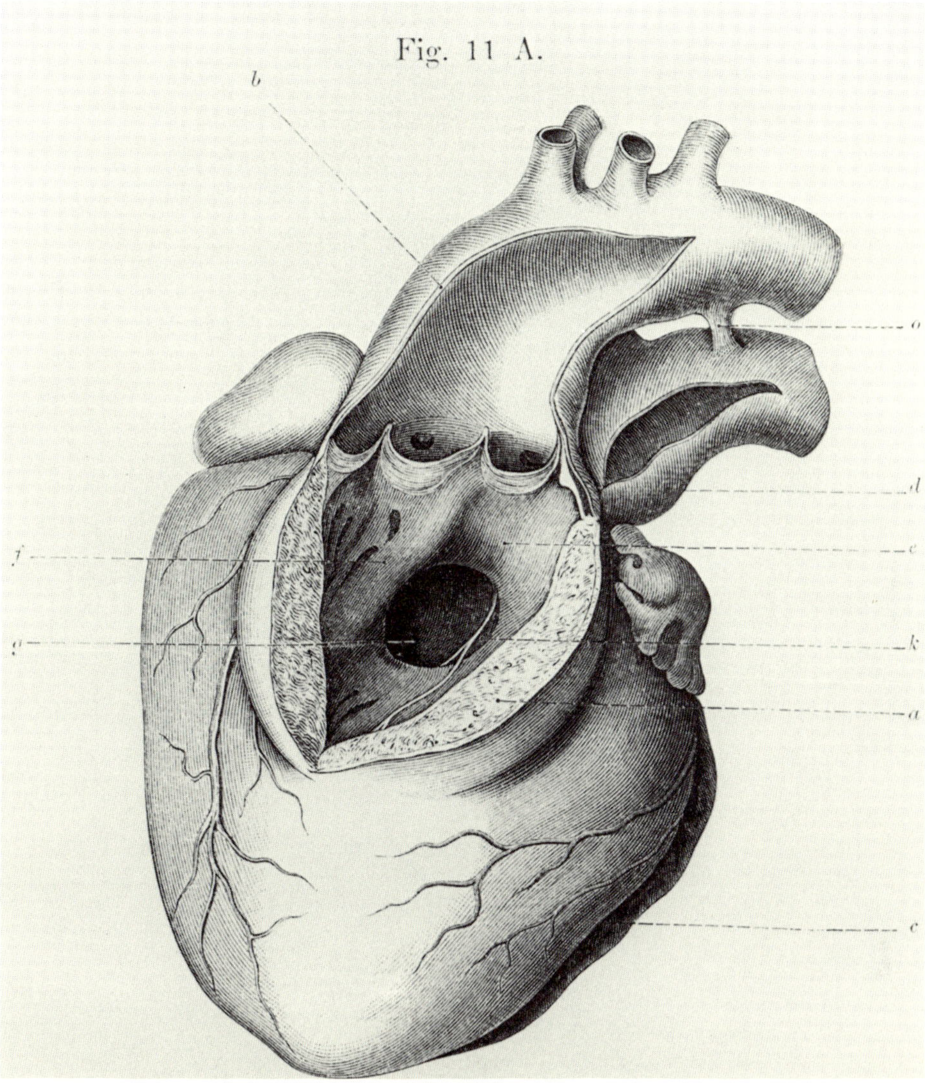

No. 921. Rokitansky. *Die Defecte der Scheidewände des Herzens.* A large congenital defect of the interventricular septem.

923. ———. ———. Philadelphia: A. Waldie, 1837. xv, 360 pp. 22.9 cm.

This first American edition, published the same year as the first Dublin edition, attests to the importance of and interest in this landmark work on the lungs.

Gift of Dr. R. N. Larimer.

924. ———. *The diseases of the heart and the aorta.* Dublin: Hodges and Smith, 1854. xvi, 689 pp. 22.2 cm. Original cloth.

Stokes confirmed his importance as a clinician in this work on the heart. His description of fatty degeneration of the heart has hardly been improved upon. He also describes the condition of slow pulse accompanied by cerebral attacks of syncope, since known as the Stokes-Adams syndrome, and he first identified the weak semi-beats of the heart between regular contractions as contractions of the auricles.

Cushing S434; Garrison-Morton 2760.

*925. Sir RICHARD OWEN (1804–1892). *Descriptive and illustrated catalogue of the physiological series of comparative anatomy contained in the Museum of the Royal College of Surgeons in London.* 5 vols. in 6. London: Printed by R. Taylor, 1833–1840. 79 plates (part fold., part col.). 28.8 cm. Original purple cloth.

Owen was the outstanding zoologist-anatomist of his time. A student of John Abernethy (see No. 731), he became Hunterian professor at the Royal College of Surgeons and later was superintendent of the Natural History Department of the British Museum. At first an anti-Darwinist, he was eventually won over to the evolutionary theory by the arguments of Thomas Huxley in its favor.

After John Hunter's (see No. 609 ff.) death, his extensive museum of anatomical specimens was cared for by his assistant, William Clift, who persuaded the British government to purchase the collection. Hunter's collection formed the basis for the collections in the Museum of the Royal College of Surgeons where Owen later became curator. The catalogue is very well illustrated, and many of the seventy-nine copperplates were drawn by William Bell (fl. 1830). The Museum was destroyed during World War II.

Garrison-Morton 326.

*926. ———. *Odontography; or, A treatise on the comparative anatomy of the teeth.* 2 vols. London: H. Baillière, 1840–1845. Vol. I: lxxiv [1] 655 pp.; Vol. II: 37 pp., 168 plates. 25.1 cm. Half morocco, uncut.

The present work on the morphology of mammalian (including human) teeth is one of the most comprehensive works ever undertaken on the subject and led Owen into the study of paleontology, in which he became an acknowledged master.

Garrison-Morton 329.

*927. ———. *On the classification and geographical distribution of the Mammalia*. London: J. W. Parker, 1859. 103 pp., illus. 22.1 cm. Maroon cloth.

Owen's mastery of vertebrate anatomy is nowhere more evident than in this little volume covering the various orders of mammals.

Osler 3596.

*928. ———. *On the anatomy of vertebrates*. 3 vols. London: Longmans, Green, and Co., 1866–1868. Vol. I: xlii, 650 pp., illus.; Vol. II: viii, 592 pp., illus.; Vol. III: x, 915 pp., illus. 22 cm.

Sir William Flower (1831–1899) considered this anatomical treatise second in importance only to Cuvier's comparative anatomy (see No. 745). The entire work was based on Owen's personal observations and includes a vast number of illustrations, many of which were drawn with the aid of the microscope, a tool which Owen helped to popularize as an instrument for naturalists. The preface contains a concise discussion of the distinction between homologous and analogous structures, a concept which Owen had introduced some years earlier.

Garrison-Morton 336; Waller 11922.

929. JOSEF ŠKODA (1805–1881). *Abhandlung über Perkussion und Auskultation*. 6th ed. Vienna: L. W. Seidel, 1864. x, 343 pp. 21.4 cm.

Škoda was another member of the New Vienna School who made lasting contributions in clinical diagnosis. Following the principles laid down by Laennec concerning the importance of physical signs and symptoms, Škoda refined the technique of percussion and auscultation, classifying various sounds according to pitch and tone. Škoda's resonance, an important sign in pneumonia, remains of value as a diagnostic aid today.

Garrison-Morton 2676 (1st ed., 1839); Osler 3989 (French ed., 1854); Waller 8978 (1st ed.).

930. SAMUEL DAVID GROSS (1805–1884). *Elements of pathological anatomy*. 2 vols. Boston: Marsh, Capen, Lyon, & Webb, and James B. Dow, 1839. Vol. I: 518 pp., illus., 4 col. fold. plates; Vol. II: 510 pp., illus., 1 col. fold. plate. 21.5 cm.

Gross, one of the best-known surgeons and teachers of his day, was one of the founders of the American Medical Association and of the American Surgical Society and taught for many years at Jefferson Medical College in Philadepia. He wrote this important treatise while professor of pathological anatomy at Cincinnati Medical College. According to Garrison, it was the first comprehensive work on the subject in English. A number of superb illustrations supplement the exhaustive text.

Garrison-Morton 2292; Osler 2842; Wellcome III, p. 170.

*931. ———. *A system of surgery; pathological, diagnostic, therapeutic and operative.* 2nd ed. 2 vols. Philadelphia: Blanchard and Lea, 1862. Vol. I: 1062 pp., illus.; Vol. II: 1134 pp. 22.9 cm.

Gross's *System of surgery* is said to be one of the greatest surgical treatises ever written and was for many years the standard text in medical schools. It went through numerous editions and was translated into several languages.

Garrison-Morton 5607 (1st ed., 1859); Osler 2842 (1882 ed.).

932. ———. *Autobiography of Samuel D. Gross . . . With sketches of his contemporaries.* 2 vols. Philadelphia: G. Barrie, 1887. Vol. I: xxxii, 407 pp.; Vol. II: viii, 437 pp., front. 22.7 cm.

Few medical histories are as engaging as this detailed and well-written autobiography. Gross's commentary on the formation and early years of the American Medical Association is particularly interesting, as are his reflections on contemporary medical figures.

Cushing G415; Osler 2843; Waller 16911.

*933. JOSEPH FRANÇOIS MALGAIGNE (1806–1865). *Traité d'anatomie chirurgicale et de chirurgie expérimentale.* 2nd ed. 2 vols. Paris: J.-B. Baillière, 1859. Vol. I: viii, 784 pp.; Vol. II: 886 pp. 20.1 cm.

One of the most respected scholars in the history of medicine, Malgaigne was equally skillful as surgeon, anatomist, and surgical historian. Written on a wide variety of subjects, his works reflect the classical training and expository skills which he nurtured throughout his life. His influence on surgery is evidenced by the great number of surgical and anatomical terms associated with his name, and by the fact that many of his descriptions and techniques remain virtually unchallenged today. Malgaigne's editions of the works of Paré (see No. 163) and his numerous other works on medical history attest to his skill as an historian. The present work on surgical anatomy, first published in 1838, is the second of Malgaigne's three works on surgery.

Garrison-Morton 5594 (1st ed., 1838); Waller 6186.

*934. ———. *Traité des fractures et des luxations.* 2 vols. and atlas. Paris: J.-B. Baillière, 1847–1855. Vol. I: vii, 842 pp.; Vol. II: 1108 pp. 21.3 cm.; Atlas: 30 plates. 44.3 cm.

This work on fractures is perhaps the best of Malgaigne's treatises on operative surgery. It includes his classic discussion of a double vertical fracture of the pelvis.

Garrison-Morton 4417; Waller 6187.

935. GUILLAUME BENJAMIN AMAND DUCHENNE (1806–1875). *De l'électrisation localisée et de son application à la pathologie et à la thérapeutique.* 3rd ed. Paris: J.-B. Baillière et fils, 1872. xii, 1120 pp., 3 plates, illus. (1 col.). 22.4 cm.

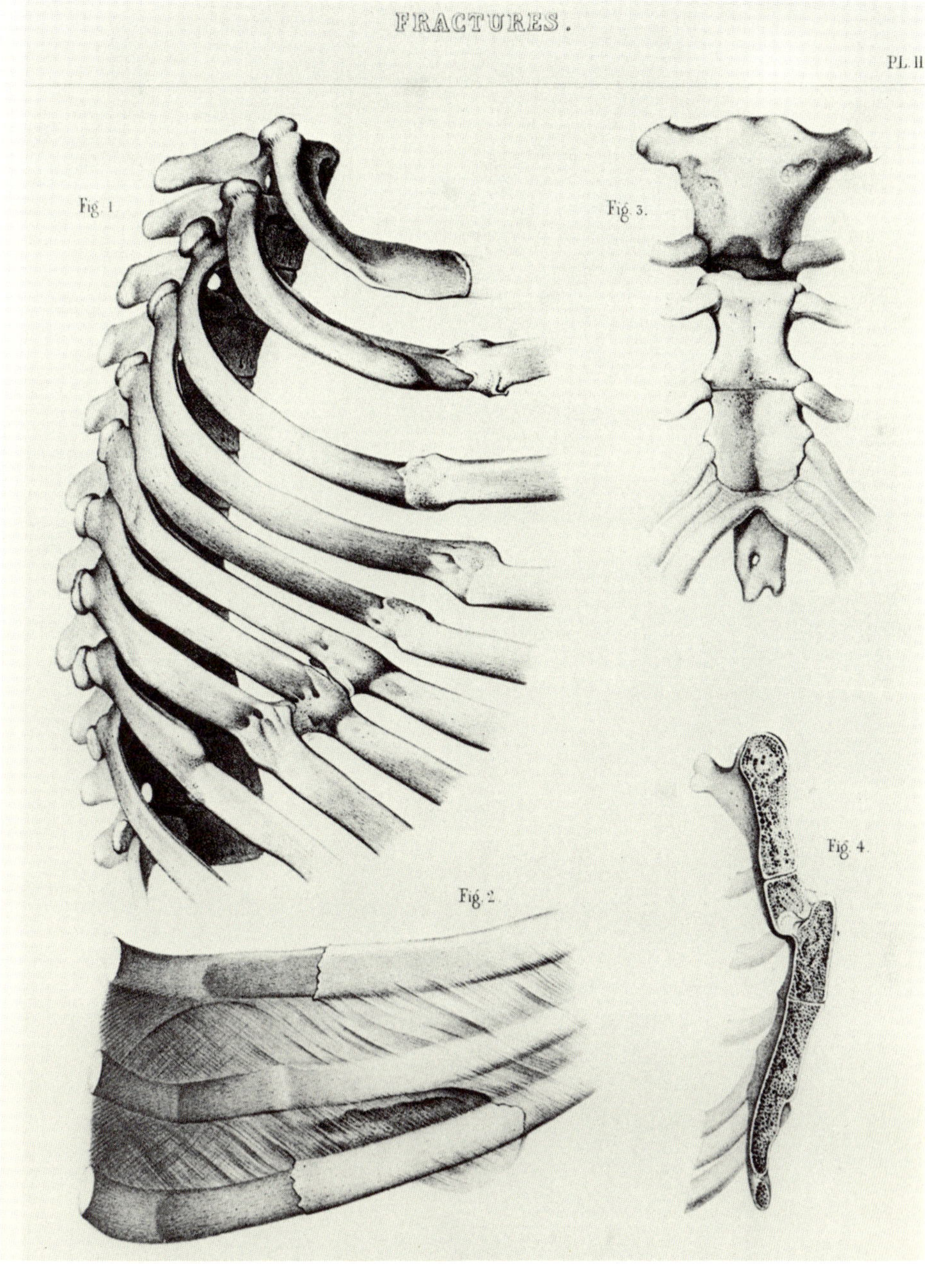

No. 934. Malgaigne. *Traité des Fractures et des Luxations.*

Eccentric, timid, ignored by contemporaries, and the subject of ridicule, Duchenne nonetheless must be regarded as one of the greatest of the early French neurologists. Though he never occupied a professorial chair or even held a hospital appointment, his personal diligence in meticulously following the course of treatment of his patients allowed him to amass a wealth of observational evidence leading to a number of fundamental discoveries in neuropathology. He was the first to describe glosso-labio-laryngeal paralysis (progressive bulbar paralysis) and progressive muscular atrophy of the upper extremities (Duchenne-Aran's disease). He was also the first to employ electrical stimulation of nerves and muscles in exploring the muscular system and in the diagnosis and treatment of neurological diseases. The results of these early experiments are summarized in this, his first major work.

Garrison-Morton 614 (1st ed., 1855); Osler 2511 (1st ed.); Waller 2604.

*936. AUGUSTE NÉLATON (1807–1873). *Elémens de pathologie chirurgicale.* 5 vols. Paris: G. Baillière, 1844–1859. Illus. 21.6 cm.

A colleague of Malgaigne at the Hôpital St. Louis, Nélaton was known as one of the finest surgeons in France and as a modest and generous man whose mild personality endeared him to his patients, students, and friends. He invented a number of surgical instruments, among them a porcelain-tipped bullet probe and a flexible rubber catheter which bears his name.

The five-volume *Elémens de pathologie chirurgicale* is Nélaton's major work and includes virtually all of his surgical innovations and discoveries.

Garrison-Morton 5597; Waller 6830.

937. MASSACHUSETTS MEDICAL SOCIETY. *Pharmacopoeia of the Massachusetts Medical Society.* Boston: Larkin, 1808. 272 pp. 18.3 cm.

The first work of its kind to be published in the United States, this early pharmacopoeia, together with those of other New England states, provided the prototype for the first *United States pharmacopeia* which was published in 1820 (see No. 1003). The purpose as stated in the Preface was "to point out those articles whose properties entitle them to be employed for the cure of diseases, with the best modes of preparing them."

Austin 1222; Cushing M192.

*938. THOMAS WHARTON JONES (1808–1891). *A manual of the principles and practice of ophthalmic medicine and surgery.* London: J. Churchill, 1847. xxxvi, 570 pp., 4 leaves of plates, illus. (4 col.). 16.9 cm.

Jones's medical versatility is reflected in his writings which include works on ophthalmology (his major field), pharmacology, ear diseases, reproductive physiology, and hematology. He is credited with discovering the amoeboid movement of leukocytes. Jones was professor of ophthalmic medicine at University College in London when he wrote this textbook of ophthalmology.

Garrison-Morton 5862; Wellcome III, p. 364.

*939. HENRY INGERSOLL BOWDITCH (1808–1892). *A brief plea for an ambulance system for the Army of the United States.* Boston: Ticknor and Fields, 1863. 28 pp. 23.7 cm.

After the death of his son in 1862 in the Battle of Centerville, Bowditch wrote this impassioned plea for a trained and organized ambulance corps to serve the Union Army. Despite his efforts and a letter of support from General McClellan (reprinted here), the request was never acted upon. Bowditch was a respected physician and teacher who made notable strides in the fields of public health and respiratory diseases. Several generations of Bowditch's family were physicians, all associated with Harvard University and well known both as clinicians and physiologists.

*940. AMÉDÉE BONNET (1809–1858). *Traité des maladies des articulations.* 2 vols. and atlas. Paris: J.-B. Baillière, 1845. Vol. I: l, 582 pp.; Vol. II: 647 pp. 21 cm.; Atlas: 16 plates. 34.9 cm.

Bonnet was physician to the Hôtel Dieu in Lyons where he held the posts of Chirurgien-majeur and Chirurgien-en-chef and established himself as a noted orthopedic surgeon. The text to this, his most famous work, details the clinical symptoms and combined medical and orthopedic treatment of diseases of the joints. The finely executed lithographs in the atlas illustrate a variety of conditions and therapeutic techniques, including immovable dressings, for which Bonnet was especially noted.

Waller 1286; Wellcome II, p. 201.

*941. ROBERT BENTLEY TODD (1809–1860). *The cyclopaedia of anatomy and physiology.* 5 vols. London: Sherwood, Gilbert, and Piper, 1836–1859. Illus. 24.3 cm.

Todd was one of the outstanding British and European scientists who, through the use of the compound microscope, brought anatomy to a fine point of accuracy. In addition to his serving for many years as professor of physiology at King's College and Westminster Medical School, Todd maintained a private medical practice in London and wrote a number of fine works on both clinical and investigative medicine. In this massive and detailed work, Todd enlisted as contributors such prominent figures as Sir Richard Owen, Richard Quain, Thomas Bell, Gilbert Breschet, and Sir James Paget.

942. THOMAS NUNNELEY (1809–1870). *A treatise on the nature, causes, and treatment of erysipelas.* Philadelphia: Barrington & Geo. D. Haswell, 1844. 235 [36] pp. 23.1 cm. Original printed boards.

Nunneley, English physician and physiologist, was a private practitioner in Leeds and was affiliated with the Leeds School of Medicine as a lecturer on anatomy and surgery. He was an accomplished eye surgeon who performed more than 1,000 cataract operations and was one of the first surgeons to achieve continuing success in excising the tongue.

This book, first published in 1841, is a comprehensive treatise on the diagnosis and treatment of erysipelas. In this first American editiion, additional information on epidemic erysipelas in Indiana and New England was included.

*943. CHARLES DARWIN (1809–1882). *On the origin of species by means of natural selection, or, The preservation of favoured races in the struggle for life.* London: J. Murray, 1859. ix, 502 pp., 1 fold. diagr. 19.7 cm. Original green blind-stamped cloth, in cloth box.

What the dropping of the first atomic bomb was to the twentieth century, the publication of Darwin's *On the origin of species* was to the nineteenth century. Battle lines were drawn on both religious and scientific grounds and the world-wide criticism and controversy attendant upon its publication lasted well into the present century.

Cushing D50; Garrison-Morton 220; Osler 1566; Waller 10786.

*944. ———. *The variation of animals and plants under domestication.* 2 vols. London: J. Murray, 1868. Vol. I: viii, 411 pp., illus.; Vol. II: 486 pp. 22.2 cm.

This work may be viewed as a detailed account of the material summarized in the first chapter of *On the origin of species.* It also contains Darwin's erroneous theory of pangenesis, a variation of Lamarckism, which taught the inheritance of acquired characteristics.

Garrison-Morton 224.1; Waller 10789.

*945. ———. *The descent of man, and selection in relation to sex.* 2 vols. London: J. Murray, 1871. Vol. I: viii, 423 pp., illus.; Vol. II: viii, 475 pp., illus., port. 19.1 cm. Original cloth.

"This is really two works. The first demolished the theory that the universe was created for Man, while in the second Darwin presented a mass of evidence in support of his earlier hypothesis regarding sexual selection" (Garrison-Morton 170). *The descent of man*, often discussed with *On the origin of species* as one of Darwin's two most important works, unduly stirred controversy and resentment well beyond the academic field. Darwin attempted to examine the mind objectively like any other phenomenon in nature.

Cushing D43; Garrison-Morton 170; Osler 1572; Waller 11799.

Sir ERASMUS WILSON (1809–1884). [*A series of anatomical drawings*].

See No. 887.

*946. JAKOB HENLE (1809–1885). *Allgemeine Anatomie.* Leipzig: L. Voss, 1841. xxiv, 1048 pp., illus., 5 fold. plates. 21.2 cm.

A follower of Bichat's pioneer work in microscopic anatomy, Henle became the greatest histologist of his day and one of the finest anatomists of any era. A man of wide interests, equally at home with the arts as with science, Henle led a life filled with politics, romance, and intrigue. After study at the University of Bonn where he became a favorite of Johannes Müller, Henle served on the faculties of the universities of Berlin, Heidelberg, and Göttingen. Henle was the first to investigate the minute structures of the epithelial system. His explanation of metastasis in cancer was the forerunner of Virchow's cellular pathology.

One of Henle's most important discoveries, several of which were first stated in the present work, was the muscular layers in the walls of the arterioles, an observation which became the starting point of the study of the vasomotor theory.

Choulant-Frank, p. 404; Garrison-Morton 543; Waller 4332.

*947. OLIVER WENDELL HOLMES (1809–1894). *Dissertations on the question How far are the external means of exploring the condition of the internal organs to be considered useful and important in medical practice?* [Boston: Printed by Perkins & Marvin, 1836]. 288 pp. 22.3 cm.

Because he is so well known for his verse and literary essays, it is often forgotten that Holmes was a physician and professor of anatomy at Harvard from 1847 to 1882. His medical writings, while offering no original discoveries, made their mark on his generation. Holmes's part in convincing obstetricians of their potential role in the transmission of puerperal fever and his introduction of the use of the microscope and stethoscope into the medical curriculum are certainly worthy of mention.

The present volume was the winning reply to the Boylston Medical Committee of Harvard, who posed the question in the title and offered a gold medal to the author of the best response. The work emphasizes the role of percussion and auscultation in diagnosis.

Osler 2987.

*948. ———. "The contagiousness of puerperal fever." (In *New England quarterly journal of medicine and surgery*. Vol. 1 (1842–1843), pp. 503–530.) 21.5 cm. Contemporary quarter calf, rebacked, in half morocco box.

This brief, lucid, and somewhat acerbic paper must be regarded as one of the most important contributions of nineteenth-century American medicine. In it, Holmes demonstrates conclusively the contagious nature of childbed fever. He showed that the dreaded disease, carried by the unwashed hands of the physician from bed to bed, could be avoided by simply washing the hands before and after pelvic examination and after postmortem examination. Like Semmelweiss, who confirmed Holmes's conclusions (see No. 992), Holmes suffered the abuse and ridicule of his fellow physicians, who only reluctantly and after many years conceded the truth.

The severity and widespread occurrence of the disease led Holmes to state in the strongest terms the obligation of the physician: "Whatever indulgence may be granted to those who have heretofore been the ignorant cause of so much misery, the time has come when the existence of a private pestilence in the sphere of a single physician should be looked upon not as a misfortune but a crime" (p. 530). The *New England quarterly journal of medicine and surgery* was published for only one year, and complete copies, such as this one, are uncommon.

Garrison-Morton 6274; Osler 2989; Waller 4852.

*949. ———. *Homoeópathy, and its kindred delusions.* Boston: W. D. Ticknor, 1842. v, 72 pp. 18.6 cm.

Holmes was quick to expose those medical systems and practices which he believed to be false. In these two lectures, originally delivered before the Boston Society for the Diffusion of Useful Knowledge, he attacks not only homeopathy (which he likens to astrology and alchemy), but four other contemporary quack claims: the royal cure of the King's Evil (scrofula), the Weapon ointment, the tar water mania of Bishop Berkeley (see No. 509), and the metallic tractors of Perkinism.

Cushing H415; Osler 2988; Waller 4850; Wellcome III, p. 293.

*950. ———. *An introductory lecture, delivered at the Massachusetts Medical College, November 3, 1847.* Boston: W. D. Ticknor, 1847. 38 pp. 22.5 cm.

Holmes's gifts as an orator caused him to be much in demand as a speaker. This lecture and the valedictory address which follows are two of many such speeches he delivered before various groups of the medical profession.

Osler 2991.

*951. ———. *Valedictory address, delivered to the medical graduates of Harvard University at the annual commencement, Wednesday, March 10, 1858.* Boston: David Clapp, 1858. 15 pp. 23.7 cm.

952. ———. *Currents and counter-currents in medical science. With other addresses and essays.* Boston: Ticknor and Fields, 1861. ix [1] 406 pp. 19.1 cm. Original cloth.

This collection of essays and lectures are good examples of Holmes's subjects and style: "Homeopathy, and its kindred delusions," "The position and prospects of the medical student," and "Mechanism of vital actions"; this last had appeared in the *North American review* for April, 1857.

Cushing H4111; Osler 2992; Waller 4849.

Gift of Dr. R. N. Larimer.

953. ———. *Border lines of knowledge in some provinces of medical science.* Boston: Ticknor and Fields, 1862. 80 pp. 18.8 cm.

Another of Holmes's many published lectures, this address was originally delivered in 1861 before the medical class of Harvard where Holmes was Parkman Professor of Anatomy and Physiology.

Cushing H408; Waller 4848.

CHARLES HUETTE (fl. 1850). *Précis iconographique de médecine opératoire et d'anatomie chirurgicale.*

See No. 970.

*954. JOSEPH MACLISE (fl. 1850). *Surgical anatomy.* London: John Churchill, 1851. [86] pp., 35 col. plates. 52.2 cm. Contemporary half calf.

Maclise was a student of Samuel Cooper (1781–1848) and a prominent London surgeon. The thirty-five large colored lithographic plates were drawn by the author. Together with the text, they represent both fine artistry and fine scholarship.

955. PAUL BECK GODDARD (1811–1866). *Plates of the arteries.* Philadelphia: Auner, 1839. vi, 49 pp., 12 col. plates. 29 cm.

Goddard, teacher of anatomy at the University of Pennsylvania and prominent medical editor, prepared this book with its twelve full-page plates for the medical student. The book was based on William E. Horner's (see No. 869) *Treatise on the special anatomy of the human body* (1826) to which the student is referred for a complete discussion of the arteries. Goddard's basic purpose was to provide the student with an up-to-date account of the principal arteries and their trunks.

Waller 3604.

956. ———. *The anatomy, physiology, and pathology of the human teeth . . . aided in the practical part by Joseph E. Parker, Dentist.* Philadelphia: Carey and Hart, 1844. 227 pp., 30 plates (incl. front.). 31.8 cm.

Goddard, together with a dentist, Joseph E. Parker, combined practical information on the treatment of dental disease based on a knowledge of pathology. The work contains much information on the use of porcelains in the making of artificial dentures. The thirty plates, showing anatomy, pathology, and dental equipment, are of special interest. There is also a brief history of earlier writing on the teeth as well as a good bibliography.

Gift of R. S. Rathbun.

*957. AMÉDÉE FORGET (1811–1869). *Recherches sur les kystes des os maxillaires et leur traitement, suivies de considérations générales sur l'amputation de la machoire inférieure.* Paris: Rignoux [1840]. 87 pp. 24.3 pp.

This book on maxillary and mandibular cysts is probably the best-known work by Forget, a respected French surgeon who contributed a number of valuable papers on surgical technique and anesthesia. The book was submitted as his doctoral dissertation to the Medical Faculty of Paris.

Wellcome III, p. 41.

958. Sir JAMES YOUNG SIMPSON (1811–1870). *Anaesthesia; or, The employment of chloroform and ether in surgery, midwifery, etc.* Philadelphia: Lindsay and Blakiston, 1849. 248 pp. 22.2 cm.

Simpson, a leading obstetrician of his time and a member of the faculty at the University of Edinburgh, introduced the use of chloroform as an anesthetic after experimenting with ether and finding it somewhat unsatisfactory. Within weeks of his demonstration in 1847 of the superiority of chloroform, it had almost universally displaced ether as a general anesthetic.

This work, which was never published in book form in Great Britain, is a collection of his writings and speeches on his experiences in the use of chloroform and ether.

Osler 1366; Waller 8959.

*959. FRANÇOIS ACHILLE LONGET (1811–1871). *Recherches expérimentales et pathologiques sur les propriétés et les fonctions des faisceaux de la moelle épinière et des racines des nerfs rachidiens.* Paris: Bechet jeune et Labé, 1841. 187 pp. 22.3 cm. Original wrappers.

Longet was one of a group of nineteenth-century French experimental physiologists who made important new discoveries concerning the nature of the nervous system. It was Longet who first demonstrated that motor impulses were transmitted in the anterior section of the spinal cord while sensory messages were confined to the posterior portion. The present work on experimental pathology of the nervous system is the first of several noteworthy contributions by Longet.

*960. ———. *Anatomie et physiologie du système nerveux de l'homme et des animaux vertébrés.* 2 vols. Paris: Fortin, Masson, 1842. Vol. I: viii, 942 pp., 4 fold. plates; Vol. II: 698 pp., 4 fold. plates. 21.3 cm. Calf-backed marbled boards.

This extensive work systematically covers the anatomy of the nervous system; and includes a particularly important discussion of the cranial nerves and the then-incompletely understood autonomic nervous system. Also presented here is the first complete description of the complex nerve innervation of the larynx.

Wellcome III, p. 544.

*961. FRIEDRICH MIESCHER (1811–1887). *De inflammatione ossium eorumque anatome generali.* Berlin: G. Eichler, 1836. xiv, 281 pp., 4 leaves of plates. 24.9 cm.

This well-known student of Johannes Müller (see No. 909) served successively as professor of pathology, anatomy, and physiology at Berlin, Bern, and Basel. Miescher discovered nuclein and was also the first to suggest the existence of a genetic code. In this book, Miescher discusses the embryology and growth of bone as well as the various inflammatory diseases that afflict the skeletal system. The work also contains Müller's *Observationes de canaliculis corpusculorum ossium atque de modo, quo terrea materia in ossibus continetur* illustrated with four very fine lithographic plates.

962. THOMAS BLIZARD CURLING (1811–1888). *A practical treatise on the diseases of the testis, and of the spermatic cord and scrotum.* Philadelphia: Carey and Hart, 1843. xiii [24]–568 pp., illus. 23 cm. Calf.

Curling, surgeon at the London Hospital for many years, was president of the Royal College of Surgeons in 1873. He was one of the first to present a clinical description of cretinism and to suggest that it was caused by a deficiency of the thyroid gland. William M. Ord (1834–1902) later coined the term "myxoedema" for this condition. This book was first published in London in 1843 and was edited for republication in the United States by Paul B. Goddard (see No. 955). Goddard made several revisions and additions to the book and, in the preface, indicated that Curling's book surpasses Sir Astley Paston Cooper's (see No. 741 ff.) earlier work on the testis.

Wellcome II, p. 420 (London ed., 1843).

Gift of H. C. Bulis and A. F. Barfoot.

ANTOINE CHARLES ERNEST BARTHEZ (1811–1891). *Traité clinique et pratique des maladies des infants.*

See No. 978.

*963. JOSEPH HYRTL (1811–1894). *Lehrbuch der Anatomie des Menschen.* Prague: F. Ehrlich, 1846. xvi, 718 pp. 23.3 cm.

Hyrtl was one of the most popular teachers in Europe and probably the most eloquent lecturer on anatomy in the nineteenth century. According to Garrison his courses were "followed by enthusiastic crowds of every race and class, even foreign nobles and consuls" (Fielding H. Garrison, *An introduction to the history of medicine.* 4th ed. Philadelphia, 1929. p. 463).

Lehrbuch der Anatomie des Menschen was written during Hyrtl's thirty-year professorship at the University of Vienna and is one of the finest unillustrated treatises on anatomy. Its deserved popularity eventually led to twenty-two editions with translations in every major language.

Garrison-Morton 413; Waller 5050; Wellcome III, p. 324.

*964. CONSTANTIN LOUIS BONAMY (b. 1812) and PAUL BROCA (1824–1880). *Atlas d'anatomie descriptive du corps humain.* 4 vols. Paris: V. Masson [1844?]–1866. 254 col. plates (some fold.). 26.8 cm. Half morocco.

Bonamy, professor of anatomy at L'École Préparatoire de Médecine de Toulouse, prepared Volume One on osteology, syndesmology, and myology as well as Volume Two on the heart, arteries, veins, lymphatics, and aponeuroses. Broca, the eminent neurosurgeon and anthropologist, prepared Volume Three on the digestive and endocrine systems and Volume Four on the genitourinary and respiratory systems. The 254 colored plates were engraved by Émile Beau (b. 1810), and each has a facing page containing the descriptive information.

Wellcome II, p. 197.

965. AUSTIN FLINT (1812–1886). *A treatise on the principles and practice of medicine.* 2nd ed. Philadelphia: Henry C. Lea, 1867. 967 pp. 23.2 cm.

After receiving his medical degree at Harvard in 1833, Flint went on to become one of the century's most brilliant leaders of clinical medicine and medical education in the United States. He taught at numerous medical schools, founded Buffalo Medical College, was active as a hospital physician, and served a term as president of the American Medical Association. His great interest was in diseases of the chest, particularly heart disease and tuberculosis. Among his best-known works are *Physical exploration and diagnosis of diseases affecting the respiratory organs* (1856), *Compendium of percussion and ausculation* (1864), *Practical treatise . . . of diseases of the heart* (1859), and *Clinical medicine* (1879).

*966. THOMAS MORTON (1813–1849). *The surgical anatomy of the groin, the femoral, and popliteal regions.* London: Taylor and Walton, 1839. [81]–207 pp., illus., 8 col. plates (6 fold.). 25.7 cm. Original cloth.

Morton was the first student of North London (University College) Hospital to be placed on the hospital staff. The present volume is one of a number of works on surgical anatomy Morton wrote during his brief lifetime. Most of the drawings, including five of the eight colored plates, were drawn by his brother, Andrew.

*967. DAVID LIVINGSTONE (1813–1873). *Missionary travels and researches in South Africa.* London: John Murray, 1857. ix, 687 pp., illus. (part fold.), 2 fold. maps, fold. plan. 21.7 cm.

Certainly one of the most remarkable men of the nineteenth century, David Livingstone almost single-handedly opened up the interior of Africa through his varied and extensive explorations of the continent. His training in Greek, theology, and medicine at Glasgow enabled him to secure a missionary station under the auspices of the London Missionary Society. His religious zeal was soon overshadowed by his revulsion at the flourishing slave trade which he termed the "running sore of Africa." The remainder of his life was devoted almost solely to exploring alternate trade routes which might undercut those based on slave labor. His journeys are recounted in this fascinating and absorbing account, which includes one of the earliest descriptions and illustrations of the tsetse fly and its role in cattle disease.

Cushing L308; Garrison-Morton 5269; Osler 5077; Waller 19917.

968. WILLIAM ACTON (1813–1875). *A complete practical treatise on venereal diseases.* 1st American ed. New York: Redfield, 1846. 334 pp., illus. (part col.). 24.1 cm.

Acton was a pupil and admirer of Philippe Ricord (see No. 906) and an internationally recognized authority on venereal diseases. This treatise, originally published in England in 1841, contains several striking colored lithographs of the various manifestations of syphilis and gonorrhea in both sexes.

969. CLAUDE BERNARD (1813–1878). *Leçons de physiologie expérimentale appliquée à la médecine.* 2 vols. Paris: J.-B. Baillière, 1855–1856. Vol. I: 520 pp., illus.; Vol. II: viii, 510 pp., illus. 21.1 cm.

Bernard, the renowned French physiologist, is regarded as the founder of experimental medicine. He had unusual literary talent but decided to devote himself to the study of medicine. Bernard became an intern under François Magendie (see No. 818 ff.) at the Hôtel Dieu in Paris in 1839 and began a fruitful association with him. Bernard assisted Magendie in his experiments, collaborated with him in his scientific papers, and later worked on his own problems and wrote his own papers. Magendie, while making great discoveries, usually went about his work in a haphazard fashion; Bernard, on the other hand, was a careful worker and observer. All of his great discoveries were based on isolated facts which he had the ability to correlate and build into larger physiological generalizations which he later verified by experiments. The Académie des Sciences awarded Bernard the *grand prix* in physiology in 1849, 1851, and 1853, for his discoveries concerning the pancreas, the liver, and the vasomotor function and other activities of the sympathetic nervous system.

This basic work on the application of experimental physiology to medicine contains, among others, his memorable work on glycogenesis and experimental diabetes.

Garrison-Morton 615; Osler 1507; Waller 954.

*970. ——— and CHARLES HUETTE (fl. 1850). *Précis iconographique de médecine opératoire et d'anatomie chirurgicale.* Paris: Méquignon-Marvis, 1856. xxvi, 495 pp., front., 113 col. plates. 18.6 cm. Contemporary green half morocco, gilt spine.

This atlas is one of the few works Bernard wrote on subjects other than physiology. It is handsomely illustrated with over 100 hand-colored steel engravings drawn from life or cadaver dissection and covers a wide range of surgical procedures.

Cushing B324 (1846 ed.); Wellcome II, p. 151 (1848 ed.).

971. CLAUDE BERNARD. *Leçons sur les effects des substances toxiques et médicamenteuses.* Paris: J.-B. Baillière et fils, 1857. vii, 488 pp. 21.4 cm.

Bernard's scientific methods were applied to good effect to the area of toxicology.

This series of lectures covers, among other subjects, the actions of poisons on the body, the physiology of toxic absorption, and the nature of toxic gases.

Garrison-Morton 1863; Waller 960; Cushing B321; Osler 1508.

*972. ———. *Leçons sur la physiologie et la pathologie du système nerveux.* 2 vols. Paris: J.-B. Baillière et fils, 1858. Vol. I: viii, 520 pp., illus.; Vol. II: 560 pp., illus. 22.3 cm. Original wrappers.

This work was the text for Bernard's course on the nervous system given at the Collége de France where he was professor of experimental physiology.

Cushing B319; Garrison-Morton 1399; Osler 1509; Waller 957.

*973. ———. *Leçons sur les propriétés physiologiques et les altérations pathologique des liquides de l'organisme.* 2 vols. in 1. Paris: J.-B. Baillière, 1859. Vol. I: xvi, 524 pp., illus.; Vol. II: 476 pp., illus. 21.2 cm.

Another of Bernard's scholarly textbooks, this work covers the physiology and pathology of blood and other body fluids.

Osler 1510; Waller 963.

*974. ———. *Introduction à l'étude de la médecine expérimentale.* Paris: J.-B. Baillière; New York: Baillière Bros., 1865. 400 pp. 21 cm.

In this significant work, Bernard presents his basic philosophy toward the analytical method in science. He illustrates his discussion of method by examples drawn from his own vast research. The work has appeared in many French editions since this first edition of 1865, and it was published in an English translation in 1927.

Osler 1511; Waller 951.

*975. ———. *Leçons sur les anesthésiques et sur l'asphyxie.* Paris: J.-B. Baillière et fils, 1875. vii, 536 pp., illus. 21 cm.

This monograph is a landmark in the history of the development of anesthesia, for Bernard did some basic work on the physiologic effects of anesthetic drugs, pointed out the dangers of such drugs, and advocated the use of pre-anesthetic depressants such as morphine.

Garrison-Morton 5673; Waller 959.

*976. ———. *Leçons sur le diabète et la glycogenèse animale.* Paris: J.-B. Baillière, 1877. viii, 576 pp., illus. 21.3 cm.

Bernard, in this work, first showed that one of the primary signs of diabetes is an excess of sugar in the blood and usually in the urine. Much of Bernard's experimentation and research had a direct relationship to clinical medicine.

Cushing B320; Garrison-Morton 3942; Osler 1515; Waller 958.

977. JAMES MARION SIMS (1813–1883). *Silver sutures in surgery*. New York: S. S. and W. Wood, 1858. 79 pp., illus. 22.7 cm.

Called to see a country woman who had incurred a retroversion of the uterus in a fall from a horse, Sims observed that examination and correction were facilitated by a lateral positioning of the patient. The adoption of this position, the subsequent invention of a special curved speculum and use of silver sutures and a silver catheter, soon allowed Sims to operate successfully for vesicovaginal fistula, a frequent and distressing complication of childbirth seen particularly among the poor. Sims's procedure (Sims's operation) was so successful that it was soon adopted worldwide.

This work was originally delivered before the New York Academy of Medicine. Sims recounts his early experience with the use of silver sutures (used to avoid sepsis) and takes full credit for their discovery and adoption.

Cushing S255; Garrison-Morton 5605.

Gift of Sara (Conn) and Harold Lincoln Thompson Foundation; James Emmett Conn Memorial Book Fund.

*978. FRÉDÉRIC RILLIET (1814–1861) and ANTOINE CHARLES ERNEST BARTHEZ (1811–1891). *Traité clinique et pratique des maladies des infants*. 3 vols. Paris: G. Baillière, 1843. Vol. I: xxxii, 850 pp.; Vol. II: [2] 782 pp.; Vol. III: [2] 743 [1] 32 pp. 21.2 cm. Dark green morocco-backed boards.

Rilliet, of Geneva, wrote this important and comprehensive work on pediatrics with his colleague Antoine Charles Ernest Barthez (1811–1891). The men had studied together at Paris and had begun this work some years before their graduation. The book received awards from a number of academies of science and medicine and is notable for its classic descriptions of pediatric diseases. One of the earliest works on pediatrics as a specialty, it contains case studies to show the etiology, clinical course, therapy, and pathology of a disease. The work went through three editions and was also translated into German.

Garrison-Morton 6333.

*979. LOUIS ALFRED BECQUEREL (1814–1862). *Séméiotique des urines*. Paris: Fortin, Masson, 1841. xvi, 576 pp. 21.7 cm.

Becquerel was an active practitioner and diagnostician and a member of the Medical Faculty of Paris as well as head physician at St. Perrine Hospital. His father, Antoine César Becquerel, was one of the founders of electrochemistry and pioneered in the field of electrolysis.

This study of the alteration of urine composition in various diseases is the younger Becquerel's first work.

Wellcome II, p. 128.

*980. ———. *Traité des applications de l'électricité à la thérapeutique médicale et chirurgicale.* Paris: Germer Baillière; New York: H. Baillière, 1857. viii, 376 pp., illus. 21.4 cm.

This monograph did much to clarify the uses of electricity in diagnosis and therapy at a time when the phenomenon was poorly understood. In spite of such scholarly works as this one, the abuse and misuse of electricity by quacks continued well into the twentieth century.

*981. ROBERT REMAK (1815–1865). *Diagnostische und pathogenetische Untersuchungen.* Berlin: August Hirschwald, 1845. viii [2] 242 pp., fold. plate. 21.5 cm.

Remak was responsible for a remarkable number of original discoveries, most notably in the areas of neurocytology and embryology. He was the first to describe non-medullated nerve fibers (fibers of Remak). He demonstrated that proliferation of tissue by cell growth was through cell division and not endogenous formation, and he introduced the three-layer concept of embryo development. Remak attended the University of Berlin and studied under the famed Johannes Müller. The son of a Polish Jew, Remak was denied a teaching career because of his religion and was forced to support himself through private practice.

The monograph on pathology and diagnosis was written as a result of research done at the clinic of Johann Schoenlein (1793–1864), noted German clinician and pathologist.

Waller 7875.

*982. Sir JOHN TOMES (1815–1895). *A course of lectures on dental physiology and surgery.* London: J. W. Parker, 1848. xii, 397 pp., illus. 21.9 cm.

The raising of the status of English dentistry from a trade to a science was largely the result of the efforts of Sir John Tomes who secured the passage of the Dental Act of 1878 providing for the mandatory education and registration of dentists. Before his reform efforts, Tomes, a surgeon, had already gained a considerable reputation through his studies of the bones and teeth and the publication of the present work, a series of lectures originally delivered at the Middlesex Hospital School of Medicine. The book covers tooth development, anatomy and pathology of the teeth, and periodontal structures and includes an account of the early use of anesthesia in dentistry. This is a presentation copy, inscribed by the author.

Garrison-Morton 3683.

*983. FERDINAND KEBER (1816–1871). *Mikroskopische Untersuchungen über die Porosität der Körper.* Königsberg: In Kommission bei den Gebrüdern Bornträger, 1854. xvi, 183 pp., 2 plates. 26.6 cm.

Keber's discovery of the micropyle, the minute opening in the ovum membrane by which sperm enter, may certainly be regarded as a major achievement in reproductive physiology. His work was supported by the eminent British embryologist, Martin Barry (1802–1855), who confirmed Keber's observations in a letter printed in this report of his research.

*984. LUDWIK MAURYCY HIRSCHFELD (1816–1876). *Traité et iconographie du système nerveux et des organs des sens de l'homme.* 2nd ed. Atlas only. Paris: G. Masson, 1866. 92 plates (part fold.). 28.1 cm.

The extensive study of neuroanatomy during the latter half of the nineteenth century resulted in a plethora of atlases of the nervous system. The exquisite plates included in this comprehensive work were drawn by J. B. Léveillé and are some of the most detailed of the time. Hirschfeld was professor of anatomy on the Faculty of Medicine at Warsaw.

Osler 2973 (1st ed., 1853).

*985. ALEXANDER ECKER (1816–1887). *The cerebral convolutions of man.* Translated by Robert T. Edes. New York: D. Appleton, 1873. 87 pp., illus. 23 cm.

Ecker was professor of anatomy at the University of Freiburg in Baden where he distinguished himself as a first-rate investigator. This work on brain convolutions and their development was first published in 1869 in Germany under the title *Die Hirnwindungen des Menschen nach eigenen Untersuchungen.*

Cushing E3 (London ed., 1873).

*986. CHARLES ÉDOUARD BROWN-SÉQUARD (1817–1894). "Recherches expérimentales sur la physiologie et la pathologie des capsules surrénales." (In *Compte rendu des séances de l'Academie des Sciences.* Vol. 43 (1856), no. 8, pp. 422–425; 542–546.) 28.2 cm.

Brown-Séquard achieved prominence in England, France, and the United States as one of the finest physiologists of his day. After meeting with little success as a writer, he turned to medicine, where his talents and curiosity found creative outlets. Frequently on the move, mainly for financial reasons, Brown-Séquard held academic appointments at various universities in England, Paris, and the United States (including Harvard and Virginia), and was always in demand for his lecturing skills. Eventually he succeeded Claude Bernard to the post of chair of experimental medicine at the Collège de France.

Brown-Séquard is best known for his research on the endocrine system, the present work being one of the most important in that field. By the simple experiment of excising the adrenal glands of animals, he proved the glands were indispensable to life. It is one of the first works to demonstrate the functions of the glands of internal secretion and is basic to the development of endocrinology.

Garrison-Morton 1140; Waller 1505a.

987. ———. *Course of lectures on the physiology and pathology of the central nervous system.* Philadelphia: Collins, 1860. xii, 276 pp., plates. 23.2 cm.

Brown-Séquard's investigation of spinal cord transection in which he defines the relative function of the posterior and anterior cord sections and their relationship to other neural pathways is one of his foremost accomplishments and is explained fully in this impressive series of lectures.

Cushing B755; Waller 1501.

*988. ———. *Lectures on the diagnosis and treatment of the principal forms of paralysis of the lower extremities.* Philadelphia: Collins, 1861. 118 pp. 22.6 cm. Original cloth.

This study of the pathway of conduction of the spinal cord and its relationship to paralysis was written shortly before Brown-Séquard accepted an appointment as physician at the National Hospital for the Paralysed and Epileptics in Queen's Square, London.

Cushing B756.

*989. ALBERT VON KÖLLIKER (1817–1905). *Handbuch der Gewebelehre des Menschen, für Aerzte und Studierende.* Leipzig: W. Engelmann, 1852. x, 637 pp., illus. 22.5 cm.

A Swiss by birth, Kölliker received his medical education by attending Müller's lectures in Berlin and studying at Heidelburg where he was graduated. After serving as prosecutor for Henle in Zurich, Kölliker was called to Würzburg where he remained for half a century. A genius, possessing remarkable powers of observation, he made enormous strides in the understanding of human and animal tissue. He was the first to apply Schwann's cell doctrine to embryology and to isolate smooth muscle fiber. Charles Sedgwick Minot (1852–1914) said that Kölliker, "knew more by direct personal observation of the microscopic structure of animals than anyone else who ever lived" (Fielding H. Garrison, *An introduction to the history of medicine.* 4th ed. Philadelphia, 1929. p. 462).

Handbuch der Gewebelehre des Menschen, one of Kölliker's most important works, may be considered the first textbook of histology.

Garrison-Morton 546; Waller 5356 (1867 ed.).

*990. ———. *Entwicklungsgeschichte des Menschen und der höheren Thiere.* Leipzig: W. Engelmann, 1861. x, 468 pp., illus. 22.5 cm. Bound with No. 873.

In this important treatise on comparative embryology, Kölliker describes the cellular segmentation and differentiation of embryonic tissue leading to the formation of complex organ systems. The text is generously supplemented with 225 woodcuts.

Cushing K167; Garrison-Morton 487; Waller 5355.

*991. JOHN WATTS (1785–1831), VALENTINE MOTT (1785–1865), and ALEXANDER HODGDON STEVENS (1789–1869). *The medical & surgical register:*

consisting chiefly of cases in the New York Hospital. Vol. I, pts. 1 and 2. New York: Collins, 1818–1820. x, 406 pp., illus., plates. 23.5 cm.

The medical and surgical register, of which only two parts were issued, is the first volume of case reports published by a United States hospital, and is one of the cornerstones in the history of American medicine, as well as one of the scarcest of medical periodicals. In it, one case report stands out as of great importance—that of Valentine Mott who first tied the innominate artery of a patient with an aneurysm of the right subclavian artery. Although this patient later died because of the excessively diseased condition of the artery, Mott performed, in all, 138 ligations for aneurysm of the great vessels, and his patients almost always recovered.

Mott received his M.D. from Columbia in 1806 and studied also in London and Edinburgh. He taught surgery in various American medical schools and carried on a tremendous surgical practice. He enjoyed an international reputation, and it was said by Sir Astley Paston Cooper that "He has performed more of the great operations than any man living, or that ever did live" (Francis R. Packard, *History of medicine in the United States*. 2 vols. New York, 1931. Vol. I, p. 415).

This copy was once owned by Willard Parker (1832–1884), another well-known American surgeon who himself performed many operations on the great vessels. His signature appears several times.

Austin 1254; Garrison-Morton 2942; Waller 10130.

*992. IGNÁC FÜLÖP SEMMELWEIS (1818–1865). *Gesammelte Werke*. Jena: G. Fischer, 1905. vi, 604 pp., plate, port. 25.6 cm. Original paper wrappers.

Medicine has witnessed few dramas as compelling as the heroic, yet tragic, career of Ignác Fülöp Semmelweis, which stands as a monument to moral and scientific courage. As obstetrician at the Vienna Krankenhaus, Semmelweis noted the high rate of deadly puerperal fever among obstetrical patients and in particular those attended by medical students who moved freely from the dissecting morgue to the wards. After instituting a strict handwashing policy, Semmelweis saw a dramatic drop in the incidence of the disease which prompted him to notify the Vienna Medical Society of his findings. In spite of his having marshaled overwhelming evidence to support his contention that the disease could be spread by attending physicians, his ideas were vehemently opposed by nearly every prominent physician of his day. A notable exception was Oliver Wendell Holmes (see No. 948) who had earlier published a paper on the contagiousness of puerperal fever. By the time that his idea finally gained acceptance it was twenty years after his definitive analysis of 1861 (included in the present work) and Semmelweis was dead, having succumbed to septicemia while a patient in a lunatic asylum.

Osler 3955; Waller 8832.

*993. AMBROISE AUGUST TARDIEU (1818–1879). *Étude médico-légale et clinique sur l'empoisonnement . . . avec la collaboration de Z. Roussin*. Paris: J.-B. Baillière, 1867. xxii, 1072 pp., illus., plates. 21.2 cm.

This exhaustive work on medico-legal toxicology was, at the time of its writing, one of the most authoritative works of its kind and is typical of the writings of Tardieu in its clarity and exactness. Covering a wide range of drugs and poisons, the book is amply illustrated with case reports and autopsies. Tardieu was professor of legal medicine at the University of Paris.

Garrison-Morton 1745; Waller 9479.

994. ———. *Étude médico-légale sur la folie*. Paris: J.-B. Baillière et fils, 1872. xxii, 610 pp., incl. facsims. 21.3 cm.

Tardieu was the foremost French medico-legal expert of his day, and his writing reflects the range of his investigations. He wrote on the legal aspects of infanticide, abortion, and hanging as well as the present work on insanity.

Waller 9480.

995. KARL VON VIERORDT (1818–1884). *Die Lehre vom Arterienpuls in gesunden und kranken Zuständen*. Braunschweig: F. Vieweg, 1855. viii, 271 pp., illus., 6 fold. plates. 21.5 cm.

Although Étienne Jules Marey (1830–1904) is usually given credit for the invention of the first practical sphygmograph in 1860, Vierordt had made, some six years earlier, an instrument designed to trace the intensity of the human pulse. A dedicated and industrious professor at the University of Tübingen, Vierordt made a number of pioneering studies in quantitative hematology including the first accurate erythrocyte count.

The present work on arterial pulse in health and disease was an expansion of a paper written one year earlier and includes Vierordt's description of his pulse measurement apparatus.

996. ———. *Die Erscheinungen und Gesetze der Stromgeschwindigkeiten des Blutes*. Frankfurt: Meidinger, 1858. viii, 208 pp., illus., 2 fold. plates. 22.2 cm.

Vierordt invented a hemotachometer by which he was able to measure the velocity of bloodflow in various arteries. In this work he describes the invention and correlates his measurements with blood volume, pulse, and respiratory rates.

Garrison-Morton 775.

*997. FRANCISCUS CORNELIS DONDERS (1818–1889). *On the anomalies of accommodation and refraction of the eye*. Translated from the author's manuscript by William Daniel Moore. London: New Sydenham Society, 1864. xvii [1] 635 pp., illus. 21.4 cm.

Probably the greatest Dutch physician of the nineteenth century and one of the finest ophthalmologists of any era, Donders was professor on the Utrecht faculty from 1848 until his death. Of his many works on the physiology and pathology of the eye, this is no doubt his finest achievement. Written in Dutch but first published in English, it contains a number of fundamental discoveries and observations on astigmatism, refraction error, and causes of strabismus and the action of the ciliary muscles. "As a contributor to physiological optics, this book ranks with the labors of Helmholtz" (Fielding H. Garrison, *An introduction to the history of medicine*. 4th ed. Philadelphia, 1929. p. 610).

Cushing D221; Garrison-Morton 5893; Waller 2521 (German ed., 1866).

*998. HENRY JACOB BIGELOW (1818–1890). "Insensibility during surgical operations produced by inhalation." (In *Boston medical and surgical journal*. Vol. 35 (1846–1847), pp. 309–317, 379–382.) 23.5 cm.

The author, for almost forty years the dominant figure in New England surgery, was quick to recognize the value of ether after witnessing Morton's celebrated demonstration at Massachusetts General Hospital on October 16, 1846 (see No. 1000). Morton's plan to patent the new agent and his unwillingness to divulge its composition prevented further experimentation until Bigelow forced the issue. Three weeks later an amputation was performed using the ether, and Morton authorized Bigelow to publish a full account of its use resulting in this fascinating paper, the first published report of the new anesthetic. This volume contains several other articles and letters on anesthesia in surgery.

Cushing B380; Garrison-Morton 5651; Osler 1355; Wellcome II, p. 166.

*999. ———. *The mechanism of dislocation and fracture of the hip. With the reduction of the dislocations by the flexion method.* Philadelphia: H. C. Lea, 1869. 150 pp., illus. 23.8 cm.

Bigelow, professor of surgery at Harvard and a pioneer in orthopedic surgery, was the first American to perform a hip joint excision. He is perhaps best remembered for his discussion of the importance of the ilio-femoral ligament (Bigelow's ligament) in the reduction of hip dislocations by the flexion method, as described in this work.

Garrison-Morton 4424; Waller 1049.

*1000. WILLIAM THOMAS GREEN MORTON (1819–1868). *Statements supported by evidence, of Wm. T. G. Morton, on his claim to the discovery of the anaesthetic properties of ether.* Washington, D.C.: [n. publ.] 1853. 582, 135 pp. 21.8 cm.

A successful Boston dentist, Morton is generally credited with the discovery of ether as a general anesthetic. His partner, Horace Wells, had used nitrous oxide with some success while Charles Jackson, Morton's preceptor during his two years of medical school, had used ether drops in filling teeth. Drawing on these experiences and after experimenting briefly with animals, Morton anesthesized a patient during a tooth extraction and less than a month later was able to make his celebrated demonstration at Massachusetts General Hospital. A long and bitter controversy ensued as to the actual discoverer of the technique, and this exhaustive mass of evidence in support of Morton was presented to a special committee selected by the Senate which, however, was never able to resolve the problem.

Cushing M538; Waller 14357.

*1001. ANTOINE FRANÇOIS ADOLPHE DELABARRE (1819–1878). *De la gutta-percha et de son application aux dentures artificielles en remplacement des plaques métalliques et des substances osseuses corruptibles.* Paris: Victor Masson, 1852. 54 pp., fold. plate. 24.2 cm.

Delabarre, son of the noted French dentist, Christophe François Delabarre (1784–1862), was a leader in introducing etherization into French dental practice and was among the early users of gutta-percha as a temporary filling material.

The present work was written only a few years after gutta-percha came into use in the late 1840's as a temporary filling and base plate material. Its use spread quickly because it was the best material available until amalgam was perfected later in the century. Delabarre discusses here the use of gutta-percha as a filler material, its use in preparing base plates and in making dentures.

*1002. FRIEDRICH THEODOR VON FRERICHS (1819–1885). *Die Bright'sche Nierenkrankheit und deren Behandlung.* Braunschweig: F. Vieweg, 1851. xii, 286 pp., 1 fold. plate. 20.4 cm.

Frerichs, a German clinician and teacher, studied medicine at Göttingen. He became widely recognized as an ophthalmologist but returned to general medicine and went on to become one of the founders of experimental pathology, eventually becoming professor of pathology at Berlin. He wrote important monographs on liver diseases and diabetes and also discovered leucin and tyrosin in the urine of patients with acute yellow atrophy. This book on Bright's disease was written early in his career when he was an associate professor at Kiel, and it laid the foundation for his subsequent achievements.

Garrison-Morton 4209; Waller 3239.

1003. *The United States pharmacopeia.* By the authority of the medical societies and colleges. Boston: C. Ewer, 1820. 272 pp. 22.5 cm.

The first official United States pharmacopoeia was a truly cooperative effort, involving delegates from all of the medical societies and colleges then in existence. It was largely a compilation and refinement of local pharmacopoeias already in use and endeavored to "select from among substances which possess medicinal power, those, the utility of which is most fully established and best understood" (Preface).

Garrison-Morton 1845; Waller 7416.

*1004. GEORGE PARKINSON (fl. 1860). *On the application of vulcanized India rubber for making artificial palates.* London: J. Churchill, 1860. 20 pp., 1 col. plate. 20 cm.

The refinement of dental and oral surgery is, for the most part, the work of American surgeons. Goodyear, in 1855, first showed the practical application of molded, vulcanized rubber (vulcanite) for correcting oral defects after removal of bony structures within the oral cavity. In this small treatise, Parkinson, an English surgeon, anatomist, and dentist, accounts his successful results of the treatment of eleven patients with defects of the hard palate, using vulcanite prostheses.

1005. HUBERT VON LUSCHKA (1820–1875). *Der Kehlkopf des Menschen.* Tübingen: Verlag der H. Laupp'schen Buchhandlung, 1871. vi, 199 pp., 10 plates (some col.). 30.9 cm.

Luschka received his medical degree at Freiburg, practiced for a time, taught at Freiburg, and eventually became professor of anatomy at Tübingen. Luschka was one of the leading anatomists of his time and made many contributions to the study of gross anatomy. He was a prolific author, writing many papers and numerous books. This book on the human larynx is representative of his anatomical studies and is a thorough work containing ten fine anatomical plates, several of which are partially colored.

Garrison-Morton 943.

*1006. Sir GEORGE MURRAY HUMPHRY (1820–1896). *A treatise on the human skeleton (including the joints).* Cambridge: Macmillan, 1858. vi [2] 620 pp., 60 plates (part fold.). 23.7 cm.

Humphry—anatomist, teacher, and surgeon—combined an active surgical practice with an academic career. He was professor of anatomy at Cambridge and later professor of surgery. He contributed widely to the scientific journals of his time and was founder and co-editor of the *Journal of anatomy and physiology.*

This, his major work, was prepared as a working anatomy for the practicing orthopedic surgeon, and his treatment of cartilages and ligaments is especially inventive. The sixty plates with their many figures were drawn on stone by Humphry's wife from preparations made by the author.

Garrison-Morton 419.

*1007. FLORENCE NIGHTINGALE (1820–1910). *Notes on nursing: what it is, and what it is not.* [1st ed., 2nd issue]. London: Harrison [1860]. 79 pp. 21.6 cm. Original cloth.

Few can fail to agree that Florence Nightingale is "the greatest figure in the history of nursing" (Garrison-Morton 1612). She was trained in France, Germany, and Egypt, and after nursing experience in England she was asked to take charge of a group of nurses being dispatched to the Crimea to care for the British wounded in the war. Her heroic efforts brought the morality rate among the soldiers there from 42 percent to 2 percent. The rest of her life was spent in the struggle to improve the care of patients and to establish nursing as a profession.

This no-nonsense book is not only a call for the establishment of training of nurses; it offers the most practical advice on the care of patients. Nursing, she says, "has been limited to signify little more than the administration of medicines and the application of poultices. It ought to signify the proper use of fresh air, light, warmth, cleanliness, quiet, and the proper selection and administration of diet."

Although this book is undated and its publication is often ascribed to 1859, it was probably not actually available to the public until 1860. The present issue is sometimes called the first issue, but as a few copies exist in which no advertisements appear on the end papers and in which a statement concerning translation rights (carried in later issues on the title page) does not appear, this must be accorded place as the second issue, before correction of several typographical errors in the text.

Cushing N98; Garrison-Morton 1612; Osler 7737; Waller 6872 (dated 1858, but certainly erroneous).

1008. ———. ———. [1st American ed.]. New York: D. Appleton and Co., 1860. 140 pp. 19.4 cm. Original cloth.

This famous book was brought out almost immediately in the United States and was reissued many times between 1860 and 1918. A second, enlarged edition was also published in England in 1860; another edition with some abridgment and some additions, called *Notes on nursing for the labouring classes,* was brought out in 1861. The work has been translated into many languages and is surely the most famous and most influential book ever written on nursing.

Cushing N101.

Gift of Dr. R. N. Larimer.

*1009. HERMANN LUDWIG FERDINAND VON HELMHOLTZ (1821–1894). *Beschreibung eines Augen-Spiegels zur Untersuchung der Netzhaut im lebenden Auge.* Berlin: A. Förstner'sche Verlagsbuchhandlung, 1851. 43 [2] pp., plate. 22.5 cm. In slipcase.

One of the scientific giants of his age, Helmholtz made fundamental advances in both physiology and physics, including the establishment of the first law of thermodynamics—that energy can be transformed from one form to another but cannot be created or destroyed. Turning his attention to neurophysiology, Helmholtz became the first to measure the speed of a nerve impulse—a feat Müller had only recently declared to be impossible. Helmholtz's extensive investigations into physiological optics led to his invention of the ophthalmoscope, now one of the most common and useful tools in clinical medicine. The present work constitutes Helmholtz's first description of his invention.

Cushing H229 (1910 ed.); Garrison-Morton 5866; Osler 1521 (1910 ed.); Waller 4294.

*1010. ———. *Handbuch der physiologischen Optik.* Leipzig: L. Voss, 1867. xiv, 874 pp., illus., 11 plates (2 fold.). 22.7 cm.

Because Helmholtz's name is linked so closely with physics and electrophysiology, it is sometimes forgotten that he was a physician who held posts at a number of prominent medical schools. It was during his tenure at Heidelberg that this monumental treatise on optics was written. Originally issued in parts between 1856 and 1866, the work provided the first real description of optical physiology including the mechanism of accommodation, the phenomenon of color vision, and the measurement of lens curvature.

Cushing H231; Garrison-Morton 1513; Waller 4299.

*1011. RUDOLF LUDWIG KARL VIRCHOW (1821–1902). *Die Einheitsbestrebungen in der wissenschaftlichen Medicin.* Berlin: G. Reimer, 1849. vi, 48 pp. 22.3 cm.

"Virchow is not only one of the most representative figures in the history of medicine of the nineteenth century, but also the greatest pathologist of all time" (Arturo Castiglioni, *A history of medicine.* New York, 1946. p. 695). Born in Pomerania, he was educated at the University of Berlin, and later taught for several years at the Pathological Institute of Charité Hospital before political activities brought about his dismissal in 1849. He then spent seven years at the University of Würzburg, but was recalled to Berlin in 1856 as director of the Charité.

This tract is a summary of Virchow's view of the relationship of medicine to social and political life.

Osler 1628; Waller 9999.

*1012. ———. *Gesammelte Abhandlungen zur wissenschaftlichen Medicin.* Frankfurt am Main: Meidinger Sohn, 1856. xiv, 1024 pp., illus., 4 plates (2 fold., 2 col.). 22.5 cm.

This work covers a wide spectrum of clinical pathology based on Virchow's experience as pathologist in Berlin and Würzburg. This copy once belonged to the Swiss histologist and anthropologist Wilhelm His (see No. 1049), whose signature is on the front flyleaf.

Osler 1629; Waller 10005.

*1013. ———. *Die Cellularpathologie in ihrer Begründung auf physiologische und pathologische Gewebelehre.* Berlin: A. Hirschwald, 1858. xvi, 440 pp., illus. 22.2 cm.

The importance of this work can scarcely be overstated; it is not only the cornerstone but the very foundation of cellular pathology and "one of the most important books in the history of medicine" (Garrison-Morton 2299). Virchow's theory that the seat of disease as well as any developed tissue could be traced back to the cell prompted his dictum "Omnis cellula e cellula" ("Every cell from a cell") to be added to Harvey's "Omne vivum ex ovo" ("Every living thing from an egg") and Pasteur's "Omne vivum e vivo" ("Every living thing from a living thing"). Although after later research the concept had to be somewhat modified, "cellular pathology" is a term which belongs to Virchow alone.

Garrison-Morton 2299; Osler 1624; Waller 9996.

*1014. ———. *Die krankhaften Geschwülste.* Vols. I–III, pt. 1 (no more published). Berlin: Hirschwald, 1863–1867. Vol. I: xii, 543 pp.; Vol. II: x, 756 pp.; Vol. III, pt. 1: 496 pp., illus. 22.5 cm.

This classic work on tumors was never completed. Intended to consist of thirty lectures, Virchow stopped after the twenty-fifth. It is a very important work on cancer, but records Virchow's erroneous conclusion that the origin of cancer is in the connective tissue, a theory that was almost immediately refuted in a paper appearing in Virchow's journal, *Archiv für pathologische Anatomie und Physiologie,* which, incidentally, is still being published and is known merely as *Virchows Archiv.*

Cushing V157; Garrison-Morton 2617; Osler 1631; Waller 10001.

*1015. MARY BAKER EDDY (1821–1910). *Science and health.* By Mary Baker Glover. Boston: Christian Scientist Publishing Company, 1875. 456 pp. 19.6 cm.

A disenchantment with orthodox medicine during years of invalidism, together with an intensive study of scripture, led Mary Morse Baker, the daughter of a New England farmer, to the conclusion that disease is mental rather than physical and that matter (and hence evil), as commonly perceived, does not exist. The phenomenal spread of her teaching resulted in the Church of Christ Scientist, with membership of nearly 100,000 members at the time of her death.

This first edition of *Science and health,* which was to be revised repeatedly throughout her lifetime, is the basic handbook of the faith.

1016. HEINRICH VON BAMBERGER (1822–1888). *Lehrbuch der Krankheiten des Herzens.* Vienna: W. Braumüller, 1857. viii, 459 pp. 20.7 cm.

Bamberger studied under both Škoda and Rokitansky and held a number of posts at the University of Vienna where he made extensive investigations on diseases of the pericardium, heart tissues, and the great vessels. This monograph is one of the earliest works to be devoted entirely to cardiac pathology.

Waller 646.

*1017. LOUIS PASTEUR (1822–1895). *Études sur la maladie des vers à soie.* 2 vols. Paris: Gauthier-Villars, 1870. Vol. I: xii, 322 pp., front., illus., plates (part col.); Vol. II: [6] 327 pp., plate. 22.3 cm. Original wrappers.

The French chemist and microbiologist Pasteur may well be the best-known scientist the world has ever known. The variety and number of his important discoveries make it difficult to select which are the two or three most important. Certainly his work on fermentation (see No. 1018), which led to the pasteurization process, had ramifications far beyond the beer and wine industries for which it was originally undertaken.

The present work is one of his most important, dealing with his studies on a disease of silkworms which was ruining the French silk industry. He isolated the bacillus causing the disease and devised the method by which it would be eliminated. From this study he turned to a study of fowl cholera and anthrax, again isolating the specific bacilli causing the diseases and finding that prevention and cure could be effected by inoculation with artificially grown cultures of the bacilli producing the disease. This led to what is perhaps his best-known discovery, a curative vaccine for hydrophobia.

Cushing P140; Garrison-Morton 2481; Osler 1549.

1018. ———. *Études sur la bière. . . . avec une théorie nouvelle de la fermentation.* Paris: Gauthier-Villars, 1876. viii, 387 pp., illus., 13 plates. 22.8 cm.

In Pasteur's important study of fermentation, he discovered that contamination of beer was caused by microorganisms found in the air and not spontaneously generated as had been previously believed. He made possible the scientific processing of beer, wine, milk, and other perishable products.

Cushing P139; Garrison-Morton 2485; Osler 1550.

1019. ———. *Examen critique d'un écrit posthume de Claude Bernard sur la fermentation.* Paris: Gauthier-Villars, 1879. xxiv, 153 pp., illus., plates. 22.6 cm.

Claude Bernard disagreed with Pasteur's (essentially correct) theory of fermentation and his notes on the subject were published in the *Revue scientifique* shortly after his death. They are reprinted here together with Pasteur's appraisal of Bernard's criticisms.

Cushing P142; Osler 1552.

*1020. ADOLF KUSSMAUL (1822–1902). *Die Störungen der Sprache.* Leipzig: F. C. W. Vogel, 1877. x, 299 pp. 20 cm.

Kussmaul was professor of medicine in various universities throughout Germany before finally settling in Strasbourg. He wrote with authority on many subjects including psychology, physiological chemistry, pathology, and neurology, and developed a number of valuable diagnostic and therapeutic procedures. This work on speech pathology, in particular his description of aphasia, is perhaps his most important contribution.

Garrison-Morton 4624; Waller 5460.

1021. Sir FRANCIS GALTON (1822–1911). *Hereditary genius: an inquiry into its laws and consequences.* London: Macmillan, 1869. vi, 390 pp., illus. 22.1 cm.

Galton was one of a handful of nineteenth-century scientists who gained prominence in a number of scientific pursuits. Born into a well-to-do family and receiving a classical education, Galton first achieved a reputation as a geographer and explorer. Later he turned to meteorology and was the first to note the importance of anticyclones in weather forecasting. In his late forties, Galton began his work in the study of human attributes, the field for which he is best known and out of which derived the science of eugenics, a term coined by Galton.

This work on the genetics of intelligence is a compilation of biographical data of

Fig. 7.

Scars and Cuts, and their Effects on the Ridges.

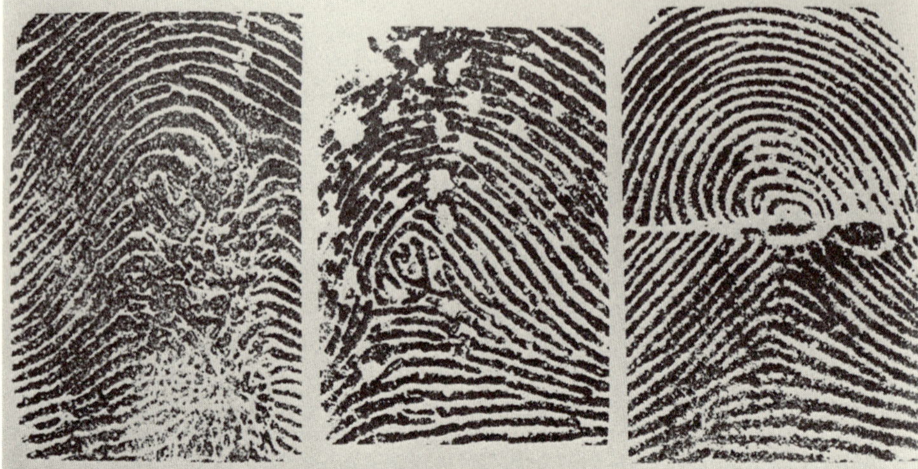

a Effect of an Ulcer. *b* Finger of a Tailor. *c* Effect of a Cut.

No. 1023. Galton. *Finger Prints.*

eminent men and their genetic history. In assessing the role of heredity, Galton unfortunately disregarded such obvious factors as socio-economic status and opportunity for education.

Cushing G82; Garrison-Morton 226; Osler 1599 (London ed., 1892); Waller 15950.

*1022. ———. *Inquiries into human faculty and its development.* London: Macmillan, 1883. xii, 387 pp., illus., plates. 22 cm.

Largely an expansion of the conclusions reached in *Hereditary genius,* this work seeks to "take note of the varied hereditary faculties of different men. . .to learn how far history may have shown the practicability of supplanting inefficient human stock by better strains, and to consider whether it might not be our duty to do so by such efforts as may be reasonable, thus exerting ourselves to further the ends of evolution more rapidly and with less distress than if events were left to their own course" (Introduction).

Cushing G83; Garrison-Morton 230; Osler 1597; Waller 3403.

*1023. ———. *Finger prints.* London and New York: Macmillan, 1892. xvi, 216 pp., illus., 16 plates (1 double col.). 22.3 cm.

The value of the fine ridges in the epidermis of the palmar surfaces of the fingers as a means of identification was known to the Chinese and others long before Galton proposed their use for such purposes. But it was Galton whose detailed studies of fingerprints led to the adoption of his classification which is still the basis for the system used throughout the world. Here a small anatomical detail is put to practical use.

Cushing G81; Garrison-Morton 186; Osler 1598; Waller 19650.

1024. HENRY HYDE SALTER (1823–1871). *On asthma: its pathology and treatment.* Philadelphia: Blanchard and Lea, 1864. viii [17]–260 pp., illus. 22 cm.

Salter distinguished himself at an early age in both academic and clinical circles, becoming in 1856 the youngest member of the Royal College of Physicians. He held the chair of physiology at Charing Cross Hospital for twelve years and afterward was named head physician. Salter's interest in asthma stemmed partly from his own affliction with the disease. This definitive work, first published in London in 1860, is generally regarded as the finest work on asthma published in the nineteenth century.

Garrison-Morton 2586 (1st ed., 1860).

Gift of Dr. Charles R. Baker.

PAUL BROCA (1824–1880). *Atlas d'anatomie descriptive du corps humain.*

See No. 964.

GUSTAVE DUGAT (1824–1894). *Études sur le traité de médicine d'Abou Djáfar Ah'mad.*

See No. 37.

*1025. HENRY GRAY (1825–1861). *Anatomy descriptive and surgical. . . . The drawings by H. V. Carter, M.D. . . . The dissections jointly by the author and Dr. Carter.* [1st ed.]. London: John W. Parker, 1858. xxiii, 750 pp., illus. (part col.). 25.4 cm. Rebound in modern buckram.

The author's opening statement in the Preface reads: "This work is intended to furnish the Student and Practitioner with an accurate view of the Anatomy of the Human Body, and more especially the application of this science to Practical Surgery." The success of that intention for more than a century could be proclaimed by generations of medical students and doctors of medicine in the English-speaking world. Gray was lecturer on anatomy at St. George's Hospital, London, and this lasting and monumental work, produced by a young man who died young, must be compared to the *Fabrica* of Vesalius, who produced his great work before the age of thirty years.

Garrison-Morton 418.

*1026. ———. *Anatomy, descriptive and surgical.* [1st American ed.]. Philadelphia: Blanchard and Lea, 1859. xxxii, 754 pp., illus. 28 cm.

The first edition of 1858 was found to have a good many errors, most of which were corrected in the 1859 edition. Gray's *Anatomy* still remains a standard textbook, and much of the original text and many of the superb anatomical illustrations have been retained throughout the thirty-four successive editions.

Garrison-Morton 418 note.

1027. JEAN MARTIN CHARCOT (1825–1893). *Leçons sur les maladies du système nerveux faites à la Salpêtrière.* [First series]. Paris: Adrien Delahaye, 1872–1873. 368 pp., illus. 22.2 cm.

"In France, Charcot was one of the greatest neurologists of his time. It was perhaps his incomparable qualities as teacher, writer, and organizer that contributed most to the great reputation of this gifted clinician. . . . He was the creator of the greatest modern neurological clinic, and a masterly describer of many disease pictures. . . . Charcot brought to his clinic at the Salpêtrière a group of devoted pupils who were among the founders of modern neurology" (Arturo Castiglioni, *A history of medicine.* New York, 1946. pp. 739–740).

Charcot was an outstanding teacher, and this course of lectures at the Salpêtrière constitutes one of the classic textbooks in the field of neurology and is his greatest work. This is the first series of lectures on nervous disorders.

Garrison-Morton 4546; Waller 1913.

*1028. ———. *Leçons sur les localisations dans les maladies du cerveau.* Paris: Progrès médical, 1876. 168 pp., illus. 21.6 cm.

Of the many works issued by Charcot, this one on the localization of functions in diseases of the brain stands out as one of the most important.

Garrison-Morton 4558; Waller 1910.

*1029. ———. *Leçons sur les maladies du foie, des voies biliares et des reins faites à la Faculté de Médecine de Paris.* Paris: Aux bureaux du Progrès médical, 1877. 380 pp., 7 leaves of plates, illus. (some col.). 21.7 cm. Contemporary half morocco.

Though best remembered as a clinical neurologist, Charcot also contributed to a more accurate knowledge of many other diseases. This classic work on diseases of the liver, biliary passages, and kidney is a fine example of his versatility.

Garrison-Morton 2228; Waller 1912.

1030. ———. *Neue Vorlesungen über die Krankheiten des Nervensystems insbesondere über Hysterie.* Autorisirte deutsche Ausgabe von Sigm. Freud. Leipzig: Toeplitz, 1886. xi, 357 pp., illus., diagrs. 22 cm.

It was as a student of Charcot that Sigmund Freud (see No. 1122 ff.) first became interested in investigating hysteria from a psychological standpoint. The present work is Freud's translation of some of Charcot's writings on the subject.

Waller 1916.

*1031. ———. *Leçons du mardi à la Salpêtrière. Policlinique 1888–1889.* Paris: Progrès médical, 1889. 579 pp., illus. 22.1 cm.

These highly readable records of Charcot's clinical sessions at the hospital where he began and ended his richly productive career show his keen insight as a clinician as well as his humor, humanity, and flair for teaching. The world-famous old hospital was named Salpêtrière because at one time it was used by King Louis XIII as a gunpowder storehouse. Another volume of the records of these courses of lectures, covering 1887–1888, was also published.

1032. ——— and ALBERT PITRES (1848–1928). *Les centres moteurs corticaux chez l'homme.* Paris: Rueff, 1895. 198 pp., illus. (part col.). 17.2 cm.

Originally a series of three papers published between 1877 and 1883, this work conclusively proved the existence of cortical motor centers in man.

Garrison-Morton 1434.

*1033. THOMAS HENRY HUXLEY (1825–1895). *Evidence as to man's place in nature.* London: Williams and Norgate, 1863. 159 pp., illus. 22.9 cm.

Eventual acceptance of the theory of evolution was due in no small measure to Thomas Huxley as the theory's strong but skeptical supporter and interpreter.

While convinced of the essential validity of the theory, he nevertheless continually questioned various facets of it. Huxley was the first to apply evolution to paleontology and in this work, perhaps his finest, he undertook the task of assessing the development of mankind. The work is particularly noteworthy for its account of the finding of the Neanderthal man and the early studies of that important specimen. Regardless of the topic, it is always enjoyable to read Huxley and appreciate his facile command of English.

Cushing H554; Garrison-Morton 165; Osler 1605; Waller 10853.

*1034. ———. *Lectures on the elements of comparative anatomy.* London: J. Churchill, 1865. xi, 303 pp., illus. 21.2 cm.

Though more than one hundred years old, the detail and clarity evidenced in this work on comparative anatomy make it worth the attention of present-day students of anatomy and zoology.

*1035. JOSEPH LISTER (1827–1912). *The collected papers of Joseph, Baron Lister.* 2 vols. Oxford: Clarendon Press, 1909. Vol. I: xliv, 429 pp., front. (port.), illus., 14 plates (part col.); Vol. II: vii, 589 pp., front. (port.). 28.6 cm.

One of the greatest of British surgeons, Lister was educated at the Universities of London and Edinburgh, and was professor of surgery at those universities as well as at the University of Glasgow. His early research on inflammation and suppuration after injuries and surgery, coupled with his interest in Pasteur's demonstration that pus formation is caused by the action of live bacteria, led him to search for a chemical means of preventing infection. He found this in carbolic acid. His system was widely and immediately adopted, thus beginning a new era in surgery leading to the universally accepted asepsis in all modern surgery. Lister was elevated to the peerage in 1897, the first medical man to be so honored.

This collection of his scientific papers contains all the papers and addresses which Lister considered to be of permanent interest and importance and was published as a memorial of the celebration of his eightieth birthday.

Cushing L289; Garrison-Morton 85; Osler 1675; Waller 5937.

*1036. JULES BERNARD LUYS (1828–1897). *Recherches sur le système nerveux cérébrospinal, sa structure, ses fonctions et ses maladies.* 2 vols. Paris: J.-B. Baillière, 1865. Text: xv, 660, 8 pp.; Atlas: 80 pp., 40 leaves of col. plates. 24.1 cm.

Luys was among the most notable of the many nineteenth-century French neurologists who made important contributions to the understanding of the anatomy and physiology of the brain. It was Luys who first delineated the four main divisions of the thalamus and described and pictured two of its structures later named for him: the subthalmic nucleus and the centre median. The forty colored lithographs in the atlas were made after Luys's own drawings and possess a clarity and three-dimensional realism hardly surpassed by modern illustrators.

Garrison-Morton 1402.

*1037. ÉTIENNE TARNIER (1828–1897). *De l'asepsie et de l'antisepsie en obstétrique.* Paris: G. Steinheil, 1894. xiv, 839 pp., 3 col. plates, illus., tables. 24.3 cm. Maroon cloth with original wrappers bound in.

Tarnier, born at Aisery, studied medicine in Paris and interned in the Maternitè Hospital at a time when puerperal fever was a major problem in its wards. He had originally intended to enter general practice, but the many obstetrical problems he encountered challenged his interest and he decided to specialize in obstetrics.

He made major contributions to solving the problem of puerperal fever at the Maternitè and, during his twenty-two years of leadership at the hospital, reduced the maternal death rate dramatically. Among his many contributions were the development of a peritoneal exclusion technique for cesarean section, design of an isolation pavilion, use of heated bassinets, the introduction of gavage feedings in his clinic, and the development of an intrauterine balloon for the induction of labor. More importantly, Tarnier is responsible for revolutionizing the obstetric forceps by adding an ingenious device of traction rods to solve the problem of how to direct traction properly in high forceps delivery. His basiotribe, still in use today, replaced Baudelocque's cephalotribe and Simpson's cranioclast combining the advantages of both in one instrument.

Tarnier was one of the earliest to introduce Lister's principles of antisepsis into obstetrics and was the first to use carbolic acid in this field. Here, in one of his major works, he outlines in detail the principles and practice of asepsis and antisepsis in the practice of obstetrics.

Garrison-Morton 5639; Waller 9490.

1038. LIONEL SMITH BEALE (1828–1906). *Disease germs; their supposed nature: an original investigation, with critical remarks.* London: J. Churchill and Sons, 1870. ix, 85 pp., 4 plates (part col.). 19.4 cm.

In this work, based on lectures he delivered at Oxford in 1868 and 1869, Beale anticipated by five years the microbe theory of disease and the concept of immunization as proposed by Pasteur. A brilliant microscopist, Beale introduced a number of important staining techniques and was the first to fix tissues for examination by injection. He also wrote several works on the microscope and did much to demonstrate its value as a diagnostic tool in clinical medicine.

*1039. JEAN HENRY DUNANT (1828–1910). *Un souvenir de Solferino.* Geneva: Imprimerie Jules-Guillaume Fick, 1862. 115 pp., col. map. 26.9 cm.

Dunant, a Swiss philanthropist, was appalled at the lack of medical care for the wounded at the battle between French and Austrian forces at Solferino in 1859. His efforts in organizing an emergency medical service and the subsequent publication of this work, in which he describes the conditions at the battle, prompted the eventual acceptance of the Geneva Convention in 1863 and the formation of the International Red Cross. In 1901, Dunant, together with the French politician and economist Frédéric Passy (1822–1912), became the first recipient of the Nobel peace prize.

Garrison-Morton 2166; Waller 2639.

1040. Sir JONATHAN HUTCHINSON (1828–1913). *A clinical memoir on certain diseases of the eye and ear, consequent on inherited syphilis.* London: Churchill, 1863. 259 pp., 1 col. plate. 22.2 cm.

The work of Jonathan Hutchinson is remarkable in both quantity and diversity. His writings reveal an encyclopedic mind conversant with virtually every area of medicine and one able to communicate effectively. As surgeon to London Hospital and later the Royal College of Surgeons, Hutchinson made numerous original observations, most notably in the areas of congenital syphilis and skin diseases. His name has been linked with a number of diseases including Hutchinson's teeth and Hutchinson's facies. In 1886, he made the first recorded observation of progeria (Hutchinson-Gilford syndrome). Much of his work is preserved in the eleven volume *Archives of surgery* (1890–1900), a journal written entirely by himself. The present work is a well-documented discussion of congenital syphilis, one of several works Hutchinson produced on the subject.

Waller 5024.

*1041. ANDREW TAYLOR STILL (1828–1917). *Autobiography of Andrew T. Still, with a history of the discovery and development of the science of osteopathy.* Kirksville, Missouri: The author [1897]. 460 pp., illus. 19.8 cm.

Although no gem of literature, this book tells the story of a man who persisted in his beliefs and who, having overcome numerous hardships, eventually founded the science of osteopathy. The son of a Methodist minister and doctor, Still had only the rudiments of a medical education when he formulated his new medical system, based on manipulative therapy and the utilization of the natural resources of the body. The early concepts of osteopathy have since undergone considerable change and expansion.

The University of Iowa copy is a presentation copy signed by the author.

*1042. CHRISTIAN ALBERT THEODOR BILLROTH (1829–1894). *Die allgemeine chirurgische Pathologie und Therapie, in fünfzig Vorlesungen.* Berlin: G. Reimer, 1863. xx, 712 pp., illus. 24.1 cm.

Billroth may be regarded as the founder of modern abdominal surgery through his pioneering work in resection of the esophagus and removal of the upper part of the stomach and portions of the bowel. For many years he was at the Vienna School of Surgery; because of his own work and that of his many eminent pupils, he must probably be considered the most important single influence on the development of modern surgical knowledge.

This scarce first edition, cheaply printed and, strangely, not in such great collections as those of Osler, Cushing, Waller, or Orr, is a landmark in the development of modern surgery and was translated into ten languages.

Garrison-Morton 5608.

1043. EDUARD FRIEDRICH WILHELM PFLÜGER (1829–1910). *Untersuchungen über die Physiologie des Electrotonus.* Berlin: A. Hirschwald, 1859. xv, 500 pp., 5 plates (1 fold.). 21.9 cm.

Pflüger studied under Johannes Müller and later succeeded Helmholtz as professor of physiology at Bonn, a post he held the remainder of his life. In 1868 he founded and directed the publication of the *Archiv für die gesamte Physiologie* (better known as *Pflüger's Archiv*), one of the most respected scientific journals in the world. This work on the physiology of nerves marks one of Pflüger's earliest investigations. Here he "first stated the laws governing the make and break stimulation of nerve with the galvanic current" (Garrison-Morton 621).

Garrison-Morton 621.

*1044. SILAS WEIR MITCHELL (1829–1914). *Injuries of nerves and their consequences.* Philadelphia: J. B. Lippincott, 1872. viii, 377 pp. 21.2 cm.

Based on his extensive experience during the Civil War at Philadelphia's Turner's Lane Hospital, where he treated hundreds of soldiers with peripheral nerve wounds, Mitchell produced this basic and time-honored work on the symptoms, signs, and treatment of nerve injuries. Together with his other major work, *Gunshot wounds* (1864), it established fundamental lines of treatment which remained essentially unchanged until World War I. Mitchell is probably as well known for his literary efforts—poems, novels, and essays—as for his famous clinical skill.

Cushing M401; Garrison-Morton 4544.

*1045. ———. *Fat and blood: and how to make them.* Philadelphia: J. B. Lippincott, 1877. 101 pp. 17.7 cm.

In this classic work, Mitchell expounded his popular "rest cure" for treatment of nervous disorders through prolonged bed rest and selective use of seclusion, massage, electricity, and diet. The work was translated into French, German, Spanish, Italian, and Russian.

Cushing M395; Garrison-Morton 4554; Osler 3418; Waller 6568 (1884 ed.).

*1046. JULIAN JOHN CHISOLM (1830–1903). *A manual of military surgery, for the use of surgeons in the Confederate Army.* Richmond, Virginia: West & Johnston, 1861. xi, 447 pp. 18.1 cm.

When the Civil War began, the Confederate Army was without any manual for the medical care of its soldiers, and this work was especially written to fill that need. It concerns itself with principles in the care of surgical emergencies, but is almost unbelievably primitive compared with modern military medicine. There is an interesting letter pasted to the front flyleaf, from George Benet, "a partially reconstructed rebel" of Columbia, South Carolina, to Dr. Elliott Cutler, who once owned this copy.

1047. ÉTIENNE JULES MAREY (1830–1904). *Physiologie médicale de la circulation du sang.* Paris: Adrien Delahaye, 1863. viii, 568 pp., 235 illus. 22.9 cm.

Marey, celebrated French physiologist, was a pioneer in the study of blood pressure and the creator of the modern sphygmograph. However, much of his work was preceded by Karl von Vierordt's (see No. 995) imperfect attempts some twenty years earlier. Marey is also credited with inventing the cine camera and with being the first scientific cinematographer. In this work, Marey presents a comprehensive treatise on the physiology of the circulatory system in its normal and diseased states.

Waller 6248.

1048. ———. *La circulation du sang à l'état physiologique et dans les maladies.* Paris: G. Masson, 1881. [4] iii [1] 745 pp. 25.1 cm. Original printed wrappers.

This work, based on Marey's earlier *Physiologie médicale de la circulation du sang* (see No. 1047), has the added benefit of nearly twenty years experience, study, and research. Marey again presents a comprehensive study of the circulatory system's physiology and pathology, and, in addition, he places special emphasis on the clinical signs of cardiac health and disease as well as the instrumentation necessary to detect and record their physiological manifestations.

Garrison-Morton 783; Waller 6245.

*1049. WILHELM HIS (1831–1904). *Die Häute und Höhlen des Körpers.* Basel: Schweighauserische Universitäts-Buchdruckerei, 1865. 34 pp. 28.5 cm.

His, a prodigious Swiss scientist, pioneered in the fields of embryology, histology, tissue origins, and anthropology. He not only developed the *Basle nomina anatomica* (see No. 1050), but he also founded the *Anatomical Gesellschaft,* the *Archiv für Anthropologie,* and the *Zeitschrift für Anatomie und Entwicklungsgeschichte.*

In the present work, His put forth the basic concepts of tissue embryology. Using serial sections and three-dimensional models to illustrate his theories, he showed that the serous spaces in the embryo are mesodermal in origin and that they are lined by the special layer which he was the first to term "endothelial."

Garrison-Morton 490; Waller 4604.

*1050. ———. *Die anatomische Nomenclatur. Nomina anatomica.* Leipzig: Verlag von Veit, 1895. vi, 180 pp., illus., 2 fold. plates. 24 cm.

This is the first appearance of the *Basle nomina anatomica* (usually called merely B.N.A.), the reform and simplification of anatomical terms suggested by and developed chiefly by His.

Garrison-Morton 432; Waller 4601.

*1051. FÉLIX GUYON (1831–1920). *Leçons cliniques sur les maladies des voies urinaires.* Paris: Librairie J.-B. Baillière et fils, 1881. xvi, 998 pp., illus. 22.3 cm.

Guyon, a native of the island of Réunion in the Indian Ocean east of Madagascar, was one of the outstanding French urologists of the nineteenth century. Professor of genitourinary surgery at the University of Paris, his clinics at the Necker hospital were attended by students from around the world. A skilled surgeon and teacher, Guyon was renowned worldwide, especially for his work with the prostate and diseases of the bladder.

The present work on genitourinary diseases is one of his most important books and is based on his lectures at Necker in 1876 and 1877. According to Castiglioni, "Felix Guyon, the greatest teacher of genito-urinary surgery of the century, with his pupil and successor, J. Albarran, inventor of the cystoscope used for urethral catheterization, were important in raising renal, vesical, and urethral surgery to a high scientific standard" (Arturo Castiglioni, *A history of medicine.* New York, 1941. p. 870).

Garrison-Morton 4177.

*1052. AXEL KEY (1832–1901) and GUSTAF RETZIUS (1842–1919). *Studien in der Anatomie des Nervensystems und des Bindegewebes.* 2 vols. Stockholm: In Commission bei Samson & Wallin, 1875–1876. Vol. I: [12] 220 pp., 39 plates (part fold., part col.), each accompanied by a leaf of descriptive letterpress; Vol. II: [6] 228 pp., 36 plates (part fold., part col.), each accompanied by a leaf of descriptive letterpress. 40.8 cm.

In this truly monumental work, Key and Retzius describe a number of very important discoveries and verifications concerning the structure of the nervous system, not the least of which is the confirmation of the existence of the foramen of Magendie. As a work of art and of scientific accuracy, the two volumes of beautifully executed colored lithographs rank with the best atlases of any age. The authors accomplished their task while at the Karolinska Institut in Sweden. Retzius (see No. 1070 ff.) was a man of great industry and versatility, the author of some 333 scientific articles as well as several volumes of poetry.

Cushing K64; Waller 5279.

1053. WILHELM MAX WUNDT (1832–1920). *Beiträge zur Theorie der Sinneswahrnehmung.* Leipzig: C. F. Winter, 1862. xxxii, 451 pp. 19.5 cm.

Generally considered the father of modern experimental psychology, Wundt was a student of Johannes Müller and later assistant to Helmholtz at the University of Heidelburg. He later held teaching posts at Berlin, Zurich, and finally Leipzig, where he established the first psychological laboratory and began the publication of *Philosophische Studien,* the first journal devoted exclusively to psychology.

This highly regarded work on sensory perception was completed only two years after Wundt's graduation from medical school.

*1054. ———. *Lehrbuch der Physiologie des Menschen.* Erlangen: Verlag von F. Enke, 1865. xiii, 661 pp., illus. 23.6 cm.

Among Wundt's important contributions to physiology are his original descriptions of isotonic curves produced by muscles under continued excitation and the effects of drugs on muscle action. This textbook on human physiology was produced while Wundt was lecturer at Heidelberg.

1055. ———. *Untersuchungen zur Mechanik der Nerven und Nervencentren.* 2 vols. in 1. Stuttgart: F. Enke, 1876. Vol. I: ix, 278 pp., illus.; Vol. II: iv, 144 pp., illus. 24.7 cm.

Wundt was one of the first to investigate the complexities of reaction time. This work on nerve transmission may be considered the basis for his later experiments on the subject.

1056. ———. *Grundzüge der physiologischen Psychologie.* 4th ed. 2 vols. Leipzig: W. Engelmann, 1893. Vol. I: xv, 600 pp., illus.; Vol. II: xii, 684 pp., illus. 22.4 cm.

Unlike other schools, which investigated and stressed the acts or functions of consciousness, Wundt's psychology dealt with the observable and the conscious mind, thus earning the label of the "content school." His two-volume classic on physiological psychology is one of the most important works of its kind. The publication of the first edition in 1874 led to Wundt's call to Zurich later that year.

Waller 10422.

1057. JOSEPH JANVIER WOODWARD (1833–1884). *Outlines of the chief camp diseases of the United States armies as observed during the present war.* Philadelphia: J. B. Lippincott & Co., 1863. xii, 364 pp. 22 cm.

Woodward, born and educated in Philadelphia, graduated in medicine from the University of Pennsylvania in 1853 and practiced medicine there until the outbreak of the Civil War. During the war, he served as assistant surgeon with the Army of the Potomac and was later in the Surgeon General's office in Washington. He was president of the American Medical Association in 1882 and also published numerous articles on microscopy, photomicrography, cancer, and other subjects. His most important work was the *Medical history of the rebellion* published in two volumes (1870–1879).

The present work is a direct result of his war experiences and was prepared to assist physicians who were not familiar with diseases common to the army. Woodward presents the chief features of such diseases as fevers, jaundice, malaria, pneumonia, and dysentery. He also includes his pathological observations as well as suggested therapies.

1058. ———. ———. [A variant issue]. Philadelphia: J. B. Lippincott & Co., 1863. xii, 364 pp. 22.1 cm.

In this variant issue, the dedication to W. A. Hammond appearing on p. [v] has been replaced by a note indicating corrections to several tables.

Presented in memory of Robert D. Gauchat.

*1059. AUGUST WEISMANN (1834–1914). *Das Keimplasma.* Jena: G. Fischer, 1892. xviii, 628 pp., illus. 27 cm. Original wrapper.

Weismann, educated at Göttingen and Giessen, practiced medicine until 1863, when he turned to biological research and zoology. Although well known for his zoological investigations, it is this classic work on heredity for which he is best known. In it he states his germ-plasm theory, the concept that although the cells of a living organism ultimately die, some portion of the protoplasm of the germ cells passes on through ovum and sperm from generation to generation. To this substance, which he named germ plasm, he assigned the task of carrying forward the elements of heredity. Weismann rejected the Lamarckian theory of the inheritance of acquired characteristics, and the influence of this landmark work led to the chromosome theory as it matured in the 1920's and 1930's.

Garrison-Morton 236; Osler 1622 (English tr., 1893).

*1060. ERNST HEINRICH HAECKEL (1834–1919). *Natürliche Schöpfungsgeschichte.* Berlin: G. Reimer, 1868. xvi, 568 pp., illus., 8 plates (2 fold.). 21.3 cm.

Apostle of Darwin and thus facing the opposition of his own teacher, Virchow, Haeckel was one of the front-ranking German biologists of his era, at a time when the entire field of biology was bursting with new discoveries.

In this work, Haeckel divides morphology into two parts: tectology, or the science of organic individuality, and promorphology, which aims to establish a crystallography of organic forms.

Garrison-Morton 224.

*1061. ———. *Anthropogenie; oder, Entwicklungsgeschichte des Menschen.* Leipzig: W. Engelmann, 1874. xvi [4] 732 pp., illus., plates (part fold., 1 col.). 23.2 cm.

This important contribution to the theory of evolution has had more influence on later biology than Haeckel's perhaps better-known work, *Natürliche Schöpfungsgeschichte* (see No. 1060). It contains a clear statement of the embryological processes, and it is in this work that Haeckel states the well-known tenet that "ontogeny recapitulates phylogeny," that is, that the formation of the individual is a repetition of the formation of the species, so graphically illustrated in Table XII of the book.

Cushing H9; Garrison-Morton 493; Waller 3917.

*1062. WILHELM VON WALDEYER-HARTZ (1836–1921). *Das Becken. Topographisch-anatomisch mit besonderer Berücksichtigung der Chirurgie und Gynäkologie.* Bonn: F. Cohen, 1899. xxvii, 690 [2] pp., illus. (part col.), plate. 26.8 cm.

This exhaustive text on the surgical anatomy of the male and female pelvis constitutes only a small part of the many contributions made by Waldeyer. A pupil of Henle (see No. 946) and later professor of anatomy at the University of Berlin, Waldeyer was the first to propose and demonstrate the germinal epithelium and the vascular layer of the ovary (Waldeyer's line). He must also be credited for his work on cancer, confirming the epithelial origin of carcinoma.

1063. MORIZ KAPOSI (1837–1902). *Handatlas der Hautkrankheiten für Studirende und Ärzte.* 3 vols. Vienna & Leipzig: W. Braumüller, 1898–1900. Vol. I: [8] pp., 114 col. plates with facing pages; Vol. II: [6] pp., 126 col. plates with facing pages; Vol. III: xiii [3] pp., 136 col. plates with facing pages. 25.4 cm.

Kaposi was born in Hungary, the son of very poor parents. Nevertheless, he eventually was able to study medicine and received his medical degree from Vienna. He was immediately appointed assistant to Ferdinand von Hebra (1816–1880), the noted Austrian dermatologist. He later married Hebra's daughter and, after Hebra's death, assumed his father-in-law's chair at the University, becoming an eminent dermatologist in his own right. Kaposi was a prolific writer and made a number of original contributions to clinical dermatology. His *Pathologie und Therapie der Hautkrankheiten* is more than ample evidence that he was a master of dermatology from the clinical, pathological, and therapeutic aspects.

The present atlas of skin diseases, with its 376 color plates, is one of the most extensive and valuable collections of illustrations in the dermatological literature.

Garrison-Morton 4001.

*1064. JOHN SHAW BILLINGS, compiler (1838–1913). *A report on the hygiene of the United States Army, with descriptions of military posts.* Washington: Government Printing Office, 1875. lix, 567 pp., illus., fold. map, plates, plans. 29.2 cm. Original cloth.

Although Billings had a distinguished career as a surgeon during the Civil War, he is better known for his achievements as a sanitary engineer, hospital planner, medical bibliographer, historian, and statistician. Billings also developed the collection of the Library of the Surgeon-General (now the National Library of Medicine), began *Index Medicus*, and served as chief executive of the New York Public Library during its early years.

In this book he reports on individual military installations around the United States and includes such information as medical statistics, climate, and plans of forts. Billings' lengthy report on the state of army hygiene is included at the beginning of the book.

*1065. JULIUS FRIEDRICH COHNHEIM (1839–1884). *Neue Untersuchungen über die Entzündung.* Berlin: A. Hirschwald, 1873. 85 pp. 24.3 cm.

A pupil of Virchow, Cohnheim was the most prominent experimental pathologist in nineteenth-century Germany. While professor of pathology at Kiel and Breslau, he investigated the inflammatory process and demonstrated, in opposition to

Virchow's theory, that pus is formed by the passage of white blood cells through the capillary walls. This short monograph contains Cohnheim's most cogent presentation of his new and essentially correct theory.

Garrison-Morton 2302; Osler 2343.

*1066. WILHELM HEINRICH ERB (1840–1921). *Handbuch der Elektrotherapie.* Leipzig: F. C. W. Vogel, 1882. vii, 738 pp., illus. 21.4 cm.

Of the many German neurologists who flourished during the later 1800's, the most significant figure was Wilhelm Heinrich Erb. Primarily known for the advances he made in identifying, classifying, and treating the muscular dystrophies, many of which still bear his name, Erb also pioneered in the use of electricity in the diagnosis and treatment of nervous disorders. This work on electrotherapy contains first descriptions of several nervous disorders and was written while Erb was professor of neurology at the University of Heidelberg, a post he held for some twenty-seven years.

1067. GERHARD HENRIK ARMAUER HANSEN (1841–1912). "On the etiology of leprosy." (In *British and foreign medico-chirurgical review.* Vol. 55 (1875), pp. 459–489.) 20.9 cm.

Hansen, a Norwegian, became interested in leprosy after joining the staff of the Leprosy Hospital in Bergen, which specialized in treating leprosy. As a result, he devoted most of his professional life to the study of the epidemiology, etiology, prevention, and management of leprosy. His discovery and demonstration of the leprosy bacillus in the early 1880's is one of the earliest reports of pathogenic bacteria. He first reported his work in the *Norsk magazin for laegevidenskaben* in 1874. The present paper in English appeared the next year as the only original communication in the April issue of the *British and foreign medico-chirurgical review.*

Garrison-Morton 2436.

*1068. ROBERT WILLIAM TAYLOR (1842–1908). *A clinical atlas of venereal and skin diseases.* Philadelphia: Lea Bros., 1889. 22, 19–427 pp., illus., 58 col. plates. 44.9 cm.

This magnificent atlas was the major work of Taylor, a prominent dermatologist and professor of genitourinary and venereal diseases at the College of Physicians and Surgeons of New York. The starkly realistic colored plates, together with a lucid text, mark the work as one of the finest atlases of its kind.

*1069. WILLIAM JAMES (1842–1910). *The principles of psychology.* 2 vols. New York: H. Holt [1890]. Vol. I: xii, 689 pp., illus.; Vol. II: vi, 704 pp., illus. 21.6 cm.

Although well known as one of the most influential thinkers of his day and as a pioneer of the new psychology in America, William James was schooled as a physician and taught anatomy and physiology at Harvard from 1872 to 1880 before transferring to the Department of Psychology and Philosophy where he remained until 1907.

In this brilliant and epoch-making work, James set for the basis of his philosophy "a world of pure experience."

GUSTAF RETZIUS (1842–1919). *Studien in der Anatomie des Nervensystems und des Bindegewebes.*

See No. 1052.

*1070. ———. *Das Gehörorgan der Wirbelthiere; morphologisch-histologische Studien.* 2 vols. Stockholm: In Commission bei Samson & Wallin, 1881–1884. Vol. I: xi, 221 pp., 35 plates; Vol. II: viii, 368 pp., 39 plates. 38.7 cm.

Retzius, professor of histology at the Karolinska Institut in Stockholm, was one of the foremost histologists of the nineteenth century. This huge work on the anatomy of the vertebrate ear did much to clarify some early problems in brain morphology.

Garrison-Morton 1566.

*1071. ———. *Das Menschenhirn; Studien in der makroskopischen Morphologie.* 2 vols. Stockholm: P. A. Norstedt, 1896. Vol. I: viii, 167 pp., illus.; Vol. II: 96 plates. 38.8 cm.

As with other works of Retzius, this massive set is an example of scholarship, accuracy, and fine printing. The ninety-six plates include both drawings and photographs depicting the minute anatomy of the brain from every possible angle.

Choulant-Frank, p. 409; Cushing R117; Garrison-Morton 1426.

*1072. ———. *Crania Suecia antiqua.* Stockholm: Gedruckt in Aftonbladets Druckerei, 1900. [6] iv, 182 pp., illus., maps, 100 plates. 41.8 cm.

Retzius' work in anthropology included detailed studies of the human skull. This large work contains data collected over four decades and includes illustrations of skulls from the stone, bronze, and iron ages with 100 superb photographic plates. This is a signed presentation copy.

*1073. ———. *Das Affenhirn in bildlicher Darstellung.* Stockholm: Centraldruckerei; Jena: G. Fischer, 1906. 31 pp., 67 plates. 39.4 cm. In slipcase.

This large atlas with its excellent plates depicting the brain of the monkey is typical of the basic contributions to neurology which this Swedish comparative anatomist made at the time of the founding of the "neurone doctrine."

1074. WILLIAM PEPPER, editor (1843–1898). *A text-book of the theory and practice of medicine.* 2 vols. Philadelphia: W. B. Saunders [1893–1894]. Vol. I: xii, 909 [24] pp., illus., 3 plates. Vol. II: xii, 1046 [28] pp., illus., 6 plates. 25.9 cm.

Pepper was a commanding figure in the evolution of American medical education. In his role as provost at the University of Pennsylvania he helped establish a standard of excellence in the training of medical students which was far ahead of its time. Among his many papers is included the first description of hyperplastic bone marrow in pernicious anemia.

As editor of the present work, Pepper drew from some of the most distinguished practitioners of his day, including Sir William Osler and John Shaw Billings.

Gift of Dr. R. N. Larimer.

*1075. ROBERT KOCH (1843–1910). "Die Aetiologie der Tuberkulose." (In *Berliner klinische Wochenschrift*. Vol. 19 (1882), pp. 221–230.) 30.5 cm.

Without doubt one of the greatest German scientists of any era, Koch was responsible for bringing the young science of microbiology to fruition. The son of a mining engineer, he was born in Klausthal, Germany. He was graduated in medicine from the University of Göttingen in 1866 and shortly thereafter served as an army surgeon during the war of 1870. After the war, he settled in Wollstein as a district physician and took up the busy routine of a country practice. In spite of the heavy demands of his practice, he continued to work actively with his microscope, having been deeply influenced by Jakob Henle (see No. 946) during his student years. His work in culturing, staining, and microscopy provided the basis for a variety of tests and procedures which are now standard practice in clinical diagnosis; his identification and isolation of specific bacteria led to new treatment modes for a number of diseases, including anthrax and cholera.

This brief journal article, in which Koch first states the actual cause of tuberculosis to be the tubercle bacillus and not nutritional deficiencies (as was widely believed), is a medical classic. His discovery helped enormously in the control of widespread affliction. For his work on tuberculosis, Koch received the 1905 Nobel prize.

Cushing K147; Garrison-Morton 2331; Waller 5338a.

*1076. ———. *Gesammelte Werke*. 2 vols. in 3. Leipzig: G. Thieme, 1912. Vol. I: 706 pp., front. (port.), 29 plates (part col.); Vol. II, pt. 1: iv, 680 pp., 11 plates (part col.); Vol. II, pt. 2: v, 681–1216 pp., 2 plates. 28.3 cm.

Koch's complete works were published two years after his death. The large volumes contain colored plates of a number of different bacteria strains and a fine photograph of Koch on the frontispiece.

Garrison-Morton 86.

*1077. Sir DAVID FERRIER (1843–1928). *The functions of the brain*. London: Smith, Elder, 1876. xv, 323 pp., illus. 23 cm.

Dedicated to John Hughlings Jackson (1834–1911), the father of English neurology, this work furnished the link between Hughlings Jackson and the later work on cerebral cortical localization by Sir Charles Sherrington (see No. 1136) and others at the turn of the century. This classic book summarizes the fundamental and startling new facts experimentally demonstrated by this remarkable neurophysiologist.

Garrison-Morton 1409.

1078. NICHOLAS SENN (1844–1908). *Principles of surgery*. Philadelphia and London: F. A. Davis, 1890. xiii, 611 pp., illus. 25.5 cm.

Senn, a native of Switzerland, came to the United States with his family in 1852. He was graduated from the Chicago Medical College, practiced in Milwaukee for a time, and went to Europe for several years to study pathology. He was professor of surgery at the College of Physicians and Surgeons of Chicago for more than ten years and eventually became professor of the principles of surgery and surgical pathology at Rush Medical College. Among his many scientific achievements were his experimental work in abdominal surgery, research into intestinal perforation, studies of surgical tuberculosis, and development of the hydrogen gas test to detect intestinal perforation. Senn wrote more than twenty books and contributed many papers to the periodical literature. This popular, comprehensive text on surgery went through four editions and was translated into Russian in 1903.

Waller 8846 (1891 ed.).

1079. Sir WILLIAM RICHARD GOWERS (1845–1915). *The diagnosis of diseases of the spinal cord*. London: J. and A. Churchill, 1880. viii, 80 pp., illus., plate. 22.1 cm.

Gowers was a prominent member of a group of British clinical neurologists who, during the latter part of the nineteenth century, made important studies in nervous system physiology and pathology. Most of Gowers' professional life was spent at University College Hospital where he developed the extraordinary powers of observation, personal study habits, and writing ability for which he was known. His works are admired almost as much for their clarity and organization as they are for content. Gowers invented the first practical hemoglobinometer and was the first to describe the bundle of nerve fibers in the spinal cord (Gowers' tract). With Sir Victor Horsley (1857–1916) he became the first to remove a spinal cord tumor successfully. Gowers was a fine artist and his *Manual and atlas of medical ophthalomology* (1879) was illustrated by his own hand.

The present work on spinal cord diseases was originally delivered in 1877 to the Medical Society of Wolverhampton. It is a fine example of the painstaking scholarship which characterizes all of his writings.

Garrison-Morton 4562; Osler 2783; Waller 3663.

*1080. IL'IA IL'ICH MECHNIKOV (1845–1916). *L'immunité dans les maladies infectieuses*. Paris: Masson, 1901. ix, 600 pp., illus. (part col.). 22.9 cm.

Mechnikov, a Russian-born zoologist and pathologist, was appointed sub-director of the Pasteur Institute in Paris in 1887 and spent the remainder of his life there. His studies on the process of intracellular digestion in invertebrates led him, step by step, to the discovery that certain white blood cells, which he callled phagocytes, have a destructive capability toward foreign bacteria in the blood stream. This was the basis of his theory of phagocytosis, giving the first definite proof of the scientific soundness of the theory of immunity and of the practice of vaccination. In 1908 he shared the Nobel prize in medicine and physiology with Paul Ehrlich.

The present book is a classic on immunity in infectious diseases and one of Mechnikov's best works.

Garrison-Morton 2555; Waller 6414.

*1081. ———. *Immunität bei Infektionskrankheiten*. Jena: G. Fischer, 1902. xi, 456 pp., col. illus. 25.7 cm.

One measure of the importance of Mechnikov's work on immunity is the appearance of a German translation just one year after the original French edition.

1082. CHARLES LOUIS ALPHONSE LAVERAN (1845–1922). "Un nouveau parasite trouvé dans le sang de plusieurs malades atteints de fièvre palustre." (In *Bulletins et Mémoires de la Société médicale des hôpitaux de Paris, (Mém.)*. Serie 2, Vol. 17(1880), pp. 158–164.) 24.1 cm.

After graduating from the University of Strasbourg in 1867, Laveran became an army physician like his well-known father. While stationed at Constantine in Algeria, he discovered the malaria parasite which he named *Oscillaria malariae*. One of the great discoveries of modern medicine, it was announced in the present paper. Laveran later served as professor of military hygiene at Val de Grâce and, resigning from the army, went to the Pasteur Institute where he devoted the remainder of his life to research and experimentation in tropical medicine and parasitology. He received the Nobel prize for medicine in 1907.

Garrison-Morton 5236.

1083. ———. *Traité du paludisme*. Paris: Masson, 1898. viii, 492 pp. [1] leaf of plates, 28 illus. (1 col.). 24 cm.

This is the last of four separate treatises on malaria published by Laveran. In it, he summarizes the long history of the study of malaria, fully describes his own discovery of the malaria parasite as well as its mosquito carrier, and places considerable emphasis on the importance and necessity of draining marshes and stagnant bodies of water. He also covers the clinical, pathological, and therapeutic aspects of malaria and concludes with material on related parasitic diseases and problems yet to be solved.

Garrison-Morton 5248; Osler 1692.

*1084. ———. *Leishmanioses: kala-azar, bouton d'orient, leishmaniose américaine*. Paris: Masson, 1917. iii, 521 pp., illus., 6 plates (2 col.). 23.9 cm. Quarter morocco.

Laveran received the Nobel prize for his work on protozoa as the cause of disease and, in particular, for his discovery of the malaria parasite in human blood. Nearly

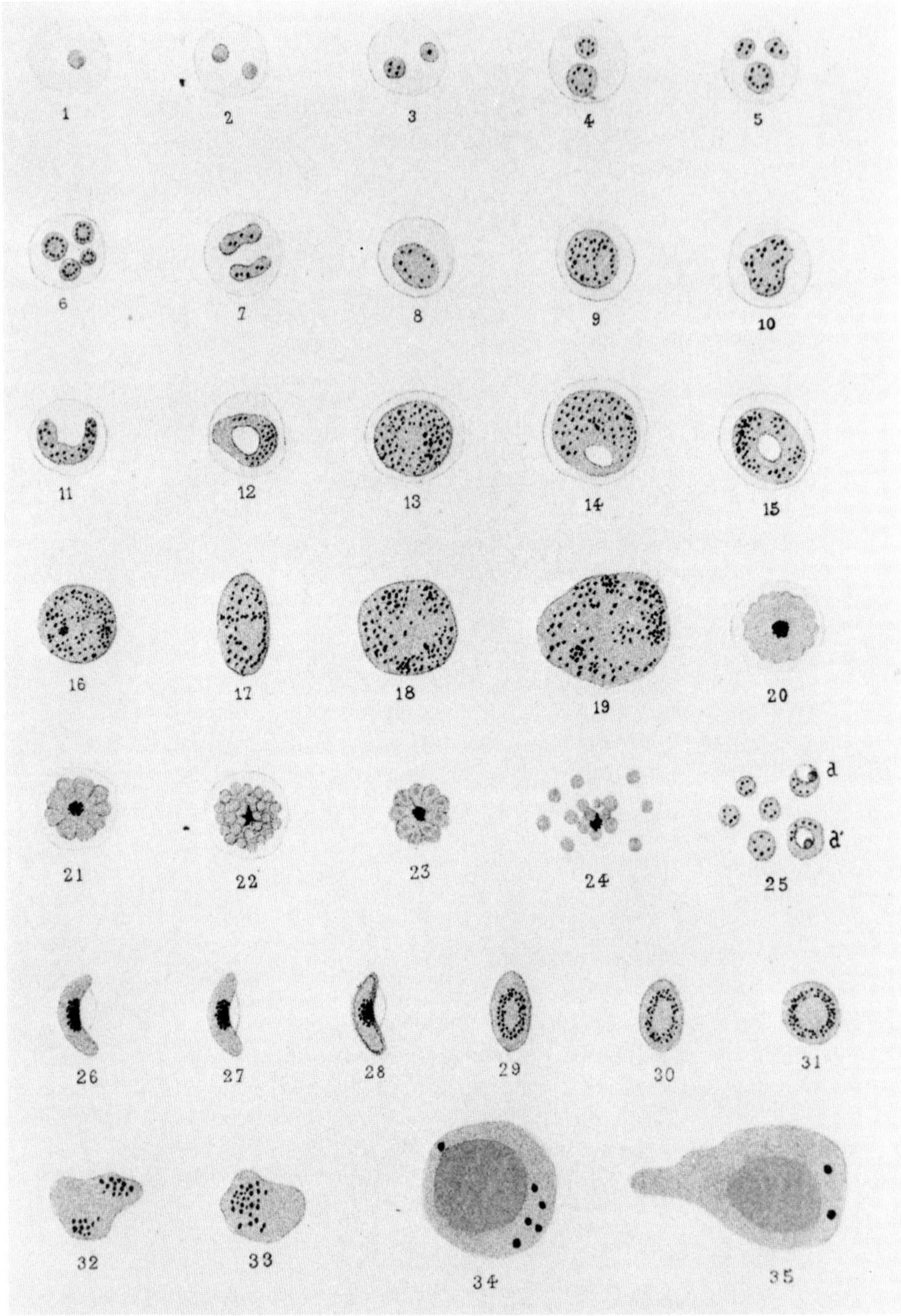

No. 1083. Laveran. *Traité du Paludisme.* The malarial parasite, called *Oscillaria Malariae* by Laveran.

all of his investigations had to do with tropical diseases as does the present treatise on Leishmaniasis, his last major work.

*1085. WILHELM CONRAD RÖNTGEN (1845–1923). "Ueber eine neue Art von Strahlen. Erste, [Zweite und Dritte] Mittheilung." (In *Annalen der Physik, Neue Folge*. Vol. 64 (1898), no. 1, pp. 1–37.) 21.1 cm.

The first report of Röntgen's discovery of the X-ray appeared in the *Sitzungsberichte der Physikalisch-Medizinischen Gesellschaft* in Würzburg in 1895. Röntgen published a second report of his research and experimentation in the same journal in 1896, and a third and final report in the *Sitzungsberichte der Koeniglichen Preussischen Akademie der Wissenschaften zu Berlin* in 1897. These three short papers, collected here for the first time, represent one of the most important advances in the history of scientific development. The importance of Röntgen's work and the resulting development of the field of radiology does not need further elaboration. Röntgen was awarded the first Nobel prize in physics in 1901.

Cushing R193, 1st report; Cushing R194, 2nd report; Garrison-Morton 2683, 1st report; Osler 1700, 1st report; Waller 8078, 1st report; Waller 8083, 2nd report.

EDWARD ORAM SHAKESPEARE (1846–1900). *Report on the origin and spread of typhoid fever in U.S. military camps during the Spanish war of 1898.*

See No. 1108.

1086. PRINCE ALBERT MORROW (1846–1913). *Atlas of skin and venereal diseases.* New York: W. Wood, 1889. 318, iv pp., illus., 75 col. plates. 41.6 cm.

Morrow, one of America's premier nineteenth-century dermatologists, was born in Kentucky and received his medical degree in 1874 from University Medical College in New York. This atlas covering the entire range of dermatological and venereal diseases is his most famous work. The colored plates, selected from the works of a number of prominent artists, effectively supplement the clearly-written text. Morrow was active in stressing the need for dissemination of information on sex hygiene to the public.

1087. GEORGE HENRY FOX (1846–1937). *Photographic illustrations of skin diseases.* 2nd ser. New York: E. B. Treat, 1889. 208 pp., col. plates. 29.3 cm.

A detailed and authoritative text supplements the nearly 100 hand-colored photographs in this fine dermatological atlas. Fox was clinical professor on diseases of the skin at the College of Physicians and Surgeons in New York.

Garrison-Morton 3996 (1880 ed.).

1088. PAUL EMIL FLECHSIG (1847–1929). *Die Leitungsbahnen im Gehirn und Rückenmark des Menschen auf Grund entwickelungsgeschichtlicher Untersuchungen.* Leipzig: Verlag von Wilhelm Engelmann, 1876. xvi, 382 pp., 20 plates (part col.). 25.8 cm.

Flechsig recognized that the understanding of the nervous system could be enhanced through the study of myelogenesis. This treatise on the pyramidal and dorsal spinocerebellar tract (Flechsig's tract) is one of the earliest and most important works on the subject. It led to Flechsig's study of nerve development in the cerebral hemispheres and the charting of the fields of the cerebral cortex. He also made notable contributions in experimental psychology and neuropathology. Most of his work was done while at the Institute of Physiology at Leipzig and the University of Leipzig.

Cushing F182; Garrison-Morton 1410; Waller 3072.

1089. SALOMON EBERHARD HENSCHEN (1847–1930). *Klinische und anatomische Beiträge zur Pathologie des Gehirns.* Vols. 1–7 (of 8 vols.) in 6. Vols. 1–4, Upsala: Almquist & Wiksell; Vols. 5–6, Stockholm: Nordiska Bokhandeln; Vol. 7, Stockholm: Selbstverlag des Verfassers; 1890–1922. Illus. 31.6 cm.

Shortly after being appointed professor of medicine at Upsala, Henschen abandoned his early work on internal medicine and became absorbed in the study of neurologic disorders. Dealing only with the gross anatomy of the brain, Henschen compiled an impressive array of observations including the discovery of the cortical visual center and important data on the visual, auditory, gustatory and olfactory pathways, shedding new light on aphasia and other brain disorders. Most of his writings may be found in this extensive treatise on which Henschen labored throughout his life.

Cushing H275; Garrison-Morton 4632.

*1090. ADOLF WEIL (1848–1916). *Handbuch und Atlas der topographischen Percussion.* Leipzig: F. C. W. Vogel, 1877. x, 183 pp., 26 col. plates. 22.3 cm.

Weil is probably best known for his original description of leptospirosis (Weil's disease) which he was able to differentiate from other types of acute jaundice. This highly regarded monograph is a detailed exposition of auscultation of the thorax in the diagnosis of intrathoracic conditions.

*1091. Sir WILLIAM MACEWEN (1848–1924). *Pyogenic infective diseases of the brain and spinal cord.* Glasgow: J. Maclehose, 1893. xxiv, 354 pp., illus., plates. 22.2 cm.

"Macewen . . . studied medicine at Glasgow, and he remained there to adorn the University and the city during the rest of his life. As an undergraduate he studied under Lister, and at the early age of twenty-eight he became a full surgeon to the Glasgow Royal Infirmary. . . . Lister was the sole architect of the antiseptic system, but Macewen must be regarded as one of the principal architects of the aseptic system. Macewen's greatest achievement is probably his foundation of neurological surgery. . . . In 1893 he published his great work *Pyogenic Infective Diseases of the Brain and Spinal Cord* . . . an incredible record of ten years' achievement. . . . There are few branches of surgery which he did not adorn" (Charles Singer and E. A. Underwood, *A short history of medicine.* Oxford, 1962. pp. 366–368).

Cushing M24; Garrison-Morton 4872; Waller 6112.

*1092. ———. *Atlas of head sections*. Glasgow: Maclehose, 1893. xiii pp., 53 plates, each accompanied by a duplicate outline plate, 4 pp. 29 cm.

This folio volume contains fifty-three copperplates drawn from photographs of sections through the head in coronal, sagittal, and transverse planes, each accompanied by a duplicate plate in outline. It was meant to supplement Macewen's *Pyogenic infective diseases of the brain and spinal cord* (see No. 1091).

Choulant-Frank, p. 409; Garrison-Morton 431.

ALBERT PITRES (1848–1928). *Les centres moteurs corticaux chez l'homme*.

See No. 1032.

*1093. AUGUSTE HENRI FOREL (1848–1931). *Die sexuelle Frage*. Munich: E. Reinhardt, 1905. viii, 587 pp. 22.8 cm.

Equally renowned as neurologist, psychiatrist, and entomologist, Forel played a large part in bringing mental health into the realm of scientific investigation. In 1875, he made the first complete section of the whole brain and, during his tenure at Zurich as professor of psychiatry, he formulated independently the concept of cellular and functional units (later termed the neuron theory). He also pioneered the use of hypnotism as a psychiatric diagnostic aid and contributed toward the understanding of alcoholism.

This classic work on "the sexual question" was published the same year as Freud's *Drei Abhandlungen zur Sexualtheorie* (see No. 1125), and is one of the first in-depth treatises on sexual hygiene. Translated into sixteen languages, it is Forel's best-known work.

Garrison-Morton 1635; Waller 3122.

*1094. HUGO DE VRIES (1848–1935). *Die Mutationstheorie*. 2 vols. Leipzig: Verlag von Veit, 1901–1903. Vol. I: xii, 648 pp., illus., 8 plates; Vol. II: xiv, 752 pp., illus., 4 plates. 23.7 cm.

Darwin, thorough as he was in marshaling evidence to support the concept of natural selection, was unable to account for the inheritance of the variations on which natural selection depends. However in 1900, De Vries, professor of botany at the University of Amsterdam, discovered the fundamental but long-unrecognized work of the Austrian monk, Gregor Mendel (1822–1884), who in 1866 had advanced a theory of genetic recombination and species variation which De Vries recognized as essentially identical to his own. De Vries gave full credit to Mendel but was able to add an observation of his own: the sudden, sometimes radical, changes in characteristics of certain plant species, which subsequently breed true, played an important role in the evolutionary mechanism, a view later supported by a wealth of evidence. The present work is De Vries' definitive treatise on mutation.

Cushing V184; Garrison-Morton 240.

*1095. GEORGE McCLELLAN (1849–1913). *Regional anatomy in its relation to medicine and surgery.* 2 vols. Philadelphia: J. B. Lippincott, 1891–1892. Vol. I: xxii, 436 pp., 53 col. plates; Vol. II: xiv, 414 pp., 44 col. plates. 28.4 cm.

The ninety-seven photographic plates included in this detailed atlas of human regional anatomy were hand-colored by the author, who was professor of applied anatomy at Jefferson Medical College and founder of the Pennsylvania School of Anatomy and Surgery.

1096. JOSEPH JULES DÉJÉRINE (1849–1917) and ANDRÉ THOMAS (1867–1963). *Traité des maladies de la moelle épinière.* Paris: J.-B. Baillière et fils, 1902. 470 pp., illus. 24 cm.

Déjérine's career included posts at La Charité, Bicêtre, and Salpêtrière. Aided by his wife and colleague, Augusta Maria Klumpke, Déjérine worked almost unceasingly, contributing numerous discoveries and observations to the growing body of literature on the physiology and pathology of the nervous system. The separation of peripheral tabes from medullary tabes, advances in the localization of brain function, and observations on expressive aphasia are among his contributions. Several diseases bear his name. As a clinician and instructor, Déjérine commanded the respect of his pupils with his communications skills and the earnest and sympathetic manner with which he treated his patients.

Déjérine wrote the present treatise on diseases of the spinal cord with his student, André Thomas. They later won the Montyon prize for their work on the subject. This is a presentation copy signed by Déjérine.

Garrison-Morton 4590.

Sir WILLIAM OSLER (1849–1919).

So great was the acclaim of his contemporaries and so continued is our appreciation of Sir William Osler that a mystique, a cult, has developed around this now legendary great clinician. Born in Canada, educated at McGill University in Montreal and later a student in several of the great European centers of medical learning, Osler first taught at McGill University from 1875 to 1884, followed by five years at the University of Pennsylvania. His career reached its peak, however, in the fifteen years (1889–1904) he spent as professor of medicine at the new Johns Hopkins Medical School in Baltimore. It was there that he introduced the bedside method of teaching; it was there that "clinical clerks," young medical students, were taken out of the lecture halls and laboratories and put in direct contact with the patient from whom they could learn, as Osler insisted, *by studying the patient.* In 1905 Osler was invited to become Regius professor of medicine at Oxford, where he spent the rest of his life.

Osler was a man of wide culture and catholic interests, a brilliant clinician, a born teacher, and a tireless student. But it was his special personality, his elusive charm, and his outgoing spirit of humanism which endeared him to his contemporaries and which continue to inspire us today. He had a passionate enthusiasm for work, for study, and for human life itself, and one may search the files of medical history without success to find another like him. His many interests and rich philosophy, the depth of his literary and historical culture, can be appreciated by a review of his writings, both medical and non-medical, and by a study of the *Bibliotheca Osleriana,* the catalogue of the great collection of books which he gave to McGill University. Osler's *Principles and practice of medicine* (see No. 1098) brought a new style to medical textbooks, with its immense store of medical information, its literary references, and its pithy, often humorous, allusions to the vagaries of the world in which we live.

Osler has been well treated by his many biographers (Thayer, 1919; Cushing, 1925; Reid, 1931; and others). The "fine machinery" of Osler's mind may be quickly appreciated by a reading of the little book, *Sir William Osler: aphorisms from his bedside teaching and writings* (New York, 1950), edited by Dr. William Bennett Bean, until recently Sir William Osler Professor of Medicine at The University of Iowa.

A long-time admirer of Osler was Dr. Robert N. Larimer, a physician of Sioux City, Iowa. For many years before his death in 1978 Dr. Larimer engaged in the pleasant and rewarding hobby of collecting as much as he could of Osler's enormous output of published materials and of selected items of Osleriana. Although Osler wrote a number of books, the largest proportion of his publications was in medical journals. He had most of these journal articles reprinted in a limited number of copies for presentation to friends and colleagues. An idea of the immensity of his published work may be gained from the list of collected reprints appearing as item No. 3576 in *Bibliotheca Osleriana,* which identifies 324 separate reprints of articles, in addition to which are scrapbooks containing an additional 161 shorter articles, letters, notices, obituaries, and pamphlets. Most of these items are elusive and many are quite rare.

Dr. Larimer was notably successful in his collecting activities and gathered nearly three hundred items of the Osler bibliography as well as additional biographical, bibliographical, and other related publications. Dr. Larimer presented his Osler collection to the University of Iowa Libraries, where it has an honored position in the Rare Book Room of the Health Sciences Library. It should be noted, too, that while Dr. Larimer's collecting activities were centered around Sir William Osler, he also collected other notable medical works, principally in the field of nineteenth century American medicine. This collection, too, has been presented to The University of Iowa. A number of these items are noted in their appropriate places in this catalogue.

The limitation of space does not permit listing more than a few of the items which seem most representative or best known of Osler's work and of the Larimer collection. All of the following works are the gift of Dr. Larimer.

1097. ———. *Aequanimitas: valedictory remarks to the graduates in medicine at the University of Pennsylvania, May 1st, 1889.* Philadelphia: Wm. F. Fell & Co., 1889. 10 pp. 23.5 cm. Original wrapper.

This farewell address to the medical graduates at the University of Pennsylvania as Osler prepared to move to Johns Hopkins University is perhaps one of the best known of all of Osler's non-clinical papers. It was frequently reprinted, beginning in 1904 in a collection of Osler's addresses called *Aequanimitas with other addresses,* which is also in the Larimer collection along with all of the later editions.

Osler 3576, No. 97.

1098. ———. *The principles and practice of medicine.* [1st ed., 1st issue]. New York: D. Appleton, 1892. xvi [1] 1079 pp., illus., diagrs. 23.5 cm. Original cloth. Inscribed by author.

"This book . . . gained and maintained a place in English, American, and even continental practice only comparable with that held by the treatise of Sir Thomas Watson (1843) in the decades preceding. The clear, concise, attractive presentation and the many citations from history and the classics, give it a unique place among scientific books with an essentially literary flavor" (Note by F. H. Garrison in Maude E. Abbott, *Classified . . . bibliography of Sir William Osler's publications.* Montreal, 1939. p. 62).

The first issue is distinguished from the second by the misspelling of Plato's *Gorgias* as "Georgias" on the verso of the third leaf. Further distinction is given to this copy of Osler's textbook by the following inscription in Osler's hand: "The Doctor's Thomas with the author's love and thanks. W. O."

The Larimer collection also contains the second issue of the same year, the third issue (1893), and no fewer than eighteen additional editions and issues.

Garrison-Morton 2231; Osler 3543 (1st issue), 3544 (2nd issue); Waller 7031 (1901 ed.).

1099. ———. *Lectures on the diagnosis of abdominal tumors.* Second reprinting. New York: D. Appleton, 1895. [5] 192 pp., illus., 21.6 cm. Original wrapper, repaired.

Osler delivered a series of lectures on abdominal tumors to the postgraduate class at Johns Hopkins in Novenber and December of 1893. They were first published in a series of articles in the *New York medical journal* during 1894. They were collected and published commercially in 1894, and republished in a new typesetting in 1895. Three other editions of this important work appear in the Larimer collection.

Osler 3564.

1100. ———. *The leaven of science.* [Philadelphia?: n. publ., 1894?]. 16 pp. 26 cm. Original wrapper.

The first separate printing of another famous address, this one delivered at the opening of the Wistar Institute at the University of Pennsylvania, May 21, 1894, and first printed in the *University medical magazine* in June, 1894.

Osler 3576, No. 148.

1101. ———. *An Alabama student.* [First separate reprinting]. Baltimore: Friedenwald, 1896. 19 pp. 20.3 cm. Original stiff wrapper.

Osler wrote a number of biographical and historical papers, and the present one is an interesting and well-known example. This biographical sketch of Dr. John Y. Bassett, an almost unknown physician from Huntsville, Alabama, who died as a comparatively young man in 1851, was based on a small packet of letters and two articles which Dr. Bassett had written. Osler makes of this slight evidence a graceful address on "a man of whom you have never heard, a humble student from a little town in Alabama." The address, presented to the Johns Hopkins Historical Club in January, 1895, was first printed in the *Johns Hopkins Hospital bulletin* in 1896. This little pamphlet is the first separate reprinting. It was later included in a popular collection of essays and addresses, *An Alabama student, and other biographical essays.*

Osler 3576, No. 166.

1102. ———. *On the association of enormous heart hypertrophy, chronic proliferative peritonitis, and recurring ascites, with adherent pericardium.* [n.p., n. publ., 1896?]. 8 pp. 24.1 cm. Original wrapper.

First separate reprinting of Osler's paper on the syndrome now known as Pick's disease, presented at the American Pediatric Society meeting in 1895 and first published in the *Archives of pediatrics* in 1896.

Osler 3576, No. 169.

1103. ———. *The Lumleian lectures on angina pectoris.* [First separate reprinting]. [London?: n. publ., 1910?]. 50 pp. 21.3 cm. Original wrapper. Inscribed by author.

While Osler was Regius professor of medicine at Oxford, he was invited to present the Lumleian lectures to the Royal College of Physicians. He gave these lectures in March, 1910, and they were immediately printed in three successive issues of *The Lancet.* The wrapper carries the unsigned inscription in Osler's hand, "With kind regards."

Osler 3575 and 3576, No. 288.

1104. PAUL MARIE LOUIS PIERRE RICHER (1849–1933). *L'art et la médecine.* Paris: Gaultier, Magnier [1902]. 562 pp., illus., plates. 28.2 cm.

Richer was one of a number of French neurologists who achieved prominence during their acquaintance with Charcot and the Salpêtrière. As the resident artist, Richer made numerous drawings and statues representing typical bodily and facial configurations of patients afflicted with various nervous and muscular diseases.

This impressive work is an historical survey of medicine as portrayed in art and includes over 300 reproductions of paintings and woodcuts.

Cushing R145; Garrison-Morton 6607; Osler 5392; Waller 14733.

*1105. IVAN PETROVICH PAVLOV (1849–1936). *Die Arbeit der Verdauungsdrüsen.* Wiesbaden: J. F. Bergmann, 1898. xii, 199 pp., illus. 24.1 cm.

The work of the Russian physiologist Pavlov in the field of the physiology of digestion led to his being awarded the Nobel prize for medicine in 1904. His demonstration of conditioned reflexes and automatic responses in dogs had consequences not only for medicine, but for political practices, the sociological sciences, and psychology as well.

This first edition in German is the first translation of this classic work on the digestive glands, published in Russia the year before.

Waller 7257.

*1106. MASSACHUSETTS. SANITARY COMMISSION. *Report of a general plan for the promotion of public and personal health.* Boston: Dutton & Wentworth, state printers, 1850. 544 pp., illus., 5 plates, maps (2 fold.). 24 cm. Original paper wrappers, in maroon cloth box.

This report to the Sanitary Commission of Massachusetts provided much of the impetus for the first organized public health measures in the United States. Prepared by a Governor-appointed committee led by Lemuel Shattuck (1793–1859), the report was based on an analysis of pre-existing health laws in ancient and contemporary Europe, and included reforms ranging from slum clearance and city planning to the protection of the health of school children and the management of rooming houses. This is a presentation copy inscribed by Shattuck.

Garrison-Morton 1609.

*1107. JAMES BLAKE BAILEY (fl. 1890). *The diary of a resurrectionist, 1811–1812.* London: Swan Sonnenschein, 1896. 184 pp., plates. 19.2 cm.

Until the passage of the Anatomy Act in 1832, which provided legal means for physicians to obtain cadavers, grave robbing by "resurrection men" was a common practice. This brutally vivid work includes firsthand accounts of the activities of the so-called "sack-em-up" men with satirical caricatures by Rowlandson, and photographs of "mortsafes," specially constructed theft-proof graves and tombs.

Cushing B32; Osler 1888.

*1108. WALTER REED (1851–1902), VICTOR CLARENCE VAUGHAN (1851–1929), and EDWARD ORAM SHAKESPEARE (1846–1900). *Report on the origin and spread of typhoid fever in U.S. military camps during the Spanish war of 1898.* 2 vols. Washington: Government Printing Office, 1904. Vol. I: xviii, 721 pp. 29.3 cm.; Vol. II: 96 maps and charts. 34.4 × 42.2 cm. Original green cloth.

Reed, a native of Virginia, received his medical degree at the University of Virginia. He was commissioned in the Army Medical Corps in 1875 and remained in the Army for the remainder of his career. Reed is perhaps best known for producing conclusive evidence that the mosquito, *Aedes aegypti,* is the vector in yellow fever, the dread disease which took so many lives in military campaigns and among the civilian population. Several years before his now-famous yellow fever studies, he headed an Army commission to study the origin and spread of typhoid fever in army camps. An abstract of the report was issued in 1900, and the present exhaustive report was published by Reed's collaborators, Victor C. Vaughan and Edward O. Shakespeare. Their work, here reported in great detail, demonstrated that flies were the major carriers of the disease, aided by dust, unclean hospital attendants, infected patients, and infected bedding and waste matter. The report was well received and had an immediate effect in the effort to develop better methods to control typhoid fever throughout the world.

VICTOR CLARENCE VAUGHAN (1851–1929). *Report on the origin and spread of typhoid fever in U.S. military camps during the Spanish war of 1898.*

See No. 1108.

*1109. ERNST FUCHS (1851–1930). *Die Ursachen und die Verhütung der Blindheit.* Wiesbaden: J. F. Bergmann, 1885. xvi, 243 pp., fold. col. diagr. 21.5 cm.

One of the most noted ophthalmologists of the nineteenth century, Fuchs practiced in Liége and later Vienna where, due to his influence, the school soon attracted students from all over Europe. Fuchs authored a number of works on eye pathology, of which this treatise on blindness is one of the most important.

Waller 3287.

1110. ———. *Text-book of ophthalmology.* Authorized translation from the 2nd enlarged and improved German ed., by A. Duane. New York: D. Appleton [1892]. xiii, 788 pp., illus. 23.2 cm.

Fuchs's textbook of ophthalmology was first published in German in 1889 and has since been translated into many languages including Japanese. It was the standard text in the field well into the twentieth century, the last English edition appearing in 1933.

Garrison-Morton 5935 (German ed., 1889).

Gift of Dr. R. N. Larimer.

*1111. ANTOINE HENRI BECQUEREL (1852–1908). *Récherches sur une propriété nouvelle de la matière; activité radiante spontanée ou radio-activité de la matière.* Paris: Firmin-Didot, 1903. 360 pp., diagrs., tables, 13 plates. 28.6 cm.

Becquerel, a French physicist, accidentally discovered the phenomenon of radioactivity in 1896, when he suffered a burn from carrying uranium in his pocket. In 1903 he shared the Nobel prize for physics with Marie and Pierre Curie, who were his pupils and friends and who were inspired by Becquerel's research in radioactivity.

Cushing B228.

1112. WILLOUGHBY DAYTON MILLER (1853–1907). *The micro-organisms of the human mouth.* Philadelphia: S. S. White Dental Mfg. Co., 1890. xx [2] 364 pp., illus. 24.5 cm.

Miller, a native of Ohio, was graduated from the University of Michigan and went to Edinburgh to study chemistry, philosophy, and mathematics. He decided to specialize in physics and went to Berlin for further studies. While in Berlin, he became interested in dentistry and returned to the United States where he received a dental degree from the University of Pennsylvania. He returned to Germany, established a dental practice, and taught at the University of Berlin. It was at Berlin that he did his notable work in bacteriology under Robert Koch. He did not return to America until 1906 and died before he could assume a teaching position at the University of Michigan. This, his most widely-recognized work, was first published in German in 1889. In it, he presents the etiology of caries and correctly explains for the first time the causative factors leading to the dissolution of enamel and dentine.

Garrison-Morton 3687.

1113. Sir JAMES MACKENZIE (1853–1925). *Diseases of the heart.* 2nd ed. London: Henry Frowde, Hodder & Stoughton, 1910. xx, 419 pp., illus., fold. plates. 24.2 cm.

Mackenzie was born in Scotland and studied medicine at the University of Edinburgh. He entered general practice in Burnley, Lancashire, and remained there for more than twenty-five years before moving to London in 1908 as a result of the acclaim he received following publication of the first edition of the present work. Mackenzie became interested in cardiac arrhythmias early in his career and developed the well-known Mackenzie Ink Polygraph to assist him with his studies. His *Study of the pulse* (1902) was the first scientific treatise on irregularities of the pulse and established his reputation as one of the leading heart specialists of the day.

The present work, first published in 1908, was an instant success and was soon translated into several foreign languages. In it, he summarized the major aspects of his work including many reproductions of tracings of abnormal pulse waves to illustrate the various types of cardiac irregularities he described and discussed. It was in this work that he first described nodal arrhythmia now known as auricular fibrillation. Mackenzie's broadly based study of heart diseases, his polygraph, and Einthoven's electrocardiograph (see No. 1145) were significant advancements in man's knowledge of the heart and prepared the way for a new era in cardiology.

Garrison-Morton 2826 (1st ed., 1908); Waller 6115 (1918 ed.).

*1114. CONSTANTIN VON MONAKOW (1853–1930). *Gehirnpathologie.* Vienna: A. Hölder, 1897. ix, 924 pp., illus. (part col.), fold. plate, fold. table. 24.6 cm.

Born in Russia but spending most of his childhood and professional life in Zurich, von Monakow was a rebellious youth and not especially promising as a student. Ousted from his home at seventeen, he decided upon a career in medicine. His studies led him to Bernhard Aloys von Gudden (1824–1886) in Munich whose investigations in neuropathology awakened von Monakow's interest. After further study in Berlin he returned to Zurich where he set up a private practice and opened a research laboratory which later became part of the University of Zurich.

Von Monakow was a prodigious worker who produced an extraordinary amount of writing in which can be found some of the most fundamental knowledge of the anatomy and physiology of the brain. His studies of the visual and acoustic pathways, his description of the rubrospinal tract, and his exploration of human behavior in relation to neurobiology all helped to foster the emergence of neuropathology as a distinct field. *Gehirnpathologie* is one of the classics of nineteenth-century German neurology. In addition to the lucid text, it is well illustrated with numerous plates and tables and includes over 3,000 references to the literature.

*1115. CHARLES EDWARD BEEVOR (1854–1908). *The Croonian lectures on muscular movements and their representation in the central nervous system.* London: Adlard, 1904. xii, 100 pp. 21.7 cm.

Beevor was physician to National Hospital at Queen's Square, London, and was most noted for his research on the localization of cerebral function which he conducted with Sir Victor Horsley (1857–1916) at the Brown Institution. This highly original work on neuromuscular physiology was first delivered before the Royal College of Physicians of London in 1903.

*1116. BYRON ROBINSON (1854–1910). *The abdominal brain and automatic visceral ganglia.* Chicago: Clinic Publishing Co., 1899. [8] 261 [3] pp., plates. 23.1 cm.

Though Robinson maintained a large practice as a clinical surgeon in Chicago, his chief contribution lies in his studies on anatomy and gross pathology. He contributed significantly to the existing knowledge of the biliary and pancreatic ducts, the ureto-ovarian circle (Robinson's circle), the ureters, and the great sympathetic nerve (the abdominal brain)—the subject to which the present work is devoted.

*1117. PAUL EHRLICH (1854–1915) and SAHACHIRO HATA (1873–1938). *Die experimentelle Chemotherapie der Spirillosen (Syphilis, Rückfallfieber, Hühnerspirillose, Frambösie).* Berlin: J. Springer, 1910. viii, 164 pp., 5 plates, tables (part fold.). 23.5 cm.

Ehrlich, director of the Institute of Serum Research at Frankfurt, was basically a chemist. He conceived the idea of creating a "magic bullet" drug to kill living organisms when he observed in his early work with dyes that bacteria would take up dye while the tissue remained unaffected. It was a first step toward the present-day extensive use of chemotherapy. Working with his Japanese assistant, he carried out 605 experiments before reaching the one compound which answered all the requirements. This was the famous "606," the magic bullet, later named Salvarsan.

Garrison-Morton 2403; Osler 1697; Waller 2707.

*1118. PAUL EHRLICH. *Grundlagen und Erfolge der Chemotherapie.* Stuttgart: F. Enke, 1911. 26 pp., 4 plates. 25.2 cm.

One of the first successful uses of Salvarsan was in the treatment of syphilis. This brief work on the basics of chemotherapy includes thirteen photographs vividly portraying the efficacy of this new therapeutic mode.

*1119. EMIL ADOLPH VON BEHRING (1854–1917). *Die praktischen Ziele der Blutserumtherapie und die Immunisirungsmethoden zum Zweck der Gewinnung von Heilserum.* 2 vols. Leipzig: G. Thieme, 1892. Vol. I: 66 pp.; Vol. II: 122 pp. 21.8 cm.

If the measure of a physician is determined by the degree to which he has contributed to the alleviation of human suffering, Behring must rank as one of the greatest. In 1890, together with his associate, Shibasaburo Kitasato, Behring discovered that the antitoxin produced in the blood of animals with diphtheria, when injected into other animals recently exposed to the diphtheria germ, provided a strong immunity to the disease. The subsequent marketing of diphtheria antitoxin in 1892 led to the control of what was once a dreaded childhood malady and to the beginning of modern immunology. In 1901 Behring received the first Nobel prize for physiology and medicine.

In this text, one of Behring's most important works, he describes the immunization process for a number of diseases including diphtheria, tetanus, and tuberculosis.

Waller 834.

1120. ALBERT LUDWIG SIEGMUND NEISSER (1855–1916). "Ueber eine der Gonorrhoe eigentümliche Micrococcusform." (In *Centralblatt für die medicinischen Wissenschaften.* Vol. 17 (1879), no. 28, pp. 497–500.) 22.7 cm.

The most significant advances in the diagnosis and treatment of venereal diseases were made in the late nineteenth and early twentieth century. The contributions of Neisser, a German-born physician educated at Breslau, to the study of gonorrhea and syphilis played a major role in this activity. Neisser was well-prepared for research in venereology having studied and trained under Heidenhain, Kohnheim, Ehrlich, Weigert, and Koch. It was known that a microscopic agent was the cause of gonorrhea and syphilis, and, in 1879, after only two years of investigation, Neisser discovered the causative organism of gonorrhea. His research and experimentation are described in the present paper in which he used the name "micrococcus" to describe the bacterium. In 1882, after additional study and research, he renamed the bacterium "gonococcus." Although his discovery was extremely important, it was not until the advent of penicillin that this widespread disease could be controlled. Neisser also studied syphilis and discovered the *Spirochaeta pallida* while working in Java just after Schaudinn and Hoffmann had isolated it in Germany. Neisser also worked with Wassermann in developing the Wassermann test for syphilis (see No. 1152).

Garrison-Morton 5208.

———. "Eine serodiagnostische Reaktion bei Syphilis."

See No. 1152.

*1121. Sir CHARLES ALFRED BALLANCE (1856–1936). *Some points in the surgery of the brain and its membranes.* London: Macmillan, 1907. xv, 405 pp., illus., ports. 22.1 cm.

Ballance, a noted English surgeon, was the youngest of four brothers who were all physicians. He received his medical education at University College, London, served with the British Expeditionary Force during World War I, and returned to the Norfolk and Norwich Hospital where he was consulting surgeon for many years. He was a skilled surgeon and, in this book on brain surgery, sets forth many ideas that were quite modern for their day. The book contains a series of three lectures on cerebral membranes, tumors, and abscesses that he prepared for the Lettsomian Lectures of the Medical Society of London in 1906.

*1122. SIGMUND FREUD (1856–1939). *Die Traumdeutung.* Leipzig: F. Deuticke, 1900. [4] 371 [4] pp. 22.4 cm.

Freud must be considered one of the most significant figures of the twentieth century. Certainly no scientist before or after him has had as much impact on the understanding of human and social behavior, and his work remains the basis for much of modern psychoanalysis and psychotherapy. His intellect and creativity remained active over a lifetime of more than eighty years during which he made striking and original discoveries, the import of which is still being felt.

Freud was born at Freiberg in Moravia and entered the University of Vienna as a medical student in 1873. He was graduated in 1881 and continued his studies at Vienna's General Hospital in order to qualify for private practice. While at the hospital he worked in the division of internal medicine and later in the psychiatric clinic under the well-known neuroanatomist, Theodor Meynert (1833–1892). In 1885, he spent several months in Paris studying under Jean Charcot (see No. 1027 ff.). As a result of his work with Charcot, Freud decided to abandon his laboratory researches into the anatomy of the nervous system in favor of clinical work on nervous disorders. During the years from 1892 to 1895, he developed his psychoanalytical method using the technique of free association. From 1895 to 1906 he worked largely in semi-isolation because he was heavily criticized and ostracized by his colleagues in the medical profession. Nevertheless, by 1906 he was beginning to attract enthusiastic followers and supporters and soon thereafter the first psychoanalytic congress was held in Salzburg. The cancer that later caused his death was first discovered in 1923, and, in 1938, Freud moved to London when the Nazis occupied Austria.

Die Traumdeutung [The interpretation of dreams] was considered by Freud to be his most significant work. It contains the beginnings of the psychoanalytic theories which he elaborated in later works, including the relationship between dreams and the deeper layers of the subconscious mind. This first edition was printed in limited numbers and is now quite scarce.

Cushing F331; Osler 2680 (English tr., 1913).

*1123. ———. ———. 6th ed. Leipzig and Vienna: F. Deuticke, 1921. vi, 478 pp. 22.7 cm.

Later editions of *Die Traumdeutung* became increasingly popular as Freud's theories gained recognition and, finally, acceptance. The sixth edition is a somewhat enlarged version with a greatly expanded list of references.

1124. ———. *Über den Traum.* Wiesbaden: J. F. Bergmann, 1901. [305]–344 pp. 25.8 cm.

This short paper on dreams includes several case studies. It was published as number eight of the series *Grenzfragen des Nerven- und Seelenlebens.*

Waller 3244.

1125. ———. *Drei Abhandlungen zur Sexualtheorie.* Leipzig and Vienna: F. Deuticke, 1905. 83 pp. 2 copies. Copy 1: 24 cm. Original paper wrappers, in quarter morocco box. Copy 2: 24 cm. Original paper wrappers, in portfolio.

While *Die Traumdeutung* was virtually ignored when first published, this work on the theory of sexuality prompted a quick and largely negative response from the scientific community. Here Freud first articulates in detail his epochal theory of infant sexuality and its effect upon later development. It has been condemned; it has been used in clinical practice; it has been idolized to the point of cultism. Accepted or rejected, the arguments presented in this work have had a deep and lasting impact upon psychiatric thinking the world over.

Garrison-Morton 4983.

Copy 1: Gift of Dr. John Martin.

*1126. ———. *Totem und Tabu.* Leipzig: H. Heller, 1913. [iii] 149 pp. 24.6 cm.

Totem und Tabu marks the entrance of Freud's theories into the anthropological and social realm. It is considered by many to be second in importance only to *Die Traumdeutung.* Freud considered primitive societies to be subject to the same influences as individuals, with the Oedipus conflict playing a dominant role in the evolution of tribal systems, religious customs and symbols. The first edition of this classic is particularly scarce.

*1127. ———. *Vorlesungen zur Einführung in die Psychoanalyse.* Leipzig: H. Heller, 1916–1917. 545 pp., plate. 22.8 cm.

Freud's popular treatise on psychoanalysis went through numerous editions and was translated into many languages including Arabic, Chinese, and Yiddish.

Garrison-Morton 4989 (English tr., 1922); Waller 3246 (1918 ed.).

*1128. ———. *Massenpsychologie und Ich-Analyse.* Leipzig: Internationaler Psychoanalytischer Verlag, 1921. 140 pp. 20.8 cm.

Like *Totem and Tabu* (see No. 1126), this work in group psychology represented a new and wholly original contribution to social psychology. By applying his "libido theory" to group structure, Freud provided new insight into such considerations as leadership, discipline, identification, love, the herd instinct, and the place and evolution of the ego within the context of group dynamics.

*1129. ———. *Das Ich und das Es.* Leipzig: Internationaler Psychoanalytischer Verlag, 1923. 77 pp. 23.7 cm.

It was in this book that Freud's far-reaching tripartite theory of personality first gained full expression, laying the groundwork for his future work and setting the stage for decades of conjecture and experimentation. In Freudian psychology the Id (Es) represents primary instincts and needs and is the source of the libido, while the Ego (Ich) is both a conscious and subconscious reaction to the social environment, mediating between the primitive id and the demands of the outside world. The Superego, which Freud earlier termed the ego-ideal, is the psychic agency that incorporates learned standards of behavior and thought, coercing the self to meet higher standards.

*1130. ———. *Zur Geschichte der psychoanalytischen Bewegung.* [First separate edition]. Leipzig: Internationaler Psychoanalytischer Verlag, 1924. 72 pp. 24.1 cm.

This historical study of psychoanalysis first appeared in *Jahrbuch der Psychoanalyse* in 1914 and again in 1922 in a collection of Freud's shorter writings.

Waller 13325.

*1131. ———. *Die Frage der Laienanalyse.* Leipzig: Internationaler Psychoanalytischer Verlag, 1926. 123 pp. 19.1 cm.

Die Frage der Laienanalyse [The question of lay analysis] is an apology in support of allowing nonmedical individuals to practice psychoanalysis. Freud lays heavy stress on the fact that psychoanalysis is a branch of psychology and not medicine and that the education required of an analyst is independent of both fields. In the process, the reader is treated to a brilliant elucidation of the theory of psychoanalysis, couched in the expository prose for which Freud was noted.

*1132. Sir JOSEPH JOHN THOMSON (1856–1940). *Rays of positive electricity and their application to chemical analyses.* London: Longmans, Green, 1913. vii, 132 pp., illus., 5 plates. 22.4 cm.

Thomson had already won the 1906 Nobel prize for his discovery of the electron when he discovered that positive ions in discharge tubes consisted of atomic and molecular particles which could be readily sorted. His find led directly to the discovery of non-radioactive isotopes and to the development of the new discipline of nuclear physics which has proven itself of vital importance in modern medicine.

*1133. GEORGES ALBERT ÉDOUARD BRUTUS GILLES DE LA TOURETTE (1857–1904). *L'hypnotisme et les états analogues au point de vue médico-légal.* 2nd ed. Paris: E. Plon, Nourrit, 1889. xv, 583 pp. 22.7 cm.

Gilles de la Tourette was a pupil of Charcot and later chief of neurology at the Salpêtrière. He is probably best known for his description of the saltatory spasm or "impulsive tic" and his treatise on hysteria. This work is on the medico-legal aspects of hypnotism, magnetism, and spiritualism which, at the time, were at the height of their popularity.

Waller 3540.

*1134. THEODOR ESCHERICH (1857–1911). *Die Darmbakterien des Säuglings und ihre Beziehungen zur Physiologie der Verdauung.* Stuttgart: F. Enke, 1886. ix, 180 pp. 26 cm. Original printed wrappers, uncut.

A native German, Escherich became professor of pediatrics at Vienna. This treatise, in which he is the first to describe the intestinal organism *Bacillus coli* (later called *Bacillus Escherichia*), can still be studied profitably today.

Garrison-Morton 1017.

*1135. FEDOR KRAUSE (1857–1937). *Chirurgie des Gehirns und Rückenmarks nach eigenen Erfahrungen.* 2 vols. Berlin: Urban & Schwarzenberg, 1908–1911. Vol. I: xii, 176 pp., illus., 25 plates (part col.); Vol. II: xxxvi, 177–823 pp., illus., 37 plates (part col.). 27.3 cm.

This work on surgery of the brain and spinal cord is richly illustrated with exceptional black and white and colored plates, which graphically depict the variety of pathological conditions of the central nervous system. Krause was professor of surgery at Berlin where he developed the first operation for extradural excision of Gasserian ganglion for trigeminal neuralgia and demonstrated the utility of whole thickness skin grafts.

*1136. Sir CHARLES SCOTT SHERRINGTON (1857–1952). *The integrative action of the nervous system.* New York: Scribner, 1906. xvi, 411 pp., illus. 21.9 cm. Original cloth.

Sherrington, educated at Cambridge and professor of physiology at Liverpool and Oxford, was a man of wide interests and accomplishments: biographer, medical historian, poet, and book collector. In this classic of modern neurology, he summed up his years of experiments and observations on the nervous system and the reflexes and developed a theory that has had a far-reaching and profound influence on modern neurophysiology and clinical neurology. Briefly, his theory was that the nervous system acts as the coordinator of various parts of the body and that the reflexes are the simplest expressions of the integrative action of the nervous system, enabling the entire body to function toward one definite end at a time. Sherrington shared the Nobel prize for medicine and physiology in 1932 with Edgar Douglas Adrian, 1st Baron Adrian (1889–1977), for their work on the nervous system.

Garrison-Morton 1432.

*1137. HERMANN OPPENHEIM (1858–1919). *Lehrbuch der Nervenkrankheiten für Ärzte und Studierende.* 5th ed. 2 vols. Berlin: S. Karger, 1908. Vol. I: xiii, 695 pp., illus. (part col.), plates (part col.); Vol. II: [696]–1641 pp., illus. (part col.), plates (part col.). 23.9 cm.

Oppenheim was the acknowledged leader of German clinical neurology during the last decade of the nineteenth century, an especially fertile period for this rapidly expanding field. After serving as assistant to Karl Westphal (1833–1890) at the Charité at the University of Berlin, he opened a private clinic which soon became an international center of neurology. Oppenheim's investigations included studies on sclerosis, syphilis, polio, alcoholism, and amyotonia congenita (Oppenheim's disease). His later work on the diagnosis and treatment of brain disease led directly to the first successful removal of a brain tumor. The present text is considered a landmark in neurology for its scholarly approach and thorough documentation. It passed through seven German editions and was translated into a number of languages, the first English edition being taken from this, the fifth German edition.

Garrison-Morton 4582 (1st ed., 1894); Waller 6990 (1894 ed.).

1138. EDGAR MARCH CROOKSHANK (1858–1928). *History and pathology of vaccination.* 2 vols. London: H. K. Lewis, 1889. Vol. I: xxiii, 466 pp., illus.; Vol. II: vi, 610 pp. 25.2 cm.

Crookshank had the rare good fortune to have studied under Lister, Pasteur, and Koch. He was an energetic teacher and noted bacteriologist, his highly regarded *Manual of bacteriology* (1886) going through four editions. This massive undertaking is both a history of smallpox vaccination and a critical inquiry into its effectiveness. Volume Two is comprised entirely of papers excerpted from other sources, ranging from Jenner's original *Inquiry* (see No. 677) to Crookshank's own observations on an 1887 outbreak of cowpox. The appearance of this volume caused no small amount of controversy within the medical ranks, owing to the fact that Crookshank saw fit to color the account with his own, quite negative, views on the efficacy of inoculation.

Cushing C494; Garrison-Morton 5435; Waller 13030.

*1139. HOWARD ATWOOD KELLY (1858–1943). *Operative gynecology.* 2 vols. New York: D. Appleton [1898]. Vol. I: xvi, 563 pp., illus. (part col.), 10 plates (part col.); Vol. II: xii, 557 pp., illus. (part col.), 14 plates (part col.). 25.9 cm.

The emergence of modern gynecology in America is due in large part to the work of Howard Kelly, professor of gynecology at the University of Pennsylvania and later at Johns Hopkins. Kelly made pioneering contributions in such areas as the use of cocaine as a local anesthetic in the treatment of uterine displacement, ureter catheterization, the diagnosis of ureteral calculi, the treatment of vesicovaginal fistula, and a host of other diagnostic and therapeutic advances. Many of these areas are included in the present work, making it one of the finest medical texts ever produced in America. The illustrations and plates are largely the work of Max

Brödel who also illustrated Kelly's later work, *Medical gynecology* (1908). Kelly was equally renowned as a medical historian and biographer, his *Cyclopedia of American medical biography* (1912) being especially noteworthy.

Garrison-Morton 6108.

*1140. PIERRE CURIE (1859–1906). *Oeuvres de Pierre Curie.* Paris: Gauthier-Villars, 1908. xxii, 621 pp., illus., 2 plates. 23.9 cm.

The tragic death of Pierre Curie at the age of forty-seven put an end to what was certainly one of the most famous scientific collaborations in history. Despite his abbreviated career and the fact that his work was sometimes overshadowed by that of his gifted wife (see No. 1156), Pierre Curie must be credited with a remarkable amount of original work of extreme importance in the understanding of radioactivity and atomic structure. He shared the 1903 Nobel prize in physics with his wife and Henri Becquerel (see No. 1111). This volume of collected writings includes works on magnetism, crystal symmetry, pyroelectric phenomena, and an account of the discovery of radium. The laudatory introduction by Marie Curie gives some interesting bits of family history.

Cushing C652; Waller 11322.

1141. ISABEL ADAMS HAMPTON ROBB (1859–1910). *Nursing: its principles and practice.* Philadelphia: W. B. Saunders, 1893. 484 pp., front., illus., plates, diagrs. 19.4 cm.

The development of nursing as a profession in the United States and Canada was greatly influenced by Isabel Hampton Robb who, while director of the nursing school at Johns Hopkins, led a number of efforts aimed at strengthening the profession. She was the first president of the Nurses Associated Alumnae of the United States and Canada (the earliest national nursing organization) and was one of the first to recommend the adoption of standards in nursing education and registration. This popular and highly regarded textbook was written during her tenure at Johns Hopkins.

*1142. WILLIAM CARNEGIE BROWN (1859–1913). *Amoebic or tropical dysentery.* London: J. Bale, 1910. viii, 271 pp., illus., plate. 20.9 cm.

Brown was a medical practitioner in Penang from 1885 to 1904, where he was able to observe firsthand the nature and variety of tropical diseases. After his return to England, he became a driving force in the formation of the Society for the Study of Tropical Diseases. This pioneer work on amoebic dysentery, together with an earlier book on sprue, constitute Brown's chief contributions to the literature of tropical medicine.

*1143. KARL LUDWIG SCHLEICH (1859–1922). *Schmerzlose Operationen: oertliche Betäubung mit indifferenten Flüssigkeiten.* Berlin: J. Springer, 1894. x, 256 pp., illus. 23.6 cm.

Although the American surgeon William Halsted (1852–1922) was the first to utilize subcutaneous infiltration anesthesia in local surgery, Schleich refined and developed the technique for making use of weak cocaine solutions and other liquids. Ironically, although Schleich's work was met with general rejection by the German Congress of Surgeons to whom it was first demonstrated, it was widely adopted in the United States. This book is Schleich's second work on infiltration anesthesia, the first being a short paper published earlier in the same year. An interesting insert has been included in this copy: a reprint from an 1891 issue of the *New York medical record* by Dr. Robert H. M. Dawborn who calls attention to Halsted's precedence in utilizing the technique but also makes the curious conclusion based on self-experimentation that water itself contains analgesic properties.

Waller 8621.

*1144. PIERRE MARIE FÉLIX JANET (1859–1947). *L'automatisme psychologique.* Paris: F. Alcan, 1889. 496 pp., illus. 22 cm.

Probably best known for his work in dissociation and psychasthenia, Janet was one of Charcot's many students who later achieved prominence in the burgeoning field of psychiatry. After receiving his doctorate in psychology from the University of Paris, he was appointed director of pathological psychology at the Salpêtrière at the request of Charcot. He later taught at the Sorbonne and the Collège de France. *L'automatisme psychologique* was Janet's first major work, and it was here that he introduced the concept of automatism, a condition in which an activity is carried out without conscious knowledge by the subject. Janet was largely responsible for the movement to reconcile the concepts of clinical and academic psychology in an attempt to find a single, unified system.

*1145. WILLEM EINTHOVEN (1860–1927). "Ein neues Galvanometer." (In *Annalen der Physik.* 4th series. Vol. 12 (1903), pp. 1059–1071.) 21.3 cm.

Causing a current to flow over a thin conducting thread stretched across a magnetic field, Einthoven discovered that the thread would deviate at right angles to the magnetic lines of force. The sensitivity of his "string galvanometer" enabled him to construct a crude electrocardiograph which could measure the small electric current produced by the action of the heart and eventually to correlate the measurements with various heart diseases. Einthoven was awarded the 1924 Nobel prize for his work.

Garrison-Morton 842.

*1146. JOHN SCOTT HALDANE (1860–1936). *Respiration.* New Haven: Yale University Press [1922]. xviii, 427 pp., illus., plates. 22.7 cm.

Much of our fundamental knowledge of the physiology of respiration is due to the work of Haldane, the Oxford physiologist whose interests in pulmonary gas exchange led him to investigate such areas as the respiration centers of the brain, the chemical regulation of respiration, gas analysis, basal metabolism, mining hygiene, gas warfare, and high altitude physiology (a study which eventually culminated in a 1913 expedition to Pike's Peak). This basic work of respiration is based on the Silliman lectures which Haldane presented at Yale University and is justly regarded as one of the finest treatises in the field of modern physiology.

Garrison-Morton 961 (1935 ed.).

1147. ELISEO CANTÓN (b. 1861). *Atlas de anatomía y de clínica obstétrica normal y patológica.* Buenos Aires: J. Peuser, 1910. [11] 174 pp., 58 plates (part col.). 67.4 cm. In portfolio.

The fifty-eight colored and black and white photographic plates in this large obstetrical atlas portray in striking detail the development of the human embryo from conception to birth in both normal and diseased states. This copy is inscribed by the author.

*1148. WILLIAM BATESON (1861–1926). *Mendel's principles of heredity.* Cambridge: At the University Press, 1909. xiv, 396 pp., illus., front., 6 plates. 23.5 cm.

Bateson is frequently called the "father of genetics" for his fundamental work in heredity. While not one of the original discoverers of Mendel's work, Bateson was one of its foremost proponents. He extended and enlarged upon Mendel's basic laws of gene segregation and assortment, noting in particular the frequent "linkage" of certain traits and the action of one gene upon another. Bateson also investigated the hereditary nature of certain diseases such as hemophilia and color blindness. The present work is a concise account of Mendelian genetics and contains an English translation of Mendel's classic work, *Versuche über Pflanzen-Hybriden* (1865).

Cushing B162; Garrison-Morton 244; Waller 10733 (1913 ed.).

1149. NICOLAS MAURICE ARTHUS (1862–1945). *De l'anaphylaxie à l'immunité.* Paris: Masson et cie, éditeurs, 1921. xxxvi, 361 [3] pp. 22.3 cm.

In 1890 Arthus established the role of calcium in blood coagulation. He later made numerous contributions to the understanding of the immune and allergic mechanisms in serum. This important work on anaphylaxis and immunity was written while Arthus was professor of physiology at the University of Lausanne.

*1150. ALBERT CALMETTE (1863–1933). *L'infection bacillaire et la tuberculose chez l'homme et chez les animaux.* Paris: Masson, 1920. vi, 619 pp., illus., 25 col. plates. 25 cm. Original paper wrappers.

Calmette, a former pupil of Pasteur, was sent to Saigon in French Indochina to direct the newly established Pasteur Institute. Finding that many people were being killed by snakebite, he developed an effective serum to neutralize snake venom. He returned to France in 1894 as director of the Pasteur Institute at Lille where he took up the study of tuberculosis and devised the conjunctival test for tuberculosis (the Calmette test). In 1924 he introduced the B.C.G. (Bacille-

Calmette-Guerin) vaccine, a living strain of bovine tubercle bacilli, for use as an immunizing agent. It was widely used at the time, especially for children. This work is a comprehensive study of the preparation and use of tuberculosis vaccines and contains a number of excellent colored plates of pathological specimens.

*1151. GREENFIELD SLUDER (1865–1928). *Concerning some headaches and eye disorders of nasal origin.* St. Louis: C. V. Mosby, 1918. 272 pp., illus. 24.8 cm. Original maroon cloth.

Sluder, a prominent otorhinolaryngologist, spent nearly his entire career in the St. Louis area and was head of the department of laryngology and rhinology at Washington University Medical School for fifteen years. He wrote nearly seventy papers and two books. In this well-illustrated book, Sluder presents his research and clinical experience with headaches and disorders of the eye that have their origin in the nasal region. It was in this work that he first described Sluder's neuralgia, neuralgia of the spenopalatine ganglion.

*1152. AUGUST VON WASSERMANN (1866–1925), ALBERT NEISSER (1855–1916), and CARL BRUCK (b. 1879). "Eine serodiagnostische Reaktion bei Syphilis." (In *Deutsche medizinische Wochenscrift.* Vol. 32 (1906), pp. [745]–746). 32 cm.

In 1905, Fritz Schaudinn's (1871–1906) discovery of the causative agent of syphilis, *Spirochaeta pallida,* was a major achievement and marked the beginning of a new era in the study of syphilis. The following year Wassermann, Neisser, and Bruck published the present article which announced their development of the Wassermann test. Wassermann received his doctor's degree at Strasbourg in the late 1880's and worked at the Robert Koch Institute for Infectious Diseases in Berlin until 1906. Prior to his work on syphilis, Wassermann had done important investigations on toxins and antitoxins. He had also developed a complement fixation test for the diagnosis of tuberculosis based on the complement fixation reaction discovered by Bordet and Gengou in 1901. The significance of the Wassermann test and its application to modern clinical medicine can hardly be overemphasized.

Garrison-Morton 2402.

*1153. JOHN WHITRIDGE WILLIAMS (1866–1931). *Obstetrics; a text-book for the use of students and practitioners.* New York and London: D. Appleton, 1903. xxii, 845 pp., front., illus. (part col.), plates (part col.). 23.5 cm. Original maroon cloth.

Williams, a native of Baltimore and a graduate of the University of Maryland, was one of the leading teachers at Johns Hopkins Medical School at the turn of the century. He was dean of the medical school from 1911 until 1923 and served many years as professor of obstetrics. Williams made important studies on the pathology of the reproductive organs, the physiology of pregnancy, and the etiology of eclampsia. His *Obstetrics* was the most popular and widely-used textbook in its field and went through seven editions before his death. Updated versions of his work are still used in many medical schools.

Garrison-Morton 6211.

1154. LUDWIG ASCHOFF (1866–1942). *Pathologische Anatomie.* 2 vols. Jena: G. Fischer, 1909. Vol. I: vi, 636 pp.; Vol. II: iv, 815 pp., illus. (part col.), 1 fold. col. plate. 24.4 cm.

Aschoff, who held the chair of pathological anatomy at Freiburg, was one of the most productive of the group of German pathologists who flourished in the late nineteenth and early twentieth centuries. He made important studies on appendicitis, gallstones and jaundice, and thrombosis, and is particularly remembered for introducing the term "reticulo-endothelial system." His outstanding textbook on pathological anatomy, here in its first edition, went through many editions and was used as a standard text until very recently.

Gift of Dr. R. N. Larimer.

*1155. SERGE VORONOFF (1866–1951). *Étude sur la vieillesse et la rajeunissement par la greffe.* Paris: G. Doin, 1926. 213 pp., plates, ports. 23.2 cm. Original printed wrappers.

Voronoff, a skilled and well-educated French surgeon, was director of the Laboratoire de Chirurgie Expérimentale at the Collège de France, where he experimented with the transplantation of various organs of the endocrine system. The clinical results of his testicular grafting for sexual rejuvenation caused a sensation in the early twentieth century, but soon faded because it was not successful in restoring sexual vigor. For substantial fees, he would transplant monkey testicles, the gonads of a young ape, or human glands. It is interesting to note that he died from syphilis contracted from one of his own monkey transplants. This book was his major work and has his signature on the flyleaf.

*1156. MARIE SKLODOWSKA CURIE (1867–1934). *Traité de radioactivité.* 2 vols. Paris: Gauthier-Villars, 1910. Vol. I: xiii, 426 pp., illus., front. (port.), 2 plates; Vol. II: 548 pp., illus., 5 plates. 25.4 cm. Original wrappers, in cloth box.

Marie Sklodowska was the fifth and youngest child of a mathematics and physics teacher in Warsaw. She completed her basic education at the age of seventeen and for the next six years served in various posts as a governess. During this time she continued to read and study the scientific literature; she entered the Sorbonne in 1891 to study for a master's degree in physics (1893) and then in mathematics (1894). She was awarded a doctorate several years later for her notable work on the nature of radioactivity. It was while she was a student in Paris that she met and eventually married Pierre Curie (see No. 1140).

In 1896 Henri Becquerel (see No. 1111) had suggested the radioactive properties of pitchblende. Inspired by this suggestion, Becquerel's pupil, Marie Curie, and her husband Pierre began the labors which led to their discovery of polonium and radium and to their sharing with Becquerel of the Nobel prize for physics in 1903. Marie was awarded the Nobel prize again for chemistry in 1911.

*1157. ———. *L'isotopie et les éléments isotopes.* Paris: Edité par la Société "Journal de physique," 1924. 210 pp., illus., plates. 23.6 cm.

Since the discovery of the radioactive substances polonium and radium by Marie and Pierre Curie, the importance of this fundamental work has developed an enlarging path through chemistry, physics, and clinical medicine. Whereas the radioactive substances were used for many years in therapeutics, isotopes have been actively used for clinical diagnostic methods for only the past three decades.

*1158. JEAN BAPTISTE AUGUSTE ÉTIENNE CHARCOT (1867–1936). *Contribution à l'étude de l'atrophie musculaire progressive, type Duchenne-Aran.* Paris: Progrès Médical, 1895. 159 pp., illus., 4 plates (part col.). 22.7 cm. Original paper wrappers, signatures uncut.

Jean Baptiste Charcot was the son of the famous Salpêtrière physician, Jean Martin Charcot (see No. 1027 ff.). He is often remembered as having led the search for the lost Antarctic explorer, Amundsen. Like his father, Jean Baptiste was a member of the Medical Faculty of Paris and was interested in degenerative diseases of the neuromuscular system. This book, dedicated to his father, is a review of the studies previously done on neuromuscular atrophy, together with reports and summaries of Charcot's own research.

Garrison-Morton 4758; Waller 1906.

ANDRÉ THOMAS (1867–1963). *Traité des maladies de la moelle épinière.*

See No. 1096.

1159. KARL LANDSTEINER (1868–1943). "Zur Kenntniss der antifermentativen, lytischen und agglutinierenden Wirkungen des Blutserums und der Lymphe." (In *Centralblatt für Bakteriologie, Parasitenkunde und Infektionskrankheiten.* Vol. 27 (1900), pp. 357–362.) 23 cm.

A native of Vienna, Landsteiner studied at the University of Vienna where he received his medical degree in 1891, after which he studied chemistry with Hantzsch in Zurich, Emil Fischer in Würzburg, and E. Bamberger in Munich. In 1900, as reported in this paper, he discovered iso-agglutinins in the human blood and demonstrated the existence of three blood groups, thereby making safe blood transfusions possible. He left Europe in 1922 and joined the staff of the Rockefeller Institute where in 1940, with Alexander S. Wiener (b. 1907), he discovered the Rh factor in human blood. Landsteiner's scientific activity was prodigious and he published more than 300 scientific articles on chemistry, pathology, serology, and immunology. He was awarded the Nobel prize for medicine in 1930 for his discovery of human blood groups.

Garrison-Morton 889.

*1160. HARVEY WILLIAMS CUSHING (1869–1939). *The pituitary body and its disorders.* Philadelphia and London: J. B. Lippincott, 1912. x, 341 pp., col. front., illus., fold. plate. 24.1 cm.

Harvey Cushing, born in Cleveland, Ohio, and educated at Harvard and Yale, taught successively at Johns Hopkins University, Harvard, and Yale, becoming the world's leading neurological surgeon. His productivity was enormous—in surgery, in research, and in publication. In addition, he was a distinguished collector of medical books which he bequeathed to Yale.

The physiology of the hypophysis, its diseases, and their treatment, were early and life-long interests of Cushing. His studies of this subject, as of most anything he touched, were exhaustive, and the textual matter, case histories, and illustrations in this pioneer work have scarcely been improved upon to this day. This book is an amplification of the Harvey Lecture of December, 1910. The front flyleaf of the University of Iowa copy carries this inscription: "Inscribed for Dr. John Martin with the regards and best wishes of Harvey Cushing, New Haven, Dec. 1, 1938."

Garrison-Morton 3896; Waller 2252.

———. *A classification of the tumors of the glioma group on a histogenic basis with a correlated study of prognosis.*

See No. 1193.

*1161. ———. *Tumors of the nervus acusticus and the syndrome of the cerebellopontile angle.* Philadelphia: Saunders, 1917. viii, 296 pp., illus. (part col.), diagrs. 24 cm. Original green cloth.

This book consists primarily of detailed and well-illustrated case histories of patients with surgically challenging lesions of the brain stem. It reveals the carefully documented case histories Cushing kept and the self-discipline with which he worked.

Garrison-Morton 4601.

*1162. ———. *Studies in intracranial physiology & surgery.* London: H. Milford, Oxford University Press, 1926. xii, 146 pp., illus. 24.1 cm. Original maroon cloth.

Cushing delivered the three papers in this book as the Cameron Prize Lectures at the University of Edinburgh in October 1925. The three lectures were: 1) "The third circulation and its channels," 2) "The pituitary gland as now known," and 3) "Intracranial tumours and the surgeon." Very little is known about the founder of these lectures, Andrew Robertson Cameron. He was born in Torland, Aberdeenshire, and completed his medical studies at Edinburgh in 1861. He emigrated to Australia, settled in New South Wales, and died there in 1878.

*1163. ——— and PERCIVAL BAILEY (1892–1973). *Tumors arising from the blood-vessels of the brain.* Springfield, Illinois and Baltimore: C. C. Thomas, 1928. x, 219 pp., illus. 24.3 cm. Original blue cloth with dust jacket.

Cushing shared the authorship of this monograph with Percival Bailey (see No. 1193). It contains the first extensive classification and description of angiomatous malformations and hemangioblastomas. The detailed and profusely illustrated case reports are, like all of Cushing's case reports, a course of instruction in themselves.

*1164. HARVEY WILLIAMS CUSHING. *Papers relating to the pituitary body, hypothalamus and parasympathetic nervous system.* Springfield, Illinois: C. C. Thomas, 1932. vii, 234 pp., illus., col. plates, diagrs. 24.2 cm. Original green cloth.

The four papers in this volume were "brought together for the convenience of those whom the general theme may interest" (Preface). The papers had all been published elsewhere and were the basis for four different lectures Cushing had given in England, Canada, and America during the years 1930 to 1932.

Garrison-Morton 3552.

*1165. ———. *Intracranial tumours; notes upon a series of two thousand verified cases with surgical-mortality percentages pertaining thereto.* Springfield, Illinois and Baltimore: C. C. Thomas, 1932. ix [3] 150 pp., illus. 25 cm. Original blue cloth.

The material covered in this book formed the basis of a report Cushing made to the International Neurological Congress in Berne, Switzerland on September 1, 1931. As usual, the case histories are clear and detailed with effective illustrations. Cushing's classification of tumors is still in use.

Garrison-Morton 4900.

*1166. ——— with the collaboration of LOUISE EISENHARDT (1891–1966). *Meningiomas, their classification, regional behavior, life history, and surgical end results.* Springfield, Illinois: C. C. Thomas, 1938. xiv, 785 pp., col. front., illus. (part col.). 25.4 cm.

"The present treatise was commenced in 1915 soon after the completion of his volume on the pituitary disorders, and it therefore represents nearly twenty-five years of work; by common consent it is regarded as Dr. Cushing's greatest clinical monograph. It is the embodiment of all the things he has stood for during his career as a clinician: his painstaking case records and photographs, his unusual artistic ability evident in his own numerous operative sketches, and his extraordinary knowledge of the day to day life of his patients" (Harvey Cushing Society, *A bibliography of Harvey Cushing.* Springfield, 1939. p. 18).

Dr. Eisenhardt, nurse, physician, brilliant neuropathologist, and devoted friend and colleague to Dr. Cushing, collaborated in the publication of the work, and her microphotographs easily support the classification used in this most exhaustive work on the subject of intracranial meningiomas.

This copy carries on the front flyleaf the following: "Inscribed for Dr. John Martin, for Dr. Harvey Cushing and Louise Eisenhardt, by L. E. December, 1939."

Garrison-Morton 4612.

1167. MAUDE ELIZABETH SEYMOUR ABBOTT (1869–1940). *Atlas of congenital cardiac disease.* New York: American Heart Association, 1936. x, 62 pp., front., 25 plates, illus., diagrs. 34.9 cm. Original maroon cloth.

In the Foreword to this book, the eminent cardiologist, Paul D. White, stated that "it was left to Maude Abbott, fired by a spark from Osler, to make the subject one of such general and widespread interest that we no longer regard it with either disdain or awe as a mystery for the autopsy table alone to discover and to solve. She has been the most important of the pioneers in establishing congenital heart disease as a living part of clinical medicine." Abbott, refused admission to the medical school of McGill University in Montreal, received her medical degree from Bishop's College. Abbott eventually was appointed to the McGill medical faculty and was later appointed curator of the McGill Medical Historical Museum. A skilled physician and pathologist, she utilized her broad clinical experience and exposure to the wide range of specimens at the museum to prepare this book on cardiac anomalies. Well-illustrated with twenty-five detailed plates, it has become a classic in its field and was reprinted in 1954.

Garrison-Morton 2865.

1168. ARTUR PAPPENHEIM (1870–1916). *Haematologische Bestimmungstafeln.* Leipzig: W. Klinkhardt, 1920. vi, 335 pp., 6 col. plates (1 fold.), diagrs. 30.9 cm.

A native of Berlin, Pappenheim initially studied mathematics and philosophy at the University, but he changed to medicine and was graduated with a medical degree in 1895. He was particularly interested in hematology and worked with several leading hematologists in Königsberg, Hamburg, and Berlin. He was a prolific author and wrote several books as well as a number of papers. Pappenheim was one of the major figures in the early days of hematology and was the founder of *Folia Haematologica.* This book on the diagnosis and detection of blood diseases was edited by Hans Hirschfeld (1873–1929) several years after Pappenheim's death.

Gift of H. P. Smith.

*1169. ALFRED ADLER (1870–1937). *Über den nervösen Charakter; Grundzüge einer vergleichenden Individual-psychologie und Psychotherapie.* Wiesbaden: J. F. Bergmann, 1912. [8] 195 [3] pp. 23.5 cm.

Adler had been a prominent member of Freud's circle in Vienna before he broke away in 1911 and established his own school of "Individual Psychology." He stressed the sense of inferiority as the motivating force in human society and saw the inability to compensate for this inferiority complex as the origin of neuroses. The present treatise is a principal work of Adler, laying the groundwork for his concept of individuality, inferiority, and compensation.

Garrison-Morton 4985.1.

*1170. ———. *Studie über Minderwertigkeit von Organen.* Munich: J. F. Bergmann, 1927. 92 pp. 24.3 cm. Original wrappers.

Adler firmly believed that somatic defects and chronic problems of health led to feelings of personal inferiority and eventually the psychoneuroses. In this book, first published in 1907, Adler introduced the concept of the inferiority complex and the method of compensation required to overcome it.

Garrison-Morton 4984.

*1171. ———. *Problems of neurosis; a book of case-histories.* London: K. Paul, 1929. xxxvii, 178 pp. 21.7 cm. Original blue buckram.

In this book of case histories Adler returns to a "consideration of the original neurological and psychotherapeutic problems in which he never lost interest. . . . We have here no formal treatise, but rather the revealing and intimate discourses of the peripatetic and philosophic physician and psychotherapist" (from the Preface). The book was written in English and editorially revised by Philippe Mairet (b. 1886), author of *A.B.C. of Adler's psychology.*

*1172. CHARLES ALBERT ELSBERG (1871–1948). *Surgical diseases of the spinal cord, membranes, and nerve roots; symptoms, diagnosis, and treatment.* [1st ed.]. [New York]: P. B. Hoeber [1941]. viii, 598 pp., illus., diagrs. 25.3 cm. Original gray cloth.

Elsberg began his career as a general surgeon and grew into neurosurgery as his career progressed. He received his medical degree at Columbia University, studied for a time in Europe, and on his return was appointed assistant pathologist at Mount Sinai Hospital in New York City. In 1909 he became neurosurgeon of the Neurological Institute of New York, which he helped found; this association continued until his retirement in 1937. From his first book in 1916, *Diseases of the spinal cord,* until his death, Elsberg's authority in neurology was greatly respected both here and abroad. This book was widely used as a standard textbook in many medical schools. It contains clear discussions of anatomy, pathology, clinical signs, and diagnostic and surgical procedures.

Garrison-Morton 4910.

*1173. RUDOLF MAGNUS (1873–1927). *Körperstellung.* Berlin: J. Springer, 1924. xiii, 740 pp., illus. 22.9 cm.

Magnus, a German, was a gifted pupil and co-worker of Sir Charles Sherrington (see No. 1136) at Liverpool. Later at the University of Utrecht, where he was professor of pharmacology, he became one of the most productive neurophysiologists of the first quarter of the twentieth century. In this monumental work on body posture, Magnus summarizes his extensive observations and experiments on the function of the otolithic organs, the nature of postural and neck reflexes, and the balancing reactions of the tonic labyrinthine reflexes.

Garrison-Morton 661.

*1174. Sir ANDREW BALFOUR, editor (1873–1931). *Report of the Wellcome Tropical Research Laboratories at the Gordon Memorial College, Khartoum.* 1st–4th. 4 vols. in

5 with 2 supplements. Khartoum: Published for the Department of Education, Sudan Government, by Baillière, Tindall & Cox, London, 1904–1911. Illus., plates (part col.), maps, diagrs. 27.4 cm.

These reports on tropical medicine, hygiene, and tropical veterinary science were edited by Balfour, who was director of the Wellcome Tropical Research Laboratories at Gordon Memorial College in Khartoum from 1902 to 1913. A Scottish physician, Balfour was an expert in tropical medicine and public health, and it was largely due to his efforts that Khartoum became a modern and sanitary city. He worked hard to improve the health of native communities in the Sudan and made a number of important discoveries in protozoology while he was in Africa. Many of his findings are included in these interesting and wide-ranging reports.

SAHACHIRO HATA (1873–1938). *Die experimentelle Chemotherapie der Spirillosen.* See No. 1117.

1175. ALEXIS CARREL (1873–1944). "Transplantation in mass of the kidneys." (In *Journal of experimental medicine.* Vol. 10 (1908), pp. 98–140.) 25.4 cm.

The replacement of diseased organs with sound ones and the restoration of amputated limbs had long been prevented because the surgeon did not have a reliable technique for re-establishing circulation in the transplanted or restored part without the danger of hemorrhage or thrombosis. It was Carrel who perfected the anastomosis of blood vessels in 1902 and, in doing so, provided the method which would revolutionize vascular surgery and make it possible to transplant organs and restore amputated limbs. It was in this paper that Carrel first described the practical application of his research, giving reports of his transplantation of the kidneys from one animal to another and the results of his experimentation.

Garrison-Morton 4235.

1176. ——— and CHARLES A. LINDBERGH (1902–1974). *The culture of organs.* New York: Hoeber, 1938. xix [3] 221 pp., illus., diagrs. 23.4 cm. Original black cloth.

Carrel studied medicine at Lyons and after graduation taught anatomy and operative surgery and did experimental work in surgery at the University. He came to Chicago in 1904 and in 1906 accepted a position at the Rockefeller Institute for Medical Research in New York. In 1908 he successfully transplanted organs, and, in 1910, Carrel demonstrated that blood vessels could be kept in cold storage for long periods of time before transplanting them. In 1912 he won the Nobel prize for his work on vascular structure and organ transplantation.

In this book, the authors describe the techniques employed in the cultivation of whole organs placed in an organ chamber apparatus developed by Lindbergh, the American aviator.

Cushing C99; Waller 1785.

*1177. JOSEPH ARNETH (1873–1956). *Die neutrophilen weissen Blutkörperchen bei Infektions-Krankheiten.* Jena: G. Fischer, 1904. 200 pp., 30 plates (part fold.). 25.6 cm. Original wrappers.

Arneth, professor of medicine at Würzburg, was an active researcher in hematology and published several books on the subject during his career. He demonstrated five groups of polymorphonuclear leucocytes in normal blood and showed how the count of their relative proportions could be used to study bone marrow reactions in disease. This is an account of his original work and the application of what is now called Arneth's formula.

Garrison-Morton 3075.

*1178. WILLIAM GEORGE MacCALLUM (1874–1944). "On the relation of the islands of Langerhans to glycosuria." (In *Bulletin of the Johns Hopkins Hospital.* Vol. 20 (1909), no. 222, pp. [265]–268.) 30 cm.

A native of Ontario, MacCallum was a member of the first class to graduate from Johns Hopkins Medical School in 1897. He subsequently became a member of the faculty and, with the exception of the period from 1909 through 1917 when he was professor of pathology at Columbia University, remained at Johns Hopkins until his death. Among MacCallum's important contributions to the health sciences were his discovery of the sexual forms of the malaria parasite in 1897, demonstration that the parathyroid glands control the metabolism of calcium in 1909, and the present paper in which he suggests a relationship between the islands of Langerhans and carbohydrate metabolism. His fundamental research on the pathology of diabetes helped lead to an understanding of the role the pancreas has in this disease.

Garrison-Morton 3962.

1179. ANTONIO EGAS MONIZ (1874–1955). *L'angiographie cérébrale.* Paris: Masson et Cie, 1934. 327 pp., illus., diagrs. 23.6 cm.

Moniz held posts at the neurology departments of both the University of Coimbra and the University of Lisbon before turning his attention to politics. He achieved a measure of fame as a statesman, serving as Portuguese ambassador to Spain and representing Portugal at the signing of the Treaty of Versailles. After his political party was deposed, he returned to the University of Lisbon where he redirected his attention to neurological research and developed the idea of utilizing X-rays to view the cerebral vessels. Using sodium iodide as a contrast medium, he successfully performed the first carotid angiogram. His technique, later refined by German and Swedish scientists, became what is now one of the most useful of neurological tests. This work on cerebral angiography is one of the best known of more than a hundred books and articles published on the subject by Moniz.

A few years later Moniz achieved even greater recognition for the development of the frontal leucotomy for the alleviation of certain anxiety states, an operation which caused no little controversy within the medical ranks owing to its radical nature and psychopathological implications. In 1949, Moniz received the Nobel prize for the operation.

Waller 6641.

*1180. CARL GUSTAV JUNG (1875–1961). *Über die Psychologie der Dementia praecox; ein Versuch*. Halle: C. Marhold, 1907. iv, 179 pp. 23.2 cm. Original printed paper wrappers.

Jung, born in a small village near Basel, Switzerland, was from a family of scholars. He was educated in his native city and was graduated in medicine from the University. Following postgraduate work in France, he worked under Eugen Bleuler at the Psychiatric Clinic and Burghölzli Hospital of the University of Zurich. He first met Sigmund Freud in 1907 and worked with him until 1912 when he departed to found his own school of psychoanalytic thought. Later he was professor of psychology at the Federal Polytechnical University in Zurich and, during the latter part of his career, professor of medical psychology at Basel.

At the Burghölzli, Jung had ample opportunity to apply his association tests to subjects with dementia praecox, and, after three years of investigation, he presented his findings in this book. In the first part, Jung gives a comprehensive survey of the theoretical literature on dementia praecox, integrating the contemporary theories about the disease. He was the first to offer a tentative psychosomatic explanation for dementia praecox in which the brain was the target organ. This meant that dementia praecox could be understood within a psychoanalytic framework, offering hope for patients who were borderline cases. It was also in this book that Jung drew international attention to Freud's fundamental theories.

*1181. ———. *Wandlungen und Symbole der Libido*. Leipzig and Vienna: F. Deuticke, 1912. 422 pp., illus. 23.5 cm.

Jung was one of Freud's early disciples and collaborators, but in 1913 he founded an independent neo-Freudian school under the name of analytic psychology. The present work was his first major statement after his break with Freud. In it he rejects Freud's concept of the libido as sexual in origin and describes it as a creative force or psychic energy. He sees the libido as expressing itself through symbols, a theory which he later developed into his concept of the collective unconscious and the archetypes. This classic in psychology is translated into English as *Psychology of the unconscious*.

Garrison-Morton 4985.2.

1182. HIDEYO NOGUCHI (1876–1928). *Serum diagnosis of syphilis and the butyric acid test for syphilis*. Philadelphia & London: J. B. Lippincott, 1910. vii [1] 173 pp., illus. (part col.), tables, col. plates. 21.9 cm. Original maroon cloth.

Noguchi, a Japanese physician, studied medicine at Tokyo and worked at the Institute for Infectious Diseases in Tokyo until 1900 when he came to Philadelphia. He worked with Simon Flexner (1836–1946) in pathology at the University of Pennsylvania until 1904 when he joined the Rockefeller Institute for Medical Research in New York. He remained at the Institute until his death from yellow fever while in Africa studying that very disease. Noguchi was the first to show that the brain tissue of paretics contained *Spirochaete pallida* and that syphilis could be transmitted from that tissue to experimental animals. In addition to his important work with snake venoms, he also cultivated several types of Spirochetes and developed a bacteria-free vaccine virus in rabbit tissues. In the Preface to this book, Noguchi states that his objectives were " . . . first to give a brief yet adequate account of the principles of serum haemolysis . . . and, secondly, to give in detail the technic of Wassermann's method and of the method recommended by the author."

Cushing N106.

Gift of Clarence Van Epps.

*1183. FRANCIS WILLIAM ASTON (1877–1945). *Isotopes.* London: E. Arnold, 1922. viii, 152 pp., illus., 4 plates. 21.6 cm. Original blue cloth.

Aston, a British physicist, worked with fellow physicist, J. J. Thomson (1856–1940), in research that led to the development of the mass spectrograph. An aircraft engineer during World War I, Aston returned to Cambridge after the war and worked under Lord Rutherford in the famous Cavendish Laboratory where he continued to work until his death, making many important contributions to the study of the chemical elements. He received the Nobel prize in chemistry in 1922 for his discovery of the isotopes of several nonradioactive elements, and he reports on that work in this basic book on nuclear physics. His work has had far-reaching effects, and refinements of it have led to the use of isotopes in nuclear medicine.

Cushing A293.

CARL BRUCK (b. 1879). "Eine serodiagnostische Reaktion bei Syphilis."

See No. 1152.

*1184. RENÉ LERICHE (1879–1955). *The surgery of pain.* Baltimore: Williams & Wilkins, 1939. xix, 512 pp., illus., plates. 21.2 cm. Modern cloth.

Leriche, an internationally known French physician, was the first surgeon to be named to the chair of experimental medicine at the Collège de France. The premier chair in France, it had been held by such famed individuals as Claude Bernard, Magendie, Brown-Séquard, and Charles Nicolle before Leriche was named in 1937. Although this is the most prestigious chair in France, the incumbent is not provided with clinical facilities in Paris, so Leriche operated at the American Hospital at Neuilly for the remaining years of his career. The occupant of the chair was required to deliver and publish a series of lectures each year and this was the first publication to result from his lectures. The book had its background in Leriche's experiences with the control of pain and surgery of the autonomic nervous system during World War I. He presents a comprehensive study of pain and its treatment in various diseases, and includes an excellent discussion of pain as an abstract concept. Initially published in French, the book went through three editions and was translated into several foreign languages. It is here translated for the first time into English by Archibald Young (1873–1939), Regius professor of surgery at the University of Glasgow.

Cushing L177 (French ed., 1937); Waller 5730 (French ed., 1940).

*1185. VITTORIO PUTTI (1880–1940). *Le fratture vertebrali.* Bologna: L. Cappelli, 1942. 383 pp., illus. (part col.). 34.3 cm.

Putti was a prominent Italian orthopedist and director of the Rizzoli Institute in Bologna. His methods were widely used and taught, and much of his work has now been incorporated into standard orthopedic procedures. This handsome publication of his writings and research was issued as a memorial to Putti.

*1186. Sir THOMAS LEWIS (1881–1945). *Clinical electrocardiography.* London: Shaw, 1913. viii, 120 pp., illus. 21.2 cm. Modern cloth.

Lewis, an English pioneer in the application of electrocardiography to clinical medicine, was one of the most prominent cardiologists of his day. He was educated in anatomy and physiology at University College, Cardiff, and in medicine at University College, London. His contributions to medicine include a classic study on the heartbeat and cardiac arrhythmias, investigations into the response of the small blood vessels of the skin, and a later series of investigations into the mechanism of referred pain. In this early work on clinical electrocardiography, Lewis concentrates on acquainting the reader with the uses of electrocardiography in the clinic and on diagnosing disorders of the heartbeat.

1187. Sir ALEXANDER FLEMING (1881–1955). "On the antibacterial action of cultures of penicillium, with special reference to their use in the isolation of *B. influenzae.*" (In *British journal of experimental pathology.* Vol. 10 (1929), no. 3, pp. 226–236.) 24.1 cm.

A native of Scotland, Fleming studied medicine at St. Mary's Hospital Medical School, University of London. In 1906, immediately after graduation, he began working in the laboratory of Sir Almroth Wright at St. Mary's Hospital. He spent his entire career at St. Mary's, becoming professor of bacteriology in 1929. A noted scientist, his major areas of research were in immunology, bacteriology, and chemotherapy. His most significant publications are those on antiseptics, the antibacterial substance lysozyme, and the present paper on penicillin which ushered in the age of antibiotics. Fleming (with Ernst B. Chain and Howard W. Florey) received the Nobel prize in 1945 for the discovery of penicillin and the subsequent investigation of its chemotherapeutic properties.

Garrison-Morton 1933.

*1188. HERMANN RORSCHACH (1884–1922). *Psychodiagnostik.* Bern: E. Bircher [1921]. 174 pp., 10 plates (part col.). 23 cm. Original printed wrappers, in portfolio.

Rorschach was born in Zurich and educated in German and Swiss medical schools. Long interested in inkblots, during his psychiatric training he made his first studies of how people react to them by trying to determine whether gifted students had more fantasies than average students. He was later introduced to psychoanalysis by Eugene Bleuler (1857–1939) and Carl Jung (see No. 1180) and continued to investigate the idea that an individual's reactions to inkblots reveal a great deal about his personality. Rorschach eventually developed a standard test of ten inkblots which he asked patients to interpret. By analyzing the patient's perceptions of each inkblot, Rorschach was able to gain valuable insights into the patient's inner life which could then be applied in therapy. This now-famous book with its portfolio of ten inkblot specimens used in the Rorschach test was based on tests given to 300 mental patients and 100 normal individuals.

Garrison-Morton 4988.1.

1189. CASIMIR FUNK (1884–1967). *Die Vitamine.* 2nd ed. Munich and Wiesbaden: J. F. Bergmann, 1922. 448 pp., illus. 24.5 cm.

Funk, the eminent Polish biochemist, studied at Geneva and Bern where he received his Ph.D. in 1904 and later, while working in London, a D.Sc. from the University of London in 1913. During his professional career he worked at various universities, research institutes, and pharmaceutical firms in France, Germany, England, and the United States.

Funk coined the term vitamin and discovered thiamine, the first vitamin to be isolated. In addition to his pioneering work in vitaminology, he investigated male and female hormones, gonadotropic hormones, antagonistic substances in the diet, deficiency diseases in cattle, and the importance of oncotine and oncostimuline in the treatment and prevention of cancer.

Funk first published the present work in 1914 and deferred publication of this second edition because of World War I. By the time this greatly revised edition was published, much of the basic work on the role of vitamin B_1 in beriberi, vitamin C in scurvy, and vitamin D in rickets had been completed. Building on Funk's basic research in vitaminology, modern-day scientists have greatly expanded our knowledge of vitamins and their vital role in growth and metabolism.

Cushing F375 (1st ed., 1914); Garrison-Morton 1051 (1st ed.).

Gift of Mrs. Ida Schlapp.

*1190. ELIZABETH KENNY (1886–1952). *Infantile paralysis and cerebral diplegia; methods used for the restoration of function.* Sydney: Angus & Robertson, 1937. xxxviii, 125 pp., plates. 21.4 cm. Original cloth with dust wrapper.

As reports of Sister Kenny's work with patients suffering from the effects of anterior poliomyelitis and cerebral diplegia began to reach America and other countries from Australia, battle lines were drawn throughout the medical profession. Some supported her work as a great therapeutic breakthrough while others disclaimed it as a fad supported with inflated claims and lacking originality. Her book reveals that she had capable professional guidance and that she was correct in her basic methodology and therapeutic approach, although she and her colleagues had some faulty ideas concerning nerve and muscle physiology. She taught the necessity and importance of both active and passive graduated exercise, hydrotherapy, the elimination of restrictive braces and splints, and the development of a positive attitude by the patient and health care team.

Garrison-Morton 4671.

ARTHUR M. WRIGHT (fl. 1930). "Acute ascending myelitis following a monkey bite, with the isolation of a virus capable of reproducing the disease."

See No. 1196.

1191. Sir FREDERICK GRANT BANTING (1891–1941) and CHARLES HERBERT BEST (1899–1978). "The internal secretion of the pancreas." (In *Journal of laboratory and clinical medicine*. Vol. 7 (1922), no. 5, pp. 251–266.) 25 cm.

Following noted service in the Canadian Army during World War I, Banting established a practice in orthopedic surgery in London, Ontario, and also served as a demonstrator in physiology at the University of Western Ontario. He developed an interest in diabetes and subsequently moved to the University of Toronto where he was joined by Best, a sophomore medical student, in the laboratory of John J. R. Macleod (1876–1935). In late 1921, only eight months after beginning their experimental studies, Banting and Best announced the discovery of insulin; and in this paper, they give a full report on their isolation of insulin from the pancreas of a dog. In 1923, Banting and Macleod received the Nobel prize for their work.

Garrison-Morton 3967.

LOUISE EISENHARDT (1891–1966). *Meningiomas.*

See No. 1166.

*1192. LESLIE BRAINERD AREY (b. 1891). *Developmental anatomy; a text-book and laboratory manual of embryology.* Philadelphia and London: W. B. Saunders [1924]. vii, 433 pp., illus. (part col.), col. plates, diagrs. 25 cm. Original cloth.

For many years professor of anatomy at Northwestern University Medical School and now an emeritus professor, the author has been recognized for decades as a leading authority in teaching and research in developmental anatomy. This textbook of embryology has gone through many editions and remains a model of clarity and accuracy.

*1193. PERCIVAL BAILEY (1892–1973) and HARVEY WILLIAMS CUSHING (1869–1939). *A classification of the tumors of the glioma group on a histogenic basis with a correlated study of prognosis.* Philadelphia: J. B. Lippincott, 1926. [5] 175 pp., illus., tables, diagrs. 22.9 cm.

Illinois-born Bailey—neurosurgeon, physiologist, philosopher, and tireless investigator—spent most of his productive life in Illinois, principally at the University of Chicago, the University of Illinois Medical School, and as director of the Illinois State Psychiatric Institute. This book is one of the first collaborative efforts of these two surgeons (for Cushing see No. 1160 ff.). Their classification of the gliomas has hardly been improved upon, though variations of it are now in use throughout the world.

Garrison-Morton 4608.

PERCIVAL BAILEY. *Tumors arising from the blood-vessels of the brain.*

See No. 1163.

*1194. JOSÉ TRUETA RASPALL (b. 1897). *Treatment of war wounds and fractures, with special reference to the closed method as used in the war in Spain.* London: Hamish Hamilton Medical Books, 1939. xiii, 146 pp., illus. 18.6 cm. Cloth.

Trueta wrote this small manual during the Spanish Civil War when he was director of the Department of Surgery at the General Hospital of Catalonia in Barcelona. The book was initially prepared in Spanish and is here enlarged and translated into English. It was first published in September, 1939, and this is the second impression of November, 1939. Trueta used the closed method of treating compound fractures which consisted of reducing the fracture, cleaning the wound, packing it with Vaseline-impregnated gauze, and immobilizing the limb in a plaster cast. The closed method was widely used by the Allied Forces early in World War II but was replaced by somewhat simpler techniques as antibiotics were introduced into use for the control of infection.

Garrison-Morton 5632; Waller 9700a (1942 ed.).

CHARLES HERBERT BEST (1899–1978). "The internal secretion of the pancreas."

See No. 1191.

*1195. PEDRO MANUEL DE ALMEIDA LIMA (b. 1903). *Cerebral angiography.* London: Oxford University Press, 1950. xiii, 221 pp., illus. 24.8 cm.

Lima, who trained under the guidance of Sir Hugh Cairns (1896–1952) at Oxford, was professor of neurology at Lisbon and head of the Neurosurgical Department at the Hospital Julio de Matos in Lisbon when this book was written. Lima had worked for more than twenty years with Egas Moniz (see No. 1179), noted neurosurgeon and winner of the Nobel prize in 1949 for the introduction of prefrontal leucotomy, to perfect the application and technique of cerebral angiography. The book gives an authoritative account of the development of cerebral angiography, the anatomy of the major cerebral vessels, and the deviations produced in these vessels by intracranial lesions. The vascular patterns of intracranial tumors revealed by cerebral angiography are also covered in considerable detail. The book is a milestone in the history of neurology although much of it has been outdated by the rapid advances in technique and the clinical knowledge of the past twenty-five years.

1196. ALBERT BRUCE SABIN (b. 1906) and ARTHUR M. WRIGHT (fl. 1930). "Acute ascending myelitis following a monkey bite, with the isolation of a virus capable of reproducing the disease." (In *Journal of experimental medicine.* Vol. 59, no. 2 (1934), pp. 115–136.) 25 cm.

A native of Poland, Sabin came to the United States when he was fifteen years old. He was graduated from New York University's College of Medicine and, after additional study, research, and training, joined the faculty at the University of Cincinnati College of Medicine. Sabin developed a life-long interest in poliomyelitis early in his career and was one of the leaders in the effort that led to the conquest of this dread disease. In the present paper, Sabin and Wright report on the research which resulted in the isolation of the Herpesvirus simiae (B virus). Sabin was one of three scientists who independently developed an oral vaccine for polio in the mid and late 1950's.

Garrison-Morton 4658.

INDEX

NOTE: The numerals in the Index refer to *entry* numbers, *not* page numbers. Italic numerals indicate primary entries; Arabic numerals indicate secondary reference(s); boldface numerals indicate the presence of an illustration in this catalogue.